OKU

Orthopaedic Knowledge Update

2

Hip and Knee Reconstruction

American Academy of Orthopaedic Surgeons

The Hip Society

The Knee Society

OKU

Orthopaedic Knowledge Update

Edited by

Paul M. Pellicci, MD
Attending Orthopaedic Surgeon
The Hospital for Special Surgery
Professor of Orthopaedic Surgery
Cornell University Medical College
New York, New York

Alfred J. Tria, Jr, MD
Associate Clinical Professor, Surgery
Robert Wood Johnson Medical School
New Brunswick, New Jersey

Kevin L. Garvin, MD
Professor of Orthopaedic Surgery
University of Nebraska Medical School
Omaha, Nebraska

The Hip Society
The Knee Society

Hip and Knee Reconstruction 2

Published 2000
by the American Academy of Orthopaedic Surgeons™
6300 North River Road
Rosemont, Illinois 60018
1-800-626-6726

The material presented in *Orthopaedic Knowledge Update: Hip and Knee Reconstruction 2* has been made available by the American Academy of Orthopaedic Surgeons™ for educational purposes only. This material is not intended to present the only, or necessarily best, methods or procedures for the medical situations discussed, but rather is intended to represent an approach, view, statement, or opinion of the author(s) or producer(s), which may be helpful to others who face similar situations.

Some drugs or medical devices demonstrated in Academy courses or described in Academy print or electronic publications have not been cleared by the Food and Drug Administration (FDA) or have been cleared for specific uses only. The FDA has stated that it is the responsibility of the physician to determine the FDA clearance status of each drug or device he or she wishes to use in clinical practice.

At the time of this writing, bone screws placed posteriorly into vertebral elements have been cleared for use in this specific manner by the Food and Drug Administration (FDA) to provide immobilization and stabilization as an adjunct to fusion in the treatment of the following acute and chronic instability or deformities of the thoracic, lumbar and sacral spine: degenerative spondylolisthesis with objective evidence of neurological impairment; fracture; dislocation; scoliosis; kyphosis; spinal tumor and failed previous fusion (pseudoarthrosis). In addition, anterior vertebral body screws (cervical, thoracic, and lumbar) are Class II devices and can be used as labeled in vertebral bodies.

Furthermore, any statements about commercial products are solely the opinion(s) of the author(s) and do not represent an Academy endorsement or evaluation of these products. These statements may not be used in advertising or for any commercial purpose.

ISBN 0-89203-218-9

Library of Congress Cataloging-in-Publication Data

Orthopaedic knowledge update. Hip and knee reconstruction 2 / edited by Paul M. Pellicci, Alfred J. Tria, Kevin Garvin; developed by the Hip Society and the Knee Society.
p.;cm
Includes bibliographical references and index.
ISBN 0-89203-218-9 (softcover)
1. Total hip replacement. 2. Total knee replacement. 3. Hip joint--Surgery
4. Knee--Surgery. I. Title: Hip and knee reconstruction 2. II. Pellicci, Paul.
III. Tria, Alfred J., IV. Garvin, Kevin. V. Hip Society (U.S.) VI. Knee Society (U.S.)
VII. American Academy of Orthopaedic Surgeons.
[DNLM: 1. Arthroplasty, Replacement, Hip. 2. Hip Joint--surgery.
3. Arthroplasty, Replacement, Knee. 4. Knee Joint--surgery. WE 860 077 1999]
RD549 .0782 1999
617.5'810592--dc21

99-059893

Acknowledgments

Contributors

José A. Alicea, MD
Assistant Clinical Professor
Texas Tech Health Sciences Center
El Paso, Texas

Deborah J. Ammeen, BS
Research Associate
Anderson Orthopaedic Research Institute
Alexandria, Virginia

Thomas P. Andriacchi, PhD
Professor, Co-chairman, Division of Biomechanics
Professor, Department of Functional Restoration
School of Engineering/School of Medicine
Stanford University
Stanford, California

John Antoniou, MD, PhD, FRCSC
Fellow in Adult Reconstructive Hip and Knee Surgery
Central DuPage Hospital/Rush-Presbyterian St. Luke's Medical Center
Chicago, Illinois

C. Lowry Barnes, MD
President
Arkansas Specialty Orthopaedics
Little Rock, Arkansas

Anuj Bellare, PhD
Instructor of Orthopaedic Surgery (Biomaterials)
Harvard Medical School
Orthopaedic Surgery
Brigham and Women's Hospital
Boston, Massachusetts

Daniel J. Berry, MD
Assistant Professor of Orthopedics
Mayo Medical School
Consultant in Orthopedic Surgery
Orthopaedics
Mayo Clinic
Rochester, Minnesota

James V. Bono, MD
Associate Clinical Professor of Orthopedic Surgery
Tufts University, School of Medicine
New England Baptist Hospital
Boston, Massachusetts

Mathias P. G. Bostrom, MD
Assistant Attending Orthopedic Surgeon
The Hospital for Special Surgery
New York, New York

Richard A. Brand, MD
Professor, Department of Orthopaedic Surgery
The University of Iowa
Iowa City, Iowa

Frederick F. Buechel, MD
Clinical Professor of Orthopaedic Surgery
Department of Orthopaedic Surgery
UMDNJ New Jersey Medical School
Newark, New Jersey

Robert L. Buly, MS, MD
Assistant Professor of Orthopaedic Surgery
Weill Medical College of Cornell University
The Hospital for Special Surgery
New York, New York

John J. Callaghan, MD
Professor, Department of Orthopaedics
University of Iowa
Iowa City, Iowa

Christopher T. Carey, MD
Orthopaedic Surgery Resident
Orthopaedic Surgery
Robert Wood Johnson—UMDNJ
New Brunswick, New Jersey

Michael J. Chmell, MD
Associate Clinical Professor
Department of Surgery
University of Illinois, College of Medicine
Rockford, Illinois

Christopher W. DiGiovanni, MD
The Hospital for Special Surgery
New York, New York

Gerard A. Engh, MD
President
Director, Knee Research
Anderson Orthopaedic Institute
Anderson Orthopaedic Research Institute
Alexandria, Virginia

Philip M. Faris, MD
Orthopaedic Surgeon
Kendrick Memorial Hospital
Mooresville, Indiana

Kevin L. Garvin, MD
Professor of Orthopaedic Surgery
University of Nebraska Medical Center
Omaha, Nebraska

Nelson V. Greidanus, MD, FRCSC
Fellow in Adult Reconstructive Hip and Knee Surgery
Central DuPage/Rush Presbyterian-St. Luke's Hospitals
Chicago, Illinois

Steven B. Haas, MD, MPH
Assistant Professor, Orthopaedic Surgery
The Hospital for Special Surgery
Cornell University Medical College
New York, New York

Armodios M. Hatzidakis, MD
Resident
Department of Orthopaedic Surgery and Rehabilitation
University of Nebraska Medical Center
Omaha, Nebraska

William L. Healy, MD
Chairman, Orthopaedic Surgery
Lahey Clinic
Burlington, Massachusetts

Gwyn Ed Howell, MD
Division of Orthopaedic Surgery
London Health Sciences
London, Ontario, Canada

Michael H. Huo, MD
Associate Professor
Department of Orthopaedic Surgery
Baylor College of Medicine
Houston, Texas

Omer A. Ilahi, MD
Assistant Professor
Department of Orthopaedic Surgery
Baylor College of Medicine
Houston, Texas

Norman A. Johanson, MD
Department of Orthopaedic Surgery
Temple University School of Medicine
Philadelphia, Pennsylvania

Michael A. Kelly, MD
Director, Insall Scott Kelly Institute for Orthopaedics and Sports Medicine
Department of Orthopaedic Surgery
Beth Israel Hospital
New York, New York

Paul F. Lachiewicz, MD
Professor
Department of Orthopedics
University of North Carolina, Chapel Hill
Chapel Hill, North Carolina

Joseph M. Lane, MD
Professor of Surgery, Orthopedics
Cornell University Medical College
Attending Orthopedic Surgeon
The Hospital for Special Surgery
New York, New York

Seth S. Leopold, MD
Major, United States Army Medical Corps
Section of Orthopaedic Surgery
Joint Replacement/Adult Reconstruction
William Beaumont Army Medical Center
El Paso, Texas

David G. Lewallen, MD
Professor of Orthopedic Surgery
Department of Orthopedic Surgery
Mayo Clinic
Rochester, Minnesota

Jay R. Lieberman, MD
Associate Professor
Department of Orthopaedic Surgery
UCLA School of Medicine
Los Angeles, California

Gregory A. Liguori, MD
Assistant Attending Anesthesiologist
Assistant Clinical Professor of Anesthesiology
The Hospital for Special Surgery
Cornell University Medical College
New York, New York

Paul M. Lombardi, MD
Adult Reconstruction Fellow
Hip/Knee Service
The Hospital for Special Surgery
New York, New York

William J. Maloney, MD
Chief, Orthopaedic Surgery
Barnes Jewish Hospital
Associate Professor
Department of Orthopaedic Surgery
Washington University School of Medicine
St. Louis, Missouri

Bassam A. Masri, MD, FRCSC
Clinical Associate Professor and Head
Division of Reconstructive Orthopaedics
Faculty of Medicine
University of British Columbia
Vancouver, British Columbia, Canada

Joseph C. McCarthy, MD
Clinical Professor of Orthopaedic Surgery
Tufts University School of Medicine
New England Baptist Hospital
Boston, Massachusetts

Thomas J. Mulvey, MD
Orthopaedic Surgeon
Midwest Orthopaedic Center, S.C.
Peoria, Illinois

Charles Nelson, MD
Assistant Attending Surgeon
Department of Orthopaedics
University of Pennsylvania
Philadelphia, Pennsylvania

Wayne G. Paprosky, MD, FACS
Associate Professor
Orthopaedic Surgery
Rush Medical College
Chicago, Illinois

Vincent D. Pellegrini, Jr, MD
Michael and Myrtle Baker Professor and Chair,
Department of Orthopaedics and Rehabilitation
Pennsylvania State University
College of Medicine
Milton S. Hershey Medical Center, Penn State
Geisinger Health System
Hershey, Pennsylvania

Paul M. Pellicci, MD
Attending Orthopaedic Surgery
The Hospital for Special Surgery
Professor of Orthopaedic Surgery
Cornell University Medical College
New York, New York

Robert Poss, MD
Professor of Orthopaedic Surgery
Harvard Medical School
Department of Orthopaedic Surgery
Brigham and Women's Hospital
Boston, Massachusetts

Hollis G. Potter, MD
Chief, Magnetic Resonance Imaging
Associate Professor of Radiology
The Hospital for Special Surgery
Cornell University Medical College
New York, New York

Chitranjan S. Ranawat, MD
Director, Department of Orthopaedic Surgery
Lenox Hill Hospital
New York, New York

Vijay J. Rasquinha, MD, FRCS(Ortho)
Department of Orthopaedic Surgery
Lenox Hill Hospital
New York, New York

Jose A. Rodriguez, MD
Department of Orthopaedic Surgery
Lenox Hill Hospital
New York, New York

Cecil H. Rorabeck, MD
Division of Orthopaedic Surgery
London Health Sciences
London, Ontario, Canada

Aaron G. Rosenberg, MD
Professor of Orthopedic Surgery
Department of Orthopedic Surgery
Rush-Presbyterian-St. Luke's Medical Center
Chicago, Illinois

Khaled J. Saleh, MD, MSc, FRCSC
Assistant Professor of Surgery and
School of Public Health
Department of Orthopaedic Surgery
University of Minnesota
Minneapolis, Minnesota

Eduardo A. Salvati, MD
Professor of Surgery (Orthopedics)
Cornell University Medical College
The Hospital for Special Surgery
New York, New York

Thomas P. Schmalzried, MD
Associate Medical Director
Joint Replacement Institute
Orthopaedic Hospital
Los Angeles, California

Richard D. Scott, MD
Associate Clinical Professor
Orthopaedic Surgery
Harvard Medical School
Boston, Massachusetts

Giles R. Scuderi, MD
Associate Chief
Adult Knee Reconstruction
Department of Orthopaedic Surgery
Beth Israel Medical Center
New York, New York

Myron Spector, MD, PhD
Professor of Orthopaedic Surgery
(Biomaterials)
Harvard Medical School
Orthopaedic Surgery
Brigham and Women's Hospital
Boston, Massachusetts

Marvin E. Steinberg, MD
Professor and Vice-Chairman
Department of Orthopaedic Surgery
University of Pennsylvania
School of Medicine
Philadelphia, Pennsylvania

Steven H. Stern, MD
Associate Professor of Clinical Orthopaedics
Northwestern University
Chicago, Illinois

Sharon Stevenson, DVM, PhD
Executive Director
Neolyte Joint Venture
Advanced Tissue Sciences
San Diego, California

Thomas S. Thornhill, MD
Chairman, Department of Orthopaedic Surgery
The Brigham and Women's Hospital
Boston, Massachusetts

Alfred J. Tria, Jr, MD
Associate Clinical Professor, Surgery
Robert Wood Johnson Medical School
New Brunswick, New Jersey

Hugh S. Tullos, MD
Professor
Department of Orthopaedic Surgery
Baylor College of Medicine
Houston, Texas

Roderick H. Turner, MD
Clinical Professor of Orthopedic Surgery
Tufts University, School of Medicine
New England Baptist Hospital
Boston, Massachusetts

Kelly G. Vince, MD, FRCSC
Associate Orthopaedic Surgeon
Kerlan-Jobe Orthopedic Clinic
Los Angeles, California

Barry J. Waldman, MD
Assistant Professor
Department of Orthopaedic Surgery
The Johns Hopkins School of Medicine
Baltimore, Maryland

Leo A. Whiteside, MD
Orthopaedic Surgeon
Director
Missouri Bone and Joint Center
Barnes Jewish West County Hospital
St. Louis, Missouri

Russell E. Windsor, MD
Professor of Clinical Orthopaedics
Weill Medical College of Cornell University
Attending Orthopaedic Surgeon
The Hospital for Special Surgery
New York, New York

Timothy M. Wright, PhD
Director, Biomechanics and Biomaterials
Professor, Cornell University Medical College
The Hospital for Special Surgery
New York, New York

Table of Contents

Contributors vii

Preface xvii

Section 1
Basic Science and General Knowledge

Section Editor

Kevin L. Garvin, MD

Chapter 1 3

Surgical Treatment of Inflammatory Arthritis
C. Lowry Barnes, MD

Chapter 2 7

Osteoarthritis
Kevin L. Garvin, MD

Chapter 3 13

Pathophysiology and Treatment of Venous Thromboembolic Disease
Vincent D. Pellegrini, Jr, MD

Chapter 4 25

Implant Materials: Metals, Polyethylene, Polymethylmethacrylate
Myron Spector, MD, PhD and Anuj Bellare, PhD

Chapter 5 35

Bone Grafts
Jay R. Lieberman, MD and Sharon Stevenson, DVM, PhD

Chapter 6 43

Application of Bone Inductive and Conductive Agents to Hip and Knee Reconstruction
Mathias P.G. Bostrom, MD and Joseph M. Lane, MD

Chapter 7 51

Perioperative Medical Management and Blood Transfusion Medicine
Armodios M. Hatzidakis, MD and Kevin L. Garvin, MD

Chapter 8 67

Anesthesia for Hip and Knee Reconstructive Surgery
Gregory A. Liguori, MD

Chapter 9 75

Imaging
Hollis G. Potter, MD

Chapter 10 83

Outcomes Assessment in Hip and Knee Replacement
Norman A. Johanson, MD

Section 2
The Hip

Section Editor

Paul M. Pellicci, MD

Chapter 11 91

Surgical Approaches and Anatomic Considerations
John Antoniou, MD, PhD, FRCSC, Nelson V. Greidanus, MD, FRCSC, and Wayne G. Paprosky, MD, FACS

Chapter 12 97

Biomechanics of the Hip and Hip Reconstruction
Richard A. Brand, MD

Chapter 13 103

Osteotomy
Robert Poss, MD

Chapter 14 109

Design Evolution—Cemented Total Hip Replacement
John J. Callaghan, MD

Chapter 15 117

Evolution of Uncemented Femoral Component Design
Daniel J. Berry, MD

Chapter 16 127

Osteonecrosis—Etiology, Pathophysiology, and Treatment
Marvin E. Steinberg, MD

Chapter 17 137

Deep Infection Complicating Total Hip Arthroplasty
Christopher W. DiGiovanni, MD, Khaled J. Saleh, MD, MSc, FRCSC, Eduardo A. Salvati, MD, Paul M. Pellicci, MD, and Bassam A. Masri, MD, FRCSC

Chapter 18 149

Dislocation
Paul F. Lachiewicz, MD

Chapter 19 155

Complications in Total Hip Arthroplasty
James V. Bono, MD, Joseph C. McCarthy, MD, and Roderick H. Turner, MD

Chapter 20 167

Mechanical Failure—Loosening and Wear
Thomas P. Schmalzried, MD

Chapter 21 175

Osteolysis
William J. Maloney, MD

Chapter 22 181

Results of Cemented Total Hip Replacement
Chitranjan S. Ranawat, MD, Vijay J. Rasquinha, MD, FRCSC (Ortho), and Jose A. Rodriguez, MD

Chapter 23 195

Cementless Primary Total Hip Arthroplasty
David G. Lewallen, MD

Chapter 24 207

Hybrid Total Hip Replacement
Charles Nelson, MD, Paul M. Lombardi, MD, and Paul M. Pellicci, MD

Chapter 25 217

Revision Total Hip Replacement
Robert L. Buly, MS, MD

Section 3
The Knee

Section Editor

Alfred J. Tria, Jr, MD

Chapter 26 **239**

Knee Joint: Anatomy and Biomechanics
Thomas P. Andriacchi, PhD

Chapter 27 **249**

Evaluating the Arthritic Knee
José A. Alicea, MD

Chapter 28 **255**

Nonarthroplasty Alternatives in Knee Arthritis
Paul M. Lombardi, MD, and Russell E. Windsor, MD

Chapter 29 **265**

Biomechanics of Total Knee Design
Timothy M. Wright, PhD

Chapter 30 **275**

Fixation in Total Knee Replacement: Bone Ingrowth
Leo A. Whiteside, MD

Chapter 31 **281**

Surgical Principles of Total Knee Replacement: Incisions, Extensor Mechanism, Ligament Balancing
Christopher T. Carey, MD, and Alfred J. Tria, Jr, MD

Chapter 32 **287**

The Knee: Rehabilitation
Steven H. Stern, MD

Chapter 33 **295**

Evaluation of Results of Total Knee Arthroplasty
Michael H. Huo, MD, Omer A. Ilahi, MD, and Hugh S. Tullos, MD

Chapter 34 **301**

Long-Term Results of Total Knee Replacement
Richard D. Scott, MD, Michael J. Chmell, MD, Aaron G. Rosenberg, MD, Seth S. Leopold, MD, Giles R. Scuderi, MD, and Frederick F. Buechel, MD

Chapter 35 **323**

Complications Associated with Total Knee Arthroplasty
Thomas J. Mulvey, MD, Thomas S. Thornhill, MD, Michael A. Kelly, MD, and William L. Healy, MD

Chapter 36 **339**

Revision Total Knee Replacement
Steven B. Haas, MD, MPH, Deborah J. Ammeen, BS, Gerard A. Engh, MD, Kelly G. Vince, MD, FRCSC, Philip M. Faris, MD, Cecil H. Rorabeck, MD, Gwyn Ed Howell, MD, Alfred J. Tria, Jr, MD, and Barry J. Waldman, MD

Index **367**

Preface

Orthopaedic Knowledge Update: Hip and Knee Reconstruction 2 builds upon and expands, while also reiterating, information contained in the first edition, published in 1995. We have tried to limit repetition as much as possible, though some is necessary to maintain a coherent text.

This resource provides the reader with the current body of knowledge pertaining to reconstruction of the adult hip and knee. It should be useful to both the specialist and generalist.

The chapters have been written by experts in each field. As much as possible, the information contained therein is rigorously objective.

We, the editors, would like to thank the authors for their efforts, and for the majority, the timely completion of their chapters. We also gratefully acknowledge the invaluable assistance of Lisa Claxton Moore, Senior Editor, and Sophie Tosta, Assistant Production Manager in the Publications Department at the American Academy of Orthopaedic Surgeons. Without their involvement, this book would not exist.

Paul M. Pellicci, MD
Alfred J. Tria, MD
Kevin Garvin, MD

Section 1
Basic Science and General Knowledge

Chapter 1
Surgical Treatment of Inflammatory Arthritis

Chapter 2
Osteoarthritis

Chapter 3
Pathophysiology and Treatment of Venous Thromboembolic Disease

Chapter 4
Implant Materials: Metals, Polyethylene, Polymethylmethacrylate

Chapter 5
Bone Grafts

Chapter 6
Application of Bone Inductive and Conductive Agents to Hip and Knee Reconstruction

Chapter 7
Perioperative Medical Management and Blood Transfusion Medicine

Chapter 8
Anesthesia for Hip and Knee Reconstructive Surgery

Chapter 9
Imaging

Chapter 10
Outcomes Assessment in Hip and Knee Replacement

Chapter 1 Surgical Treatment of Inflammatory Arthritis

Introduction

The many forms of arthritis produce similar consequences in the involved joints: pain, loss of motion, and deformity. Reconstructive surgery may be indicated to treat any of these sequelae and may be necessary as a preventive measure. Pain relief is the most attainable result of reconstructive surgery and should be the primary indication of most operations. Restoration of motion and function is less predictable, and careful preoperative assessment of each patient's impairment and disability must be performed before level of improvement can be predicted.

There are significant differences between osteoarthritis and rheumatoid arthritis; however, the end result, arthritic damage to the joint, is the same. There are unique aspects to the surgical treatment of rheumatoid arthritis and other types of inflammatory arthritis that may place the patient at increased risk.

Patients with inflammatory arthritis, especially those with rheumatoid arthritis, often have special surgical needs because of multiple joint involvement. A multidisciplinary team, comprised of an arthritis surgeon, rheumatologist, nurses, therapists, and social workers, is important to assist the patient. The patient, also an integral part of this team, should be involved in any decision-making and planning of surgical events so that there is a better understanding of the staging of surgical procedures, duration of treatment, and rehabilitation. It is also important for the team to assist the patient in establishing realistic goals from surgery. Because the patient may have preconceived expectations regarding the outcome of surgery, it is important that the team help the patient establish realistic goals. The surgical patient with rheumatoid arthritis or an inflammatory arthritic variant is often discouraged or depressed because a series of operations may be needed before functional independence is achieved. For this reason, proper education of the patient before surgery is imperative.

Preoperative Evaluation

The first consideration is whether a painful joint in a patient with rheumatoid arthritis requires surgery. Continued nonsurgical management with medication and physical therapy may be appropriate if synovitis is the main cause of the patient's pain and disability. Surgical, chemical, or radioactive synovectomy may be appropriate if synovitis fails to respond to medication and there is no significant structural damage to the joint. It is unrealistic to expect treatment of synovitis to be sufficient in the presence of significant structural damage to the joint. Even so, it is often appropriate to try anti-inflammatory medications and use of a walker or crutches to alleviate symptoms from a lower extremity weightbearing joint. If these measures fail and structural damage is documented, surgical intervention with arthrodesis or arthroplasty may be indicated.

It is better to perform surgery in a staged fashion, as joints are structurally destroyed, rather than wait until the patient has numerous significantly involved joints in order to avoid prolonged hospitalization, multiple anesthetics, and several operations over a short time period. The patient should be in optimal medical condition. If on glucocorticoids, the patient should be on the lowest possible maintenance dose because these agents are suggested to increase the risk of infection. Other sources of infection should be identified and treated; for example, carious teeth should be filled or extracted before surgery on the joints, and patients with urinary tract infections should be treated prior to surgery. Many female patients have asymptomatic bacteria, and it is therefore recommended that women have a urine culture performed prior to surgery. If males have significant prostatic hypertrophy and nocturia, they may be candidates for preoperative treatment prior to total joint replacement surgery. It may be useful to determine before surgery if the patient is able to void in the supine position.

Most patients with rheumatoid arthritis or other significant inflammatory arthritis should be evaluated preoperatively by physical and/or occupational therapists. The rehabilitation team may help assess the patient's motivation and ability to participate in the postoperative program and also determine what specific requirements may be necessary following surgery. Instruction and use of a walker or crutches prior to surgery may shorten the postoperative instruction period.

If multiple operations are planned, it is often useful to perform a more simple operation initially to get a better understanding of how the patient will respond to surgical intervention. For instance, if both the hip and knee require arthroplasty treatment, it is better to treat the hip prior to the knee for a number of reasons. Compared to total knee replacement, total hip replacement is characterized by less pain postoperatively, and the rehabilitation requires much less patient cooperation. If a patient does not respond well to total hip replacement, it can be predicted that he or she will have a worse response to total knee replacement.

There are certain characteristics shared by patients with rheumatoid arthritis or inflammatory arthritis that affect recovery. For instance, most of these patients have multiple joint involvement, with other joints affecting the function of the joint being operated. The rheumatoid patient having joint replacement surgery is usually approximately 10 years younger than the patient with osteoarthritis. For this reason, the prosthetic joints of these patients not only need to last longer, but they are also at increased risk for late complications such as delayed infections, late loosening, and compressed wear.

Much has been written about the increased susceptibility to infection in rheumatoid arthritis patients. It has been documented that the patient with rheumatoid arthritis who undergoes total hip replacement does have a significantly increased rate of late hematogenous infection of the joint. As mentioned previously, many patients with inflammatory arthritis are also on glucocorticoids, which are also suggested to increase the risk of infection. Aspirin and anti-inflammatory medication, used by almost all patients with inflammatory arthritis, may also produce difficulties with intraoperative and postoperative bleeding.

Management of antirheumatic medications in the perioperative period are important. Nonsteroidal anti-inflammatory medications should be discontinued at least 5 half-lives prior to surgery and aspirin should be discontinued at least 7 to 10 days prior to surgery to decrease bleeding. The anti-inflammatory medication should be discontinued during hospitalization and during the immediate postoperative period if the patient is to receive Coumadin for deep vein thrombosis prophylaxis. Nonacetylated salicylates may be substituted for other anti-inflammatory medications because they have no significant effect on platelet activity.

Antimalarials, auranofin, parenteral gold salts, sulfasalazine, and penicillamine may be continued during the preoperative as well as the immediate postoperative period.

It is recommended that methotrexate be temporarily discontinued during the immediate preoperative period and during hospitalization because of fluid balance alterations that may affect risks of side effects. Methotrexate is generally discontinued for approximately 2 weeks.

Azathioprine may be continued in the preoperative period as long as the patient's leukocyte count is greater than 3,500 mm^3, but should be temporarily discontinued during hospitalization. Rheumatologic consultation is recommended for all patients receiving azathioprine and who are scheduled for surgery.

Corticosteroids are continued during the preoperative period and stress dosages are usually given perioperatively. Many regimens have been described to provide stress coverage the day of surgery, and must include 100 mg hydrocortisone given prior to the surgery and subsequent fewer doses for the first 24 hours. Corticosteroid replacement therapy is usually recommended even if steroids have been discontinued in the past year. Others, however, have suggested that patients receiving glucocorticoids may not require stress doses to undergo orthopaedic operations.

Treatment

Rheumatoid Arthritis

In addition to the systemic problems associated with rheumatoid arthritis, multiple joint involvement often creates special difficulties for the surgical patient. A walker or crutches is necessary after lower extremity surgery, which may pose unique problems for the patient with multiple joint involvement. Extensive arthritic involvement at the shoulder, elbow, or wrist may require the use of forearm crutches or platform walkers during the postoperative period. In addition, it may be necessary to surgically treat the upper extremity prior to the lower extremity. For instance, it may be necessary to perform wrist arthrodesis so that the patient can use forearm crutches after surgery.

In patients who do not have 100° of knee flexion, maximal assistance is required from the upper extremities in rising from a seated position. If the upper extremities cannot withstand these forces, maximal hip and knee flexion must be a goal for surgery in order to minimize the need for upper extremity assistance.

There is significant cervical spine involvement in 30% to 40% of patients with rheumatoid arthritis. Although the patient is usually asymptomatic, preoperative evaluation with lateral flexion and extension views of the cervical spine is necessary to document the presence of C1–C2 instability.

Juvenile Rheumatoid Arthritis

Patients with juvenile rheumatoid arthritis present certain challenges that may influence the result of surgical intervention. The temporomandibular joint is frequently involved; when combined with micrognathia, certain difficulties may be encountered with intubation and respiration following extubation. Fiberoptic intubation may also be necessary.

The range of motion achieved after hip and knee joint replacement in juvenile rheumatoid arthritis is usually less than would be predicted at the time of surgery. Special measures such as serial casting may be necessary to correct knee flexion contracture following total knee replacement. Patients with juvenile rheumatoid arthritis often have total joint replacement at a very young age, require revision surgery, and are at increased risk for late complications.

Ankylosing Spondylitis

Patients with ankylosing spondylitis have diminished chest excursion and are at greater risk for postoperative pulmonary problems. Intubation may also be extremely difficult because of cervical spine rigidity. Fiberoptic intubation may be necessary, and sometimes even preoperative tracheostomy is required. Ossification in the anulus fibrosus and spinal ligaments may also make administration of spinal anesthetic very difficult.

Patients with ankylosing spondylitis frequently fail to regain the same range of motion following total hip replacement as would be expected in patients with rheumatoid arthritis or osteoarthritis. Although this range of motion may be less, it is often enough to significantly improve the patient's ability to perform activities of daily living. Patients with ankylosing spondylitis may have an increased risk of heterotopic ossification. Endomethacin or perioperative irradation may be used to decrease the risk of heterotopic ossification.

Psoriatic Arthritis

Patients with psoriatic arthritis may have skin involvement in the area of the proposed surgical incision. Microbacterial contamination may lead to an increased risk of infection. It is therefore recommended that the skin be treated aggressively with topical agents or ultraviolet light prior to any surgical procedure. In addition, patients are asked to use antimicrobial soaps prior to surgery.

Enteropathic Arthropathy

Arthropathies related to chronic inflammatory intestinal disease have an increased risk of infection when joint replacement is performed. There may be increased infection from the close proximity of the colostomy and there is also an increased risk of late hematogenous seeding.

Systemic Lupus Erythematosus

Patients with systemic lupus erythematous may develop metabolic bone disease and osteonecrosis of the femoral head at a very early age. These patients may require joint replacements, putting them at increased risk for early loosening and multiple revision arthroplasties. These patients are often on glucocorticoids and may be at increased risk of infection as well.

Summary

Although total joint arthroplasty has dramatically improved the function of patients with arthritis, these procedures must still be considered evolutionary. Changes in surgical technique, prosthetic design, and biomaterials continue. Because of continuing advance, surgery should be delayed in patients who continue to function at a satisfactory level with discomfort that is tolerable. Procedures such as fusion and osteotomy should be used when appropriate, especially in younger patients. An abiding principle of reconstructive surgery is that preservation of bone stock by timely early performance of nonprosthetic procedures is preferable to joint replacement, particularly in young, active patients.

Experience has revealed that the more anatomic the joint replacement, the greater the likelihood for long-term success. The technical expertise of the arthritis surgeon is correlated with the early functional result and complication rate.

Long-term outcome studies of large numbers of patients will help determine the appropriate choice of prosthetic designs. Appropriate clinical judgment in selecting patients for surgery and the use of precise surgical techniques, however, will remain the dominant aspects in the surgical management of arthritis.

Annotated Bibliography

Chmell MJ, Scott RD, Thomas WH, Sledge CB: Total hip arthroplasty with cement for juvenile rheumatoid arthritis: Results at a minimum of ten years in patients less than thirty years old. *J Bone Joint Surg* 1997;79A:44–52.

Eighteen percent of femoral components and 35% of acetabular components are revised at an average of 12.8 and 11.8 years, respectively. Long-term durability of components in these young patients remains a concern.

Connor PM, Morrey BF: Total elbow arthroplasty in patients who have juvenile rheumatoid arthritis. *J Bone Joint Surg* 1998;80A: 678–688.

In 23 total elbow replacements followed for 2 or more years, results were excellent in 12, great in 8, and poor in 3. The improvement in range of motion was not as consistent as that of pain relief.

Friedman RJ, Schiff CF, Bromberg JS: Use of supplemental steroids in patients having orthopaedic operations. *J Bone Joint Surg* 1995;77A:1801–1806.

Twenty-eight patients receiving chronic exogenous glucocorticoids were given their baseline dose of steroid instead of perioperative stress dosing. No evidence of adrenal insufficiency was detected.

Laskin RS, O'Flynn HM: Total knee replacement with posterior cruciate ligament retention in rheumatoid arthritis: Problems and complications. *Clin Orthop* 1997;345:24–28.

This award-winning article compared the results of posterior cruciate ligament (PCL)-retaining total knee replacement (TKR) in patients with rheumatoid arthritis and osteoarthritis. Patients with rheumatoid arthritis had an increased rate of failure and were noted at revision to have abnormal PCLs. It was concluded that patients with rheumatoid arthritis should be treated with a posterior stabilized design of TKR.

Schemitsch EH, Ewald FC, Thornhill TS: Results of total elbow arthroplasty after excision of the radial head and synovectomy in patients who had rheumatoid arthritis. *J Bone Joint Surg* 1996;78A:1541–1547.

This review suggests that results were adversely affected and complications increased in these rheumatoid patients having capitellocondylar elbow replacement following failed radial head excision and synovectomy. A more constrained prosthesis may be indicated in some of these patients.

Terrono AL, Feldon PG, Millender LH, Nalebuff EA: Evaluation and treatment of the rheumatoid wrist. *J Bone Joint Surg* 1995;77A:1116–1128.

This instructional course lecture gives an excellent summary of rheumatoid wrist surgery, including prophylactic and reconstructive procedures.

Wattenmaker I, Concepcion M, Hibberd P, Lipson S: Upper-airway obstruction and perioperative management of the airway in patients managed with posterior operations on the cervical spine for rheumatoid arthritis. *J Bone Joint Surg* 1994;76A:360–365.

This article discusses the many challenges of airway management in patients with rheumatoid arthritis. In the patients having posterior cervical spine surgery, significant benefit is shown from fiberoptic intubation while the patient is awake.

Weinblatt ME: Antirheumatic drug therapy and the surgical patient, in Sledge CB, Ruddy S, Harris ED Jr, Kelley WN (eds): *Arthritis Surgery*. Philadelphia, PA, WB Saunders, 1994, pp 669–673.

This chapter presents an excellent review of the perioperative management of antirheumatic medicines.

Wolfe F, Zwillich SH: The long-term outcomes of rheumatoid arthritis: A 23-year prospective, longitudinal study of total joint replacement and its predictors in 1,600 patients with rheumatoid arthritis. *Arthritis Rheum* 1998;41:1072–1082.

Twenty-five percent of rheumatoid patients will undergo total joint replacement within 21.8 years of disease onset. After primary total joint replacement, 25% will have a record joint replacement within 1 year and 50% within 7 years.

Classic Bibliography

Burton KE, Wright V, Richards J: Patients' expectations in relation to outcome of total hip replacement surgery. *Ann Rheum Dis* 1979;38:471–474.

Collins DN, Barnes CL, FitzRandolph RL: Cervical spine instability in rheumatoid patients having total hip or knee arthroplasty. *Clin Orthop* 1991;272:127–135.

Huo MH, Salvati EA, Browne MG, Pellicci PM, Sculco TP, Johanson NA: Primary total hip arthroplasty in systemic lupus erythematosus. *J Arthroplasty* 1992;7:51–56.

Jergesen HE, Poss R, Sledge CB: Bilateral total hip and knee replacement in adults with rheumatoid arthritis: An evaluation of function. *Clin Orthop* 1978;137:120–128.

Kilgus DJ, Namba RS, Gorek JE, Cracchiolo A III, Amstutz HC: Total hip replacement for patients who have ankylosing spondylitis: The importance of the formation of heterotopic bone and of the durability of fixation of cemented components. *J Bone Joint Surg* 1990;72A:834–839.

Perhala RS, Wilke WS, Clough JD, Segal AM: Local infectious complications following large joint replacement in rheumatoid arthritis patients treated with methotrexate versus those not treated with methotrexate. *Arthritis Rheum* 1991;34:146–152.

Sledge CB: Joint replacement surgery in juvenile rheumatoid arthritis. *Arthritis Rheum* 1977;20(suppl 2):567–572.

Sledge CB, Zuckerman JD, Shortkroff S, et al: Synovectomy of the rheumatoid knee using intra-articular injection of dysprosium-165-ferric hydroxide macroaggregates. *J Bone Joint Surg* 1987;69A:970–975.

Stern SH, Insall JN, Windsor RE, Inglis AE, Dines DM: Total knee arthroplasty in patients with psoriasis. *Clin Orthop* 1989;248:108–111.

Walker LG, Sledge CB: Total hip arthroplasty in ankylosing spondylitis. *Clin Orthop* 1991;262:198–204.

Chapter 2
Osteoarthritis

Osteoarthritis occurs with increased frequency in older individuals; however, the interrelationship between aging and osteoarthritis is less clear. Although osteoarthritis may begin at a relatively young age, it progresses to become clinically apparent and, accordingly, "more prevalent" with aging. Alternatively, osteoarthritis may result when changes in cartilage brought about by aging predispose the joint to degeneration in response to external factors such as biomechanical stresses.

It is known that hypertrophic arthritis could develop in response to a variety of different insults. Almost any form of injury or disease of a joint can initiate the process that results in osteoarthritis. Osteoarthritis can follow a mechanical insult, such as a meniscectomy, or an inflammatory joint disease, such as rheumatoid arthritis. This knowledge led to the differentiation of osteoarthritis into 2 main types: secondary, when a causative actor can be identified, and primary, when no such cause is apparent. However, it is now apparent that such a scheme is too simple, because the development of some forms of secondary disease, such as postmeniscectomy knee osteoarthritis, depends on a multitude of risk factors, including age, sex, and family history, in addition to the identified cause. Studies comparing the prevalence of a disease in different populations often provide insights about the disease's etiology. Caucasian populations from well-developed countries have similar rates of osteoarthritis in the hands and knees. Black American women had higher rates of knee osteoarthritis than did white Americans in the U.S. National Health and Nutrition Examination Survey (NHANES I), even after adjustment for age and weight. No racial differences in osteoarthritis rates were found in men. Black Jamaican women also have high rates of knee osteoarthritis. Furthermore, the expression of osteoarthritis depends on the insult: in osteoarthritis secondary to rheumatoid arthritis, for example, osteophyte formation is suppressed.

Diagnostic Evaluation/Epidemiology

Because osteoarthritis is a heterogeneous condition, the different ways in which it is expressed has hampered the development of diagnostic criteria. This great heterogeneity is explained by the new concept of an overlapping group of osteoarthritis disorders that have variable degrees of degradation, repair, and bone reaction. It also helps in the development of a framework for the description of osteoarthritis. However, there is no one way to recognize osteoarthritis, and no clear dichotomy exists between those with and without the condition. Furthermore, there are several different potential uses for any diagnostic criteria that might be developed (Outline 1). These diagnostic criteria must be standardized so that direct comparison of different investigations of patients with osteoarthritis is possible.

The main clinical symptoms and signs in symptomatic osteoarthritis include use-related joint pain, stiffness of joints after inactivity, restricted range of motion, bony swelling, and joint crepitus of the joint. Other features, including pain at rest or at night, instability, and joint deformity, may be present.

There are 3 main problems with any attempt to define osteoarthritis clinically. (1) Many of the key clinical features, such as pain, do not persist and depend on factors such as general health, in addition to joint pathology. (2) Many of the symptoms and signs are subjective and/or cannot be reproduced. (3) Many of the clinical features are nonspecific; for example, pain, restricted movement, stiffness, deformity, and instability can be present in any form of chronic arthritis.

In spite of these difficulties, some clinical features can be helpful and discriminative. For example, the presence of palpable Heberden's nodes of the distal interphalangeal joints is a fairly reproducible physical sign, which correlates well with radiographic changes. Similarly, bony swelling and crepitus at the knee joint are signs that have relatively low interobserver or intraobserver error, which helps differentiate between osteoarthritis and inflammatory forms of chronic arthritis.

The history and common pathologic definition of osteoarthritis both emphasize focal loss of articular cartilage and increased activity of the subchondral and marginal bone. In the majority of epidemiologic and clinical studies of the disease over the past 40 years, plain radiographs have been used to confirm the presence of these features. The atlas-based Kellgren and Lawrence criteria, which differentiate 4 grades of disease, have been the most widely used until recently. Different studies have used different definitions of

Parts of this chapter have been adapted from Kuettner KE, Goldberg VM (eds): Osteoarthritic Disorders. *Rosemont, IL, American Academy of Orthopaedic Surgeons, 1995.*

Outline 1
Possible uses and types of diagnostic criteria for osteoarthritis

Possible uses for diagnostic criteria*

- Population studies (cross sectional/longitudinal)
- Case control studies
- Studies of disease process
- Patient-based studies of natural history
- Intervention studies

Types of diagnostic criteria†

- Radiographic changes
- Other imaging modalities
- Symptoms and/or physical signs
- Body fluid tests (synovial fluid, blood, urine)
- Histopathology

*It is unlikely that a single set of diagnostic criteria will be applicable to all uses

†It is likely that a combination of different aspects will be used in most criteria

(Reproduced with permission from Dieppe P: The classification and diagnosis of osteoarthritis, in Kuettner KE, Goldberg VM (eds): *Osteoarthritic Disorders*. Rosemont, IL, American Academy of Orthopaedic Surgeons, 1995, pp 5–12.)

osteoarthritis, and this inconsistency has frequently created confusion. In most studies, cases are defined as those with at least definite osteophytes by radiograph (grade 2 changes). Scandinavian studies have used a definition that requires at least joint space narrowing, and clinical studies have used subjects in whom symptoms are present.

There are 3 reasons why plain radiographs can be difficult to interpret when detecting osteoarthritic features. The first is that they lack sensitivity; joint damage needs to be extensive before changes are seen on the plain radiographs. Second, the emphasis is on bone changes; bony abnormalities are easier to see and grade than the changes in the joint space that constitute the only way cartilage disease can be detected. Third, radiographic scoring is subjective and has poor reproducibility. Until recently, measurement was hardly ever attempted, and little or no attempt was made to assess the reproducibility of the findings recorded by different observers.

Radiographic evaluation has been further complicated because the findings do not always correlate with the patient's findings. Five hundred patients were studied over a 3-year period in Bristol, England; 415 (average age, 65.6 years) completed the study. Although 193 of these patients had knee joint disease at the onset, a correlation between radiographs and clinical changes during the period of study could not be identified.

Over the last few years, several advances have been made in understanding the role of plain radiographs in assessment of osteoarthritis. The reliability of new and old grading scales has been discussed, and ways of measuring the interbone distance or volume have been described. It is clear, then, that the quality and value of information that can be obtained improves immensely with attention to detail with patient positioning, careful grading of the individual features of osteoarthritis on radiographs, and measurement of the cartilage space.

Arthritic Changes and Pathology

Cartilage degeneration during osteoarthritis is characterized by profound changes in the articular surface (fibrillation), the deeper zones (fissuring), and in partial or complete loss of the tissue (erosion). In addition, more subtle early changes occur in chondrocyte biosynthetic activity and biochemical composition. On the basis of the understanding of the structure-function relationships of normal articular cartilage, it is known that these structural and compositional changes in osteoarthritis cartilage will influence the mechanical behavior and intrinsic material properties of this tissue.

Proteoglycans (PGs), found in cartilage, form a diverse family of glycoproteins with the common characteristic that they possess at least 1 glycosaminoglycan (GAG) chain attached to a core protein. Chondrocytes synthesize and secrete into the extracellular matrix a number of PGs, including aggrecan, a member of the large PG family; the small PGs biglycan, decorin, and fibromodulin; and the α2-chain of type IX collagen, which can be substituted with a chondroitin sulfate/dermatan sulfate GAG chain.

The characteristic large PG species of cartilage consists of a highly substituted monomeric core protein of about 220 kd; the mature molecular weight is approximately 2,500 kd. There are approximately 100 chondroitin sulfate and 20 keratan sulfate GAG chains covalently bound to the core protein. The aminoterminal end of the core protein noncovalently binds along strands of hyaluronate, resulting in aggregates of up to 250×10^6d. The aggregates are stabilized by a third component, link protein. These hydrophilic supramolecular aggregates are responsible primarily for the low-friction surface and compressive resilience of articular cartilage, properties embodied in the recently coined name for the large aggregating PG of cartilage-aggrecan.

A panel of monoclonal antibodies that recognize subtle changes in the biochemistry of cartilage PGs has been identified. The changes result from either anabolic or catabolic processes in cartilage metabolism that lead to the eventful onset of arthritis. These monoclonal antibodies recognize new epitopes (called neoepitopes) that are produced as a result of specific anabolic or catabolic processes in metabolism. Two classes of monoclonal antibodies that recognize neoepitopes generated during the pathogenesis of arthritis have been produced and characterized. These antibodies can be used to monitor changes in the biochemistry of cartilage PGs in the early stages of the disease process. Antibodies that recognize anabolic neoepitopes in cartilage PGs detect changes in PG biochemistry that parallel switching of the chondrocyte phenotype in its attempt to repair the tissue. In contrast, antibodies recognizing catabolic neoepitopes detect specific PG degradation products, which result from the actions of matrix proteinases (catabolic agents) that cause cartilage destruction. Both classes of monoclonal antibodies show potential for the development of diagnostic procedures for monitoring the progression of cartilage's attempts at repair and also its eventual destruction in arthritis. Furthermore, they have potential for the discovery of therapeutic agents that may stop or slow the progression of the disease.

Mechanical forces can induce change in the form and structure of many biologic materials in vivo, including articular cartilage. This effect, called Wolff's Law, has been most widely studied in the field of bone remodeling. Recent studies have shown that when the mechanical loading regimen of a joint is changed, for example in immobilized or overused joints in vivo, there are significant changes in the composition, molecular structure, and mechanical properties of the articular cartilage. These changes seem to be reversible, and, therefore, represent an active remodeling process on the part of the chondrocytes to maintain homeostasis. However, certain in vivo changes, for example, those induced by joint instability secondary to the rupture of an anterior cruciate ligament (ACL) or by injury or removal of the medial meniscus in the knee, appear irreversible. These changes include damage to the microstructure, altered chondrocyte metabolism and biochemical composition, and deleterious changes in the material properties and load-carrying behavior of the articular cartilage. Clinically, it is a combination of early and subtle changes that progress and ultimately result in cartilage degeneration and osteoarthritis. A canine model of osteoarthritis (transection of the ACL) was used to demonstrate that such changes lead to progressive damage of the articular cartilage, which proceeds inexorably toward the development of true osteoarthritis.

A group of patients with hip arthritis were studied to determine the amount of synovial fluid present in the hip. Chondroitin-6-sulfate and chondroitin-4-sulfate concentrations were studied in relation to age and radiologic stage of the disease. Chondroitin-6-sulfate was predominant in all disease stages, and there was a negative correlation with advanced age. Chondroitin-4-sulfate and chondroitin-6-sulfate concentrations were lower with advanced disease than in earlier stages of arthritis. Although these isomers may serve as markers reflecting extracellular matrix (ECM) metabolism, the mechanism to turn on the process may be critical to the treatment of osteoarthritis.

In matrix-depleted osteoarthritic cartilage, the chondrocyte may undergo repair-specific changes in the amounts and types of expressed gene products. Although there have been a number of studies on chondrocyte metabolism and matrix biosynthesis in osteoarthritic cartilage, it is not yet clear whether attempts at cartilage matrix repair represent an elevation of normal turnover or whether wound healing in cartilage involves the production of a matrix that differs biochemically and biomechanically from normal cartilage.

What is the rationale for the presence of gene products not normally found in adult cartilage? Chondrocytes in osteoarthritic cartilage might, like other tissues undergoing stress, downregulate normally expressed gene products and produce stress proteins, which might give the cell a survival advantage. Although construction of an ECM occurs outside the cell, it probably is not a completely random entropy-driven assembly of macromolecules. During normal maintenance and repair of cartilage, regulatory molecules, such as decorin, are produced that may influence ECM assembly. Only a small fraction of the total repertoire of the chondrocyte has been discovered, and other proteins regulating matrix assembly during development may be re-expressed during repair. Furthermore, ordered matrix assembly may be directed by a specific program of gene expression, which involves turning genes on and off in a temporal sequence. Such an ordered program of expression has been observed during callus formation following bone fracture.

Cartilage Repair

Cartilage repair in defects extending through the subchondral bone is initiated by an influx of pluripotent mesenchymal cells that undergo differentiation. Expression of cartilage-specific messenger RNA (mRNA) is not completely restricted to cartilage; it has been observed in cells recruited during cartilage repair. For example, cells in the inner cambial layer of developing periosteum have been shown to express type II collagen mRNA, which could indicate the state of readiness of this cell population to differentiate into chondrocytes. Similarly, expression of aggrecan and link protein mRNA by cultured mesenchymal stem cells obtained from rabbit bone marrow has been observed. These cells rapidly differentiate into chondrocytes when placed into defects in rabbit articular cartilage. Differentiating mesenchymal cells may express matrix components, alternatively spliced forms of cartilage proteins, and growth factors known to be produced during embryonic chondrogenesis. Insights into cartilage repair at the level of gene expression are likely to emerge from studies of chondrogenesis during development. Conversely, novel gene products specific to repair may shed light on developmental processes.

Surgical Treatment

The goal of surgical treatment of patients with osteoarthritis is to decrease or eliminate pain and improve function. The great success of joint replacements in achieving these goals has stimulated substantial investment in refinement of joint implants and techniques of joint replacement and led the public and many physicians to view these procedures as the only effective methods of treating osteoarthritis. Optimal current practice and future development of the surgical treatment of osteoarthritis require a broader perspective. In particular, procedures that decrease pain and improve function by restoring the joint instead of resecting and replacing it would have great advantages, especially for young patients and for patients with less advanced joint degeneration who want to maintain a high level of activity.

Procedures performed with the intent of treating osteoarthritis by preserving or restoring articular cartilage surfaces include osteotomies and muscle releases; joint debridement including shaving fibrillated cartilage; resection or perforation of subchondral bone; resection arthroplasty; and periosteal, perichondral, and osteochondral autografts and allografts. Although surgeons have reported series of patients treated by these procedures, in many instances it is difficult to evaluate the results. The studies lack control or comparison groups or randomization of patients among treatments, length of follow-up is often short, the methods of measuring outcomes vary among surgeons and often are not well defined, and most studies consist of retrospective reviews rather than prospective clinical trials. Despite these limitations, evaluating the results of current practices contributes to understanding of the potential for surgical treatment of osteoarthritis.

Promising experimental methods of stimulating formation of a new joint surface include growth factors, cell transplants, and artificial matrices. Thus far, none of these approaches has been shown to regenerate tissue that duplicates the structure, composition, mechanical properties, and durability of articular cartilage in an osteoarthritic joint, and it is unlikely that any one of these methodologies will be generally successful in the treatment of human osteoarthritis. Instead, the available clinical and experimental evidence indicates that future optimal surgical treatments of osteoarthritic joints will begin with a detailed analysis of the structural and functional abnormalities of the involved joint and the patient's expectations for future joint use. Based on this analysis, the surgeon can develop a treatment plan that potentially combines correction of mechanical abnormalities (including malalignment, instability, and intra-articular causes of mechanical dysfunction), debridement that may or may not include limited penetration of subchondral bone, and applications of growth factors or implants that may consist of a synthetic matrix that incorporates cells or growth factors followed by a postoperative course of controlled loading and motion.

Annotated Bibliography

Dieppe P, Cushnaghan J, Shepstone L: The Bristol 'OA500' study: Progression of osteoarthritis (OA) over 3 years and the relationship between clinical and radiographic changes at the knee joint. *Osteoarthritis Cartilage* 1997;5:87–97.

This study concluded that radiographic change may not be a good indicator for clinical outcome in established, symptomatic osteoarthritis.

Guilak F, Ratcliffe A, Lane N, Rosenwasser MP, Mow VC: Mechanical and biochemical changes in the superficial zone of articular cartilage in canine experimental osteoarthritis. *J Orthop Res* 1994;12:474–484.

In a canine model of early osteoarthritis generated by transection of the anterior cruciate ligament, changes in tensile mechanical properties and biochemical composition of the superficial zone of the articular cartilage were studied. Disruption and remodeling of the collagen network was observed in the superficial zone of the articular cartilage.

Muller FJ, Setton LA, Manicourt DH, Mow VC, Howell DS, Pita JC: Centrifugal and biochemical comparison of proteoglycan aggregates from articular cartilage in experimental joint disuse and joint instability. *J Orthop Res* 1994;12:498–508.

In 2 canine models involving altered joint loading, the effects on the biochemical composition and proteoglycan aggregate structure of articular cartilage were compared. The most interesting contrast between the 2 models was the approximately 80% decrease in hyaluronan content after transection of the anterior cruciate ligament.

Setton LA, Mow VC, Muller FJ, Pita JC, Howell DS: Mechanical properties of canine articular cartilage are significantly altered following transection of the anterior cruciate ligament. *J Orthop Res* 1994;12:451–463.

In this study, compressive, tensile, and swelling properties of articular cartilage were evaluated at 2 time periods after transection of the anterior cruciate ligament in greyhounds. It was noted that the pattern and extent of changes in these properties indicate that altered joint loading severely compromises the overall mechanical behavior of the articular cartilage.

van der Kraan PM, Vitters EL, Meijers TH, Poole AR, van den Berg WB: Collagen type I antisense and collagen type IIA messenger RNA is expressed in adult murine articular cartilage. *Osteoarthritis Cartilage* 1998;6:417–426.

The authors studied the reparative process in murine articular cartilage after moderate proteoglycan depletion to determine if the process is accompanied by a change in chondrocyte phenotype. It was concluded that the absence of changes in collagen mRNA expression indicates that a change in chondrocyte phenotype does not occur during the repair process after moderate proteoglycan depletion.

Wotton SF, Dieppe PA, Duance VC: Type IX collagen immunoreactive peptides in synovial fluids from arthritis patients. *Rheumatology* 1993;8:338–345.

The authors studied whether type IX collagen-related peptides can be detected in the synovial fluid of patients with arthritis in order to determine if these peptides can serve as molecular markers of arthritis.

Yamada H, Miyauchi S, Hotta H, et al: Levels of chondroitin sulfate isomers in synovial fluid of patients with hip osteoarthritis. *J Orthop Sci* 1994;250–254.

Levels of chondroitin sulfate isomers in the synovial fluid of hip osteoarthritis patients were studied to determine their significance as markers of extracellular matrix metabolism. The results indicate that the concentration of these isomers in synovial fluid varies with disease severity.

Classic Bibliography

Doherty M, Watt I, Dieppe P: Influence of primary generalised osteoarthritis on development of secondary osteoarthritis. *Lancet* 1983;2:8–11.

Felson DT: Epidemiology of hip and knee osteoarthritis. *Epidemiol Rev* 1988;10:1–28.

Grover J, Roughley PJ: Versican gene expression in human articular cartilage and comparison of mRNA splicing variation with aggrecan. *Biochem J* 1993;291:361–367.

Anderson JJ, Felson DT: Factors associated with osteoarthritis of the knee in the first national Health and Nutrition Examination Survey (HANES I): Evidence for an association with overweight, race, and physical demands of work. *Am J Epidemiol* 1988;128: 179–189.

Davis MA, Ettinger WH, Neuhaus JM, Barclay JD, Segal MR: Correlates of knee pain among US adults with and without radiographic knee osteoarthritis. *J Rheumatol* 1992;19:1943–1949.

Hart DJ, Spector TD, Brown P, Wilson P, Doyle DV, Silman AJ: Clinical signs of early osteoarthritis: Reproducibility and relation to x-ray changes in 541 women in the general population. *Ann Rheum Dis* 1991;50:467–470.

Mörgelin M, Paulsson M, Hardingham TE, et al: Cartilage proteoglycans: Assembly with hyaluronate and link protein as studied by electron microscopy. *Biochem J* 1988;253:175–185.

Mow VC, Ratcliffe A, Poole AR: Cartilage and diarthrodial joints as paradigms for hierarchical materials and structures. *Biomaterials* 1992;13:67–97.

Howell DS, Treadwell BV, Trippel SB: Etiopathogenesis of osteoarthritis, in Moskowitz RW, Howell DS, Goldberg VM, Mankin HJ (eds): *Osteoarthritis: Diagnosis and Medical/Surgical Management*, ed 2. Philadelphia, PA, WB Saunders, 1992, pp 233–252.

Mankin HJ, Brandt KD: Biochemistry and metabolism of articular cartilage in osteoarthritis, in Moskowitz RW, Howell DS, Goldberg VM, Mankin HJ (eds) *Osteoarthritis: Diagnosis and Medical/Surgical Management*, ed 2. Philadelphia PA, WB Saunders, 1992, pp 109–154.

Doege K, Rhodes C, Sasaki M, Hassell JR, Yamada Y: Molecular biology of cartilage proteoglycan (aggrecan) and link protein, in Sandell LJ, Boyd CD (eds): *Extracellular Matrix Genes*. San Diego, CA, Academic Press, 1990, pp 137–155.

Carney SL, Billingham ME, Muir H, Sandy JD: Demonstration of increased proteoglycan turnover in cartilage explants from dogs with experimental osteoarthritis. *J Orthop Res* 1984;2:201–206.

Brandt KD, Braunstein EM, Visco DM, O'Connor B, Heck D, Albrecht M: Anterior (cranial) cruciate ligament transection in the dog; A bona fide model of osteoarthritis, not merely of cartilage injury and repair. *J Rheumatol* 1991;18:436–446.

Kellgren JH, Lawrence JS: Radiological assessment of osteoarthrosis. *Ann Rheum Dis* 1957;16:494–502.

Chapter 3
Pathophysiology and Treatment of Venous Thromboembolic Disease

The Problem

Venous thromboembolic disease (VTED) presents the most significant perioperative threat to the life of the total joint replacement patient; as such, it remains one of the most controversial and emotional topics in contemporary orthopaedics. Historically, the unprotected patient incurred a risk of deep vein thrombosis (DVT) between 70% and 84% after total hip (THA) or knee (TKA) arthroplasty, with a frequency of symptomatic pulmonary embolism (PE) approaching 15% and fatal PE of 1% to 3.4%. A fatal PE rate of 3.4% was reported for 2,012 consecutive THAs performed from 1969 to 1971 when the average duration of surgery was 2.4 hours, the blood loss was 1,650 cc, patients remained on bed rest for 1 week before ambulation, and the mean postoperative hospital stay was 3 weeks. There is no argument that several prophylactic regimens, both pharmacologic and mechanical, as well as improvements in surgical technique and anesthetic management alone, have reduced the prevalence of DVT following total joint replacement; demonstrating a similar reduction in the rate of fatal PE is a statistically more difficult task because of its rarity.

Some recent information from the environment of earlier postoperative mobilization and decreasing hospital stay suggests a fatal PE rate as low as 0.35% in 1,162 THA patients with 6 month follow-up in 1 study and 0.12% in 3,432 THA in another series with only 3 month follow-up in the absence of any chemoprophylaxis. On the other hand, the overall perioperative mortality following 7,959 THA in the absence of VTED prophylaxis was reported to be 1.68% in 1977. Twenty years later, 2 series involving a total of 12,769 THA patients accounted for an overall mortality rate of 1.71% without VTED prophylaxis, suggesting that little had changed in the intervening 2 decades. Not surprisingly, current management of VTED risk is as varied as these disparate perceptions of the prevalence of VTED.

New knowledge of the basic science of coagulation has better elucidated the mechanisms of and predisposition to venous thrombosis. At the same time, the relative risks and benefits of prophylaxis, the choice of specific agent and its optimal duration of use in the face of abbreviated hospitalization, the role of routine diagnostic surveillance, and guidelines for treatment of established VTED have all come under renewed scrutiny. These timely issues form the basis of this review.

Current Epidemiology of VTED

Both DVT and PE remain major health problems in contemporary medicine; PE can be fatal and DVT is the common precursor to PE. PE frequently escapes detection, and its prevalence is difficult to quantitate; in the general population, the frequency of autopsy-proven fatal PE is 2.5 times that of symptomatic nonfatal PE. Alternatively, DVT may be solely responsible for morbidity related to chronic venous insufficiency. Postthrombotic syndrome is evident in 35% to 70% of patients with previous DVT at 3 years, and 50% to 100% at 10 years, depending on the extent of initial thrombosis. Analysis of patients with venogram-confirmed asymptomatic DVT showed 67% to have signs and symptoms of postthrombotic syndrome 5 years postoperatively compared with only 32% who had negative postoperative venograms. Popliteal or more proximal involvement increases the frequency and severity of chronic venous insufficiency; up to 8% of patients with proximal thrombosis will eventually develop skin ulceration. Postthrombotic morbidity is even more common following " idiopathic" than after postoperative DVT.

Routine prophylaxis has become the standard of care in North America following THA and TKA since the recommendations of the National Institutes of Health (NIH) Consensus Conference in 1986, and low-intensity warfarin the most common agent used by orthopaedists over the past 2 decades. Nonetheless, while warfarin has considerably reduced the prevalence of DVT, it remains between 15% and 25% after THA and between 35% and 50% after TKA. The frequency of clinically significant bleeding events with warfarin has been reduced from 8% to 12% with a prothrombin time index of 2.0 to 1% to 2% with acceptance of low inten-

The author or the departments with which he is affiliated has received something of value from a commercial or other party related directly or indirectly to the subject of this chapter.

sity anticoagulation to maintain the prothrombin time index between 1.3 and 1.5 (International Normalized Ratio [INR] between 2.0 and 2.5). Although these figures indicate that VTED is more refractory to standard prophylaxis following TKA, most (85% to 90%) of those thrombi occur below the venous trifurcation in the deep calf veins and, therefore, carry less immediate risk of embolization. In contrast, the distribution of DVT after THA was historically a nearly equal split between proximal (40%) and distal (60%) thrombi, but in more recent trials with contemporary prophylactic agents there were fewer than 10% proximal thrombi after THA, with the remainder occurring in the calf. Therefore, under the influence of current prophylaxis, 85% to 90% of all DVT following both THA and TKA occur in the calf, focusing greater attention on distal thrombotic disease. Furthermore, longitudinal surveillance studies have demonstrated that 17% to 23% of these distal thrombi extend to the more proximal veins of the thigh where they acquire considerable embolic potential.

Four reports, including 2 in the past 2 years, account for a total of 4 deaths (0.05%) attributed to PE during a 6-month follow-up of 7,687 THA patients on perioperative Coumadin prophylaxis. The corresponding overall death rate was 0.32% (21/6,588) for 3 of the reports with these figures available. Although not derived from the same clinical trial, these death rates are lower than the 6-month 0.35% PE mortality cited for unprophylaxed THA patients and the corresponding 1.71% overall mortality rate reported by investigators from the United Kingdom. This reduction in both fatal PE and overall mortality substantiates the value of routine prophylaxis and, consequently, supports the strategy of warfarin prophylaxis for VTED after THA.

Pathogenesis of Venous Thromboembolism

Virchow's triad remains the basis of the conceptual understanding of the mechanism of coagulation, and perturbations in those pathways are responsible for the abnormalities of thrombosis following total joint replacement. Recent discoveries concerning the clotting cascade form the basis of new therapeutic approaches to thrombotic disease.

Familial Thrombophilia and Factor V Leiden

Familial thrombophilia, the heritable tendency to develop severe and recurrent VTED, often spontaneously, has been inadequately explained by any deficiency of circulating anticoagulants; levels of proteins C and S as well as antithrombin III were rarely found to be low in these patients. Mutations in genetic material encoding proteins C, S, and antithrombin III were found in aggregate to account for less than 5% of all cases of familial thrombophilia. In 1994, a single amino acid substitution of glutamine for arginine in the protein C cleavage region of factor V was reported to occur in 50% of familial thrombophilia cases compared with only 3% to 7% of the general population (Fig. 1). This single nucleotide substitution, known as Factor V Leiden, is responsible for resistance of activated factor V to activated protein C inactivation, which normally provides a physiologic checkrein on the clotting cascade.

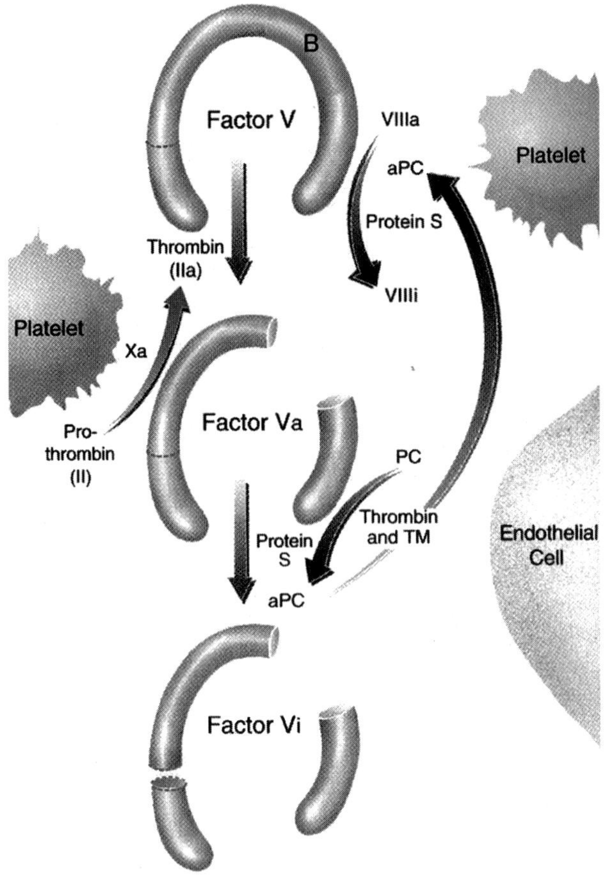

Figure 1

Procoagulant and anticoagulant actions of factor V. Before activation (top) factor V is a single chain polypeptide that may serve, in concert with protein S, as a cofactor in the inactivation of factor VIIIa by activated protein C. Factor V is activated (middle) to become a 2-chain polypeptide, factor Va, when its B domain is excised by thrombin (factor IIa). On the platelet surface, factor Va in turn greatly accelerates the activation of prothrombin (factor II) by factor Xa. Activated protein C (aPC) inactivates factor Va to factor Vi (bottom) in the presence of protein S by cleaving a single Arg-Gly peptide bond in factor Va. This is the site of the Factor V Leiden mutation, substituting glutamine for arginine, that imparts resistance of Factor Va to aPC cleavage. (Reproduced with permission from Hajjar KA: Factor V Leiden—An unselfish gene? *N Engl J Med* 1994;331:1586.)

Variable phenotypic expression of Factor V Leiden subsequently has been shown to be responsible for a range in severity of a host of clinical disease states related to thrombosis. More than half of all persons with Factor V Leiden will develop DVT in the presence of a single additional risk factor, such as a long-bone fracture or a total joint arthroplasty. In the obstetric population, the presence of Factor V Leiden predicts a 60% occurrence of DVT in the first trimester. In a study in which nearly 15,000 men were followed for cardiovascular events, an equal 4% to 6% prevalence of Factor V Leiden was observed among those experiencing no events, myocardial infarction, or stroke; in contrast, Factor V Leiden was found among 11.6% of those with PE or DVT for a relative risk of 3.5. Similarly, among men over age 60 with primary spontaneous DVT, the prevalence of Factor V Leiden was 26%. In 2 preliminary studies of THA and TKA patients, there has been no correlation between the presence of Factor V Leiden, or depletion of any of the other circulating anticoagulants, and the occurrence of VTED. This negative observation may be explained by the preliminary nature of the findings, or by a thrombogenic stimulus associated with violation of the medullary canal during total joint arthroplasty that is so intense that it overshadows any heritable predisposition to thrombosis that Factor V Leiden might impart.

Thrombogenesis Following Musculoskeletal Injury

It has long been recognized that orthopaedic VTED is more refractory to standard prophylaxis than that occurring after general surgical procedures. This was first made evident by the inefficacy of subcutaneous heparin in preventing DVT after THA and has subsequently been shown to be secondary to a decline in antithrombin III levels after skeletal injury or manipulation of the medullary canal as occurs during total joint arthroplasty.

A recent study of a population of multiply injured patients with an Injury Severity Score of greater than 9 serves to underscore the important influence of skeletal trauma on the clotting cascade. In 349 patients studied using contrast venography, the overall DVT prevalence was found to be 58% with a proximal DVT rate of 18%. As in VTED following total joint arthroplasty, the majority of these patients were asymptomatic; DVT was clinically evident in only 3 of 201 patients. The overall prevalence of DVT associated with specific single-system trauma was 41% for injury to the face, chest, or abdomen and 39% for closed head injury compared with 66% for lower extremity fracture and 68% for spinal cord injury. The overwhelming influence of fracture on the development of DVT was shown by DVT prevalences of 61% with pelvic fracture, 77% with tibial shaft fracture, and 80% with femoral shaft fracture. Femoral or tibial shaft fracture was associated with a relative risk of DVT of nearly 5 times that of the overall group. Spinal cord injury was associated with an 81% prevalence of DVT and an odds ratio of 8.5 compared with the total group.

The same investigators subsequently studied the impact of VTED prophylaxis in this patient population, and 2 years later they reported on a series of 344 polytrauma patients randomized to 2 anticoagulant protocols. They observed an overall DVT prevalence of 44% in 60 patients on unfractionated heparin compared with 31% in 40 patients on enoxaparin ($p = 0.014$); corresponding rates for proximal DVT were 15% and 6% ($p = 0.012$), respectively. Major bleeding complications were 5 times more frequent with enoxaparin (2.9%) than heparin (0.6%; $p = 0.12$). Caution is indicated with use of fractionated heparins for VTED prophylaxis in the polytrauma patient, especially those with closed head trauma, visceral injury, or those expected to undergo delayed surgical fracture repair, especially involving the pelvis.

Thrombogenesis During Anesthesia and Total Hip Arthroplasty

Increasing evidence suggests that the principal thrombogenic stimulus associated with THA occurs intraoperatively. More specifically, the time of femoral preparation has been shown to be closely linked with intense activation of the clotting cascade as well as torsion, and even complete obstruction, of the femoral vein. Pioneers in the investigation of the effects of anesthesia and intraoperative events on the process of thrombogenesis measured markers of thrombin generation and fibrin formation in circulating blood during THA. They demonstrated that the process of thrombosis does not begin with the start of the operation, but rather is delayed until preparation of the femoral canal. Elevation in prothrombin F1.2, thrombin-antithrombin complexes, fibrinopeptide A, and D-dimer was most pronounced during insertion of the cemented femoral component and continued to increase through 1 hour postoperatively. Mean values for 3 of the 4 markers were significantly higher after insertion of cemented compared with cementless femoral components. Mean pulmonary artery pressures peaked, and central venous oxygen tension reached a nadir after reduction of the hip, attesting to the delayed collection of embolic medullary contents in the lung because of kinking of the femoral vein during component insertion. Mechanical manipulation of the vein during positioning of the limb for femoral preparation likely also causes local intimal injury, which completes Virchow's triad in this high-risk scenario of hypercoagulability and stasis.

The efficacy of short-acting anticoagulants on blunting the intraoperative activation of the clotting cascade during THA was subsequently investigated. Ten units/kg of standard heparin given intravenously following implantation of the socket significantly inhibited fibrin formation, and 20 units/kg completely suppressed formation of fibrin. With a half-life of 30 to 40 minutes, this dose of unfractionated heparin provided only a brief risk of bleeding, and no additional intraoperative bleeding was evident. This strategy targets anticoagulation as a means to prevent intraoperative clot formation rather than retarding extension of existing thrombi postoperatively. In clinical trials, an average intraoperative dose of 1,200 U heparin was administered intravenously to 212 primary THA patients in conjunction with hypotensive epidural anesthesia before preparation of the femur. The overall DVT rate was 6.4% with a proximal thrombus prevalence of only 3.2% as determined by ultrasonography. No untoward bleeding was observed. All patients also received either postoperative aspirin (80%) or warfarin (20%) as VTED prophylaxis. Controlled trials in which the effects of intraoperative heparin are isolated from those of other anticoagulants and with venogram end point are necessary to better define the role of this approach to VTED prophylaxis.

The effects of epidural anesthesia have similarly benefited VTED prophylaxis. The mechanism of reduction of venous thromboembolism with epidural anesthesia/analgesia has been the subject of much conjecture. Inhibition of platelet and leukocyte adhesion or stimulation of endothelial fibrinolysis have been proposed, but controlled studies have not substantiated these as valid mechanisms. Rather, the sympathectomy effect of epidural blockade resulting in increased lower extremity blood flow is likely responsible for the reduction in venous thrombosis by mitigating the adverse effects of stasis. A 40% to 50% reduction of overall DVT is observed with regional as compared with general anesthesia, irrespective of the type of anticoagulant prophylaxis used. Fatal PE also is reduced by epidural anesthesia. Authors of a retrospective review of THA and TKA report an in-hospital fatal PE rate of 0.12% (7/5,874) with general anesthesia between 1981 and 1986 compared with 0.02% (2/9,685; $p = 0.03$) with epidural anesthesia between 1987 and 1991. The addition of hypotension to the epidural anesthetic reduces blood loss and secondary vasoconstriction. An overall venographic DVT rate of 10.3% and a proximal DVT rate of 4.3% have been reported in 2,037 THA patients also receiving either aspirin or Coumadin prophylaxis. Fatal PE occurred in a single patient (0.04%); of 22 PEs (1.1%), 11 (0.54%) occurred after hospital discharge, with 10 in patients with negative screening venograms. Continuation of the epidural catheter for postoperative analgesia has been purported to further extend benefits of VTED prophylaxis. In 322 consecutive THAs with epidural anesthesia and 48-hour postoperative epidural analgesia, the overall venographic DVT rate was 8.9% with proximal thrombi in 2.3%; all of these patients received concurrent coumadin prophylaxis for VTED.

With the exception of a few centers, anesthetic type has received limited attention for its role in modifying expression of VTED, and the role of the anesthetic method deserves further study. Most importantly, it must be acknowledged as a variable and controlled in future trials comparing efficacy of different methods of prophylaxis of VTED.

Diagnosis of Venous Thromboembolism

Deep Vein Thrombosis

It is well established that the clinician cannot rely solely on the physical examination and findings such as swelling, pain in the calf, palpable cords, or a positive Homan's sign to reliably diagnose DVT. Unfortunately, fatal PE may be the first manifestation of VTED, underscoring the importance of early and accurate diagnosis. A number of diagnostic tools are available to recognize DVT, but at the present time only contrast venography and ultrasonography are widely used in practice.

Ascending contrast venography remains the most reliable and sensitive method for detection of asymptomatic and nonocclusive venous thrombi in the high-risk postoperative arthroplasty patient. It is equally effective in identification of proximal and distal thrombi. The disadvantages of venography include local discomfort at the injection site, hypersensitivity reaction, and thrombosis secondary to the contrast agent. The recent introduction of more expensive nonionic iso-osmolar contrast agents has reduced the risk of iatrogenic venous thrombosis to acceptable rates well below 1%. The utility of venography as a routine surveillance tool has been suggested but its cost efficacy remains to be definitively proven.

Ultrasound is a noninvasive diagnostic imaging technique that allows visualization of venous channels and graphic presentation of flow; the coupling of Doppler technology allows determination of flow directionality. Duplex ultrasound and color flow Doppler ultrasound have been sensitive in identifying spontaneous onset thrombi in symptomatic patients but have had variable sensitivity in the postoperative patient. Notwithstanding isolated institutions with demonstrated expertise, the sensitivity of color Doppler ultrasound compared with venography ranges from 38% to 100% in detecting silent postoperative proximal DVT and 10% to 88% for calf DVT (Fig. 2). The largest venogram-controlled trials investigating calf thrombi reported sensitivities of color flow

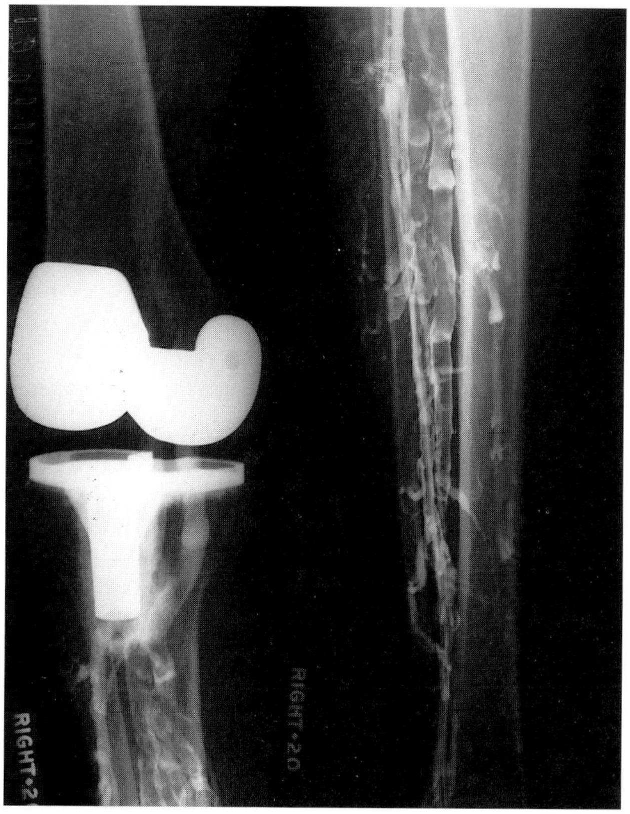

Figure 2

Distal deep vein thrombosis (DVT) after total knee arthroplasty. Extensive DVT of the paired deep peroneal veins of the calf with contiguous extension into a duplicated popliteal vein above the venous trifurcation. Color flow Doppler screening was negative when performed in the morning before this afternoon contrast venogram.

Doppler of only 10% and 33%. Although noninvasive and easily repeated in serial screening, ultrasound is not sufficiently sensitive for general application in routine postoperative surveillance of the arthroplasty patient as a means to guide prophylaxis or selective treatment of DVT.

Pulmonary Embolism

The clinical signs of PE also are often nonspecific and include pleuritic chest pain, tachycardia, pleural rub, tachypnea, and dyspnea. Patients with proximal DVT may complain of pain or swelling in the thigh. In general, as with the diagnosis of DVT, these clinical signs are unreliable. Objective testing is necessary to establish the diagnosis of PE.

Ventilation-perfusion scanning, when used with a baseline preoperative scan as in clinical trials, is a reliable screening test for PE. However, in the absence of a comparison study, a single ventilation-perfusion scan incorrectly predicts PE in 15% of the high probability scans and incorrectly rules out PE in 15% of the low probability scans compared with pulmonary angiography. This degree of reliability is not sufficient to institute therapeutic anticoagulation in the postoperative patient in view of the consequences and frequency of bleeding complications. The practical clinical value of nuclear scanning is that a normal perfusion scan essentially rules out the possibility of meaningful PE. Pulmonary angiography remains the best method to positively establish the diagnosis of PE.

There remains an unfulfilled need to reliably establish the diagnosis of DVT and PE by reproducible noninvasive means. Magnetic resonance (MR) venography has shown promise in the study of pelvic venous thrombosis and MR angiography may prove equally valuable in the evaluation of PE. Helical or spiral computed tomography allows direct viewing of all but small peripheral lung emboli. Before either of these modalities is adopted as standard practice, more extensive clinical trials to establish efficacy and cost are needed.

Prophylaxis of VTED

Routine prophylaxis for VTED following THA and TKA was recommended as standard practice by the NIH Consensus Conference in 1986. An understandable preoccupation with bleeding complications was then responsible for the slow acceptance of anticoagulant prophylaxis. Nonetheless, increasing use of warfarin has been documented, and the literature bespeaks a favorable impact on thromboembolism-related mortality.

Subsequent groups have modified the recommendations of the NIH Consensus Conference based on the availability of newer agents and methods of prophylaxis, but none have recommended the abandonment of routine chemoprophylaxis. Despite the real reduction in the prevalence of DVT and fatal PE inherent in the recent advances of surgical technique and anesthetic management, there remains demonstrable benefit to routine prophylaxis of VTED as measured by reduction of both overall and PE-related mortality following total joint arthroplasty. Moreover, venous thromboembolism remains the most common reason for emergency readmission following total joint replacement. Current prophylaxis following THA results in venographically documented DVT in 15% to 26% of patients on warfarin and 6% to 21% of patients on low molecular weight heparin, with proximal DVT rates of approximately 2% to 5% on either regimen. The contemporary questions concerning VTED prophylaxis center around choice of agent relative to risk-benefit ratio, largely as it reflects bleeding complications, and duration of prophylaxis in the face of shorter and shorter periods of postoperative hospitalization.

Warfarin

Coumadin is the most commonly used single agent for prophylaxis of thromboembolic disease after THA. In a landmark study the start of prophylactic anticoagulation was delayed until the fifth postoperative day, presumably because of a concern over bleeding problems in the early postoperative period, and untoward bleeding was still observed in 4.1% of patients on warfarin. In a similar report, administration of warfarin prophylaxis for 3 weeks postoperatively resulted in overall bleeding complications in 1.5% of 3,000 THAs. A bleeding rate of 4.7% was noted in the first 405 cases; closer monitoring and lowering of the target prothrombin time from 18 to 20 seconds to 16 to 18 seconds resulted in a reduction in bleeding problems to 1% in the next 2,595 cases. Of the 44 major bleeding complications, 36 were wound hematomas and 8 involved the gastrointestinal or genitourinary tracts. Cementless stems were associated with a bleeding rate of 2.3%.

Early studies with bleeding rates of 8% to 12% suggest that concern over hemorrhagic complications of routine prophylaxis was justified. More recent recommendations favoring reduced intensity anticoagulation with a prothrombin time ratio of 1.3 to 1.5 times control or an INR of 2.0 to 2.5 have been associated with lower rates of bleeding. One series of 1,079 consecutive patients undergoing primary or revision THA produced a bleeding complication rate of 1.2% using a target range of 1.3 to 1.5 for the prothrombin time index. Several additional studies have documented overall in-hospital bleeding events of clinical significance in the 1% to 2% range in the absence of any hemorrhage-related mortality. Nonwound related bleeding complications in orthopaedic patients on anticoagulant therapy predominantly involve the gastrointestinal and genitourinary tracts, as demonstrated in these studies. Orthopaedic studies of a few hundred patients are designed to have adequate statistical power to investigate thromboembolic disease with a venographic prevalence of 20%. However, because of the lower prevalence of bleeding complications (in the range of 1% to 5%), statistically significant conclusions relative to bleeding rates associated with various anticoagulant therapies cannot be made in studies of this size.

Outpatient anticoagulant use introduces prolonged exposure to bleeding risk. In one study, there were 3.7% (10 of 278) major bleeding episodes in-hospital (9 wound hematomas and 1 gastrointestinal bleed); including "minor" bleeds, there was an overall in-hospital bleeding rate of 6%. Following discharge and during the 12-week period of extended warfarin prophylaxis, an additional 5% (13 of 268) experienced "minor" bleeding. In a similar study with a structured program of outpatient warfarin prophylaxis after THA, there was a bleeding complication rate of 3.2% in 125 patients managed on warfarin for 4 weeks after surgery. No patient required readmission for bleeding.

Predictors of major bleeding in medical patients on warfarin anticoagulation in the same age range as those undergoing THA have been investigated. The most common site of bleeding is the gastrointestinal tract. Investigators have identified risk predictors of major bleeding episodes in 565 patients on outpatient warfarin therapy that emphasize comorbid medical conditions and the intensity of anticoagulant therapy. They observed a major bleeding rate of 3% in the first month following discharge in patients on outpatient warfarin therapy with an incremental rate of 0.8% per month for each subsequent month on anticoagulant therapy. These data, from considerably larger study populations than those commonly used in orthopaedic trials, suggest a major outpatient bleeding rate of 4% to 5% in patients on warfarin for 3 months. These outpatient bleeding complications often escape recognition in clinical and cost-efficacy studies, because their cost is not directly attached to the index hospitalization during which the total joint replacement was performed.

Recent evidence suggests that a combination of continuous epidural anesthesia and postoperative epidural analgesia in conjunction with warfarin is associated with greater efficacy in prevention of DVT than traditional use of warfarin alone. There have been no wound hematomas requiring reoperation, epidural hematomas, or other morbid bleeding events. Indeed, the prevalence of DVT (overall 8.9%, proximal 2.3%) with combined warfarin and epidural anesthesia compares favorably to published results with any pharmacologic regimen, including fractionated heparins, without the associated bleeding complications. Both epidural anesthesia and analgesia, which were recently contraindicated with use of fractionated heparins, and early mobilization likely contribute to the low prevalence of DVT and improve on the 20% DVT prevalence with warfarin alone. A provocative observation is that segmental proximal thrombosis, which accounts for as much as 50% of all DVT after THA, was rare with this combined prophylaxis. Warfarin, in conjunction with continuous epidural anesthesia and analgesia and early patient mobilization after THA, is an effective strategy of VTED prophylaxis without the associated bleeding risk of newer fractionated heparin preparations. All trials using these newer agents should have concurrent control groups and stratify for anesthetic type and length of stay because both may affect the prevalence of TED.

Aspirin

Aspirin has witnessed a roller coaster pattern of enthusiasm and lack thereof, related to its utility in prophylaxis of VTED after total joint arthroplasty. The NIH Consensus Conference found no justification of the efficacy of aspirin in this setting and did not include it among 3 recommended agents with demonstrated efficacy in reducing rates of DVT and PE. The greatest attribute of aspirin is its safety, and recommendations for its use are usually predicated on the lack of associated bleeding complications rather than its proven efficacy.

A large scale meta-analysis of antiplatelet prophylaxis for VTED recently has been published. A pooled analysis of 53 surgical trials (including only 9 with aspirin, studied during elective orthopaedic procedures) demonstrated a reduction in fatal PE from 0.9% to 0.2% ($p = 0.0001$) with aspirin when compared to control subjects. In elective orthopaedic patients (studied in a total of 13 trials, only 9 of which used aspirin) the prevalence of DVT was reduced to 37.5% from 53.2% in controls.

The efficacy of aspirin in VTED prophylaxis following total joint arthroplasty remains poorly demonstrated and inconclusively proven. Better studied, equally safe, and more effective interventions are available.

Mechanical Modalities

External pneumatic compression devices increase venous return, decrease stasis, and enhance endothelial derived fibrinolysis without bleeding risk and are therefore inherently attractive. Calf and thigh sleeves have been associated with a reduction in calf DVT but a greater prevalence of high-risk proximal DVT after THA compared with warfarin. Plantar foot compression in combination with aspirin reduces the prevalence of proximal DVT after TKA when compared with aspirin alone. External pneumatic devices alone have not been shown to be as or more effective than pharmacologic prophylaxis after either THA or TKA, but may offer some advantage used in combination with these agents. Although the value of elastic compression stockings is widely accepted, a recent study suggests their influence after THA was only to shift the distribution of DVT from distal to proximal with no effect in reducing absolute DVT prevalence.

Fractionated Heparins

The introduction of fractionated heparin with molecular weight in the range of 5,000 d, in comparison to the mean 15,000-d molecular weight of unfractionated heparin, has provided another alternative to conventional oral anticoagulants in prophylaxis of thromboembolism following total joint replacement. With an enhanced steric affinity for antithrombin III and activated factor X, the fractionated heparin molecule provides a more active agent at an earlier point in the clotting cascade than conventional heparin (Fig. 3). Furthermore, by virtue of less plasma protein binding, the fractionated heparins are more bioavailable, require no monitoring, and have been associated with a lower frequency of both idiosyncratic and autoimmune-mediated thrombocytopenia. All of these factors, including an ambitious marketing program by commercial parties, have contributed to their initial popularity.

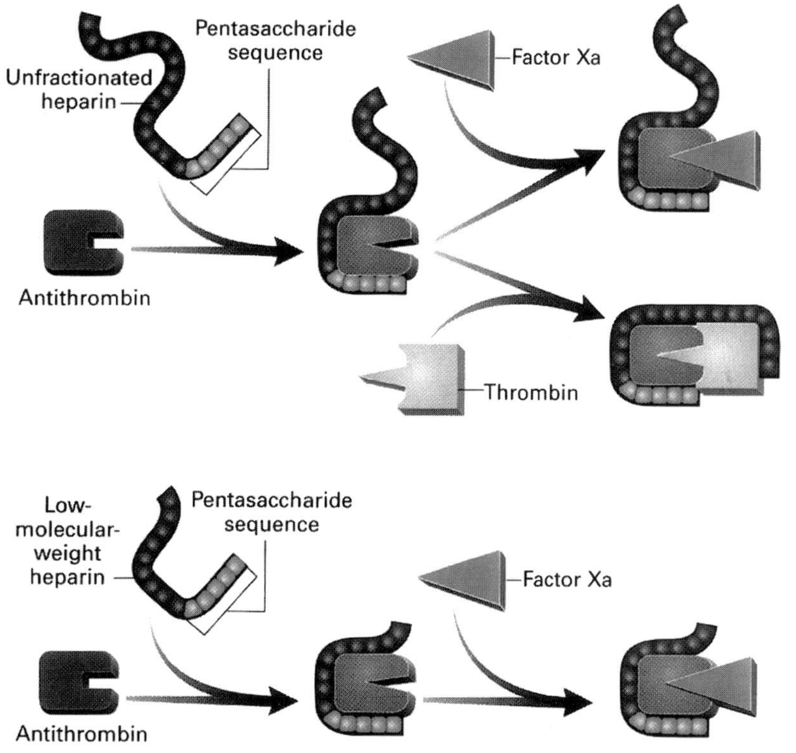

Figure 3

Catalysis of antithrombin mediated inactivation of thrombin or factor Xa by unfractionated heparin or low-molecular weight heparins. The interaction of both unfractionated (UFH) and fractionated heparins (FH) with antithrombin III (ATIII) is mediated by the pentasaccharide sequence of the drugs. Binding of either to ATIII causes a conformational change at its reactive site that accelerates its reaction with factor Xa; therefore both UFH and FH catalyze the inactivation of factor Xa by ATIII. In contrast to FH, UFH also catalyzes the inactivation of thrombin by forming a ternary complex with thrombin that requires a pentasaccharide chain at least 18 units in length. FH saccharide chains are too short to bind with ATIII and thrombin, thereby explaining the relatively selective inhibitory action of the fractionated heparins at factor Xa. (Reproduced with permission from Weitz JI: Low-molecular-weight heparins. *N Engl J Med* 1997;337:689.)

Numerous clinical studies have proven the efficacy of fractionated heparins in reducing the frequency of thromboembolism compared to placebo and unfractionated heparins following THA and TKA. Increased efficacy in prevention of DVT has been demonstrated primarily in controlled trials against unfractionated heparin in both THA and TKA. However, it is noteworthy that recent studies report reduced prevalence of DVT when compared with warfarin, especially after TKA. Current prophylaxis following THA has resulted in venographically documented DVT in 15% to 26% of patients on warfarin and 6% to 21% of patients on low-molecular weight heparin, with proximal DVT rates of approximately 2% to 5% on either regimen. Overall frequency of DVT with fractionated heparins as low as 6% following THA and 25% following TKA both represent statistically significant reductions in prevalence as compared with warfarin. On the other hand, bleeding complications, especially related to the surgical site, with major and overall bleeding rates of 4% and 12%, respectively, have been as much as 2 to 4 times more frequent with fractionated heparin than with warfarin.

While low-molecular weight heparins offer anticoagulant prophylaxis without need for attendant monitoring and periodic phlebotomy, notwithstanding the need to teach self-injection on an outpatient basis, the fractionated heparins are associated with a frequency of bleeding complications that exceeds that associated with warfarin therapy.

In a meta-analysis of methods used for prevention of DVT after hip replacement, a sixfold greater risk of "clinically important" bleeding was associated with the use of low-molecular weight heparins than with controls, and 50% greater than with warfarin. In the largest published direct comparison of a low-molecular weight heparin (logiparin) with warfarin after total joint replacement, 795 THA and 641 TKA patients were studied. The authors observed modest reductions in DVT after THA from 23.2% in the warfarin group to 20.8% in the logiparin group (p = not statistically significant) and after TKA from 54.9% with warfarin to 45% with logiparin ($p = 0.02$). Proximal DVT was increased in the THA group with logiparin from 3.8% with warfarin to 4.8%. After TKA, proximal DVT was reduced with logiparin from 12.3% to 7.8%. Pooled analysis demonstrated a reduction of overall DVT from 37.4% with warfarin to 31.4% with logiparin ($p = 0.03$). These modest reductions in DVT prevalence were offset by an increase in bleeding complications. Major bleeding complications were observed in 6 of 397 warfarin patients (1.5%) as compared with 11 of 398 logiparin patients (2.8%) after THA and 3 of 324 warfarin (0.9%) compared with 9 of 317 logiparin patients (2.8%) after TKA. Wound hematomas were more than twice as common in the logiparin THA group (23 of 398 [5.8%] versus 10 of 397 [2.5%], $p = 0.03$) while also increased with logiparin after TKA (5.9% versus 8.8%). Pooled analysis of major bleeding episodes demonstrated a significantly greater prevalence with logiparin (2.8% versus 1.2%, $p = 0.04$).

Other studies with similar categorization of major and minor bleeding complications have reported a greater frequency of bleeding events associated with the use of fractionated heparins. These studies of smaller groups of patients had insufficient statistical power to determine significance between treatment groups. In a prospective controlled trial with dalteparin versus warfarin in 580 patients undergoing THA, overall venographic DVT prevalence was 15% in the dalteparin group compared with 26% in the warfarin group ($p = 0.006$) while proximal DVT prevalence was 5% and 8% in these 2 groups ($p = 0.185$), respectively. Overall rates of major bleeding events were not significantly different between the groups (2.2% with dalteparin versus 1.4% with warfarin, p = not statistically significant), but more patients on dalteparin required red cell transfusion (48% versus 31%, $p = 0.001$) and surgical side bleeding complications were more than 4 times more frequent in the dalteparin group (4.4% versus 1%, $p = 0.03$). One dalteparin patient experienced transient thrombocytopenia and required reoperation for evacuation of a draining hematoma.

Clinically evident VTED after THA was compared between groups receiving either adjusted dose warfarin (1,494) or 30 mg every 12 hours enoxaparin (1,517) prophylaxis. All clinically suspected events were confirmed by objective testing. Pharmacologic prophylaxis was administered for an average of 6.5 days in each group and VTED events were monitored for 3 months after hospital discharge. Confirmed VTED was noted in 3.6% of enoxaparin and 3.8% of warfarin patients at final follow-up. Thromboembolic events were more common in-hospital in the warfarin group (1.1% warfarin versus 0.3% enoxaparin) and more frequent following hospital discharge in the enoxaparin group (2.7% warfarin versus 3.3% enoxaparin). Clinically significant bleeding occurred in 20 (1.3%) enoxaparin and 8 (0.5%) warfarin patients. Analysis of adverse bleeding events revealed that 78% of enoxaparin patients with a notable bleed had either received the initial enoxaparin dose within 12 hours of the operation or had the drug administered twice a day rather than on a daily schedule. Similarly, in a case-control study of 152 patients each receiving either enoxaparin or pneumatic compression prophylaxis for VTED increased bleeding was associated with fractionated heparin. The postoperative drop in hematocrit was significantly greater in the enoxaparin group, and major bleeding events occurred in 3.3% of enoxaparin compared with a 1.3% of pneumatic compression patients. Patients in this study who received their initial enoxaparin dose more than 10 hours postoperatively had significantly fewer complications than those receiving the drug within 10 hours of the operation.

The published literature, therefore, presents a clear dose-response relationship between increasing doses of fractionated heparin and decreasing incidence of DVT associated with a trade-off of increasing hemorrhagic complications. This point is well illustrated in a dose-response study of a series of 568 THA patients in whom 3 different regimens of enoxaparin were used for DVT prophylaxis (10 mg every day, 40 mg every day, 30 mg every 12 hours). Associated with increasing success in reduction of DVT prevalence to 25%, 14%, and 11%, respectively, in these 3 groups with increasing dose of enoxaparin were statistically significant increases in overall hemorrhagic events at rates of 5%, 11%, and 13%, respectively ($p < 0.05$). It has become increasingly evident that bleeding complications, especially those related to the surgical wound, associated with the use of fractionated heparins at a dose sufficient to significantly reduce the prevalence of DVT occur at rates considerably greater than those observed with low dose warfarin regimens.

Recently the association of epidural or spinal anesthesia, epidural hematomas, and the use of fractionated heparins has come under serious scrutiny. In December 1997 the United States Food and Drug Administration (FDA) issued a Public Health Advisory based on more than 30 spontaneous safety reports of patients who developed epidural or spinal hematomas with concurrent use of enoxaparin and epidural or spinal puncture. Many of the hematomas were reported to have caused neurologic injury, including long-term or permanent paralysis. Approximately 75% of the patients were described as elderly females undergoing elective orthopaedic procedures. In June 1998, a subsequent report from the FDA described 43 patients with epidural or spinal hematomas after receiving enoxaparin as the basis of the Public Health Advisory. Emergency decompressive laminectomy was performed in 28 patients and permanent paraplegia occurred in 16 patients. Thirty-six patients had received enoxaparin for VTED prophylaxis associated with THA or TKA procedures carried out under spinal or epidural anesthesia. In view of these events, the concurrent use of neuraxial anesthesia, especially with an indwelling epidural catheter, and fractionated heparins of any type should be avoided.

Further clinical study remains to determine the risk-benefit profile of this family of agents and their ultimate utility in joint replacement surgery. The rapid onset and reversal of action and ease of use in the intensive care unit has already established their place in the management of VTED in polytrauma patients with long-bone and pelvic fractures. Market-driven establishment of drug cost will be the major determinant of cost efficacy of these agents. In considering the many years necessary for surgeons to accept routine warfarin prophylaxis of VTED along with an attendant bleeding complication rate of 1% to 2%, it is difficult to endorse fractionated heparin regimens associated with significantly greater bleeding rates during inpatient hospitalization. It would appear that adopting fractionated heparin as the standard in VTED prophylaxis after THA or TKA is not justified at this time; caution should be exercised even with its selective use in this patient population.

Thrombin Inhibitors

A new class of agents that tightly bind and directly inhibit the many actions of thrombin has recently begun testing in clinical trials. In contrast to heparin, these agents even neutralize thrombin entrapped within established clots and bring the potential of even greater efficacy in VTED prevention. As always, the concern over increased bleeding risk accompanies the promise of greater efficacy, and it will be incumbent upon clinical trials to answer this question.

In 1 study of 1,587 THA patients, recombinant hirudin (desirudin) decreased overall and proximal DVT rates compared with enoxaparin from 25.5% to 18.4% ($p = 0.001$) and 7.5% to 4.5% ($p = 0.01$), respectively. Major bleeding events occurred with comparable frequency in enoxaparin and hirudin groups (2.0% versus 1.9%), as did wound hematomas (7.9% versus 8.3%). However, this trial used enoxaparin at a less efficacious dosing schedule (40 mg subcutaneously every day), which has also been shown to be associated with a lower frequency of the bleeding complications responsible for the decreased popularity of the fractionated heparins at the current time.

Managing Extended Risk of Thromboembolic Disease

The risk of late postoperative DVT after total joint arthroplasty is recognized to continue for 3 months, long beyond the contemporary 5-day hospital discharge. Two viable strategies include extended outpatient thromboembolic prophylaxis for all patients or routine surveillance and selective treatment of identifiable DVT.

Fractionated heparin therapy compared with placebo in patients with a normal venogram at hospital discharge reduced the prevalence of new asymptomatic DVT from 19.3% to 7.1% as identified by venogram 3 weeks later. Similarly, in several other studies extending fractionated heparin prophylaxis beyond hospital discharge after joint replacement, the incidence of new venogram-positive asymptomatic DVT was 12% to 20% in the absence of continued anticoagulation. The clinical significance of these findings is unclear in the context of observed readmission rates of less than 1% for symptomatic thromboembolic events in venogram-negative patients discharged after a 7- to 10-day hospitalization for THA or TKA without further anticoagulation. Moreover, continued routine outpatient anticoagulation increases total exposure to bleeding risk and would likely be accompanied by incremental bleeding events in this elderly population.

Alternatively, a strategy of routine postoperative surveillance and selective treatment of DVT reduces outpatient anticoagulation and is accompanied by a similar frequency of 0.8% readmission for TED, but requires a reliable screening test with better patient acceptance than venography. Although current opinion in North America supports continued VTED prophylaxis beyond the acute hospitalization, specific guidelines for this practice have not yet been established.

Treatment of Established VTED

The principal objective in treatment of VTED is to prevent occurrence of fatal PE, with secondary goals to reduce the morbidity of acute and recurrent DVT as well as to minimize the risk of late postphlebitic syndrome.

Proximal DVT and PE

Treatment for proximal DVT is initiated with full intensity intravenous heparin to prolong the activated partial thromboplastin time (aPTT) to 2.0 times control. However, full heparinization within 5 days of joint replacement was accompanied by major bleeding events in more than one third of patients in 1 study. Avoidance of a heparin bolus to initiate therapy is recommended. Furthermore, the critical decision to institute therapeutic intensity heparin in this setting should be justified by reliable findings of PE or high risk proximal DVT on angiography or contrast venography. A high probability ventilation/perfusion scan alone is insufficient evidence to institute therapeutic intensity heparin anticoagulation in the first postoperative week following joint replacement; the risks of pulmonary angiography to confirm the diagnosis of PE are less than the risk of bleeding into the surgical wound with its attendant complications in this early postoperative period. Unnecessary anticoagulation should be avoided. Alternatively, intermittent subcutaneous fractionated heparin has been shown to be effective in treatment of proximal DVT or PE in place of conventional heparin, and it may be equally safe and more cost-effective than traditional therapy. Although this development will potentially move anticoagulation to the outpatient setting for medical patients with VTED, postoperative patients continue to be better managed in-hospital at this time in view of their greater risk of bleeding at the surgical site and the lack of any data to suggest that the risk of major perioperative bleeding with fractionated heparins is reduced in this setting.

An inferior vena cava filter is reserved for specific circumstances when full anticoagulation is absolutely contraindicated or in the event of recurrent PE despite intravenous heparin and a therapeutic aPTT. The filter is not itself without hazards, frequently requires long-term oral anticoagulation, and has not been clearly shown to significantly reduce the frequency of fatal PE.

Conventional wisdom holds that subsequent warfarin treatment, maintaining the INR at 2.0 to 2.5, is recommended for 6 weeks for calf thrombosis, 3 months for proximal DVT, and 6 months for PE. Recent studies suggest that more protracted oral anticoagulant therapy of established DVT reduces risk of thromboembolic complications and late recurrence during a 2-year follow-up; 6 months of warfarin reduced second events by 50% (9.5% versus 18.1%) compared with the conventional 6-week therapy, with an identical frequency of bleeding complications. Similarly, indefinite oral anticoagulation following a recurrent VTED event reduced the likelihood of subsequent recurrence from 20.7% with 6-month anticoagulation to 2.6% when followed for a 4-year period. Bleeding complications were elevated by more than threefold in the indefinite treatment group.

Distal DVT

Management of isolated calf DVT in the postoperative setting is equally controversial. Newer data demonstrate that untreated calf DVT following THA has been precursor to either proximal clot propagation or symptomatic embolic events in 17% to 23% of patients; oral anticoagulant (warfarin) therapy for this condition is recommended for 6 to 12 weeks in the postoperative patient.

Annotated Bibliography

Bergqvist D, Benoni G, Bjorgell O, et al: Low-molecular-weight heparin (enoxaparin) as prophylaxis against venous thromboembolism after total hip replacement. *N Engl J Med* 1996; 335:696–700.

Continuation of enoxaparin for 3 weeks after discharge reduced DVT rates from 39% (placebo after discharge) to 18%; proximal DVT was reduced from 24% to 7%, and PE occurred in 2 placebo and no enoxaparin patients.

Colwell CW Jr, Spiro TE, Trowbridge AA, et al: Use of enoxaparin, a low-molecular-weight heparin, and unfractionated heparin for the prevention of deep venous thrombosis after elective hip replacement: A clinical trial comparing efficacy and safety. Enoxaparin Clinical Trial Group. *J Bone Joint Surg* 1994; 76A:3–14.

Among 604 valuable patients, the prevalence of DVT was 6% with twice daily dosing compared with 15% with daily dosing and 12% for unfractionated heparin. Major bleeding occurred in 4%, 1%, and 6%, respectively, in these same groups.

Eriksson BI, Wille-Jorgensen P, Kalebo P, et al: A comparison of recombinant hirudin with a low-molecular-weight heparin to prevent thromboembolic complications after total hip replacement. *N Engl J Med* 1997;337:1329–1335.

Desirudin compared with 40 mg daily of enoxaparin was found to reduce overall and proximal DVT rates from 25.5% to 18.4% and 7.5% to 4.5%, respectively, with comparable bleeding complication rates (2% major and 8% wound hematomas).

Francis CW, Pellegrini VD Jr, Totterman S, et al: Prevention of deep-vein thrombosis after total hip arthroplasty: Comparison of warfarin and dalteparin. *J Bone Joint Surg* 1997;79A: 1365–1372.

Greater efficacy in prevention of DVT with dalteparin (15% versus 26%) was at the expense of greater wound-related bleeding complications (4% versus 1%, $p = 0.03$) and more frequent need for postoperative transfusion (48% versus 31%, $p = 0.001$).

Geerts WH, Code KI, Jay RM, Chen E, Szalai JP: A prospective study of venous thromboembolism after major trauma. *N Engl J Med* 1994;331:1601–1606.

Venographic prevalence of DVT in polytrauma patients was 58% with 18% proximal thrombi; nearly all were asymptomatic. Skeletal injury predicted the greatest DVT risk; pelvic fracture 61%, tibia fracture 77%, femur fracture 80%.

Leclerc JR, Geerts WH, Desjardins L, et al: Prevention of venous thromboembolism after knee arthroplasty: A randomized, double-blind trial comparing enoxaparin with warfarin. *Ann Intern Med* 1996;124:619–626.

Among 417 patients, enoxaparin reduced overall DVT from 51.7% to 36.9% compared with warfarin. There was no difference in proximal DVT, 10.4% versus 11.7%. Major bleeding occurred in 1.8% on warfarin and 2.1% on enoxaparin.

Lieberman JR, Wollaeger J, Dorey F, et al: The efficacy of prophylaxis with low-dose warfarin for prevention of pulmonary embolism following total hip arthroplasty. *J Bone Joint Surg* 1997;79A:319–325.

In 1,099 THA patients receiving low intensity warfarin (prothrombin time [PT] index 1.3 to 1.5) an average of 15 days there were 12 (1.1%) symptomatic PE and major bleeding events, associated with a PT over 17 seconds, after 32 (2.9%) procedures.

Oishi C, Grady-Benson JC, Otis SM, Colwell CW Jr, Walker RH: The clinical course of distal deep venous thrombosis after total hip and total knee arthroplasty, as determined with duplex ultrasonography. *J Bone Joint Surg* 1994;76A:1658–1663.

Of 41 patients with distal DVT, 7 (17%) evidenced asymptomatic extension to proximal veins on serial duplex ultrasonography at 14 days postoperatively, and 1 patient (3%) manifested symptomatic proximal DVT 11 months after THA.

Pellegrini VD Jr, Clement D, Lush-Ehmann C, Keller GS, Evarts CM: Natural history of thromboembolic disease after total hip arthroplasty. *Clin Orthop* 1996;333:27–40.

Six-month readmission rate for VTED was 0% in 55 patients treated for a positive venogram, 1.1% in 269 with a negative venogram and no further prophylaxis, 1.6% in 732 patients without screening venography, and 17.4% in 23 patients with a false negative venogram who received no warfarin therapy.

Planes A, Vochelle N, Darmon JY, Fagola M, Bellaud M, Huet Y: Risk of deep-venous thrombosis after hospital discharge in patients, having undergone total hip replacement: Double-blind randomised comparison of enoxaparin versus placebo. *Lancet* 1996;348:224–228.

Venogram negative patients at hospital discharge received enoxaparin or placebo for 3 weeks; overall DVT was reduced by continued prophylaxis (7% versus 19%), nearly entirely by decrease in calf DVT. No PE occurred in either group.

Schulman S, Rhedin AS, Lindmarker P, et al: A comparison of six weeks with six months of oral anticoagulant therapy after a first episode of venous thromboembolism: Duration of Anticoagulation Trial Study Group. *N Engl J Med* 1995;332: 1661–1665.

During a 2-year follow-up of 897 patients, the recurrence rate of VTED was 18.1% with 6 weeks and 9.5% with 6 months of coumadin therapy for established DVT; mortality and major hemorrhage were the same in both groups.

Sharrock NE, Go G, Harpel PC, Ranawat CS, Sculco TP, Salvati EA: Thrombogenesis during total hip arthroplasty. *Clin Orthop* 1995;319:16–27.

Intraoperative activation of the clotting cascade and changes in pulmonary pressures and venous oxygenation were found to coincide with preparation of the femoral canal and were most intense with a cemented as compared with a cementless stem.

Warwick D, Williams MH, Bannister GC: Death and thromboembolic disease after total hip replacement: A series of 1162 cases with no routine chemical prophylaxis. *J Bone Joint Surg* 1995;77B:6–10.

Among 1,152 consecutive THA the total VTED morbidity in 6 months was 3.4%; 0.34% fatal PE, 1.2% clinically apparent PE (0.7% readmission), and 1.89% venographically confirmed clinically apparent DVT (1.13% readmission). The authors consider evidence insufficient to recommend postdischarge prophylaxis.

Wells PS, Lensing AW, Davidson BL, Prins MH, Hirsh J: Accuracy of ultrasound for the diagnosis of deep venous thrombosis in asymptomatic patients after orthopedic surgery: A meta-analysis. *Ann Intern Med* 1995;122:47–53.

Of the 17 studies reviewed, the sensitivity for detection of asymptomatic proximal vein thrombosis ranged from 38% to 100%; only 2 had adequate venogram control for analysis of distal DVT and sensitivity ranged from 20% to 88%.

Classic Bibliography

Amstutz HC, Friscia DA, Dorey F, Carney BT: Warfarin prophylaxis to prevent mortality from pulmonary embolism after total hip replacement. *J Bone Joint Surg* 1989;71A:321–326.

Hirsh J: Oral anticoagulant drugs. *N Engl J Med* 1991;324: 1865–1875.

Hirsh J, Levine MN: The optimal intensity of oral anticoagulant therapy. *JAMA* 1987;258:2723–2726.

Hirsh J, Levine MN: Low molecular weight heparin. *Blood* 1992;79:1–17.

Hull RD, Raskob GE, Hirsh J, et al: Continuous intravenous heparin compared with intermittent subcutaneous heparin in the initial treatment of proximal-vein thrombosis. *N Engl J Med* 1986;315:1109–1114.

Hull R, Raskob G, Pineo G, et al: A comparison of subcutaneous low-molecular-weight heparin with warfarin sodium for prophylaxis against deep-vein thrombosis after hip or knee implantation. *N Engl J Med* 1993;329:1370–1376.

Johnson R, Green JR, Charnley J: Pulmonary embolism and its prophylaxis following the Charnley total hip replacement. *Clin Orthop* 1977;127:123–132.

NIH Consensus Development: Prevention of venous thrombosis and pulmonary embolism. *JAMA* 1986;256:744–749.

Patterson BM, Marchand R, Ranawat C: Complications of heparin therapy after total joint arthroplasty. *J Bone Joint Surg* 1989;71A:1130–1134.

Sikorski JM, Hampson WG, Staddon GE: The natural history and aetiology of deep vein thrombosis after total hip replacement. *J Bone Joint Surg* 1981;63B:171–177.

Chapter 4
Implant Materials: Metals, Polyethylene, Polymethylmethacrylate

Introduction

The principal materials employed in hip and knee arthroplasty include cobalt-chromium alloy, titanium alloy, ultrahigh molecular weight polyethylene, and polymethylmethacrylate. When considering how the behavior of these materials relates to the performance of total knee and hip replacement prostheses, it is polyethylene wear that continues to be the most evident cause of failure. The often rapid and extensive destruction of bone attributable to polyethylene wear particles is so dramatic, and so challenges revision arthroplasty, that it has commanded the most attention in recent years. However, the actual incidence of this problem remains somewhat in question. The prevalence of polyethylene wear particle-induced osteolysis is great enough to warrant changes in how the material is processed so as to improve its resistance to wear. Extrinsic factors that contribute to the wear of polyethylene, such as prosthetic designs that reduce stresses in the polymer, prosthetic designs and manufacturing processes that reduce the number of particles released from modular junctions that can participate in 3-body wear of polyethylene, and materials that may allow the production of more scratch-resistant metallic counterfaces, are also being addressed.

Less evident than polyethylene wear and particle-induced osteolysis is the loosening of prostheses that also ultimately necessitates revision arthroplasty. In the case of the cemented device, fractures in the cement sheath can lead to destabilization. Such failure is less dramatic than polyethylene wear and can occur over a longer time scale. Laboratory investigations continue to test new forms of bone cement that are of higher strength and that may elicit more favorable biologic responses.

The failure of metallic components due to their breakage has not been a problem in recent years. However, for specific types of devices, corrosion and wear processes play a role in failure as they generate particulate debris that can affect wear of the articulating surfaces and that may provoke inflammatory reactions. The role of metals in total joint arthroplasty is being expanded as metal-on-metal articulations are being reintroduced in response to the polyethylene problem. It is much too early to determine the benefit-risk ratio for such prostheses and what place they will occupy in the repertoire of devices available to orthopaedic surgeons for joint arthroplasty.

Metals

The breakdown of the metallic component of total joint prostheses as a result of corrosion, wear, or fracture has not proved to be the principal cause of failure of joint arthroplasties in recent years. Therefore, there has been little impetus for the investigation of new metals for this application. Recent findings with selected prostheses indicate that inadequate manufacturing processes and injudicious design can predispose certain metallic modular components to corrosion and wear.

Particles resulting from the corrosion of metals are the product of the precipitation of implant-derived metal ions with inorganic or organic molecules from the biologic milieu. These particles are to be distinguished from the metallic debris resulting from wear processes. Little is known about the mechanisms by which the corrosion products precipitate and their role in inciting an inflammatory response. Most implant-derived metal particles are the result of wear rather than corrosion processes. However, while the metallic ions resulting from corrosion may not be evident in the form of precipitated particles, they can affect biologic processes. Moreover, they can enter the circulatory system and become distributed throughout the body. There have been no studies that definitively relate an adverse systemic response to prosthesis-released metal ions.

One or more of the authors or the departments with which they are affiliated have received something of value from a commercial or other party related directly or indirectly to the subject of this chapter.

Corrosion and Wear Processes Associated With Modular Devices

The primary problem involving the corrosion of metals in total joint replacement prostheses has been associated with the taper connections of certain modular joint replacement components. Recent retrieval studies have shown examples of severe corrosion at the head-neck taper connection of certain designs of hip replacement prostheses. This corrosion process increases the release of metal ions that can directly elicit a biologic response or form a precipitate. Particulate corrosion products themselves can provoke other biologic responses as they are phagocytosed and can promote 3-body wear of the articulating surfaces.

The corrosion of certain designs of devices comprising cobalt-chromium alloy heads on stems manufactured from the same metal may be related to an angular mismatch between the taper on the male aspect of the connection and the bore on the female component. This condition favors fretting corrosion in which the relative micromotion between the components results in the abrasive wear of the passivation-oxide layer on the components, subsequently predisposing them to corrosion. Implementation of manufacturing processes with the high tolerances that can be achieved using current methods can so reduce the mismatch to greatly diminish this corrosion process.

Crevice corrosion in association with titanium alloy hip replacement prostheses has also been identified as a source of particles. Corrosion products comprising titanium oxides and hydroxides were found in the interface between the metallic stem and the surrounding bone cement. These corrosion products were also found in the peri-implant tissues in macrophages and in multinucleated foreign body giant cells.

It is often difficult to definitively determine the process responsible for the generation of particles. In particular, particles from the junction between cobalt-chromium alloy femoral heads and titanium stems has been attributed to both galvanic (mixed metal) corrosion and fretting wear. Regardless of the process, it is clear that modular devices introduce some risk of particle generation. Fortunately, problems attributed to them have not yet become so prevalent that the advantages of such prostheses need to be yielded.

Particulate Corrosion Products Recent studies of retrieved components have demonstrated that when they form, solid corrosion products can migrate through the periprosthetic tissues, subsequently becoming engulfed by macrophages and multinucleated foreign body giant cells or becoming lodged in the polyethylene bearing surface. The particles resulting from corrosion of certain total hip replacement prostheses comprising cobalt-chromium alloy heads on titanium alloy or cobalt alloy stems were identified as a chromium-orthophosphate hydrate-rich material. That such particles in vivo could be found in the surface of the polyethylene acetabular liners suggested their participation in 3-body wear of the articulating couple. Despite these observations, the generation of corrosion products of this type has not been found to be a principal cause of failure of the majority of prostheses that come to revision arthroplasty. Moreover, the most severe cases of corrosion appear to be related to certain designs of devices, perhaps because of suboptimal manufacturing of the modular junctions. Corrosion per se is not a principal factor in the performance of prostheses fabricated using the currently employed metals.

Local and Systemic Response to Corrosion Products When administered to monocytes and macrophages in vitro, particles or certain corrosion products were found to serve as potent activators of the cells with the capacity to stimulate bone resorption in a dose-dependent manner.

While adverse tissue reactions to implant-derived particles do not appear to be principally caused by metallic corrosion products, it is important to note that such reactions can occur. An unusual foreign body reaction to particulate corrosion products was recently found in the tissue around a failed total knee implant comprising several different cobalt alloys. The same patient displayed ipsilateral inguinal lymphadenopathy. Both the tumor and lymph nodes appeared to contain sarcoid-like, noncaseating granulomas associated with the extensive cobalt-alloy debris. Although this finding was restricted to a single patient, it demonstrates the severity of the reaction that can occur.

Recent studies have also reported the presence of implant-derived metallic particles at autopsy in the end organs of implant patients. The highest levels of metal were found in a cadaver that had a loose, worn device. Another study using tissues obtained from autopsy found increased levels of titanium in the spleens of individuals implanted with titanium alloy total hip replacement prostheses. Selected specimens also had an increased concentration of titanium in the liver. Longitudinal data have also been obtained that demonstrate increased levels of titanium in the spleen, despite the fact that concentrations of titanium and aluminum in the serum had not increased. This finding demonstrated that deposition of metal can occur in end organs in patients with well-functioning devices, even though there may not be any measurable increase in the level of the metal in the serum.

Cobalt has been found in the serum and chromium in the urine in patients with failed modular implants. The elevated metal ion levels have been associated with devices that display moderate to severe corrosion at the modular junction. Such elevated levels generally have not been found in patients who had no corrosion or mild corrosion and in a control population.

Although there has been no pathology associated with the elevation of implant-derived metal ions, or corrosion or wear particulates, incidental findings of granulomatous lesions have been reported. An awareness of the generation of metallic ions and particles by joint replacement prostheses and their dissemination throughout the body is important, so as not to miss the documentation of periprosthetic or distant organ lesions that may be associated with these agents.

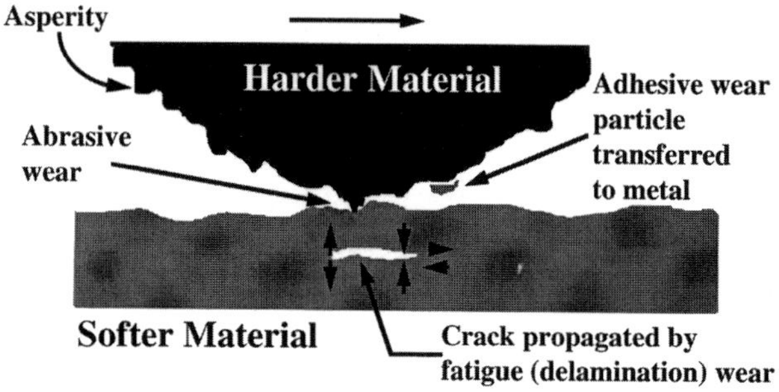

Figure 1

Schematic demonstrating the wear processes that apply to the metal-on-polyethylene articulation of total hip and knee replacement prostheses.

Tribology of Metal-on-Polyethylene Articulation

Several wear processes can occur in total hip and knee replacement prostheses (Fig. 1 and Table 1). Questions persist as to the contribution of particles from the coatings to 3-body wear of polyethylene. Some studies have documented a higher wear rate of the polyethylene liner in uncemented total hip arthroplasties when compared to cemented prostheses. There appears to be an overlap in the range of wear rates of cemented and uncemented acetabular components. Many radiographic investigations have demonstrated detachment of elements of the coating. It has been concluded that the 3-body wear caused by the presence of the loose metal beads from the coating is a possible reason for the severe wear of the polyethylene insert, the associated osteolysis, and the higher revision rate.

Direct evidence for the participation of metal particles, derived from the coating of uncemented devices, in wear occurring at the articulating surface must be determined from the direct examination of retrieved acetabular liners and the mated femoral heads. Although several such studies have been performed on cemented prostheses, showing cement particles in the polyethylene liner and their effect in roughening the femoral head, there have been relatively few such reports for uncemented components. As part of an analysis of retrieved components from modular prostheses, polyethylene liners were found that had embedded metallic debris that could be traced to a plasma-sprayed coating. Another study of other types of noncemented devices also found metallic debris in cup devices examined using stereomicroscopy. In that study it was observed that scanning electron microscopy can detect metallic debris in components in which no debris can be found at the light microscope level.

An indirect approach to obtaining information about the importance of particles embedded in the acetabular liner, as third bodies, in the wear of cups has been to evaluate the topography of the metallic femoral head counterface. A recent study found an increase in the roughness of most modular heads retrieved from prostheses with porous metallic and hydroxyapatite coatings. No significant difference, however, in overall surface roughness was found between the porous coated and cemented groups. In this investigation, the heads from the hydroxyapatite-coated prostheses displayed significantly lower values for certain parameters of roughness. It was of some interest to note that elemental analysis of 4 polyethylene liners from the hydroxyapatite-coated femoral stem group, while displaying no evidence of embedded ceramic particles, displayed the presence of silica, which may be traced to the agents used for surface treating of the prostheses by the manufacturer.

Table 1

Wear processes and the resulting particle size

Type	Mechanism	Particle size
Adhesive	Chemical adhesion	nm to µm
Abrasive (2-body)	Plowing of asperity through softer material	µm
Abrasive (3-body)	Entrapment and plowing of particle	µm
Fatigue/Delamination	Propagation of subsurface cracks to the surface by cyclic compression, tension, shear	µm to mm

Several authors have investigated the effect of the roughness of a metal counterface on the wear of polyethylene in laboratory tests. These investigations show how wear of polyethylene is greatly affected by the roughness of the counterface, generally quantified by the measurement of the averaged length from a reference line to the peaks and valleys comprising the topography, the factor R_a (Fig. 2). In some novel laboratory wear tests, the effect of individual scratches in a metal counterface on polyethylene wear was investigated. In experiments initially performed with water as the lubricant, and more recently with bovine serum, individual scratches, 10-µm wide, in the metal counterface—equivalent to a single scratch on a 22-mm diameter femoral head—increased the wear of polyethylene by as much as 70-fold, in a reciprocating wear test. It is of importance that these individual scratches were not adequately reflected in the R_a measurement, which while increasing from 0.007 to 0.013 mm, was still well within the specifications for a femoral head. It was found that the scratch feature that was the major determinant of the amount of wear was the height of the ridge of metal bordering the scratch and raised above the surface, R_p-peak (Figs. 2 through 4). This ridge of piled-up material was formed as metal was displaced when the groove was plowed. The amount of pileup can be related to depth and width of the scratch, with deeper, wider scratches correlating to higher pileup. The laboratory testing demonstrated an order of magnitude increase in the wear factor as the scratch depth increased from 1 to 7 µm, corresponding to an increase in width from 20 to 55 µm. There was an additional 30% increase to a plateau value for the wear factor as the scratch width increased to 200 µm. The authors concluded that in the case of transverse scratches, once the scratch depth has achieved a value of about 10 µm, the wear factor becomes insensitive to deeper cuts. Scratches with this critical depth of 7 to 10 µm and width of 55 to 200 µm could be produced by the metal particles originating with the porous metal coating (approximately 100 µm and greater in diameter), allowing these particles to have a significantly greater influence on

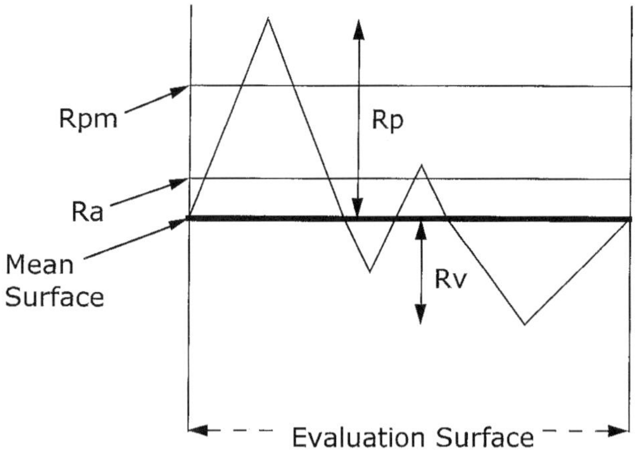

Figure 2

Diagram showing the parameters that can be used to describe a scratch. R_a, average roughness that takes into consideration the valleys as well as the peaks; R_p, the maximum peak height above the mean surface; R_v, the depth of the valley; R_{pm}, the mean value for peaks.

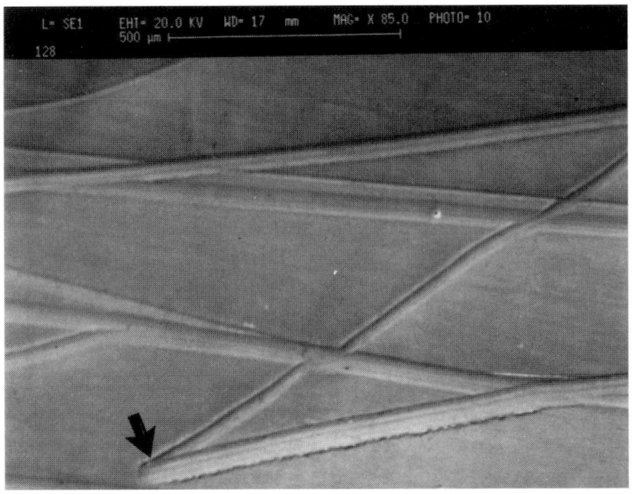

Figure 3

Scanning electron micrograph showing the scratches on a retrieved cobalt-chromium alloy femoral component.

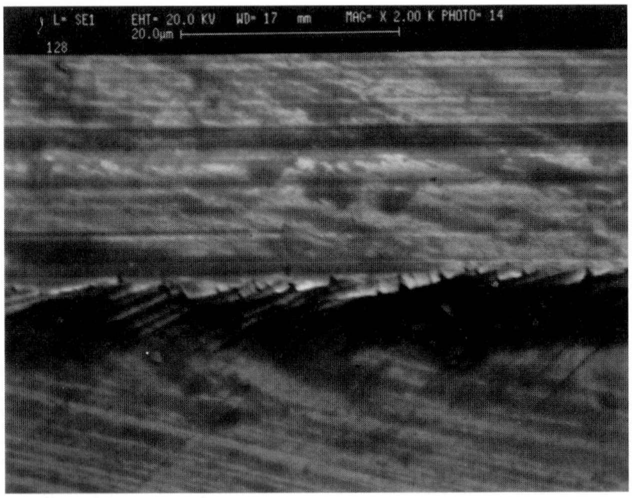

Figure 4

Scanning electron micrograph of a single scratch showing the pileup of metal forming a ridge along its length.

wear of polyethylene than particles of 1 to 10 μm in diameter, from other sources. Scratches of this width have been detected on retrieved femoral heads and condyles.

Also of importance in the laboratory study was the finding that when the piled-up material was removed by remedial lapping, the wear rate returned to its initial value corresponding to the isotropic roughness of the undisturbed counterface. In vivo, during continuing articulation, wear of the ridges of the scratches in the cobalt-chromium femoral head occurs simultaneously with wear of the polyethylene.

Because metal counterface roughness is an important factor in polyethylene wear, the parameters used to assess the surface roughness need to be carefully considered. The average roughness, R_a, is frequently used to define the metallic surface quality in total knee and hip arthroplasty. However, surfaces can have the same R_a but a greatly different appearance. More useful parameters may be those that define height of the highest ridge of metal (R_p) or the mean value for the peak heights, R_{pm} (Fig. 2).

That particles from porous coatings can play a role in the wear processes occurring at the articulation of total hip arthroplasties emphasizes the importance of implementing technologies that produce robust coatings. Moreover, new forms of polyethylene, and also other types of articulation, should be evaluated in laboratory experiments that expose the articulation to the types of particles that could be expected to migrate to the joint space from coatings for uncemented components. Although further investigation of the effect of counterface roughness on failure of total knee arthroplasty is needed, current findings support the implementation of a more scratch-resistant surface.

Metal-on-Metal Articulation

Concerns about the wear of polyethylene have prompted reintroduction of metal-on-metal articulation for total hip arthroplasty. With renewed interest in this articulation has come additional laboratory testing that has begun to identify factors that influence its tribology. Long-term clinical follow-up of metal-on-metal prostheses revealed a linear wear rate of approximately 6 μm or less per year, with approximately 0.6 mm^3 of metallic wear debris per year. This is an order of magnitude less than the wear rate of metal-on-polyethylene devices. However, because of the small particle size of the metal debris, the number of particles can be substantial.

Cobalt-chromium-molybdenum alloys have been employed in the fabrication of metal-on-metal devices because of their relative corrosion resistance and hardness. The high-carbon, wrought form of this alloy has been recommended for this application on the basis of the presence of small, finely distributed carbides at the surface. Moreover, the wrought form generally has less surface roughness and a lower coefficient of friction than couples using the cast alloy. In addition, it can undergo a strain-induced microstructural transformation that results in a more wear-resistant crystallographic structure.

Another important factor that influences the tribology of metal-on-metal articulations is the clearance between the femoral head and acetabular cup. It is important that the radii be such that there be polar contact of the head with the cup (instead of an equatorial contact). This articulation allows for the ingress and egress of lubricating fluid. The contact area is proportional to the diameter of the components and inversely proportional to the clearance (the difference between the head and cup diameters). The effective radius has been defined as the radius of the sphere in contact with a flat surface, where the contact area is the same as that for the corresponding head-cup combination. As the head and cup become congruent with reducing clearances, conditions favor high frictional torque and equatorial seizing.

As with other articulating couples, the nature of the lubrication of metal-on-metal articulation profoundly influences the potential for wear. Fluid film lubrication resulting in the separation of the articulating surfaces and preventing wear is a function of the topography of the counterfaces, the lubricant viscosity, and the relative movement of the articulating surfaces and may occur with metal-on-metal prostheses. Such lubrication is obviated in metal-on-polyethylene couples as a result of the large asperities on the polymeric component (such as machine marks). Boundary lubrication related to the adsorption of molecules from the synovial fluid onto the surfaces is generally the mode of lubrication that occurs in total joint arthroplasty.

The prospect of the more widespread clinical implementation of metal-on-metal couples has raised the question of the articulation as a source of significant metal ion release. Patients in whom McKee-Farrar total hip implants had been clinically successful for more than 20 years were found to have a ninefold increase in the level of chromium in the serum, a 35-fold increase in the level of chromium in the urine, and at least a threefold increase in the level of cobalt in the serum of the individuals. Even higher elevations were found in another group of patients who had metal-on-metal surface replacement prostheses for less than 2 years. Recent investigations of the tissues retrieved with metal-on-metal hip prostheses have revealed unremarkable tissue response to metallic ion release and wear debris. However, continuing investigations are warranted to provide assurance that untoward biologic reactions will not result from the use of metal-on-metal devices.

Polyethylene

It is well known that polyethylene components of total joint replacement prostheses undergo wear process that produce polyethylene wear debris as a result of the articulation of the harder metallic component, usually a cobalt-chromium alloy, against the softer polyethylene component (Fig. 1). The generation of wear debris not only damages the surface of the polyethylene component but is also known to elicit a biologic response that often results in bone resorption. This bone loss (referred to as osteolysis) can eventually lead to loosening of the prosthetic device. The location and size of polyethylene particle-induced osteolytic lesions often greatly complicate revision surgery. Work in recent years has focused on processing parameters that serve as the determinants of the resistance of polyethylene to wear. The reduction of the amount of wear debris from, and surface damage to, polyethylene would prolong the lifetime of such prostheses.

Effects of Gamma-Radiation Sterilization on Polyethylene Components

A few years ago, laboratory investigations of unimplanted as well as retrieved polyethylene components began to reveal alterations in the material that could be traced back to the gamma irradiation method of sterilization (Figs. 5 through 8). The most dramatic changes in polyethylene acetabular and tibial components were found in sections microtomed from the devices. The fragility of the polymer at certain locations could be clearly seen as a result of its fragmentation during sectioning. This breakdown of the polymer at certain sites also revealed itself as an opaque, whitish region when specimens were examined by transmitted light. That the breakdown generally occurred at a particular location below the surface led to the formation of what was referred to as a "white band." Infrared spectroscopy analysis revealed that these locations in the polymer were sites of high oxidation. Associated testing demonstrated the expected substantial alteration in the mechanical properties. The location of the white band at approximately 1 mm below the surface in tibial components coincided with the depth at which delamination of polyethylene is frequently seen in the device.

These findings of changes in the molecular structure and properties of polyethylene resulting from gamma irradiation were consistent with what had been known for many decades about the effect of ionizing radiation on polymers. In fact, the question is why attention was not drawn earlier to the problem of gamma irradiation of polyethylene orthopaedic components. Perhaps an answer lies in the fact that a large percentage of components sterilized in this fashion performed flawlessly during the lifetime of many patients. In fact, although the adverse effects of gamma irradiation of polyethylene parts are undisputed, the question remains as to the contribution of the gamma radiation-induced breakdown of polyethylene to the failure of the arthroplasty procedure in many patients.

That the principal culprit in the gamma radiation-induced

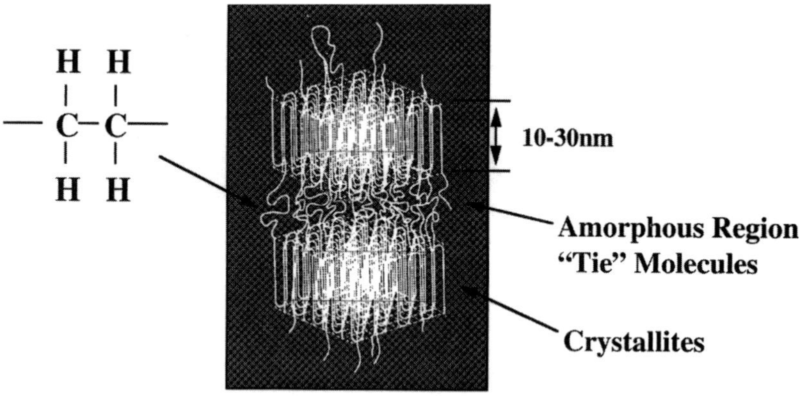

Figure 5
Schematic showing the molecular structure of ultrahigh molecular weight polyethylene.

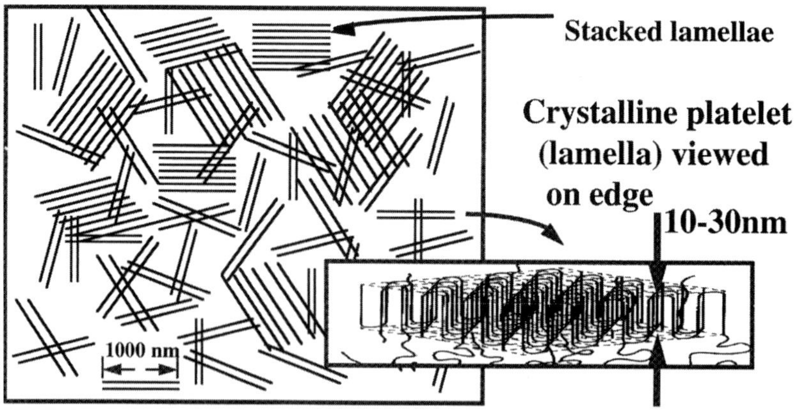

Figure 6
The nanometer level structure of polyethylene comprising the stacked crystallite lamellae.

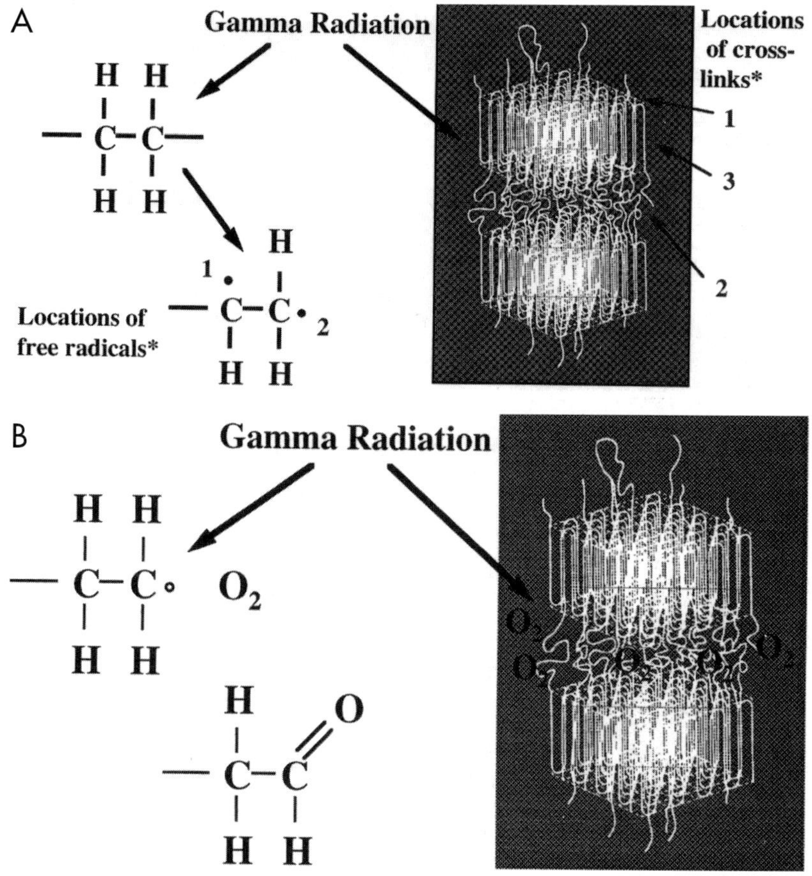

Figure 7

The free radical production by gamma radiation (**A**), and the ensuing oxidation (**B**).

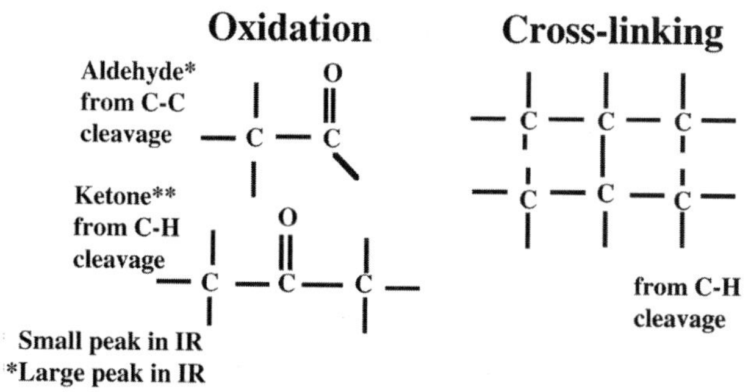

Figure 8

The molecular structures that result from gamma irradiation.

breakdown of polyethylene was oxygen led to changes in the sterilization method. Parts to be gamma irradiated are contained in environments free of oxygen: in a vacuum or in packages in which the oxygen had been replaced by a neutral gas such as argon or nitrogen. Other approaches have been to forego the use of gamma irradiation altogether and to use other methods of sterilization such as ethylene oxide gas and gas plasma. Altering the environment during the process of gamma irradiation of polyethylene components addressed the initial binding of oxygen to the free radicals produced by exposure to the ionizing radiation. However, these free radicals are long-lived, and this factor raised questions about the oxidation that would proceed after the parts were removed from their oxygen-free environment. This scenario led to the implementation by certain manufacturers of poststerilization methods to eliminate free radicals produced by gamma irradiation. Certain thermal processing of parts after gamma irradiation can result in the combination of free radicals and a reduction in their number.

Several methods are currently being used for the sterilization of polyethylene components in ways that will disfavor oxidation. It is not yet possible, however, to determine if there are substantial differences in the clinical wear performance of parts sterilized with these different processes.

Investigation into the effects of gamma radiation of polyethylene not only revealed the unfavorable oxidative process, but that cross-linking also occurs (Fig. 8). Again, these findings merely confirmed what had been know for decades about the use of ionizing radiation to cross-link polymers. The question that arose in the case of the use of gamma irradiation of polyethylene for sterilization was: Is there a substantial benefit to the gamma radiation cross-linking polyethylene that was overshadowed by the adverse effects of oxidation? Laboratory investigation of cross-linked polyethylene yielded such promising results that processes to cross-link the polymer have been implemented and the resulting cross-linked polyethylene parts are on the threshold of being introduced into the clinic.

New Forms of Polyethylene

The problems associated with wear of polyethylene components in joint replacement prostheses has prompted work directed toward the development of new forms of polyethylene to improve wear resistance.

One approach used to reduce surface damage and subsurface crack growth in knee components is through development of new prosthetic designs that increase the contact area between components, thereby reducing stress in polyethylene. Such methods, based on measurements and calculations of contact stress on components, have led to the development of thicker and more conformal polyethylene components that are expected to reduce catastrophic failure and delamination wear.

Other approaches to reduce wear rates in polyethylene have involved alteration of the number or size of the crystallites or the molecular bonding of the molecular chains in the noncrystalline domains of the polymer. Methods used to realize this goal include processing techniques that apply high pressure to the polymer and the use of cross-linking chemistry.

High Pressure Forms of Polyethylene A few years ago, high-pressure crystallization was used to produce polyethylene components with an increase in mechanical properties such as yield stress and modulus of elasticity (Table 2). Two forms of high-pressure polyethylene that vary in certain mechanical properties (such as modulus of elasticity) have been introduced into the clinic for total hip and knee arthroplasty. The primary difference in the bulk structure of conventional and high-pressure forms of polyethylene is that in conventional polyethylene the degree of crystallinity is 50% to 55%, and 68% to 75% in the latter. The high-pressure process facilitates thickening of crystallites in polyethylene from 0.025 μm in conventional processes to approximately 0.2 μm in the high-pressure form. Although the high-pressure polyethylene is more resistant to deformation by creep and fatigue crack growth, it has never been shown to have a substantially higher wear resistance in laboratory wear tests.

Table 2
Properties of new forms of polyethylene relative to conventional polyethylene

	High Pressure	X-Linked
Crystallinity	↑	↓
Yield strength	↑	↓*
Modulus of elasticity	↑*	↓
Strain to break	↑	↓*
Fracture toughness	↑	↓*
Creep	↓*	?
Hip simulator wear	No difference	↓

Recent clinical results indicate that the linear wear rate and consequential incidence of osteolysis and revision rate for the high-pressure form of polyethylene are greater than for conventional polyethylene. Why the clinical wear rate for this modification of polyethylene might be greater than for conventional polyethylene, despite the improvement in certain mechanical properties, is not entirely clear. It may be that the high-pressure form is less resistant to oxidation than previously appreciated. If so, implementation of sterilization methods that do not favor oxidation may result in improved performance of this form of polyethylene. However, that wear of polyethylene devices is as multifactorial as it is indicates that additional laboratory investigations of high-pressure forms of polyethylene will be required before their wear performance can more fully be explained.

Cross-Linked Polyethylene

Cross-linking is currently being used in an attempt to improve the wear performance of polyethylene in the hip joint. Cross-linking of polyethylene converts the otherwise linear, high molecular weight polyethylene macromolecule into an interpenetrating, networking structure of polymer chains. This type of molecular structure is often quantitatively characterized by the molecular weight between cross-links (usually referred to as M_c), that is, the higher the M_c, the lower the density or degree of cross-linking junctions. Cross-linking of polyethylene can be performed using cross-linking agents such as peroxides and silanes, and by the use of gamma or electron beam radiation (Outline 1). Laboratory hip simulator wear tests have shown that there is a decrease in wear rate with an increase in degree of cross-linking of polyethylene. These studies, and the clinical results of a few trials that employed cross-linked polyethylene acetabular cups several years ago, provide compelling evidence that cross-linking can reduce wear rates in acetabular components.

Although cross-linking has been found to improve the performance of polyethylene components, the trade-off in other mechanical properties (Table 2) has raised questions about the potential problems with such an approach and focused attention on the indications that might best benefit from its use. With an increase in cross-linking density comes an undesirable reduction in mechanical properties such as reduced elongation to failure, which occurs largely in the case of radiation cross-linking but to a lower extent with peroxide cross-linking. Associated with this reduction in the elongation to break is a reduction in the energy required to propagate a crack and the resistance of cross-linked parts to cyclic load-

Outline 1
Methods for cross-linking polyethylene

Chemical
- Peroxide
  - Residual peroxide permits oxidation

Physical
- γ-Radiation
  - Irradiate at room temperature, then melt to initiate x-linking and remove free radicals, then cool
  - Heat polyethylene to melting and then irradiate

Electron Beam
  - Heat polyethylene to just below melting and then irradiate

ing. It is possible that while cross-linking may improve wear resistance it may place components at greater risk of fracture. In addition, there is a reduction in the degree of crystallinity with increasing cross-link density, which suggests that there will be an increased amount of deformation by creep in such components. Finally, it was observed using laboratory uniaxial, reciprocating wear tests that cross-linked polyethylene had a larger increase in wear rates when a rougher counterface was used compared to non-cross-linked polyethylene. It is not yet known whether this increased susceptibility to a rough counterface is caused by a reduced degree of crystallinity in cross-linked polyethylene or to a reduced elongation to failure.

Because of the questions related to the change in certain properties with cross-linking, only an intermediate degree of cross-linking (an equivalent radiation dose of 50 to 100 kGy rather than 200 kGy) is being used by many, so that there is a balance between increase in wear resistance and reduction in mechanical properties. Some have shown that although there is a strong effect of radiation dose (or cross-link density) on wear resistance in hip simulator tests, similar doses led to less improvements in wear rates using a knee simulator. One reason for lower sensitivity of wear to cross-linking in the knee simulator is that linear wear tracking does not lead to high volumetric wear rates even for conventional polyethylene, and it is difficult to conclude whether cross-linking is appropriate for knee components using smooth counterface, linear tracking; some believe that a low level of cross-linking may be beneficial for the knee prosthesis.

Understanding of the wear behavior of polyethylene components has increased over the past few years as the adverse effects of gamma irradiation (in air) sterilization have become clear. This understanding has led to methods to improve the wear performance of the polymer using cross-linking methods. However, it will still be several years before the clinical benefits of new methods of processing polyethylene are elucidated, and the benefit-risk ratio established.

Polymethylmethacrylate

Polymethylmethacrylate (PMMA) bone cement continues to be the gold standard for stabilization of total joint replacement prostheses. The material, as it is currently used in the clinic, has been substantially unchanged over the past 2 decades. Persisting questions, however, about how certain limitations in the material properties may impact its long-term performance, have continued to prompt investigations of modified forms of cement.

It is well known that the cement sheath surrounding joint prostheses can crack. Such fractures, however, have never been directly demonstrated to be the cause of failure of the system. Despite this lack of direct correlation of fracture of the cement to arthroplasty longevity, efforts continue to address ways of increasing the static and dynamic (fatigue) strengths of the material.

The principal efforts directed toward the improvement of the performance of cement have addressed its handling intraoperatively. The newer generation of cement techniques has addressed issues related to the preparation of the canal for the insertion of cement and the technology for its delivery and pressurization.

Of the work directed toward improving the mechanical properties of PMMA, the methods for reducing voids through mixing are the only ones that have found their way into the clinic. Methods involving centrifugation or vacuum mixing have been shown to reduce the voids in the cement. While studies have shown concomitant increases in the strength of cement specimens in laboratory testing, questions persist as to the benefit of such approaches to improving the performance of the cement sheath in vivo. While the benefits of certain techniques for handling cement can be seen in well controlled laboratory tests, the operating room handling of the material and the lack of control in its insertion into the bony cavity raise questions about the benefit of certain cement preparation techniques.

Current laboratory investigations are addressing the improvements in cement performance by fiber or particulate reinforcement, and monomers other than methylmethacrylate. The addition of metallic, polymeric, and carbon fibers to

PMMA as reinforcement has been demonstrated to improve mechanical performance. However, questions remain about the ability of the reinforcing fibers to intrude the interstices of cancellous bone and their ultimate contribution to improving the performance of the cement sheath in vivo. The clinical performance of hydroxyapatite particles as filler to improve the mechanical properties of bone cement has not yet been demonstrated.

Other forms of acrylic bone cement currently undergoing investigation include poly (ethyl methacrylate)/*n*-butyl methacrylate. Introduction of other monomers is directed toward improving the biologic response to the cement and its mechanical properties. Monomers other than methylmethacrylate that are currently used for PMMA bone cement have been reported to elicit more favorable biologic responses and mechanical properties (lower modular elasticity). However, the clinical performance of these cements has not yet been demonstrated.

Another issue recently raised regarding the behavior of conventional PMMA relates to shrinkage of the material during its polymerization. Does this shrinkage lead to separation of the cement sheath from the metallic stem or from the bone? Laboratory studies in progress are investigating modifications of the cement and its handling to reduce such shrinkage.

Annotated Bibliography

Metals

Chan FW, Bobyn JD, Medley JB, Krygier JJ, Yue S, Tanzer M: Engineering issues and wear performance of metal on metal hip implants. *Clin Orthop* 1996;333:96–107.

Factors affecting the wear of metal-on-metal prostheses were reviewed and wear test results using a laboratory hip simulator presented.

Dowson D, Taheri S, Wallbridge NC: The role of counterface imperfections in the wear of polyethylene. *Wear* 1987;119: 277–293.

A single scratch on a metal counterface was shown to have a profound effect on polyethylene wear in laboratory testing, depending on the pile-up of metal on the edge of the scratch.

Fisher J, Firkins P, Reeves EA, Hailey JL, Isaac GH: The influence of scratches to metallic counterfaces on the wear of ultra-high molecular weight polyethylene. *Proc Inst Mech Eng [H]* 1995; 209:263–264.

Scratches on metal counterfaces were found to substantially increase wear in laboratory testing.

Hailey JL, Ingham E, Stone M, Wroblewski BM, Fisher J: Ultra-high molecular weight polyethylene wear debris generated in vivo and in laboratory tests: The influence of counterface roughness. *Proc Instr Mech Eng [H]* 1996;210:3–10.

The effect of counterface roughness on polyethylene wear was demonstrated in this laboratory study.

Jacobs JJ, Gilbert JL, Urban RM: Corrosion of metal orthopaedic implants. *J Bone Joint Surg* 1998;80A:268–282.

This review reported the contribution of corrosion products from certain types of prostheses on wear at the articulating surface and described the biologic response to the debris.

Polyethylene

Oonishi H, Ishimaru H, Kato A: Effect of cross-linkage by gamma radiation in heavy doses to low wear polyethylene in total hip prosthesis. *J Mater Sci Mater Med* 1996;7:753–763.

Gamma radiation cross-linking of polyethylene cups was found to reduce wear in a laboratory hip simulator study.

Polymethylmethacrylate

Demian HW, McDermott K: Regulatory perspective on characterization and testing of orthopedic bone cements. *Biomaterials* 1998;19:1607–1618.

This review noted the types of testing necessary to provide a meaningful characterization of bone cements.

Lewis G: Properties of acrylic bone cement: State of the art review. *J Biomed Mater Res* 1997;38:155–82.

The properties of bone cements were thoroughly reviewed.

Chapter 5
Bone Grafts

Introduction

Bone grafting is an essential tool for the restoration of bone stock that is often necessary to obtain a stable reconstruction during revision total hip or knee arthroplasty. The number of revision total hip and knee arthroplasties has increased steadily over the past decade. In addition, as the number of multiple revision procedures increases, bone loss problems will increase as well. Therefore, a thorough understanding of bone graft biology, options, and limitations is necessary.

There are 3 biologic processes that influence bone graft function and use: osteogenesis, osteoinduction, and osteoconduction. Osteogenesis refers to bone formation with no indication if the cellular origin is from the host or the graft. Osteogenesis requires viable osteoblasts that form new bone. This process is most often associated with transplantation of viable autologous cancellous bone or vascularized bone (for example, vascularized fibula or ilium).

Osteoinduction refers to the recruitment of host mesenchymal cells from the surrounding soft tissue or bone that then differentiate into bone-forming cells. Bone morphogenetic protein (BMP) is one of the most well studied osteoinductive agents. BMP is present in fresh autografts and even in allografts if they are properly preserved. Osteoconduction is the process of ingrowth of blood vessels, perivascular tissue, and osteoprogenitor cells from the host bed into the graft structure. The graft serves as a scaffold for the ingrowth of new bone.

It is essential that specific terminology be used when defining bone grafts. Grafts may be defined by their origin, placement, viability (vascularized or nonvascularized) at surgery, and whether or not the graft is fresh or preserved. An autograft is one that is moved from one site to another in the same individual. An allograft refers to tissue transferred between 2 genetically different individuals of the same species. Xenografts are tissues from one species transferred to a member of a different species; the use of these grafts with present technology is limited. There is also a special situation of grafting called the isograft, which is tissue transplanted between 2 genetically identical individuals (identical twins) or inbred laboratory animals. Bone grafts may be further defined as cancellous or cortical, vascularized or nonvascularized. These grafts may be preserved by freezing, freeze-drying, or radiation.

Biology of Autografts and Allografts

Bone graft incorporation is a complex multifaceted process, and the rate, pattern, and completeness by which it is achieved is influenced by the inherent biologic activity of the graft (the presence of living cells and their products), its osteoinductive potential (ability of the graft to induce an osteogenic response from the host tissue), and its osteoconductive potential (ability of the graft to support the host osteogenic response).

The role of the graft in the incorporation process is quite variable. For instance, a vascularized autograft does not require as much support from the perigraft environment because it has its own blood supply and living cells. However, nonvascularized cancellous or cortical grafts and allografts are more dependent on the perigraft environment to either respond to cellular signals (osteoinduction) or provide an adequate blood supply from the surrounding soft tissue.

In general, the less inherent biologic activity that a particular graft, such as frozen allograft, possesses, the more dependent the graft is on the perigraft environment. The graft's biomechanical stresses are also important because graft incorporation is influenced by mechanical stability, particularly if the graft is also providing structural support. If the graft is unstable, vascularization will be delayed or inhibited. Morcellized allograft chips have been used successfully to treat contained defects in the acetabulum. In these cases, the surrounding host bone is usually well vascularized and mechanical support is not required by the graft.

The pattern of bone formation after grafting, the revascularization of various types of grafts, and the factors influencing host/graft union has been studied in different animal

One or more of the authors or the departments with which they are affiliated have received something of value from a commercial or other party related directly or indirectly to the subject of this article.

models. The presence or absence of living histocompatible committed, bone-forming cells is the principal determinant of the rate and amount of new bone formation associated with a bone graft. Fresh autogenous bone grafts contain live osteogenic cells and are therefore osteogenic and osteoinductive. Fresh autografts, either cancellous or cortical, demonstrate rapid formation of new bone. The presence or absence of a vascular pedicle affects the pattern of new bone formation.

In nonvascularized cancellous autografts, new bone forms on the surface of trabeculae. The incorporation of a cancellous graft involves a dynamic equilibrium between inflammation, revascularization, and osteoinduction. Vascularization of the graft may occur several days after implantation. Growth factors such as BMP are active in the early stages after implantation and induce host mesenchymal cells to migrate into the graft. Host vessels, osteoblasts, and osteoblast progenitor cells infiltrate the graft. Thus, the early stages of grafting include inflammation, revascularization, and osteoinduction. The graft subsequently undergoes remodeling and osteoconduction. A final phase of cancellous autograft incorporation is integration of the graft into the surrounding host bone. This whole process may take 6 months to 1 year.

The rate of revascularization of a cortical autograft is markedly slower when compared to cancellous autografts. Significant centripetal vessel invasion is observed in the substance of stable nonvascularized fresh cortical autografts 4 weeks after surgery in rats, and 7 weeks after surgery in dogs. Furthermore, even under optimal circumstances bone resorption will dominate over bone formation in the early phases of cortical graft incorporation, and extensive osteonal remodeling occurs. Cortical autografts will eventually incorporate with the host bone but the process is prolonged. Cortical autografting is generally limited to the fibula but are now in limited use as vascular grafts have become more popular.

In vascularized cortical autografts a small amount of periosteal new bone forms and normal osteonal remodeling is maintained. The newly formed bone eventually becomes integrated with the original graft. The most common sources of vascularized grafts are the fibula, iliac crest, and ribs. Recently, vascularized fibula grafts have been used to treat osteonecrosis of the hip. Successful microvascular repair and stable fixation are essential in graft incorporation whenever a vascularized graft is used. Vascularized autografts are harvested with a vascular pedicle and are reanastomosed to the host blood supply at the time of surgery. Although technically demanding, these grafts are being used more frequently with improvements in microvascular techniques over the past decade. The use of these types of grafts should be reserved for treatment of large defects or instances when the surrounding soft tissue has limited blood supply secondary to trauma, radiation, or osteonecrosis. In these situations, a graft that does not have its own blood supply will have a limited chance of success.

Over the past decade vascularized fibula grafts have been adapted to treat osteonecrosis of the hip. Although the results look promising, more studies are required to determine the specific indications because of cost and complications noted. In a study of 247 vascularized fibula grafts (198 patients), either objective motor weakness, subjective ankle weakness, or sensory abnormalities was noted in 19% of the limbs; at 5-year follow-up, one of these conditions was noted in 18 of 78 limbs (24%) studied.

Allogenicity adds another level of complexity to successful incorporation of allograft bone. Fresh allografts elicit a host immune system response that can either delay graft incorporation or even result in significant graft resorption. In order to attenuate the immune response and for convenience, bone allografts are processed. Grafts are usually either frozen or freeze-dried. Although these techniques decrease the immunogenicity of the graft, they also decrease biologic potential because all live cells are removed.

Grafts can be either structural or nonstructural. Structural grafts may be either cortical, cancellous, or osteochondral. Nonstructural grafts are either cancellous or morcellized chips. The structural grafts have limited biologic activity. Revascularization and remodeling occur to a limited extent in processed allografts. In both animal experiments and human retrievals, union was noted at the host-graft junction via external callus from the host. In general, internal remodeling is limited and is restricted to the superficial ends of the graft. Soft tissue becomes attached to the graft by a seam of new bone.

There is another method of processing that has demonstrated interesting clinical potential. Chemosterilized autolysed, antigen extracted, allogeneic bone (AAA bone) preserves BMP and other osteoinductive factors while limiting the immunogenicity of the graft. This type of bone graft has been used successfully in treating recalcitrant fracture nonunions. However, because this bone construct is demineralized it cannot be used as a weightbearing strut.

Immunology

It is well documented that fresh allograft will invoke a host immune response that leads to failure of the graft. In order to reduce graft immunogenicity most grafts in current use are either frozen or freeze-dried. Although this processing reduces the host immune response it does not completely eliminate it.

The response of the host to an allograft is predominantly a cell-mediated response to cell-surface antigens. The major histocompatibility complex (MHC) contains genes that encode for class I and II antigens that elicit the immune response to allograft bone. Class I antigens are designated as HLA-A, B, and C; class II antigens are called HLA-DR, DP, and DQ. T lymphocytes in the host are activated by these class I and class II antigens. However, the exact mechanism of rejection of allograft bone has not been delineated. A recent animal study assessed the influence of histocompatibility matching and freezing of a cortical bone graft on incorporation in a rat segmental femoral defect model. Fresh or frozen cortical bone grafts were implanted in the bone defects and were matched for both MHC and non-MHC antigens (syngeneic grafts), or matched for MHC but not for non-MHC antigens (minor mismatch), or mismatched for both MHC and non-MHC antigens (major mismatch). Freezing markedly attenuated the systemic antibody response. However, freezing also reduced the biologic activity of the graft. The decrease in both immunologic and biologic activity was probably secondary to cell death that occurs as a result of the freezing process.

Histocompatible antigen mismatching had a profound impact on graft revascularization. In general, the frozen mismatched allograft that is most commonly used today in clinical practice had the least predictable process of incorporation.

Recently, attention has focused on the potential influence of human leukocyte antigen (HLA) matching in humans and the immune response to allograft bone. A multicenter study was performed to assess the immunologic responses in human recipients of massive frozen (-80° C) osseous and osteochondral grafts. After grafting, 49 of 84 recipients (58%) showed evidence of sensitization to class I antigens and 46 of 84 recipients (55%) showed evidence of sensitization to class II antigens. The influence of sensitization on graft incorporation and clinical outcome could not be ascertained.

In another study assessing the potential relationship between HLA matching and radiographic incorporation of allografts, there was a trend toward better graft incorporation with HLA matching but no statistically significant difference with mismatched recipients.

Therefore, there is an immune response to allograft implantation that may influence graft incorporation. However, the incorporation of a nonvascularized graft is a complex process that in addition to the immune reaction of the recipient, is influenced by several factors, including perigraft environment, graft stability, and the biomechanical loads of the graft. The biologic activity of a graft may be improved by the addition of growth factors. Successful results with AAA bone grafts suggests that additional research in this area is necessary.

Allografts in Total Hip Arthroplasty

Bone loss may be a significant problem when trying to revise a total hip arthroplasty. In general, the surgeon must assess the extent of bone loss and determine if some type of bone grafting will be necessary. Because there is no general agreement with regard to the use of various types of grafts, the surgeon should be aware of all the bone graft options that are available. Morcellized allograft chips have been used successfully to fill cavitary defects. These grafts have also been used in conjunction with antiprotrusio cages and to supplement structural allografts. These grafts are osteoconductive and incorporate in a manner similar to cancellous autografts, but at a decreased rate. It is essential that the surrounding bone is well vascularized.

The indications for structural allografts for revision of acetabular components remains controversial. Long-term clinical results with this technique have been variable and the data is difficult to analyze because of inconsistencies in the classification of the acetabular defects. The success of a graft is dependent on a variety of factors such as the type of graft (for example, femoral head versus distal femur), the rigidity of fixation between the graft and the host, and the mechanical stresses placed on the graft. Graft lysis over time with subsequent loosening of the cup has been a problem. In 30 hips treated with femoral head allografts with 10-year follow-up, 47% of the acetabular components failed. However, in 8 of 10 hips, bone stock was sufficient to enable revision without further segmental grafting. These authors recommended structural bone grafting only as a salvage procedure.

However, 2 more recent series suggested that there may be a specific role for structural allografts. In one series, 31 hips were treated with major structural allografts screwed to the pelvis and fitted with uncemented cups. At an average follow-up of 5.7 years there was a 19% rate of acetabular loosening. However, the only failures in this series were noted in hips in which the allograft supported more than 50% of the acetabular component. In another study of 33 hips treated with bulk acetabular allografts, the authors reported restoration of bone stock in 76% of hips. When the graft was noted to support more than 50% of the cup it was recommended that a reconstruction ring with cement also be used.

Bone stock restoration is the major goal of segmental acetabular allografts. Bone stock restoration is initially dependent on graft union and subsequently on the state and degree of graft resorption. It remains controversial whether or not incorporated allograft bone truly represents restored bone stock. Graft lysis does increase with time. There are certain general guidelines for using structural allograft in the acetabulum that may improve long-term results: (1) The graft and host must be carefully prepared and an excellent fit with rigid fixation must be obtained. (2) Less than 50% of the acetabular component should be supported by graft alone. (3) Cemented cups should be used when 50% of the cup area is supported by graft and the use of a reinforcement ring should be considered.

Allografts of the proximal femur usually involve proximal femoral allografts, cortical strut grafts, or impaction grafting with morcellized bone. In general, bulk proximal femoral allografts are used when there is extensive proximal bone loss and the graft is providing partial replacement of the femur. It is recommended that femoral components be cemented into the allograft implant for increased stability; both cemented and cementless stems have been used for distal fixation. It is essential that rigid fixation be obtained between the implant-allograft composite and the distal host bone. The type of fixation selected will be determined by the extent and quality of the remaining host bone. Fixation options include a distal press fit, cement, or distal interlocking screws. A step cut may also be made in the distal aspect of the graft to increase rotational stability. The allograft host junction should be bone grafted with autograft if possible.

Cortical strut allografts are used to enhance bone stock and provide stability when the bone stock of the femur is insufficient. These strut grafts may be fixed to the femur with wires or cables. These grafts typically unite, revascularize, and remodel. Animal studies have confirmed the incorporation of these grafts.

Another treatment option for restoring femoral bone stock is impaction bone grafting with morcellized allograft bone and a cemented stem. The goal with this technique is to reconstitute the bone stock of the proximal femur. There have been several reports in the literature highlighting this technique. One study reported satisfactory results with short-term follow-up (18 to 49 months) of 56 revision total hip arthroplasties. None of the hips required another revision. In a more detailed analysis of 34 patients with an average follow-up of 32 months, the authors noted incorporation of the allograft in 94% of femurs. However, the authors were concerned about the high rate of fracture of the femur (18%) and the high rates of subsidence (38%) with an average of 10.1 mm (range 4 to 31 mm) in these patients. This technique requires further study.

Unfortunately, data from human retrievals is limited. In 1 postmortem analysis, an inner zone containing fragments of dead bone and cement, an interface zone, and an outer zone of regenerated cortical bone were identified. More detailed analysis of retrieved specimens will be necessary to determine if this allograft becomes truly revascularized, an essential factor if the construct is to have long-term durability.

Allografts in Total Knee Arthroplasty

Loss of bone stock on both the femoral and tibial sides of the knee joint is now a fairly common problem when revising a failed primary total knee arthroplasty. Unfortunately, at present there is no classification system that surgeons use to classify bone loss associated with revision total knee arthroplasty. Therefore, it is difficult to outline specific indications for the use of allograft bone in a revision total knee arthroplasty.

In general, the type of total knee arthroplasty system used for a revision procedure will be influenced by the quality of soft tissues, specifically the ligamentous stability and extent of bone loss. Bone defects can be classified as contained, which means having an intact surrounding cortex, and uncontained, which means having a cortical defect combined with a deficiency of the metaphyseal trabecular bone. Morcellized allograft bone is used to treat contained defects. These defects are usually limited to 1 side of the tibial plateau or to a single femoral condyle. In addition, the prosthesis must be stabilized on the host bone. Structural allografts are usually reserved for treatment of large uncontained defects, specifically where the bone loss is so extensive that knee stability and the joint line cannot be maintained with either standard augments or extra-thick polyethylene inserts.

On the femoral side, structural allografts are usually required when the defects are greater than 1 cm distal and/or posterior. Femoral head allografts can be used to treat large defects involving 1 condyle, and can be secured to the femoral bone and then cut down using the standard cutting blocks. In instances where there is extensive loss of both condyles, a distal femoral allograft may be necessary.

On the tibial side, extensive defects greater than 1 cm that cannot be treated with metallic wedges may be stabilized with allograft bone. The type of allograft used will depend on the shape of the defect. Femoral head allografts can be used for small or intermediate-sized proximal uncontained defects, whereas a proximal tibia may be necessary for extensive proximal bone loss. In one series, 35 bulk allografts were used for both primary and revision total hip and knee arthroplasty in 30 patients. No revisions were required at an average follow-up of 50 months. The authors recommended the use of cemented components with cementless stems. In another study, 30 total knee arthroplasties in 28 patients were revised with allograft bone and stemmed components. At an average follow-up of 50 months, 7 of 30 knees (23%) were considered either failures secondary to infection, or had tibial component loosening, fracture of the graft, or nonunion at the allograft-host joint.

In general, it is recommended that bulk allografts be used in conjunction with cemented components with stems to attain a stable construct. Stability at the junction between the graft and the host bone is essential. In some cases, additional fixation with plates and screws may be necessary. Finally, careful handling of the surrounding soft-tissue envelope is critical.

Annotated Bibliography

Biology/Autografts

Garbuz DS, Masri BA, Czitrom AA: Biology of allografting. *Orthop Clin North Am* 1998;29:199–204.

This article is a review of the biology of allograft bone.

Stevenson S, Li XQ, Davy DT, Klein L, Goldberg VM: Critical biological determinants of incorporation of non-vascularized cortical bone grafts: Quantification of a complex process and structure. *J Bone Joint Surg* 1997;79A:1–16.

Fresh and frozen cortical bone grafts were implanted in a rat segmental femoral defect model. The grafts were either matched for both major and nonmajor histocompatibility complex and non-MHC antigens (syngeneic grafts), matched for MHC but not for non-MHC antigens (minor mismatch) and mismatched for both MHC and non-MHC antigens (major mismatch). Revascularization was influenced by histocompatibility–antigen matching. Syngeneic grafts revascularized more quickly and to a greater degree than the grafts with a major or minor mismatch. Frozen mismatched allograft (similar to one used clinically) had the least predictable process of incorporation.

Stevenson S, Emery SE, Goldberg VM: Factors affecting bone graft incorporation. *Clin Orthop* 1996;324:66–74.

This article reviews the data from several animal models used to study the factors that influence bone graft incorporation, including revascularization, new bone formation, processing (freezing), and histocompatibility antigen disparities.

Urbaniak JR, Coogan PG, Gunneson EB, Nunley JA: Treatment of osteonecrosis of the femoral head with free vascularized fibular grafting: A long-term follow-up study of one hundred and three hips. *J Bone Joint Surg* 1995;77A:681–694.

This article presents a retrospective review of patients with osteonecrosis of the hip treated with a free vascularized fibular graft. The most successful results were seen in patients without subchondral collapse of the femoral head.

Vail TP, Urbaniak JR: Donor-site morbidity with use of vascularized autogenous fibular grafts. *J Bone Joint Surg* 1996;78A: 204–211.

This article discusses a retrospective study of 247 vascularized fibula grafts in 198 patients. Forty-seven (19.0%) of the 247 lower limbs developed either objective motor weakness, subjective ankle discomfort, or sensory abnormalities in the leg. At a minimum 5-year follow-up, 18 of the 74 limbs (24.3%) had at least 1 of these findings. The prevalence of pain in the ankle and lower limb increased with time.

Allografts

Stevenson S, Shaffer JW, Goldberg VM: The humoral response to vascular and nonvascular allografts of bone. *Clin Orthop* 1996;326:86–95.

Rat and dog models were used to assess a donor-specific antibody response to nonvascularized and vascularized grafts. Nonvascularized segmental femoral grafts were analyzed in the rat, and nonvascularized fresh and cryopreserved massive osteochondral allografts and vascularized and nonvascularized fibula allografts were evaluated in dogs. Massive grafts elicited a more sustained antibody response than smaller grafts, and freezing the graft reduced the antibody response. The potential benefits of tissue antigen matching require further study.

Immunology

Muscolo DL, Ayerza MA, Calabrese ME, Redal MA, Santini-Araujo E: Human leukocyte antigen matching, radiographic score, and histologic findings in massive frozen bone allografts. *Clin Orthop* 1996;326:115–126.

The study assessed the influence of HLA matching on the radiographic incorporation of allografts. Patients with 1 or more HLA class I antigen matches had higher radiographic scores than patients with grafts that were totally mismatched. However, the differences in radiographic scores were not statistically significant.

Strong DM, Friedlaender GE, Tomford WW, et al: Immunologic responses in human recipients of osseous and osteochondral allografts. *Clin Orthop* 1996;326:107–114.

A multi-institutional study was performed to evaluate the immunologic responses for human recipients of massive frozen (-80° C) osseous and osteochondral allografts. Sensitization before transplant was shown in 33 of 84 patients (39%). After grafting, 49 of 84 recipients (58%) showed evidence of sensitization to class I antigens and 46 of 84 recipients (55%) showed evidence to sensitization to class II antigens. However, no clear relationship has been established between the degree of HLA matching and incorporation of massive frozen allografts.

Tomford WW: Transmission of disease through transplantation of musculoskeletal allografts. *J Bone Joint Surg* 1995;77A: 1742–1754.

A review of the diseases previously transmitted in clinical cases, the risk of disease transmission, and methods used to reduce the risk of disease transmission when using musculoskeletal allografts are presented.

Allografts and Revision Total Hip Arthroplasty

Garbuz D, Morsi E, Gross AE: Revision of the acetabular component of a total hip arthroplasty with a massive structural allograft: Study with a minimum five-year follow-up. *J Bone Joint Surg* 1996;78A:693–697.

The authors reported on 33 hips that had a major, noncontained defect of an acetabular column in which 50% of the acetabulum was involved. Eighteen of 33 hips had a successful result at an average follow-up of 7 years. In 7 hips (21%) the graft united but the component loosened. All of these hips had a successful revision procedure (average follow-up 4 to 6 years), and the graft was fixed to support the cup at repeat revision. Eight hips had failure of both the prosthesis and the allograft. The authors recommend the use of a reconstruction ring and a cup inserted with cement is recommended when the graft supports more than 50% of the cup.

Garbuz DS, Penner MJ: Role and results of segmental allografts for acetabular segmental bone deficiency. *Orthop Clin North Am* 1998;29:263–275.

This article presents a review of the published literature related to treatment of acetabular bone deficiency and its treatment with structural allografts.

Head WC, Malinin TI, Mallory TH, Emerson RH Jr: Onlay cortical allografting bone grafting for the femur. *Orthop Clin North Am* 1998;29:307–312.

A review of the indications, surgical technique, and results of cortical strut allografts used to treat femoral bone stock loss is presented. The authors report on 265 patients with a graft union rate of 99%. Only 3% of these patients required femoral revision surgery with a minimum follow-up of 7.5 years.

Meding JB, Ritter MA, Keating EM, Faris PM: Impaction bone-grafting before insertion of a femoral stem with cement in revision total hip arthroplasty: A minimum two-year follow-up study. *J Bone Joint Surg* 1997;79A:1834–1841.

This article presents a review of 34 revision total hip arthroplasties using a collarless polished tapered stem and impaction bone grafting only. Complications included 4 intraoperative and 2 postoperative fractures of the femur at an average follow-up of 30 months. Two patients (6%) needed a repeat revision for aseptic loosening and subsidence was noted in 38% of patients (average 10.1 mm). The authors recommended impaction bone grafting when proximal femoral osteopenia was extremely severe.

Nelissen RG, Bauer TW, Weidenhielm LR, LeGolvan DP, Mikhail WE: Revision hip arthroplasty with the use of cement and impaction grafting: Histological analysis of four cases. *J Bone Joint Surg* 1995;77A:412–422.

A histologic analysis of 4 cases after revision hip arthroplasty with impaction bone grafting was performed. Three relatively ill-defined zones were identified from biopsy specimens: an inner zone consisting of bone cement, fibrous tissue, and necrotic trabeculae, a middle zone consisting of viable trabecular bone, and an outer zone consisting of viable cortex.

Shinar AA, Harris WH: Bulk structural autogenous grafts and allografts for reconstruction of the acetabulum in total hip arthroplasty: Sixteen-year-average follow-up. *J Bone Joint Surg* 1997;79A:159–168.

The authors reviewed 70 hips (62 patients) treated with bulk structural autogenous grafts and allografts with an average follow-up of 16.5 years. Graft lysis was noted in 32 of 70 hips (46%).

Schreurs BW, Slooff TJ, Buma P, Gardeniers JW, Huiskes R: Acetabular reconstruction with impacted morsellised cancellous bone graft and cement: A 10- to 15-year follow-up of 60 revision arthroplasties. *J Bone Joint Surg* 1998;80B:391–395.

In 60 revision acetabular components using impacted morcellized bone allografts and a cemented polyethylene cup, there were 37 cavitary defects and 23 combined defects. The overall survival rate at an average follow-up of 11 years (average, 10 to 15 years) was 90%. Five hips required a re-revision for either aseptic loosening (3) or infection (2).

Allografts and Total Knee Arthroplasty

Engh GA, Herzwurm PJ, Parks NL: Treatment of major defects of bone with bulk allografts and stemmed components during total knee arthroplasty. *J Bone Joint Surg* 1997;79A:1030–1039.

The authors reviewed the results of 35 allografts in 30 patients an average of 50 months after implantation. Long-stemmed components were used in all cases. There were no revisions and 26 of 30 patients (87%) had a good or excellent result.

Ghazavi MT, Stockley I, Yee G, Davis A, Gross AE: Reconstruction of massive bone defects with allograft in revision total knee arthroplasty. *J Bone Joint Surg* 1997;79A:17–25.

A review of 30 knees (28 patients) who had a revision total knee arthroplasty with allograft bone is presented. At an average follow-up of 50 months, the success rate was 77% (23 knees). There were 7 failures: infection (3), loosening (2), graft fracture (1), and nonunion of the graft host junction (1).

Harris AI, Poddar S, Gitelis S, Sheinkop MB, Rosenberg AG: Arthoplasty with a composite of an allograft and a prosthesis for knees with severe deficiency of bone. *J Bone Joint Surg* 1995;77A:373–386.

Fourteen patients were treated with a massive allograft and a standard total knee prosthesis for severe bone loss. At an average follow-up of 43 months there were 13 satisfactory results. Five principles for the use of massive allografts were outlined: (1) allograft tissue can transmit disease; (2) the allograft should be fixed with instrumentation; (3) the prosthesis should be cemented to the allograft; (4) the graft should not be trimmed; and (5) the soft-tissue envelope must be handled with care.

Classic Bibliography

Anderson AF, Green NE: Residual functional deficit after partial fibulectomy for bone graft. *Clin Orthop* 1991;267:137–140.

Emerson RH Jr, Malinin TI, Cuellar AD, Head WC, Peters PC:

Cortical strut allografts in the reconstruction of the femur in revision total hip arthroplasty: A basic science and clinical study. *Clin Orthop* 1992;285:35–44.

Enneking WF, Mindell ER: Observation on massive retrieved human allografts. *J Bone Joint Surg* 1991;73A:1123–1142.

Gie GA, Linder L, Ling RS, Simon JP, Slooff TJ, Timperley AJ: Impacted cancellous allografts and cement for revision total hip arthroplasty. *J Bone Joint Surg* 1993;75B:14–21.

Hooten JP Jr, Engh CA Jr, Engh CA: Failure of structural acetabular allografts in cementless revision hip arthroplasty. *J Bone Joint Surg* 1994;76B:419–422.

Johnson EE, Urist MR, Finerman GA: Resistant nonunions and partial or complete segmental defects of long bones: Treatment with implants of a composite of human bone morphogenetic protein (BMP) and autolyzed, antigen-extracted, allogeneic (AAA) bone. *Clin Orthop* 1992;277:229–237.

Kwong LM, Jasty M, Harris WH: High failure rate of bulk femoral head allografts in total hip acetabular reconstructions at 10 years. *J Arthroplasty* 1993;8:341–346.

Nather A, Goh JC, Lee JJ: Biomechanical strength of non-vascularised and vascularised diaphyseal bone transplants: An experimental study. *J Bone Joint Surg* 1990;72B:1031–1035.

Paprosky WG, Magnus RE: Principles of bone grafting in revision total hip arthroplasty: Acetabular technique. *Clin Orthop* 1994;298:147–155.

Schreurs BW, Buma P, Huiskes R, Slagter JL, Slooff TJ: Morsellized allografts for fixation of the hip prosthesis femoral component: A mechanical and histological study in the goat. *Acta Orthop Scand* 1994;65:267–275.

Stevenson S, Horowitz M: The response to bone allografts. *J Bone Joint Surg* 1992;74A:939–950.

Chapter 6
Application of Bone Inductive and Conductive Agents to Hip and Knee Reconstruction

Over the last decade there has been a rapid development of various new synthetic products that are designed not only to serve as bone graft substitutes but also to enhance the fixation of noncemented implants to bone. The synthetic materials and coatings can be defined as combinations of osteoconductive matrices, osteogenic cells, and/or osteoinductive materials. In discussing the application of osteoinductive and osteoconductive materials to the field of total joint arthroplasty, the various products will be described according to their use as bone graft substitutes or enhancers of implant fixation. Experimental and practical experience in animal studies and in human clinical area will be reported.

Osteoconductive and Osteoinductive Materials as Bone Graft Substitutes

Autogenous bone grafting remains the preferred means of augmenting bone healing throughout a broad spectrum of orthopaedic disorders. The ideal bone graft or bone graft substitute should provide 3 elements: (1) an osteoconductive matrix that provides a scaffolding amenable for bone ingrowth; (2) osteoinductive factors that can be chemical or physical components that induce the various stages of the bone repair process; and (3) osteogenic cells that have potential to differentiate and carry forth the various stages of bone regeneration. Autogenous cancellous bone graft contains all 3 components: (1) hydroxyapatite and collagen, which are well suited to serve as an osteoconductive framework; (2) numerous stromal cells within the cavity lining, which have osteogenic potential; and (3) cancellous bone and the adjacent hematoma, which contain a family of growth factors, most notably bone morphogenetic proteins (BMPs) and transforming growth factor-β (TGF-β), which have the ability to induce and to augment the regenerative processes.

Although autogenous cancellous bone grafts have all of these elements, they are present to a more limited extent in autogenous cortical bone. The advantage of cortical grafts is that their structure confers compressive strength and, thus, provides mechanical support. In addition to the osteoinductive, osteoconductive, and osteogenic properties of these autogenous grafts, they are histocompatible, do not transport disease, and retain viable osteoblasts that participate in the formation of bone.

Although autogenous bone grafting is effective, it has several shortcomings and potential complications. An important disadvantage, especially in the field of total joint reconstruction, is that a limited quantity of bone is available for harvest. In addition, there is significant donor site morbidity, with rates as high as 25%, including surgical donor site infections and pain, increased anesthesia time, and significantly increased surgical blood loss.

Allograft bone provides an alternative to the use of autogenous bone grafts. Unfortunately, allograft bone grafts have a number of potential problems, including immunogenicity, risk of viral and bacterial disease transmission, and limited osteoconductive and osteoinductive properties. Because of the disadvantages of both autogenous and allograft bone grafts, there is a true need for osteoconductive and osteoinductive bone graft substitute products.

Demineralized Bone Matrix

Demineralized bone matrix (DBM), although technically a processed allograft, is a bone graft substitute with enhanced biologic properties. DBM is produced from acid extraction of bone, leaving noncollagenous proteins, bone growth factors, and collagen. Demineralized materials have no structural strength, but have enhanced osteoinductive capability afforded most notably by BMP. DBM is currently prepared by bone banks, and special chemically processed forms such as Grafton (Osteotech, Shrewsbury, NJ) are now available. DBM has been used in clinical settings to promote bone regeneration, mainly in well-supported, stable skeletal defects. Excellent results from preliminary clinical use have been presented but the data to support its widespread use are limited. Despite the enhanced osteoinductive potential, the actual functionally accessible BMP within these demineralized grafts is exponentially less than that used in recombinant BMP studies.

The bone banks have not provided the actual amount of BMP that is available from the various graft preparations. Some commercially available DBM preparations cannot induce bone in the Urist biologic mouse muscle test. All the DBMs are easy to mold intraoperatively; however, they do not provide intrinsic strength. The clinical applications of DBMs in hip and knee reconstruction include augmentation of traditional autogenous bone grafts and of cancellous allografts so as to enhance the osteoinductive properties of the composite graft.

At this time the United States Food and Drug Administration (FDA) requires sterilization of the DBM as prepared by bone banks, and this step may, in fact, decrease some of the viability of the available BMP within the preparation. DBM does afford the potential of enhanced osteoinduction and to date has been used as an adjunct to more traditional grafting materials. When successful in achieving union, DBM develops bone with comparable mechanical strength to that of autograft. DBM is currently available freeze-dried and processed from cortical and/or cancellous bone in the form of powder, crushed, as chips, or as Grafton® gel.

Grafton gel (Osteotech, Shrewsbury, NJ) is processed from human bone by a patented technique that incorporates a permeation treatment that does not expose tissue to ethylene oxide or gamma radiation, thus possibly protecting larger amounts of native BMP. It is processed into a gel consistency and packaged in a syringe from which it can be applied directly during surgery. It has no structural strength and has been used most successfully in conjunction with internal fixation or as an adjunct of other grafting materials. Two additional forms of the Grafton gel formulation are currently under development. One is in the form of a collagen mat retaining the noncollagenous proteins and the other as a woven collagen mass that has the appearance of steel wool.

Bone Marrow and Stem Cells

Autogenous bone marrow also can be used to enhance bone healing. The osteogenic capabilities of bone marrow have been well known since Boujon's original observation in 1869. Bone marrow contains osteoprogenitor cells on the order of 1 per 50,000 nucleated cells in the young to 1 per 2 million in the elderly, and certain concentration techniques have increased that number fivefold. When grown in porous ceramic, bone marrow can bring osteoprogenitor cells to a deficient grafting bed. Using a rat model of femoral segmental defect, investigators have been able to demonstrate that autogenous marrow has the osteogenic capability to heal a bone defect. Following bone marrow implantation, woven bone occurred initially, progressed to early lamellar bone, and subsequently molded in a volumetric fashion. When placed in a fresh femoral defect and given in sufficient amounts, the bone marrow produced a rate of union comparable to that of autogenous bone graft. The bone formed by marrow demonstrated comparable biomechanical properties to that of a cancellous bone graft. Significant bone formation occurred when the marrow was percutaneously injected into femoral nonunions. These studies, as well as those by other investigators, have indicated that bone marrow can lead to structurally competent bone regeneration in an orthotopic location.

Clinically, it has been demonstrated that, when provided in adequate amounts, bone marrow can successfully treat nonunions in patients. Bone marrow should be harvested in aliquots of approximately 2.5 ml per site. If gathered in larger amounts, the marrow would be diluted with blood. The marrow should be used immediately to maintain its viability. Although it has limited use in hip and knee reconstruction, bone marrow, like DBM, offers the ability to augment all currently used synthetic grafts and allografts. There is essentially no morbidity from obtaining bone marrow.

It is desirable for the osteoprogenitor cells to be easily increased in number and in concentration. To achieve this goal, investigators have isolated bone marrow and grown it under special culture conditions to specifically expand mesenchymal stem cells. These cells, when given in an appropriate composite mixture including ceramics and collagens, have been able to heal osseous defects in a series of animal models. They are still in preclinical trials at this time but offer further opportunities for the use of an expanded marrow stem cell population.

Biosynthetic Graft Materials

Ceramics Ceramics have been used solely as osteoconductive bone graft matrices. Most calcium phosphate ceramics currently under investigation are synthetic and composed of either hydroxyapatite (HA), tricalcium phosphate (TCP) or a combination of the two. These biomaterials are being produced commercially as porous implants, nonporous dense implants, or granular particles with pores. Most calcium phosphate ceramics are created using a high temperature process called sintering and high-pressure compaction techniques. Another form of ceramics, called replamineform, is produced from marine coral specimens using a hydrothermal exchange method that replaces the original calcium carbonate of the coral with a calcium phosphate replicate. In contrast to the random pore structure created in totally synthetic porous materials, the pore structure of the coralline calcium phosphate implants is highly organized, similar to that of human cancellous bone.

Cancellous bone itself has a complex trabecular pattern in which approximately 20% of the total matrix is bone and the remaining area is marrow space interconnected through pores. Synthetic ceramics have various sized pores, but lack pore-to-pore connectivity. Therefore, when used as graft material the osteogenic material must resorb the bone to gain access to the interior pores. The exception is ceramics derived from materials such as coral that have a biologic pore interconnectivity mesh network. There are some new materials currently under development in which a collagen matrix mesh network is initially established, and then is covered with a thin layer of highly carbonate enriched HA ceramic so that the pores remain interconnected.

The chemical composition of ceramic profoundly affects its rate of bioresorption. TCP undergoes biologic resorption 10 to 20 times faster than HA. In clinical trials, TCP has been reported, in some circumstances, to have been totally resorbed, but in most others it persists for years. Once in the body, TCP is in part converted chemically to HA which is degraded slowly. The resorbing cell for HA is the foreign body giant cell, not the osteoclast. It resorbs 2 to 10 mm of HA and then ceases further resorption. Consequently, segments of HA ceramic will remain in place in the body for up to 7 to 10 years. In clinical applications TCP remodels more readily because of its porosity, but is weaker; it provides significantly less compressive strength than HA. The combination of the two is used clinically to offer both advantages. Material factors such as surface area affect the biologic degradation, and, in general, the larger the surface area the greater the bioresorption. Dense ceramic blocks with small surface areas biodegrade slowly when compared to porous implants. Thus, the shape and architecture of the ceramic will have a profound effect on resorption rates.

The ceramics are brittle and have very little tensile strength. Use of ceramics in applications requiring significant torsion bending or shear stress seems impracticable at present. However, mechanical properties of porous calcium phosphate materials are comparable to those of cancellous bone once the materials have been incorporated and remodeled. Ceramics must be shielded from loading forces until bony ingrowth has occurred. Rigid stabilization of surrounding bone and nonweightbearing are required during this period because the ceramics can tolerate minimal bending and torque load before failing.

The optimal osteoconductive pore sizes for ceramics appear to be between 150 and 500 µm. Ceramics appear to have no early adverse effects such as inflammation, and foreign body responses to ceramics are practically nonexistent when the ceramics are in a structural block arrangement. However, small granules of material have been shown to elicit a foreign body giant cell reaction. When ceramics are used, the radiographic findings demonstrate a continued presence of the ceramic for a prolonged period of time because of the failure of complete remodeling. Persistent dense radiographic imagery creates difficulty in determining the degree of bony growth and incorporation into the implant. The TCP, which is more biodegradable, loses more of its radiodensity and appears to be more fully incorporated into the bone.

The replamineform ceramics are a porous HA material derived from the calcium carbonate skeletal structure of sea coral. The pore size of these is determined by the genus of the coral used. The coral genus *Gonipora* has a microstructure similar to human cancellous bone. The coralline HA derived from *Gonipora* has large pores measuring from 500 to 600 µm in diameter with interconnections of 220 to 260 µm. The coral genus *Porites* has a microstructure that appears similar to that of an interstitial cortical bone, with a smaller pore diameter of 200 to 250 µm, parallel channels interconnected by 190-µm fenestrations, and a porosity of 66%. Coralline HA are available as Pro Osteon (Interpone, Irvine, CA) implant 500 and Pro Osteon 200 respectively, with the latter providing greater compressive strength.

A ceramic that forms in vivo has been created under the name of SRS (Norian, Cupertino, CA). This ceramic has a high carbonate substitution within the HA. When injected or placed in a bony cavity it will create a very firm cera ic mass within hours, and most of its compressive strength is achieved within 24 hours. However, there is little control over the porosity of this material. There is some demonstration that extraosseous forms can be resorbed. However, the SRS that is injected within bony cavities remain stable for long periods of time because of the high density of the newly formed ceramic. This injectable ceramic is undergoing clinical trials in metaphyseal fractures, most notably intertrochanteric fractures.

Other forms of calcium products have been used in the past, most notably calcium sulfate or plaster of Paris. This material can form within the site and was first used clinically over 30 years ago. It has a very rapid turnover, and most of it is resorbed within weeks to months. New forms of commercially available calcium sulfate are currently being introduced to the market under the trade name Orthoset (Wright Medical Technology, Arlington, TN).

Experimental animal studies have consistently demonstrated superior performance of autologous bone graft when compared to ceramic implants alone. However, some studies have yielded promising results when certain specific conditions are met. Clinically, the first successful results with ceramics were reported in dentistry and reconstructive craniofacial surgery. In orthopaedics, efficacy of coralline HA ceramics and autogenous grafts has been demonstrated for certain applications, particularly tibial plateau fractures that are under compression. In a random trial using coralline HA versus cancellous bone in the tibia, no differences in functional outcome were reported. Histologic analysis of the newly formed bone at the time of hardware removal revealed bony growth into and around the ceramic, with both cortical and cancellous bone in appropriate locations. Investigators also have studied TCP and found it comparable to autogenous bone when filling defects secondary to trauma and benign tumors. Although ceramics readily can be used to fill contained defects about the hip or knee, when placed in a structural position, because of their brittle nature, the ceramics must be protected by the orthopaedic implant fixation or they can fail. If particulate ceramics arc used, care must be taken to prevent the migration of the graft material into the bearing surface of a total joint replacement because significant third body wear may occur.

When used as filling to restore volume in cavities, the osteoconductive HA bonds well to bone. Bone ceramics alone do not have osteoinductive property. However, there is some suggestion that HA has sufficient affinity for local growth factors that serve in the regeneration process. Coralline HA, when placed in a muscle pouch, will demonstrate onlay bone growth. Investigators have demonstrated that ceramics can be filled with bone marrow and that bone marrow grows well within the ceramics and results in a composite. In addition, when used in animal models, mesenchymal stem cells work best in conjunction with ceramic HA. The composite of ceramics and bone marrow has not been reported in human trials to date. It can be concluded that ceramics can serve as a bone graft expander and/or filler material, particularly in compressive application. Because the ceramic is brittle and has no initial hoop strength or shear strength, the bone must be protected while the ceramic is being incorporated.

Composite Grafts Collagraft (Zimmer, Warsaw, IN, and Collagen Corporation, Palo Alto, CA) is a commercially prepared composite consisting of suspended deantigenated bovine fibrillar collagen and porous calcium phosphate ceramic of which 65% is HA and 35% is TCP. The mixture is not osteoinductive, and the addition of autogenous bone marrow provides osteoprogenitor cells and a limited amount of growth factors such as platelet-derived growth factor and TGF-β within the bone marrow clot. Calcium phosphate consists of granules having 70% porosity and a pore diameter ranging from 500 to 1,000 μm. The collagen is purified from bovine dermis and is 95% type I collagen and 5% type III collagen. A prospective randomized multicenter trial recently compared the composite graft with a cancellous iliac bone graft in acute long-bone fractures. The composite graft consisting of Collagraft plus autogenous marrow showed no significant differences in functional result or radiographic appearances when compared to autogenous bone graft. The use of the Collagraft significantly shortened the surgical time and avoided the complications and morbidity of autograft harvesting. However, the study did not include a control group treated without any grafting, and additional trials against such controls are needed, particularly in the face of markedly improved trauma instrumentation and methodology.

Collagraft is currently available only as a paste or in soft strips; therefore, it provides no structural strength. In addition, it has a tendency to flow if there is continued bleeding at the site of the fracture. Care must be taken to maintain its location until the clot has formed. Biopsies of patients with the Collagraft demonstrated slight inflammation at the site of the granules, but there were significantly fewer infections in patients treated with Collagraft as compared to patients treated with autogenous graft. This appears to be a material that can be used as a bone graft expander or a graft substitute for stabilized fractures that are protected for internal fixation but require grafting as a result of extensive comminution or segmental bone loss. It is contraindicated in intra-articular fractures because of the potential migration of granules into the joint. Caution is likewise indicated when Collagraft is used around a total joint arthroplasty, because the HA granules may result in third-body wear. If there is a contained defect, its use may be considered in the joint arthroplasty setting.

Osteoinductive Growth Factors

Growth factors have become an important area of investigation in an effort to enhance fracture healing, but there has been little application of these factors in the field of hip and knee arthroplasty. Although much of the research done with growth factors has been done in the setting of fracture healing, most of the biologic events are similar to those of bone-graft healing seen in total joint arthroplasty.

Bone healing is a complex interaction of many local and systemic regulatory factors. This interaction causes primitive undifferentiated mesenchymal cells to migrate, proliferate, and differentiate at the site of bone healing. These local mediators, along with the microenvironment, also influence genes coding for the type of matrix that the repair cells will form. As recent studies have furthered the knowledge of cellular proliferation, chondrogenesis, and osteogenesis, a number of mediators have been implicated as the predominant growth factors in fracture healing. Some of these factors include acidic and basic fibroblast growth factor, platelet-derived growth factor, TGF-β, and BMP.

The BMPs are low molecular weight glycoproteins that function as morphogens. They belong to an expanding TGF-β superfamily. The BMPs have a pleomorphic function that ranges from extracellular and skeletal organogenesis to bone generation and regeneration. BMP-induced bone in postfetal life recapitulates the process of embryonic and endochondral ossification. Through recombinant gene technology, BMP is available in large amounts for basic research and clinical trials. Recombinant human BMP (rhBMP) induces structurally sound orthotopic bone in a variety of experimental systems, including porous ingrowth in rats, femoral defects in rats, femoral defects in rabbits, femoral defects in sheep, mandibular defects and spinal fusions in dogs, and long-bone defects and spine fusions in monkeys.

Clinically, BMP has been used for the treatment of established nonunions and spine fusions. To date there have not been any reports of tumorigenesis and any untoward events. The initial clinical BMP preparation represents a mixture of BMPs, although it is highly concentrated (300,000 ×). It has resulted in a success rate of more than 93% in failed nonunions and a 100% success rate in spinal fusions to date. This product, however, is not recombinant BMP, and in addition to containing a number of different BMPs, this mixture also contains osteocalcin.

Studies with rhBMPs have been largely related to animals, although clinical trials are currently underway in the United States and Europe. The application of rhBMP-2 in adult sheep resulted in structurally intact and rigidly healed femoral defects by 12 months. Both woven and lamellar bone bridged the defect site, and, apparently, the normal sequence of ossification, modeling, and remodeling events had occurred. These reports using rhBMP-2 confirm prior reports by others that BMP-2 can heal skeletal defects in a wide range of animals. The healing of large segmental defects in primates has also been shown. Similar healing of spinal fusions in a number of animals has been demonstrated, and there now appears to be adequate evidence that both rhBMP-2 and 7 used in pharmacologic doses in various animal models are quite efficacious and superior to autogenous grafts in achieving spinal fusion.

Other growth factors have been evaluated as to their efficacy in biologic enhancement. The effect of exogenous TGF-β in a rabbit fracture model has been investigated. In this study, TGF-β was injected into the developing calluses of rat tibial fractures healing under stable or unstable mechanical conditions 4 days after fracture. The fractures were examined for 4 to 14 days after fracture. A large amount of edema developed around the injection site. The fractures healing under stable mechanical conditions consisted almost entirely of bone. The effects of 16-μg injections of TGF-β were minimal, but the 600-μg dose led to a small increase in the size of the callus. Callus fractures healing under unstable mechanical conditions had a large area of cartilage over the fracture site, with bone on each side. On unstable fractures, TGF-β retarded and reduced bone and cartilage formation in the callus. The overall size of the callus was not affected. In conclusion, it was believed that TGF-β does not stimulate fracture healing under either stable or unstable mechanical conditions during the initial healing phase. It was further argued that agents that stimulate callus proliferation may retard bone remodeling.

Currently none of the recombinant growth factors have been approved for use by the FDA, and human trials are ongoing. However, the clot associated with bone marrow and the noncollagenous mixture in demineralized bone available from the bone bank and from processed allografts do contain small amounts of biologically active factors. More comprehensive studies are warranted to demonstrate the actual efficacy of these factors in providing true augmentation to the healing process.

Conclusions About Current Biosynthetic Bone Grafting Materials

For the orthopaedic surgeon in general and the total joint surgeon in particular, a number of grafting materials are available as alternatives to autogenous bone graft for use in a wide range of clinical applications.

Ceramics are available in powders, granules, and blocks. The ceramic blocks provide compressive strength and can confer critical structural support. However, they are brittle and until they are incorporated into the existing adjacent bone they are mechanically weak when exposed to shear and tension forces. Because ceramics are exclusively osteoconductive, they are contraindicated for use by themselves. They must be combined with autograft or have access to a rich bone marrow, and as such are effective graft fillers or expanders.

DBM offers a limited source of BMP and can be used as an adjunct in the regeneration process because of its limited osteoconductive potential. DBM provides no immediate torque or compressive strength and thus would be contraindicated as the sole material when grafting large cortical segmental defects. Its clinical applications include augmentation of autogenous and allograft bone.

Bone marrow is best used as an adjunct to existing allograft or biosynthetic ceramics to provide osteoprogenitor cells to compromised grafting beds. It provides no structural strength; it is strictly an adjunct to other grafts and works well to "jump start" nonunions.

Composite grafts including ceramic, collagen, and bone

marrow have been used successfully, but again they are in a form without structure and have to be protected until they are osseointegrated. They have a role in augmenting limited autogenous bone grafting.

BMP is not currently available in highly purified or recombinant form, but the closest alternative is DBM, which is readily available from bone banks. Although rhBMP is still in clinical trials, it is anticipated that it will be easily available to orthopaedic surgeons in the near future. In the setting where the grafting site is compromised and all 3 components of osteoconduction, osteoinduction, and osteoprogenitor cells are required, autogenous graft is probably superior. However, a composite of particulate, ceramic, bone marrow, and DBM, which incorporates all 3 regenerative components, may be just as effective.

Enhancing Fixation of Implants

Achievement of optimal biologic fixation of orthopaedic implants to bone requires minimizing the initial interface gap between the bone and implant, minimizing the initial micromotion between the bone and implant, and enhancing bone growth on the prosthesis. The first 2 variables are controlled by surgical technique and implant design. Enhancement of biologic fixation requires the optimal surface on the implant.

Bone has been demonstrated to heal onto and into a variety of porous metal surfaces. Work done during the 1980s and early 1990s has demonstrated that pore sizes and surface finishes can be created so as to optimize the healing of bone onto and into the surface. Much work has been done on establishing the optimal pore size of the surface. The surface finish also contributes to the initial fixation of the implant, with the rougher, higher-friction surfaces clearly creating a better initial fixation than smoother surfaces. It is now clear that some metals, such as titanium, are more likely to have bone grow on the surface than others. Yet despite significant advances in the development of metal surfaces of noncemented implants, the reported incidences of bone ingrowth from autopsy retrieval series remains low, and improvement of the long-term fixation of the implant requires the use of biologically active coatings.

Osteoconductive Coatings

Although during the late 1980s there was increasing experimental evidence that treatment of implants with osteoconductive coatings such as HA or HA/TCP by plasma flame spraying enhanced bone ingrowth, only recently have there been any clinical data to support the use of these surfaces. The data to support their use on the femoral components of total hip arthroplasties and the tibial component of total knee arthroplasties is currently the most compelling. However, the evidence to support their use on acetabular components is weak.

Osteoconductive Coatings on Total Hip Replacements There have been several clinical reports of the use of HA-coated femoral components. In 2 series of both older and young patients using a proximally coated femoral component, it has recently been reported that there was an extremely low failure rate resulting from mechanical and aseptic failure at a minimum of 5 years' follow-up. Although the authors do not directly analyze the results of their acetabular components, a 15% revision rate of the acetabular components, with most of the implanted cups being HA coated, indicates that the HA-coated acetabular components are not performing as well as the femoral stems. The results using a different HA-coated femoral component in young patients have also been reported, with encouraging results at early follow-up of around 5 years. Once again, the results of the acetabular components were not as good.

In both of these designs, there were radiographic signs of bone ingrowth and of remodeling of the bone around the implant. At this relatively early time, intramedullary osteolysis remained rare. It has been argued by proponents of HA coatings that the cirumferential coating provides a protective barrier for intrusion of articular wear debris into the bone-implant interface, and there are canine data to support these claims.

Osteoconductive Coatings on Total Knee Replacements A number of studies support the use of HA coatings on the tibial component of total knee arthroplasties. Recently, it was reported that radiostereometric analysis techniques indicated a significantly greater amount of migration of porous-coated tibial components compared to HA-coated components. In this well-controlled, single-blind randomized series there was no difference in migration between HA-coated implants and cemented tibial implants. In a less accurate study of HA-coated versus grit-blasted titanium noncemented implants, there were fewer radiolucencies at the bone-implant interface under the HA-coated implants than under the grit-blasted implants. Based on these studies, many believe that a cementless HA-coated implant should be considered for young, more active patients.

What precisely happens to HA coating on the implants over time remains controversial, with some experimental evidence suggesting that its resorption depends on the loading environment. Others argue that debonding of the ceramic from the metal may prove to be a significant weakness of these coatings and may result in particulate debris. Although the use of these particular coatings may enhance bone ingrowth, third-body wear due to HA particles may cause accelerated wear of the bearing surface. The presence of HA in the bearing surfaces of total hip replacements has been reported, as has a case of severe osteolysis caused by third-body wear in an implant with HA coating. The extent to which this third-body wear issue will become a clinical problem is unknown.

Osteoinductive Coatings

Although in most clinical situations the use of standard porous coating is sufficient to achieve stable biologic fixation of implants, there continue to be clinical situations in which fixation of cementless prosthetic components is compromised. These include osteoporosis, situations with micromotion in which gaps exist between the bone and the implant, and during revision of failed prostheses. There are clinical data on the use of osteoconductive coatings, but to date there have been no published clinical series using osteoinductive coatings on total joint implants. However, compelling preclinical data support the use of several of these agents as enhancers of biologic fixation of total joint implants.

In 1994, TGF-β1 was used to enhance the fixation of bone to an unloaded metal mesh implant. In this model, fibrous metal implants were inserted in the cancellous bone beds of canine humeri. The implant was designed so there was a 3-mm gap between the metal and the surrounding bone. Using 2 different doses of TGF-β, this group was able to demonstrate both histologically and biomechanically enhanced bone ongrowth, on the implants when they were coated with TGF-β. This bone ongrowth was dose-dependent, with a lower dose causing a stronger bond than the higher dose coatings. One of the shortcomings of this study was that these implants were unloaded and rigidly fixed.

A subsequent series of canine studies by another group addressed this deficiency. They demonstrated that TGF-β enhanced the ongrowth of bone on both unloaded and loaded TCP-coated implants. In this series, TGF-β was absorbed onto TCP-coated titanium alloy implants. The implants were then inserted in the medial and lateral femoral condyles of canine knees. In the initial experiments on unloaded implants, there was a dose-related enhancement of histologically determined bone ongrowth, with the higher dose (3.0 μg/implant) coating demonstrating a threefold increase in bone ongrowth. Mechanical testing showed a threefold increase in fixation in the intermediate-dose group (0.3 μg/implant). This increase in fixation, however, was not as dramatic in implants that were loaded initially. Although there was a 59% increase in bone-implant contact, mechanical push-out tests failed to show a difference between TGFβ-coated implants and untreated ceramic-coated implants.

In addition to coating implants with TGF-β, other investigators have been using BMPs in an attempt to stimulate bone healing. A rat model was used to demonstrate that bone ongrowth could be enhanced by coating porous-coated titanium implants with rhBMP-2. This effect appeared to be dose related. However, no mechanical testing was performed. These investigators subsequently have demonstrated enhanced bone ongrowth in an unloaded implant in a rabbit model. Although histologic analyses demonstrated enhanced ongrowth based on histomorphometric analyses, no improvement in mechanical push-out testing could be demonstrated.

In addition to promoting bone growth in gaps between the implant and native bone, osteoinductive factors may be of significant value in improving bony fixation of implants with marginal initial bony stability. In such a setting, the bone-implant interface is subjected to micromotion. Using a unique rabbit model in which fibrous tissue is formed as a result of tissue deformation, it was demonstrated that rhBMP-2 could form bone in the setting of this tissue deformation-micromotion.

Thus, implants coated either with osteoinductive coatings alone or with a combination of osteoinductive and osteoconductive coatings can enhance bone ongrowth based on histomorphometric parameters. Furthermore, it appears that bone healing can be enhanced in the setting of micromotion through the use of BMPs. Whether these osteoinductive agents enhance mechanical stability has not yet been demonstrated, and, more importantly, whether these coatings will be of clinical utility remains to be determined.

Annotated Bibliography

Bone Graft Substitutes

Bruder SP, Kraus KH, Goldberg VM, Kadiyala S: The effect of implants loaded with autogenous mesenchymal stem cells on the healing of canine segmental bone defects. *J Bone Joint Surg* 1998;80A:985–996.

When compared to an osteoconductive carrier, the use of mesenchymal stem cells significantly enhanced healing of a critical-sized long bone defect. There was a substantially higher union rate of the native bone to the carrier in the implants loaded with the mesenchymal stem cells. The importance of osteogenic stem cells in the development of bone graft substitutes was stressed.

Constantz BR, Ison IC, Fulmer MT, et al: Skeletal repair by in situ formation of the mineral phase of bone. *Science* 1995;267: 1796–1799.

The development of a process for the in situ formation of the mineral phase of bone was described. Inorganic calcium and phosphate sources were combined to form a paste that is surgically implanted by injection. Under physiologic conditions, the material hardened in minutes with an ultimate compressive strength of 55 mPa. The composition and crystal morphology of the material formed were similar to those of bone. A novel approach to skeletal repair is being tested in human trials for various applications; in one of the trials the new biomaterial is being percutaneously placed into acute fractures.

Cook SD, Baffes GC, Wolfe MW, Sampath TK, Rueger DC, Whitecloud TS III: The effect of recombinant human osteogenic protein-1 on healing of large segmental bone defects. *J Bone Joint Surg* 1994;76A:827–838.

A rabbit segmental model was used to demonstrate the effect of recombinant human bone morphogenetic protein 7 (BMP-7) in enhancing healing. Osseous union was achieved in all but the lowest dose groups treated with BMP-7. Biomechanically the new bone formed had strengths comparable to intact bones. Histologically the bone appeared to be remodeling normally. This and other studies emphasize the important role osteogenic growth factors play in bone graft substitutes.

Enhancement of Biologic Fixation

Bostrom MP, Aspenberg P, Jeppsson C, Salvati EA: Enhancement of bone formation in the setting of repeated tissue deformation. *Clin Orthop* 1998;350:221–228.

In a setting of tissue deformation that otherwise favors the formation of fibrous tissue bone morphogenetic protein-2 significantly augmented bone formation. Thus, osteogenic growth factors may be of value in the future to enhance bony stabilization of orthopaedic implants.

Capello WN, D'Antonio JA, Feinberg JR, Manley MT: Hydroxyapatite-coated total hip femoral components in patients less than fifty years old: Clinical and radiographic results after five to eight years of follow-up. *J Bone Joint Surg* 1997;79A: 1023–1029.

Use of hydroxyapatite-coated total hip femoral components in 152 hips demonstrated no aseptic or mechanical failure at a minimum of 5 years of follow-up. Four stems (2.6%) were revised because of pain. Serial radiographs revealed mechanically stable implants with osseous ingrowth and minimal endosteal osteolysis.

Cole BJ, Bostrom MP, Pritchard TL, et al: Use of bone morphogenetic protein 2 on ectopic porous coated implants in the rat. *Clin Orthop* 1997;345:219–228.

Bone morphogenetic protein-2 demonstrated appositional bone formation on porous coated implants in an ectopic nonweightbearing in vivo assay.

Lind M, Overgaard S, Nguyen T, Ongpipattanakul B, Bunger C, Soballe K: Transforming growth factor-beta stimulates bone ongrowth: Hydroxyapatite-coated implants studied in dogs. *Acta Orthop Scand* 1996;67:611–616.

Use of transforming growth factor-beta on ceramic-coated implants demonstrated significantly increased bone ongrowth compared to untreated implants. Mechanical pushout tests, however, failed to demonstrate a difference between groups.

Loupasis G, Hyde ID, Morris EW: The Furlong hydroxyapatite-coated femoral prosthesis: A 4- to 7-year follow-up study. *Arch Orthop Trauma Surg* 1998;117:132–135.

Forty-five Furlong hydroxyapatite-coated total hip replacements showed no aseptic loosening of the stems but 2 acetabular failures at an average of 71 months follow-up.

Onsten I, Nordqvist A, Carlsson AS, Besjakov J, Shotts S: Hydroxyapatite augmentation of the porous coating improves fixation of tibial components: A randomized RSA study in 116 patients. *J Bone Joint Surg* 1998;80B:417–425.

At 2 years, fixation of tibial components of total knee arthroplasties was enhanced by use of hydroxyapatite-coated implants as demonstrated by radiostereometric analysis. Fixation of the hydroxyapatite-coated implants was comparable to cemented implants. Porous coated implants demonstrated significantly higher migration rates than cemented or hydroxyapatite-coated implants.

Sumner DR, Turner TM, Purchio AF, Gombotz WR, Urban RM, Galante JO: Enhancement of bone ingrowth by transforming growth factor-beta. *J Bone Joint Surg* 1995;77A:1135–1147.

In an unloaded canine model, porous implants coated with transforming growth factor-beta showed a threefold increased amount of bone ingrowth than untreated implants. Higher doses did not enhance bone ingrowth.

Classic Bibliography

Bucholz RW, Carlton A, Holmes R: Interporous hydroxyapatite as a bone graft substitute in tibial plateau fractures. *Clin Orthop* 1989;240:53–62.

Cornell CN, Lane JM, Chapman M, et al: Multicenter trial of Collagraft as bone graft substitute. *J Orthop Trauma* 1991; 5:1–8.

Johnson EE, Urist MR, Finerman GA: Bone morphogenetic protein augmentation grafting of resistant femoral nonunions: A preliminary report. *Clin Orthop* 1988;230:257–265.

Peltier LF: The use of plaster of Paris to fill defects in bone. *Clin Orthop* 1961;21:1–31.

Urist MR: Bone: Formation by autoinduction. *Science 1965*; 150:893–899.

Wozney JM, Rosen V, Celeste AJ, et al: Novel regulators of bone formation: Molecular clones and activities. *Science 1988*;242: 1528–1534.

Chapter 7
Perioperative Medical Management and Blood Transfusion Medicine

Introduction

Medical management of total joint arthroplasty (TJA) patients has been quite successful, despite common complicating medical conditions. Intraoperative mortality is almost nonexistent, and perioperative mortality is extremely low, even for patients older than 85 years. The standard of care in TJA results in minimal complications and expeditious discharge to home for most patients. Decisions in perioperative management must be made with the surgeon's thorough understanding of the risks, benefits, and costs involved. Perioperative and postoperative complications are minimized with careful preoperative evaluation, diligent perioperative management, and rational blood conservation strategy.

Preoperative Evaluation/ Perioperative Medical Management

Performing an adequate preoperative evaluation and choosing the proper consultations preoperatively are critical to the success of the operation. The American Society of Anesthesiology has used the Dripps' stratification system to assess perioperative mortality (Table 1). A complete history and physical examination is the most important component of preoperative assessment. Signs of cardiovascular, thromboembolic, cerebrovascular, pulmonary, and urologic disease are significant indicators of risk for increased intraoperative and postoperative morbidity and/or mortality. In addition, conditions such as diabetes mellitus, rheumatoid arthritis, corticosteroid dependence, obesity, and hematologic or endocrine disease should be thoroughly evaluated and treated before, during, and after surgery to ensure success. Selected laboratory and radiographic tests and clinical care pathways are also instrumental in providing optimal perioperative care.

Cardiovascular Disease

Significant cardiovascular disease can predispose patients to perioperative myocardial infarction (MI) or sudden cardiac death. The American College of Cardiology and the American Heart Association Task Force on Perioperative Cardiovascular Evaluation in 1996 compiled a list of predictors helpful in determining cardiovascular risk (Outline 1). The American College of Cardiology now recommends a wait of at least 4 to 6 weeks after MI to perform elective surgery, in contrast to the 6-month waiting period accepted previously. Perioperative MI often presents with arrhythmia, confusion, hypotension, or congestive heart failure. Only 50% of patients exhibit typical chest pain.

Well-controlled stable angina is a relatively minor risk factor for total joint replacement. Unstable angina, however, must be evaluated and treated aggressively. Severe left ventricular dysfunction entails an increased risk for perioperative cardiac failure and death if the ejection fraction is 25% or less. Patients with severe failure should have their cardiac function optimized preoperatively and should be monitored

Table 1
Preoperative assessment classification

ASA status	Examples of preoperative patients
Class 1: No disease	Healthy 25-year-old
Class 2: Mild to moderate systemic disease	65-year-old with well-controlled DM type 2
Class 3: Severe systemic disease	70-year-old with CHF and rest angina
Class 4: Life-threatening systemic disease	30-year-old with DM type 1 in ketoacidosis
Class 5: Morbidly ill	70-year-old with angina and mesenteric ischemia

E is added to each class if surgery is an emergency

ASA, American Society of Anesthesiology; DM, diabetes mellitus; CHF, congestive heart failure. (Reproduced with permission from Fiorillo AB, Solaro FX Jr: Preoperative medical evaluation, in Callaghan JJ (ed): The Adult Hip. Philadelphia, PA, Lippincott-Raven, 1998, pp 601–632; and from Dripps RD: New classification of physical status. *Anesthesiology* 1963;24:111.)

Outline 1

Clinical predictors of increased perioperative cardiovascular risk (myocardial infarction, congestive heart failure, death)

Major

Unstable coronary syndromes
- Recent myocardial infarction* with evidence of important ischemic risk by clinical symptoms or noninvasive study
- Unstable or severe† angina (Canadian class III or IV)‡

Decompensated congestive heart failure

Significant arrhythmias
- High-grade atrioventricular block
- Symptomatic ventricular arrhythmias in the presence of underlying heart disease
- Supraventricular arrhythmias with uncontrolled ventricular rate

Severe valvular disease

Intermediate

Mild angina pectoris (Canadian class I or II)

Prior myocardial infarction by history or pathologic Q waves

Compensated or prior congestive heart failure

Diabetes mellitus

Minor

Advanced age

Abnormal EKG (left ventricular hypertrophy, left bundle branchblock, ST-T abnormalities)

Rhythm other than sinus (eg, atrial fibrillation)

Low functional capacity (eg, inability to climb 1 flight of stairs with a bag of groceries)

History of stroke

Uncontrolled systemic hypertension

EKG indicates electrocardiogram
*The American College of Cardiology National Database Library defines recent myocardial infarction as greater than 7 days but less than or equal to 1 month
†May include "stable" angina in patients who are unusually sedentary
‡Campeau L: Grading of angina pectoris. *Circulation* 1976;54:522–523
(Reproduced with permission from Eagle KA: Guidelines for perioperative cardiovascular evaluation for noncardiac surgery. *J Am Coll Cardiol* 1996;27:910–948.)

perioperatively with a Swan-Ganz catheter and arterial lines. Valvular dysfunction, especially aortic and mitral stenosis, can cause significant perioperative morbidity and/or mortality. Patients with mechanical valves should discontinue warfarin therapy 3 to 5 days before surgery. Intravenous heparin is then administered for anticoagulation, and is discontinued 4 to 6 hours before surgery. Heparin and/or warfarin administration is resumed within 24 hours postoperatively. Patients on warfarin therapy for atrial fibrillation should also discontinue its use for 3 to 5 days before surgery, and resume anticoagulation the evening of the operation.

Patients with hypertension controlled by medication should take their regular dose of medication perioperatively, either orally or intravenously. Patients on diuretics should have a serum potassium level obtained preoperatively to assess potential hypokalemia, which must be corrected before surgery. Uncontrolled hypertension with diastolic pressure above 110 mm Hg or systolic pressure above 200 mm Hg should delay surgery until corrected. Morbidity and mortality in these patients occur as a result of wide swings in blood pressure occurring at induction of anesthesia, in the immediate postoperative period, and between postoperative days 3 and 5 when third space fluids are mobilized.

History and physical findings of significant peripheral vascular disease should alert the physician to the potential for cardiovascular disease and compromised wound healing. Patients predisposed to deep vein thrombosis (DVT) or pulmonary embolism have an increased likelihood of occurrence after TJA, and should be anticoagulated in standard fashion. Suspicion of DVT in this group of patients may warrant studies to evaluate the deep venous system.

Cerebrovascular Disease

Previous cerebrovascular accident (CVA) or neurologic compromise can be temporarily or permanently exacerbated as a result of an operation or general anesthetic. It is important to fully document neurologic status preoperatively. Residual paresis and/or spasticity after CVA can lead to decreased function and/or increased dislocation rates after total hip replacement. Recent history of transient ischemic attack (TIA) should prompt thorough investigation, because most associated cerebrovascular accidents occur within 1 year of TIA. Auscultation for carotid bruit is an important aspect of the initial physical examination. Patients with symptomatic or hemodynamically significant (> 75%) carotid stenosis as determined by carotid Doppler studies should have carotid endarterectomy performed well in advance of TJA. If carotid stenosis is less than 70%, TJA may prudently be performed 4 to 6 weeks after TIA.

Pulmonary Disease

The presence of significant restrictive or obstructive pulmonary disease can lead to perioperative respiratory failure and inability to be weaned from the ventilator after general anesthesia. Lung function in patients with restrictive lung disease is better than in patients with obstructive disease, because respiratory drive is preserved in the former. Patients with restrictive lung disease secondary to significant obesity or skeletal/neuromuscular disorder, however, are at risk for pulmonary complication. Patients with smoking history, chronic obstructive pulmonary disease (COPD), and asthma must have their lung function optimized before TJA. COPD patients should refrain from smoking several weeks in advance of surgery. COPD and asthmatic patients' perioperative pulmonary function should be medically optimized with bronchodilators (theophylline, beta-agonists, anticholinergic inhalers) and inhaled corticosteroids on a continuous basis. Arterial blood gas should be determined when significant pulmonary disease is suspected, because a P_{CO_2} greater than 45 mm is a predictor of increased perioperative pulmonary morbidity. Epidural or spinal anesthesia is preferred for patients with significant pulmonary disease, as intubation and mechanical ventilation are avoided. Respiratory therapy should be added to the standard pulmonary regimen of incentive spirometry, coughing, deep breathing exercises, and early ambulation used in all patients.

Diabetes Mellitus, Uropathy

Patients with diabetes mellitus should be evaluated for quality of blood sugar control and presence of associated conditions. Perioperatively, blood sugar levels should be kept below 240 mg/dl to prevent glycosuria, dehydration, and hyperglycemia-induced impairment of phagocytosis and wound healing. A postoperative sliding scale of subcutaneous regular insulin can be used to maintain blood glucose levels between 100 and 240 mg/dl until the patient is eating regularly. Blood glucose can then be stabilized with the patient's normal insulin/oral hypoglycemic schedule. Moderate hyperglycemia is tolerated well, but hypoglycemia should be avoided. Blood glucose levels should be checked preoperatively and every 4 to 6 hours perioperatively. Most oral agents should be held the day of surgery, but chlorpropamide is longer acting and should be held the day before surgery.

Diabetes-associated cardiovascular, gastrointestinal, and renal involvement should be assessed carefully preoperatively and treated aggressively perioperatively. Auscultation of vascular bruits should prompt evaluation by a specialist. Autonomic neuropathy with perioperative gastroparesis is common and is well treated with 10 to 30 mg of metaclopramide given intravenously every 6 to 8 hours. Studies have shown that if cephalosporin prophylaxis and clean air laminar flow rooms are used, there is not increased deep wound or prosthetic infections after TJA in patients with diabetes. Less problematic infectious complications such as superficial wound or urinary tract infections do occur more often in patients with diabetes and must be diagnosed and treated appropriately. Urinary tract infections identified preoperatively are treated with oral antibiotics. Before TJA is performed, success of therapy must be confirmed by a repeat urinalysis and culture that is negative for infection. A history or presence of chronic urinary tract infections or obstructive uropathy can lead to high rates of prosthesis infection, and these problems must be adequately resolved before the operation is undertaken.

Rheumatoid Arthritis

Patients with rheumatoid arthritis (RA) often suffer from anemia of chronic disease. Augmentation of their red cell indices with erythropoietin should be considered, for reasons that will be discussed later.

Heart murmurs should prompt antibiotic prophylaxis. Patients on significant chronic hydrocortisone treatment (> 7.5 mg prednisone equivalent per day) for any diagnosis should be given a stress dose of glucocorticoid preoperatively. One appropriate dosing schedule uses hydrocortisone 100 mg given intravenously one half to 1 hour before surgery, followed by 2 more 100-mg doses 8 hours apart.

Patients with RA should also be carefully evaluated for cervical spine subluxation, which is characterized by pain at the C1 and C2 nerve root levels. Radiographically, C1-2 subluxation is characterized by atlantoaxial translation on flexion or extension views of the cervical spine. If atlantoaxial subluxation is diagnosed, special precautions are taken during intubation to avoid spinal cord injury.

Obesity

TJA patients often exhibit varying degrees of obesity. Morbid obesity is empirically associated with complications, such as increased pulmonary dysfunction, atelectasis, wound dehiscence, and infection, although these associations have not been well proven scientifically. A recent retrospective review of 190 total hip replacement patients comparing nonobese, obese, and morbidly obese patients found no difference in the incidence of perioperative and postoperative complications at an average follow-up of 48 months. Another review, comparing 50 morbidly obese primary total knee patients to 1,539 patients who were not, found a significantly increased incidence of wound complications and avulsed medial collateral ligament. At a mean follow up of 5 years, knee functional scores were significantly lower in morbidly obese primary total knee patients than in nonobese patients. Cardiovascular disease, sleep apnea, and decreased pulmonary reserve are common in morbidly obese patients and should be assessed thoroughly.

Hematologic or Endocrine Disease

Anemias, coagulopathies, and blood dyscrasias should be identified preoperatively and treated. Patients with anemia of chronic disease, hemophilia, and sickle cell disease should be given special attention. Administration of erythropoietin is recommended for patients with anemia of chronic disease who exhibit a hemoglobin (Hgb) concentration between 10 and 13 g/dl (hematocrit [Hct] between 30% and 39%). Severe anemia as characterized by an Hgb concentration less than 10 g/dl (Hct < 30%) usually does not respond as well to erythropoietin secondary to the severity of underlying hematologic disease. For all patients, aspirin and nonsteroidal anti-inflammatory medications should be discontinued for a full week before surgery to ensure optimum platelet function.

In hemophiliacs, levels of factors VIII or IX should be determined and, if deficient, supplemented with intravenous factor. White cell CD4 counts are depressed in hemophiliacs with acquired immunodeficiency syndrome. If counts are less than 200×10^9 cells per liter, surgery should be postponed to avoid postoperative infection. Patients with sickle cell disease exhibit high intraoperative blood loss and infection rates. In these patients, epidural or spinal anesthesia is preferred, and strict attention should be paid to adequate hydration, prophylactic antibiotics, and thromboembolic prophylaxis.

Before TJA is performed, signs and symptoms of endocrine disease should be identified, including exophthalmos, hyperreflexia, delayed reflexes, cushingoid facies, striae, buffalo hump, and excess skin pigmentation, which should provoke a thorough endocrine evaluation.

Laboratory Tests/Radiography

Baseline laboratory tests include anteroposterior and lateral chest radiographs, an electrocardiogram (EKG), and a complete blood count to assess preoperative red cell and platelet indices. A microscopic urinalysis with culture is also obtained

Patient:__________ **Date Admitted:**__________ **Expected Length of Stay:**__________ **Diagnosis:**__________

Identification #__________ **Date Pathway Begun:**__________ **Actual Length of Stay:**__________ **Procedure:**__________

Days/Dates	Pre-Op	Day of TJA	POD #1	POD #2	POD #3	POD #4	Discharge Day	Post operative check 6 weeks
Consults Evaluation	History and Physical Physical Therapy (RT) Occupational Therapy (OT) Blood Conservation Discussion Anesthesia Internal Medicine (if needed)	-	Occupational and Physical Therapy	Rehabilitation unit evaluation	-	-	-	-
Diagnostic Studies	Routine: CBC, UA with Micro, C&S XR: Chest, Hip and Pelvis EKG PRN's: ESR, CRP, Hip aspiration Type and Cross	Hgb/hct in recovery Hip XR in recovery	Protime Hgb/hct	Protime Hgb/hct	Protime	Protime	Protimes 1-2 times per week per Home Health Agency, Rehab unit as ordered	XR's: AP Pelvis & Lateral hip
Activity	As Tolerated	Bedrest Reposition every 2 hours	Up to chair BID Ambulate with assistive device per PT Instruct for exercises	OT: functional transfers Reinforce ADL equipment usage Progress exercises	OT: Provide ADL equipment prn Progress ambulation with assistive device per PT	Transfer with minimal assist Continue ambulation increasing distance	Ambulate with assistive device minimal assistance Transfers independent	Ambulate with assistive device independently
Treatments	Hibiclens scrub to leg evening before and morning of surgery	Overhead frame with trapeze Eggcrate mattress, thigh high Thigh high TED hose bilaterally (remove every 4 hr/inspect skin) Hemovac, Foley, I&O's q8hrs. Incentive spirometer q2hrs Vital Signs/Neurovasc q4hrs Abductor pillow Pulse oximetry Inspect hip dressing, skin	same	Discontinue hemovac Straight cath prn Vitals/Neuro checks to q8 hrs DC epidural per anesthesia Change hip dressing	Discontinue I&O's Change dressing prn		Dressing change Assess incision Continue TED hose	DC TED hose Assess wound healing
Diet	NPO after midnight	Clear liquids, advance as tolerated	Regular or Pre-hospital	same	same	same	same	same
Medications	Iron supplementation if participating in PAD, erythropoietin	IV Fluids, Ancef IV q8hrsX3 doses Coumadin10mg po Analgesia, anti-emetic, epidural per Anesthesia Routine and home medications No NSAIDS / ASA	Heplock IV Coumadin as written daily	IV heplock if not done Oral pain meds, anti-emetics per Ortho Coumadin as written	DC heplock Adjust coumadin	Coumadin as written	Anticoagulation therapy followed by Ortho clinic Oral pain meds	Discontinue Coumadin Primary hip: 3 weeks Revision hip: 6 weeks
Patient Education	Purpose and preparation for total hip Arthroplasty, Blood conservation Booklets and handouts	Orientation to nursing unit Pain management Total hip precautions	Coumadin teaching	Reinforce: coumadin teaching, pain mgmt hip precautions ADL equipment usage	Meds Home care/rehab unit arrangement Wound care	Reinforce: wound care Coumadin teaching Discharge instructions		
Discharge Planning	Assess and identify home care needs Identify home care agency			Discuss discharge needs with patient and family	Review discharge plans with patient/family Notify rehab unit of pending discharge	Discharge home/rehab unit. Notify community agency, Ortho clinic of post hospital arrange. anticoagulation treatment	Discharge to home from rehab facility	

Figure 1

Clinical care pathway for total hip replacement. (Developed by Kerby Selmer, RN, MS, ONC; Mary Peterson, RNC, MS; Mary Kay Gamble, RN, MC, and Kevin Garvin, MD.)

preoperatively because occult urinary tract infections are quite common, especially in elderly patients. Obtaining a prothrombin, partial thromboplastin, and/or bleeding time is necessary only if the patient has a history of easy bruising or bleeding. Other laboratory tests are ordered to assess specific diseases identified in the preoperative evaluation. Appropriate consultation of medical and surgical specialty services should be obtained preoperatively for further evaluation and optimization of the complicated patient's condition before and after TJA.

Clinical Care Pathways

For complicated and healthy patients alike, the use of a standard protocol for perioperative management improves quality and efficiency of care. Clinical care pathways have been developed to fulfill this need. These pathways are organized according to the day in reference to the date of surgery (preoperative, day of surgery, postoperative day 1, 2, etc) and the type of evaluation or order performed (consults, diagnostic studies, activity, treatments, diet, medications, patient education, and discharge planning). The use of clinical care pathways provides substantial uniformity of care, decreased lengths of stay, decreased total costs, and opportunity for systematic follow-up of results for TJA patients. An example for total hip replacement is demonstrated in Figure 1.

Blood Loss and Replacement in Total Joint Arthroplasty

TJA often entails significant blood loss, making the patient's potential to require transfusion an important component of the preoperative evaluation. To avoid intraoperative or postoperative complications, red cell indices must be maintained at acceptable levels to ensure adequate oxygenation of the heart, brain, and peripheral tissues.

Total blood loss represents both intraoperative estimated blood loss and postoperative wound drainage. Its magnitude depends on the joint replaced (knee or hip), and the type of procedure (primary, bilateral, or revision operation). In a retrospective review of almost 500 TJA patients from 1995 to 1997, estimated blood loss, postoperative drain outputs, autologous donation participation, and transfusion requirements (Table 2) were calculated. These figures are comparable to recent reports in the literature. Blood loss was least with primary total knee replacement, greater in revision knee and primary total hip replacement, and greatest with revision hip and 1-stage bilateral knee replacement. Intraoperative estimated blood loss was greatest in total hip revision, but postoperative drain output was greatest in bilateral total knee replacement. However, the accuracy of estimated surgical blood loss and postoperative drain output in reflecting total perioperative red cell loss is questionable. Intraoperative red blood cell loss estimates are unreliable secondary to inaccuracy of estimated blood volume loss, intercompartmental shifts, the dilutional effect of administered crystalloid fluids, and intraoperative irrigation. Postoperatively, red blood cell losses are overestimated, because most postoperative wound drainage is serosanguinous effusion rather than overt bleeding. Investigations have therefore shown wide ranges in total blood loss. The effect of cement has also varied from study to study, causing a decrease in average total blood loss of 0 to 200 cc.

Calculations of red blood cell loss from postoperative measurement of red cell indices are probably more accurate. There is empiric and scientific evidence that relatively consistent postoperative decreases in Hgb can be expected depending on the type of operation. In a recent study of 299 patients,

Table 2
Blood loss, preoperative autologous donation participation and transfusion rates in total joint arthroplasty patients

Operation Type	Number of Patients	Estimated Blood Loss (cc) Standard Deviation	Postoperative Drain Output (cc) Standard Deviation	Autologous Blood Donation Rate (percent of patients)	Percent of Patients Transfused
Primary total knee	157	185 106	491 103	46%	23%
Revision total knee	32	310 308	407 312	44%	47%
Bilateral total knee	29	340 211	718 406	72%	72%
Primary total hip	167	522 377	388 245	61%	35%
Revision total hip	104	827 538	391 308	52%	60%

Hgb losses as a result of primary and revision total hip arthroplasty were calculated to be 3.7 ± 1.7 g/dl and 4.8 ± 2.4 g/dl, respectively. These consistent losses coupled with knowledge of the patient's preoperative red blood cell index values can greatly assist the surgeon in recommending a particular red blood cell conservation strategy. For example, patients undergoing primary TJA with a preoperative Hgb level of 15 g/dl or greater rarely require transfusion, because perioperative blood loss usually is not great enough to cause transfusion-requiring anemia.

Total blood loss in joint replacement surgery has decreased significantly in the 1990s due to improved surgical technique. Specific techniques include use of tourniquets (for total knee arthroplasty), gentle tissue handling, anatomic dissection, and minimization of blood loss with use of electrocautery and epinephrine-soaked sponges. The elimination of postoperative wound drains has also been attempted, with less significant effect in decreasing blood loss and transfusion rates. Eliminating postoperative drains does not seem to cause decreased range of motion or increased superficial or deep infection rates, and does not affect long-term results after TJA. Some still believe that elimination of surgical drains results in a significant increase in wound hematoma, ecchymosis, and drainage, making drain placement after TJA a matter of surgeon preference. Drains should be discontinued by postoperative day 2, because bacterial colonization becomes significant within 48 hours postoperatively.

In the past, higher intraoperative and postoperative blood losses and less stringent transfusion indications made perioperative blood transfusion necessary in a large proportion of TJA patients. In response to significant viral contamination of the allogeneic blood supply, the standard of care for TJA patients is to minimize allogeneic transfusion. This has been accomplished by using various blood conservation techniques, predominantly the donation of autologous blood. As the requirements for blood transfusion after TJA have decreased, the safety of the allogeneic blood supply has improved markedly and significant risks of autologous donation have been elucidated. For TJA at the turn of the 20th century, hematologic management necessitates that the surgeon understand the physiology of anemia, proper indications for transfusion, and the benefits and risks of allogeneic blood, autologous donation, and other strategies used to avoid allogeneic transfusion. Only through this knowledge can the perioperative complications and cost of allogeneic transfusion and its alternative strategies be minimized.

Physiology of Anemia

Significant blood loss during and after TJA often creates acute hypovolemia and decreased blood oxygen-carrying capacity. At the time of surgery, blood loss, urine output, and insensible losses can cause significant hypovolemia. Physiologic signs and symptoms, usually a response to hypovolemia alone, are often erroneously attributed to surgicaly induced acute anemia. In response to hypovolemia, stimulation of the adrenergic nervous system and a release of vasoactive hormones cause peripheral vasoconstriction and increased venous return to the heart. This results in increased cardiac output via increased stroke volume and/or heart rate. In addition, resorption of fluids from the interstitial/intracellular compartments and renal conservation of fluids and electrolytes increase intravascular volume. Peripheral vasoconstriction leads to metabolic acid accumulation and resultant hyperventilation, which also results in increased cardiac output via increased negative intrathoracic pressure. As a result, increased heart and respiratory rate occur in an attempt to increase intravascular volume. These signs are often misconstrued as signs of insufficient oxygen-carrying capacity.

Healthy patients can tolerate blood losses of up to 35% of their estimated blood volume without requiring transfusion if kept normovolemic with adequate fluid replenishment. In addition, moderate normovolemic anemia has not been shown to adversely affect wound healing or length of hospital stay in TJA patients. Correction of hypovolemia by administration of crystalloid fluids alone is adequate for most healthy patients with an Hgb > 7 g/dl (Hct > 21%). However, patients with significant systemic illness (cardiopulmonary, peripheral vascular, and cerebrovascular disease) have a decreased ability to adequately compensate for hypovolemia/anemia-induced oxygen deficit. This increases the risk of perioperative myocardial ischemia, angina, claudication, TIAs, and seizures in these patients, requiring more liberal transfusion indications.

Transfusion Indications

Better understanding of the physiologic response to hypovolemia and anemia has led to significantly better defined transfusion indications in the perioperative period. The clinical practice of keeping a patient's Hgb level > 10 g/dl and Hct > 30% with transfusion, regardless of the patient's clinical condition, was first introduced in the early 1940s. This so-called "10/30 rule" was the standard of practice until the late 1980s. In 1988 the National Institutes of Health Consensus Conference on Perioperative Red Blood Cell Transfusion significantly changed this philosophy. There is no evidence that mild-to-moderate anemia contributes to perioperative morbidity. No single measure can replace good clinical judgment as the basis for decision making regarding perioperative transfusion. Despite this landmark change, there has been a marked heterogeneity between hospitals and individual physicians in regard to the proportion of TJA patients given transfusions, secondary to the lack of clearly defined transfusion criteria practiced for autologous and allogeneic blood.

Transfusion should be based on the patient's risks of developing complications of inadequate oxygenation. Intraoperative transfusion for an Hgb < 7 g/dl (Hct < 18%) is almost always indicated, but transfusion for an Hgb > 10 g/dL (Hct > 30%) is rarely necessary. Patients who have an Hgb between 7 and 10 g/dl and are demonstrating myocardial ischemia electrocardiographically, have unexplained tachycardia, have hypotension unresponsive to intravenous fluids or have a significant history of cardiovascular disease should undergo transfusion to prevent MI.

Postoperatively, the indications for transfusion should also be clinically based. Patients can tolerate surprisingly low red blood cell indices, as evidenced by low mortality after TJA for Jehovah's Witnesses, who for religious reasons refuse transfusions. Transfusion strategy not only should minimize mortality, but also should result in optimization of red cell indices so that morbidity associated with inadequate tissue oxygenation is minimized. Postoperatively, an Hgb of ≤ 7 g/dl ≤ (Hct < 18%) should prompt transfusion. Hypovolemia and anemia-induced shortness of breath, fatigue, malaise, and orthostatic hypotension can interfere significantly with the patient's mobility and activity. Therefore, prudent transfusion is indicated for TJA patients if they demonstrate these signs (in addition to anemic red cell indices) and are refractory to treatment with intravenous fluids. Patients with significant cardiovascular, pulmonary, and cerebrovascular disease must be observed vigilantly for signs and symptoms of decreased oxygenation and should be treated aggressively with prudent fluid and red blood cell administration. With these indications, patients actively participate in physical therapy and can be discharged home expeditiously with safe hemodynamic reserve.

Discarding liberal red blood cell index triggers and focusing on treating hypovolemia first with crystalloid fluids have resulted in significantly reduced transfusion needs in TJA patients. In addition, the maxim that at least 2 units of blood need to be transfused to show benefit is no longer accepted. One unit of packed red blood cells (PRBCs), red blood cell concentrate separated from plasma and platelets, generally increases a patient's Hgb by 1.0 g/dl (Hct 3%) and often is sufficient to increase oxygen delivery to acceptable levels. Transfusing only 1 unit decreases transfusion exposure for patients with symptomatic marginal anemia.

Benefits and Risks of the Allogeneic Blood Supply

Allogeneic transfusion is the receipt of volunteer blood donated for the local or national blood pool. This blood is necessarily different from the patient's own but is typed and matched properly for A, B, and Rh, the major antigens responsible for blood compatibility and rejection. In addition, a cross match in which the patient's blood is mixed with donor blood is performed before transfusion. The donor's blood is transfused only if there is no reaction. Allogeneic blood provides the benefit of increased oxygen-carrying capacity with simplicity and convenience. Transfusion of allogeneic blood is usually in the form of PRBCs. Typing, cross matching, and administration of 2 units of allogeneic PRBCs costs less than $200 at most centers. The risks of allogeneic blood, however, have caused a significant fear shared by both physicians and patients. Adverse outcomes secondary to allogeneic transfusion can be divided into those causing minor and those causing major consequence.

The most common adverse reactions to allogeneic PRBC transfusion are minor febrile and allergic reactions, which occur at a frequency of approximately 1% to 4%. Minor febrile nonhemolytic transfusion reactions are characterized by chills or rigors and a temperature increase of 1°C or greater. It is a diagnosis of exclusion, and other causes of postoperative and posttransfusion fever should be ruled out. Minor allergic urticarial reactions are characterized by a pruritic rash, edema, headache, and dizziness and are treated with an antihistamine such as diphenhydramine (50 mg by mouth or intramuscularly). Only patients with a history of allergic transfusion reaction need be premedicated with an antihistamine.

Major adverse consequences from allogeneic transfusion are very rare and include infectious transmission of viruses, bacteria, and parasites; anaphylactic reactions; acute lung injury; immunomodulation; transfusion error; and hemolytic reaction. Historically, high rates of transfusion in TJA and a higher prevalence of human immunodeficiency virus (HIV) and viral hepatitis in the allogeneic blood supply have resulted in the development of elaborate and expensive alternative strategies designed to avoid the use of allogeneic blood. However, with the advent of better screening tests over the past 10 years, the allogeneic blood supply is remarkably safe in regard to infectious contamination. In the 1980s and early 1990s the rate of HIV transmitted per unit of transfused blood was as high as 1 in 100 units in some urban areas, and the transmission of non-A, non-B hepatitis (now recognized as hepatitis C) was as high as 1 in 10 units transfused. As a result of highly improved, rigorous donor screening and sensitive serologic testing of allogeneic blood, these risks have been minimized. As of 1996, the estimated rates of transmission of HIV, hepatitis C, hepatitis B, and human T-cell lymphoma virus (HTLV) are, respectively, 1 in 680,000, 1 in 100,000, 1 in 63,000, and 1 in 641,000 units. Most transfusion experts agree that the transmission of viral disease via allogeneic blood is currently a minimal risk. Other pathogens (bacteria, parasites) probably have even smaller transmission rates.

The estimated prevalence of bacterial contamination of allogeneic or autologous red blood cells is approximately 1 in 31,000 units. The most common contaminant is *Yersinia enterocolitica*, a gram-negative coccobacillus that can cause asymptomatic bacteremia or bacteremia with only mild gastroenteritis symptoms. At 3 weeks of standard storage temperature (4°C), *Y enterocolitica* is able to replicate sufficiently and produce enough endotoxin to cause significant reaction when transfused. This type of reaction should be suspected if there is an onset of fever and shaking chills within 2 hours of transfusion, with subsequent nausea and vomiting, diarrhea, oliguria, and hypotension. Shock, respiratory symptoms, and bleeding secondary to disseminated intravascular coagulation can occur, causing an estimated mortality rate of 1 in 1 million. However, these reactions are underreported and often not diagnosed correctly, prompting a recent review to conclude that bacterial contamination is likely the most common microbiologic problem in transfusion medicine. Parasitic disease, including malaria, Chagas disease, babesiosis, leishmania, and toxoplasmosis, has also been reported to occur as a result of transfusion, but because of the exclusion of donors with significant travel histories, these pathogens are almost nonexistent in the United States blood supply today.

Patients with history of previous transfusion or immunoglobulin A (IgA) deficiency are susceptible to anaphylactic reactions at a rate of approximately 1 in 150,000 units transfused. These rare reactions occur immediately after transfusion of only a few milliliters of blood and are characterized by nausea and vomiting, difficulty breathing, coughing, bronchospasm, respiratory arrest, shock, and loss of consciousness. Transfusion should be immediately stopped and 0.5 to 1.0 cc of epinephrine at 1:1000 dilution should be administered subcutaneously, followed by aggressive supportive care. Patients with severe IgA deficiency should be given only washed cellular blood components and IgA-deficient plasma products to prevent these reactions.

Transfusion-related acute lung injury (TRALI) is a rare but life-threatening complication that occurs in approximately 1 in 500,000 units transfused. It is characterized by acute respiratory distress with severe bilateral pulmonary edema and severe hypoxemia in response to a recent transfusion. Associated fever and hypotension unresponsive to fluid administration can occur. Although the acute clinical presentation is similar to adult respiratory distress syndrome, TRALI usually improves substantially within 48 to 96 hours if the patient is given prompt and vigorous respiratory support, including intubation and mechanical ventilation.

Transfusion-associated graft-versus-host disease (GVHD) occurs with extreme rarity in predisposed individuals, including lymphoma patients, immunocompromised patients, patients who have had bone marrow transplantation, and patients receiving directed donor units from a blood relative. Approximately 1 week after transfusion, affected patients have fever, cutaneous eruption, diarrhea, and liver function abnormalities. Treatment is notoriously unsuccessful, with death occurring 3 to 4 weeks after transfusion. GVHD can be prevented by irradiation of transfused cellular components for at-risk patients and counseling patients to not participate in directed donation from blood relatives.

One of the more controversial consequences of allogeneic blood transfusion is its immunologic consequence. Allogeneic transfusion has been suspected empirically to suppress immune function, leading to increased allograft survival in renal transplant patients, and increased cancer recurrence and postoperative infection. In vitro studies have demonstrated suppression of T-helper lymphocytes, natural killer (NK)-cell function, and cytokine production after allogeneic blood exposure. Although it is not as pronounced, in vitro suppression of NK-cell function and cytokine production also occurs after autologous donation and transfusion.

Investigators of the immunologic potential of allogeneic blood have not unanimously agreed on the existence of a clinically relevant effect. Some retrospective reviews have claimed a twofold to elevenfold increase in postoperative infections for patients receiving allogeneic blood. In contrast, the most recent meta-analysis of cancer patients receiving allogeneic, autologous, and leukocyte-depleted blood could not prove a significant difference in cancer recurrence or postoperative infection rate. A recent retrospective review of 300 total hip arthroplasty patients also could not prove a significant increase in infectious complications secondary to allogeneic transfusion. This topic will remain controversial until large prospective studies confirm that the effect is clinically relevant. If allogeneic blood transfusion is proven to significantly increase postoperative infection, there is promise in leukocyte depletion by filtration, an effective and inexpensive technique shown to decrease allogeneic blood's immunogenicity.

Given the current rarity of infectious transmission and other complications, the most significant adverse outcome of allogeneic blood is probably transfusion error. Managerial and clerical errors result in the administration of the wrong unit of blood in approximately 1 in 12,000 units transfused, resulting in approximately 800 to 900 transfusion errors per year. These types of errors result in ABO incompatible transfusions and hemolysis, with fatal reactions occurring in 1 per 100,000 to 1 per 1 million units transfused. Signs and symptoms of acute hemolytic transfusion reaction include hypotension, tachypnea, tachycardia, fever, chills, chest and/or flank pain, and a burning sensation at the infusion site. If these occur in association with transfusion, blood infusion should be stopped immediately, the blood bank notified, and proper steps in further therapy and investigation taken.

Alternative Strategies to Allogeneic Transfusion

Since 1985, the focus of public concern and medical practice has been on minimizing transfusion-linked viral disease, specifically that caused by HIV and hepatitis virus. Currently, acquiring an infectious disease from the allogeneic blood supply is a very low risk, but nonetheless still occurs. Alternative measures can be taken preoperatively, intraoperatively, and postoperatively to boost or maintain red cell indices so that exposure to allogeneic blood is minimized. Preoperative methods to decrease exposure to the allogeneic blood pool include directed donation, preoperative autologous donation, and erythropoietin. Intraoperative means of red blood cell conservation include hypotensive anesthesia, acute normovolemic hemodilution (ANH), and cell salvage. Cell salvage also can be used in the immediate postoperative period. The nature of benefits of these strategies and their attendant risks must be understood to ensure rational and cost-effective hematologic care.

Directed Donation Secondary to the fear of viral contamination, patients sometimes wish to choose their own donors from among family or friends, a practice called recipient-selected transfusion or directed donation. Directed donor blood is therefore allogeneic with its inherent complications, and studies have shown that directed donor units actually exhibit a significantly higher incidence of anti-hepatitis B core antigen than found in the national allogeneic blood supply. Patients desiring directed donation blood should be counseled of this increased risk for transfusion-transmitted hepatitis, and should also be made aware that their risk for GVHD is higher with transfusion of related donor blood.

Preoperative Autologous Donation Preoperative autologous donation (PAD) is the donation, before surgery, of a patient's own blood. Blood is collected preoperatively at 1-week intervals to obtain a predetermined number of units, with the first unit obtained no sooner than 5 weeks before TJA (shelf-life of 1 unit of autologous blood is 35 to 42 days) and the last unit obtained at least 4 days before TJA. The patient should take iron supplementation during autologous procurement, either ferrous sulfate 325 mg by mouth 3 times a day or ferrous gluconate 325 mg by mouth 5 times a day, to allow maximal recovery of red blood cell indices via erythropoiesis. Red blood cell indices are obtained before each donation, and donation is not allowed if a patient's Hgb is < 11 g/dl (Hct < 33%). In addition, patients weighing < 50 kg and patients with severe coronary artery disease may not predonate. Because of a more labor-intensive collection process, 1 unit of autologous blood is about $50 more expensive than a unit of allogeneic blood. The total price of 2-unit PAD and transfusion is approximately $200 to $400, depending on the institution.

Several studies have shown that having TJA patients uniformly donate 1 to 4 units of blood significantly reduces the need for allogeneic blood. In classic studies from the late 1980s and the early 1990s, uniform PAD, the recommendation of autologous donation to all TJA patients, was practiced. The risk for hepatitis in the allogenic blood supply at that time was reported to be 1% to 10%. Transfusion indications were dictated by the "10/30" transfusion trigger in some studies and by clinical indications in others. Autologous donors were exposed to allogeneic blood significantly less often than nondonors. However, most collected units were eventually returned to the donors, exposing most of them to transfusion events. This practice made good sense, because the risks of viral transmission at that time were much greater than the risks of transfusion error. A current retrospective review of 489 TJA patients who practiced uniform PAD recommendation but had stricter transfusion criteria, also showed PAD's benefit. Only 10% of the autologous donors needed allogeneic transfusion as opposed to 26% of nondonors. However, exposure to either allogeneic or autologous blood was higher (50%) in donors. Recent investigations of radical prostatectomy, total abdominal hysterectomy, and TJA patients unanimously conclude that patients participating in autologous donation are at significantly higher risk for transfusion of any type.

Higher rates of transfusion in autologous programs are a result of less stringent transfusion indications for autologous blood and the capacity of donation to create anemia. Studies have shown a consistent predonation to preoperative hemoglobin drop of approximately 1.3 g/dl. PAD, therefore, exacerbates existing anemia and makes some nonanemic individuals anemic at the time of surgery, necessitating the use of their predeposited blood. As overall transfusion rates are increased, so is the aggregate risk of transfusion error and hemolytic reaction. In addition, acute hemolysis has been reported to occur after the correct administration of autologous blood. Significant bacterial proliferation occurs in autologous units as a result of increased storage times, because donation occurs as early as possible to ensure recovery of erythropoiesis. Recommending PAD to all TJA patients therefore becomes more risky as the viral contamination of blood declines.

PAD also entails significant inconvenience, risk for donation reactions, and wastage leading to increased costs. Considerable time commitment is required from patients because they need to travel to the blood bank, remain there for testing and donation, and are restricted from heavy activity on the day of donation as a result of the acute loss of fluid and red blood cells. Many TJA patients are at risk for significant donation reactions because of their underlying cardiopulmonary and vascular disease. Minor vasovagal reactions occur in 2% to 5% of autologous donors, and serious reactions requiring hospitalization also occur at a rate of 1 in 16,700. Most reactions resulting in hospitalization are a result of vasovagal attack, with occasional anginal exacerbation, hypotension, arrhythmias, syncope, MI, compartment syndromes, arteriovenous fistula, phlebitis, and pseudoaneurysm. Surgical repair of damaged blood vessels is sometimes required. Oxygen-carrying capacity is also decreased in autologous blood, because levels of 2,3-diphosphoglycerate are significantly decreased after 1 week of storage.

The risks of bacterial contamination and adverse donor reactions in uniform autologous donation and transfusion protocols are comparable to the risks of these complications in allogeneic transfusion. In the meantime, the risks of transfusion error and acute hemolysis are approaching the risk of viral contamination of allogeneic blood (Fig. 2). Therefore, more rigorous indications are being implemented for autologous transfusion, and fewer patients are actually requiring return of their own blood. Despite higher rates of transfusion in autologous donors than nondonors, over half of autologous units collected for TJA are not transfused. In most American blood banks and hospitals, autologous donors do not meet the stringent health criteria required for allogeneic donation. In addition, autologous units have a very short shelf life by the time the patient is discharged from the hospital. Therefore, autologous units that are not used are discarded, resulting in a significant loss of valuable blood and health care dollars.

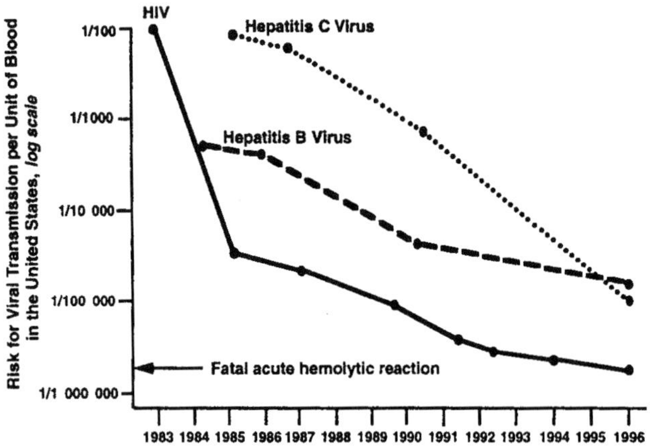

Figure 2

Decrease in per unit risk for transmission of hepatitis B virus (broken line), hepatitis C virus (dotted line), and HIV (solid line) by blood transfusion in the United States. The arrow shows the current risk for death from acute hemolysis for comparison. (Reproduced with permission from Aubuchon J, Birkmeyer J, Busch M: Safety of the blood supply in the United States: Opportunities and controversies. *Ann Int Med* 1997;127:904–909.)

More than 300,000 lower extremity arthroplasties per year are performed in the United States. If every TJA patient donates 2 units, total autologous blood donation would amount to 600,000 units per year. Because 50% of autologous blood units for orthopaedic patients are not used, approximately 300,000 units would be discarded. At $100 to $200 per unit, this would result in about $30 million to $60 million wasted per year. Many insurance companies will not pay for predonation unless the units are actually used, shifting the burden of this cost to the patient and health care provider. Many cost analysis studies have recently concluded that uniform PAD in TJA patients is not cost effective. These studies take into consideration the increased overall safety of the blood supply. In contrast, some cost analyses assume hypothetical increases in infections and length of stay for patients receiving allogeneic blood, finding collection of autologous blood more efficient. As the immunomodulatory effect of allogeneic blood is still controversial, cost analyses regarding PAD are inconclusive. The high rate of wastage caused by overcollection and increased risk for transfusion for PAD participation, however, are unequivocal.

It is logical, in terms of cost and safety, to make the collection of autologous blood more efficient. More selective PAD guidelines should be followed, which result in the avoidance of any transfusion event, either allogeneic or autologous. PAD should not be recommended to patients with low likelihood of transfusion. Alternative strategies should be recommended if proven to be of equal or greater benefit and equal or less risk in individual patients. Recommending against PAD is potentially difficult, because patients tend to assume hyperinflated risk estimates of allogeneic blood and currently are willing to pay above the price for autologous units. The lay media is partly responsible for this, tending to focus on the worst and most dramatic adverse complications of medical practice. However, counseling patients with low likelihood of transfusion against autologous donation has potential, because physician recommendation is the most consistent factor in a patient's decision to donate.

To be effective, discussions of inflated perceptions of associated risk should first be seriously considered, not ignored or disparaged, and followed by provision of information regarding the actual incidence of transfusion complications. To place low risk estimates into perspective, mortality estimates of everyday activities can be compared to the incidence of complications of allogeneic blood and PAD. As of 1997, the risks of being involved in a fatal car accident or having a fatal accident at home were greater than the fatal complications of receiving allogeneic blood (Fig. 3). Rational discussion of individualized risks and benefits of preoperative autologous donation may result in many patients deciding to accept a low risk of allogeneic transfusion to avoid the complications of PAD. Anticipation of transfusion need according to preoperative risk factors can aid the surgeon in these discussions.

The type of operation and preoperative Hgb and Hct levels are very important risk factors for transfusion and good determinants of ability to tolerate surgery without transfusion. For example, in primary total knee arthroplasty the blood loss is usually low and transfusion is not normally required, provided that the patient has nonanemic red blood cell indices. Even procedures that incur greater blood loss, such as total hip revision, can be performed without need for transfusion, if the patient's preoperative red blood cell indices are robust and alternative strategies are used.

TJA patients with a preoperative Hgb ≥ 15 g/dl undergoing primary TJA rarely require transfusion. In addition, primary TJA patients younger than 65 years old exhibit minimal transfusion rates if their preoperative Hgb is > 13 g/dl. Younger patients presumably have less severe concomitant cardiopulmonary disease and are more capable of compensating for moderate anemia. In a recent study, approximately 25% of all TJAs performed at the institutions fit either of these criteria. Counseling these patients to not participate in PAD could substantially improve the efficiency and safety of PAD before TJA on a nationwide basis. In addition, logically chosen alternative strategies, including erythropoietin administration, hypotensive anesthesia, ANH, and intraoperative and/or postoperative red blood cell salvage can be used alone or in combination to reduce the error risk of allogeneic or autologous transfusion.

Erythropoietin Erythropoietin alpha is a recombinant form of the glycoprotein hormone produced by the human kidney to stimulate red blood cell production and maturation in the bone marrow. The subcutaneous injection of recombinant erythropoietin has long been used to boost the red blood cell indices of cancer and chronic renal failure patients who suf-

Adverse Transfusion Outcomes	Estimated Frequency
Allogeneic blood (only)	
Febrile Non-Hemolytic Reaction	1:25 - 1:100
Allergic reaction	1:25 - 1:100
Anaphylactic reaction	1:150,000
Infectious transmission	
Hepatitis B	1:63,000 - 1:200,000
Hepatitis C	1:103,000
HIV	1:493,000 - 1:800,000
HTLV	1:641,000
Parasites	1:1,000,000 - 1:4,000,000
Transfusion Related Lung Injury	1:500,000
Graft vs Host Disease	rare
Increased postoperative infection (compared with leukocyte reduced or autologous blood)	0 - 25%
Autologous blood (only)	
Minor donor reaction (vasovagal)	1:20 - 1:50
Donor reaction requiring hospitalization	1:16,800
Allogeneic and Autologous blood	
Clerical error	1:12,000 - 1:50,000
Acute hemolysis	1:6,000 - 1:25,000
Acute hemolysis & death	1:100,000 - 1:1,000,000
Bacterial contamination	1:31,390
Sepsis/shock	1:1,000,000
Mortality from Unintentional Injury (U.S. 1996)	
All	1:2,860
Motor Vehicle Accidents	1:6,250
Accident at home	1:10,000
Falls	1:20,000
Poisonings	1:27,000
Drownings	1:66,700
Fires/Burn	1:83,300
Riding a bicycle	1:330,000
Collision with railroad train	1:500,000
Mortality from all accidents, by age (years)	
45-54	1:3,450
55-64	1:3,270
65-74	1:2,260
75 and greater	1 in 720

Estimated Adverse Transfusion Events per Year	
Transfusion error	800-900
ABO incompatible error	460-520
Fatal hemolytic reaction	20-30
HIV transmission	8 to 18
Malaria transmission	3

Number of accidental deaths per year in U.S 1996 due to:	
Natural/Environmental accidents	1474
Commercial airline crashes	1132
Recreational boating accidents	716
Lightning	84

Accident mortality statistics from National Safety Council (1997). *Accident Facts, 1997 edition.* Itasca, IL.

Figure 3

Current risks of allogeneic and autologous blood compared with unintentional injury deaths in the United States. (Reproduced with permission from Aubuchon J, Birkmeyer J, Busch M: Safety of the blood supply in the United States: Opportunities and controversies. *Ann Int Med* 1997;127:904–909.)

fer from symptomatic anemia. Administration of erythropoietin alpha can also increase the preoperative red blood cell indices of moderately anemic TJA patients preoperatively, decreasing the need for transfusion postoperatively. This has proven to be a safe practice with minimal complications. The United States Food and Drug Administration (FDA) has approved the administration of erythropoietin alpha to patients undergoing orthopaedic surgery who exhibit a preoperative hemoglobin level between 10 and 13 g/dl. The approved regimen is 600 units/kg given subcutaneously on preoperative days 21, 14, 7, and the day of surgery, incurring a cost to the patient of approximately $700 to $1,000. In many states Medicare currently offers full reimbursement for this indicated use.

Recent investigations show that use of recombinant erythropoietin during the 3 weeks before surgery results in increased Hgb and Hct levels and decreased need for postoperative transfusion in TJA patients, without significant adverse complications. Erythropoietin especially benefits anemic patients whose red blood cell indices are too low to donate sufficient autologous blood, the group at highest risk for allogeneic transfusion. Erythropoietin provides a more effective reduction in allogeneic transfusion than PAD for these selected patients, justifying its cost.

Erythropoietin stimulates red blood cell production, placing an increased demand on iron stores. Therefore, patients should take iron supplementation (iron sulfate 325 mg by mouth 3 times a day) to prevent iron deficiency. Vitamin C 250 mg taken orally 3 times a day and folic acid 1 mg taken orally once a day are also recommended. Erythropoietin's use is contraindicated in those patients with uncontrolled hypertension, known hypersensitivity to mammalian cell-derived products, or known hypersensitivity to human albumin. A slightly higher incidence of DVT occurs in individuals with a Hgb level > 15 g/dl. In addition, erythropoietin's use in patients with chronic renal failure causes a slightly increased risk for thrombotic events and seizures, presumably secondary to increased proliferation of platelet cell lines and increased viscosity of blood, with resultant hypercoagulability. This effect, however, has not been reproduced in TJA patients. Nonetheless, due to these slight increases in risk, patients with an Hgb level > 13 g/dl or history of recent proximal DVT, MI, or cerebrovascular accident should not be given erythropoietin. If screening Hgb levels determined before each administration become > 15 g/dl (Hct ≥ 45%) during treatment, administration of erythropoietin should be deferred.

Hypotensive Anesthesia Hypotensive anesthesia, the deliberate intraoperative lowering of a patient's blood pressure, results in decreased blood loss during TJA. It is routinely and safely used for most patients and has been shown to decrease transfusion requirements. Mean average blood pressure is kept at approximately 60 mm Hg, using a combination of volatile anesthetics, narcotics, and vasodilators. Blood pressures are recorded by automated tracings, which assure that the degree of hypotension is consistent and adequate.

Hypotensive anesthesia has proven to be safe alone or in conjunction with PAD and ANH. Patients with significant cardiovascular, cerebrovascular, or renal disease should be excluded because their underlying disease may be exacerbated by sustained hypotension. Patients with these conditions should not be given hypotensive agents. Screening should include EKG, careful history and physical examination, and determination of preoperative blood urea nitrogen and creatinine. If high-risk patients are thus excluded, hypotensive anesthesia is a safe, inexpensive, and effective procedure for TJA patients that should be used whenever possible.

Acute Normovolemic Hemodilution ANH involves withdrawing a patient's own blood at the time of surgery before incision and replacing the volume with crystalloid or colloid fluid to maintain intravascular volume. The patient's blood is more dilute, theoretically decreasing total red blood cell loss during surgery. The whole blood is then returned to the patient after the operation, when blood loss has ceased. A volume previously is determined by standard formulas to decrease the patient's Hgb/Hct to a desired level; 3 to 4 units of whole blood are withdrawn by the time a urinary bladder catheter is placed, and positioning, scrubbing, and draping of the patient have occurred. The blood is maintained at room temperature to preserve platelet function and is gently agitated periodically to prevent coagulation. Blood is administered in reverse order from its withdrawal so the most concentrated blood is returned last. Transfusion occurs after wound closure, if the patient's Hgb decreases below a previously determined critical level (usually 6 g/dl) during the case, if EKG signs of myocardial ischemia develop (eg, ST depression), or if unexplained severe hypotension or tachycardia unresponsive to intravenous fluids occurs. A small amount of Lasix (0.25 to 1.0 mg/kg) is administered intravenously during transfusion to prevent fluid overload.

ANH has been shown to be a safe and effective method for reducing allogeneic blood requirements after elective surgery, including coronary artery bypass and spinal fusion. A recent prospective study showed that ANH was as effective as 2-unit PAD in preventing allogeneic transfusion in radical prostatectomy patients. Another study combined the practice of moderate hemodilution with PAD in total hip replacements, significantly reducing autologous transfusion requirements. Beneficial hemodynamic effects of ANH include increased cardiac output and increased peripheral tissue oxygen delivery secondary to decreased viscosity and increased venous return. ANH blood is of higher quality than preoperatively donated or allogeneic blood, because its platelets, coagulation factors, and 2,3-diphosphoglycerate levels are preserved. In ANH, there also is virtually no risk of transfusion error or bacterial contamination. Cost is incurred only for the extra tubing, collection bags, and a small amount of anticoagulant. If performed efficiently, no extra time in surgery is incurred, resulting in a total cost of approximately $80 for withdrawal and transfusion of 2 ANH units.

Moderate hemodilution to a Hgb level of 9 g/dl has been shown to be safe in elderly patients with no history of severe preexisting disease. Because the acute reduction in Hgb decreases overall oxygen-carrying capacity, an increase in cardiac output and, therefore, cardiac blood flow is required. Thus, this technique has the potential to increase the risk of myocardial ischemia or infarction in patients with significant decrease in cardiac reserve. Patients with a history of significant previous coronary artery disease, recent MI (within 2 months), severe aortic stenosis, and significant myocardial hypertrophy should not undergo hemodilution. In addition, TJA patients sometimes have underlying significant cardiac disease in the absence of previous documentation, history, or EKG changes. To prevent complications, patients' EKG tracings are closely monitored from the onset of phlebotomy and anesthesia induction to the end of surgery. Blood should be promptly reinfused to patients exhibiting these signs to restore myocardial oxygenation. Adequate lung function is also required to ensure adequate oxygenation; therefore, patients with acute or chronic pulmonary disease should not be hemodiluted. Patients with significant renal, liver, coagulation, or infectious disease should also be excluded.

A recent meta-analysis of ANH hypothesized that its apparent significant effect in decreasing allogeneic transfusion requirements in several studies may actually have been due to flawed study design. ANH is logistically challenging, and requires a dedicated and skilled anesthesia team to be successful. Nonetheless, ANH has many potential benefits over PAD and allogeneic blood, including increased safety and decreased cost, and has promise as a technique that may supplement or supplant PAD for some TJA patients. The efficacy, safety, and efficiency of ANH needs to be studied in large, well-designed, randomized prospective trials if it is to achieve general acceptance for TJA.

Intraoperative Salvage Intraoperative red blood cell salvage ("Cell Saver", Sorin Biomedical Inc, Irvine, CA) entails salvage of shed blood from wound drainage during surgery. The drainage blood is washed, and the red blood cells are isolated and returned to the patient, devoid of free Hgb, debris, clotting factors, or platelets. Intraoperative salvage has been shown to significantly decrease the requirement of allogeneic blood if expected intraoperative blood loss is approximately 1,000 cc. Therefore, intraoperative cell salvage is standard in the care of revision hip arthroplasty patients. Device, materials, and personnel costs total approximately $200 to $400 for 2 units. Air embolism and transfusion errors occur very rarely, but have resulted in mortality.

Postoperative Salvage Devices have also been invented to collect and reinfuse postoperative wound drainage. Some studies have shown that postoperative drainage reinfusion is beneficial in decreasing allogeneic transfusion after TJA, but others have not demonstrated significant efficacy. Because of the serosanguinous nature of postoperative wound drainage, the volume of red blood cells salvaged is often insufficient to provide benefit. Postoperative reinfusion is not efficacious in decreasing allogeneic exposure in primary total knee replacement or in primary total hip replacement if autologous blood is available. Mild adverse reactions, which presumably are due to increased cytokines in reinfused blood, also occur, including fever, hypotension, and upper airway edema. The devices for unwashed reinfusion cost approximately $150. New devices wash postoperative drainage free of cytokines and debris, but are more expensive. Therefore, postoperative cell salvage probably is cost-effective only for operations with high postoperative wound drainage, such as 1-stage bilateral total knee replacement. It may also be beneficial in patients with bleeding diatheses or in patients whose medical conditions prohibit them from alternative therapies.

Experimental Alternatives Reduction of blood loss using aprotinin, desmopressin, collagen pads, fibrin glue, and cold compressive dressings has been attempted with equivocal benefit. In addition, blood substitutes, such as perfluorocarbons and free-hemoglobin containing solutions, are currently in the experimental phase.

Legal Considerations Because serious complications can occur from transfusion or its alternative strategies, legal informed consent is important. The patient must be objectively informed of the benefits (avoiding serious risk of inadequate oxygen-carrying capacity and death), common minor risks (febrile transfusion reaction, etc), and less common but serious risks (transfusion error, hemolytic transfusion reaction, and viral contamination) of allogeneic transfusion. The risks and benefits of available alternatives to allogeneic transfusion (directed donation, PAD, cell salvage, ANH, erythropoietin, etc) must also be fully explained to the patient. The informational discussion should take place far enough in advance of surgery to allow for participation in alternatives. After full discussion of benefits and risks of all therapy options, individuals have the right (within medical limits) to participate in whichever blood conservation technique they choose, even if their choice goes against physician recommendation. The patient's voluntary, uncoerced choice should be documented in the chart. A transfusion consent form may be used for this purpose, but a well-written, witness countersigned progress note documenting the full discussion may also suffice.

Transfusion-related malpractice or negligence suits usually occur as a result of inadequate informed consent or the unnecessary administration of blood products. Therefore, the elements of informed consent, understanding of the physiology of anemia, and adherence to proper transfusion indications are essential to sound medicolegal care. An objective and thorough discussion of transfusion and alternatives also contributes to enhanced rapport and a mutually supportive treatment relationship.

Table 3
Algorithm for blood conservation for TJA*

Operation Type	Hemoglobin ≥ 15 g/dL or Hemoglobin ≥ 13 g/dL and Age < 65	Hemoglobin < 15 g/dL but ≥ 13 g/dL and Age ≥ 65	Hemoglobin < 13 g/dL
Primary Total Knee	Hyp Anes	Hyp Anes PAD and/or ANH	Hyp Anes Epo PAD and/or ANH
Revision Total Knee	Hyp Anes PAD and/or ANH	Hyp Anes PAD and/or ANH	Hyp Anes Epo PAD and/or ANH
Bilateral Total Knee	Hyp Anes Postop CS PAD and/or ANH	Hyp Anes Postop CS PAD and/or ANH	Hyp Anes Postop CS Epo PAD and/or ANH
Primary Total Hip	Hyp Anes	Hyp Anes PAD and/or ANH	Hyp Anes Epo PAD and/or ANH
Revision Total Hip	Hyp Anes Intraop CS PAD and/or ANH	Hyp Anes Intraop CS PAD and/or ANH	Hyp Anes Intraop CS Epo PAD and/or ANH

* Hyp Anes = hypotensive anesthesia; ANH = acute normovolemic hemodilution; PAD = preoperative autologous donation;

Conclusion

Medical management of TJA has been quite successful, with a very low incidence of complications. Improved preoperative evaluation, treatment of associated complicating conditions, and clinical care pathways have contributed to this success. Improved surgical technique, better understanding of the physiologic effects of surgically induced hypovolemia and anemia, and more physiologic transfusion criteria have decreased the overall transfusion rate and its attendant complications. Allogeneic blood is beneficial and inexpensive. The risk of viral contamination is markedly decreased, and the risk for transfusion reaction secondary to transfusion error is probably as or more significant.

PAD has been shown to decrease allogeneic exposure. However, uniform recommendation of PAD regardless of risk factors for transfusion has resulted in higher overall transfusion rates and voluminous waste of autologous blood. Because of the frequency of donation-induced anemia and increased overall transfusion rates, the aggregate risk of donation reaction, bacterial contamination, transfusion error, and hemolytic reaction in uniform PAD protocols approximates or exceeds the risks of judicious allogeneic blood transfusion. Consideration of preoperative red blood cell indices, patient age, and type of operation can make PAD programs more efficient by identifying patients at low risk for transfusion. Refraining from PAD in these patients can significantly decrease waste, inconvenience, risk, and cost to the patient without appreciably increasing allogeneic exposure. In appropriately selected patients, alternative methods of red blood cell optimization can decrease overall transfusion exposure in a cost-effective manner with minimal complications. A proposed algorithm for perioperative hematologic optimization using these alternatives is presented in Table 3.

Currently, the orthopaedic surgeon is able to make more judicious decisions regarding the advantages, disadvantages, and risks of transfusion and its alternative strategies. Patients should be well informed of these advantages, disadvantages, and risks, because they are more active in the medical decision-making process and must provide informed consent for their transfusion-related care. Rational consideration of these facets of management coupled with effective patient communication will result in care that improves on the success of TJA through the turn of the century and beyond.

Annotated Bibliography

Eagle KA, Brundage BH, Chaitman BR, et al: Guidelines for perioperative cardiovascular evaluation for noncardiac surgery: Report of the American College of Cardiology/American Heart Association Task Force on Practice Guidelines (Committee on Perioperative Cardiovascular Evaluation for Noncardiac Surgery). *J Am Coll Cardiol* 1996;27:910–948.

This is the consensus report of the 1995 American College of Cardiology/American Heart Association Task Force on Practice Guidelines and the Committee on Perioperative Cardiovascular Evaluation for Noncardiac Surgery on the current standard of care for perioperative cardiovascular management.

Fiorillo AB, Solano FX Jr: Preoperative medical evaluation in, Callaghan JJ, Rosenberg AG, Rubash HE (eds): *The Adult Hip.* Philadelphia, PA, Lippincott-Raven, 1998, pp 601–613.

This comprehensive chapter describes in detail guidelines in the care of medically complicated TJA patients. The authors discuss proper ordering of laboratory tests and assessment of cardiovascular, pulmonary, cerebrovascular, and other systemic disease.

Transfusion Medicine

Indications for Transfusion

Practice Guidelines for Blood Component Therapy: A Report by the American Society of Anesthesiologists Task Force on Blood Component Therapy. *Anesthesiology* 1996;84:732–747.

This task force concluded that transfusion indications in the perioperative period should be based on the patient's risks of developing complications of inadequate oxygenation. They determined that 18% to 57% of transfusions are given for inappropriate indications.

Risks of Allogeneic Blood

Schreiber GB, Busch MP, Kleinman SH, Korelitz JJ: The risk of transfusion-transmitted viral infections: The Retrovirus Epidemiology Donor Study. *N Engl J Med* 1996;334: 1685–1690.

The authors analyzed over 2 million blood donations and estimated the frequency of donors with HIV, hepatitis B and C, and HTLV who gave tainted blood during the window period following a recent undetected infection, thus passing all screening tests.

Vamvakas EC, Moore SB, Cabanela M: Blood transfusion and septic complications after hip replacement surgery. *Transfusion* 1995;35:150–156.

This retrospective review of the incidence of postoperative septic complications of 420 total hip arthroplasties found an infection rate of 9.5% in allogeneic recipients, compared to 6.4% in unexposed patients (p = 0.226).

Preoperative Autologous Donation

Blumberg N, Kirkley SA, Heal JM: A cost analysis of autologous and allogeneic transfusions in hip-replacement surgery. *Am J Surg* 1996;171:324–330.

The authors analyzed the cost effectiveness of PAD for total hip arthroplasty, including the controversial effect of increased postoperative bacterial infection. They concluded that allogeneic transfusion was $1,000 to $1,500 more expensive than no transfusion or the receipt of 1 to 5 units of autologous blood.

Etchason J, Petz L, Keeler E, et al: The cost effectiveness of preoperative autologous blood donations. *N Engl J Med* 1995;332: 719–724.

The authors analyzed the cost-effectiveness of PAD for total hip arthroplasty, calculating a quality adjusted life year (QUALY) of over $235,000 per autologous unit. In comparison, recent studies calculate the QUALY of total hip replacement overall to be $2,000 per QUALY.

Forgie MA, Wells PS, Laupacis A, Fergusson D: International Study of Perioperative Transfusion (ISPOT) Investigators: Preoperative autologous donation decreases allogeneic transfusion but increases exposure to all red blood cell transfusion. Results of a meta-analysis. *Arch Intern Med* 1998;158: 610–616.

This meta-analysis of randomized and cohort studies regarding PAD showed that autologous donors were 3 to 12 times more likely than nondonors to receive transfusion of any type, suggesting that surgical technique and transfusion protocols may be as important as PAD in decreasing allogeneic blood exposure.

Lee SJ, Liljas B, Churchill WH, et al: Perceptions and preferences of autologous blood donors. *Transfusion* 1998;38:757–763.

This investigation gave surveys to 647 autologous donors. The authors found that patients expressed a strong preference for PAD and indicated that they would be willing to pay substantial amounts of money even if PAD was not covered by insurance.

National Heart, Lung, and Blood Institute Expert Panel on the Use of Autologous Blood: Transfusion alert: Use of autologous blood. *Transfusion* 1995;35:703–711.

This consensus conference outlined the indications for autologous blood collection and transfusion. It was concluded that autologous blood should be collected only for patients with a 10% or greater chance of transfusion. Alternatives to PAD are discussed.

Popovsky MA, Whitaker B, Arnold NL: Severe outcomes of allogeneic and autologous blood donation: Frequency and characterization. *Transfusion* 1995;35:734–737.

The authors studied over 3.8 million allogeneic and 218,000 preoperative autologous donations, discovering 33 donation reactions requiring hospitalization due to autologous donation. Autologous donors were 11 times more likely than allogeneic donors to have a reaction.

Risk Factors for Transfusion

Hatzidakis A, Mendlick RM, Reddy R, McKillip T, Garvin K: Preoperative autologous donation in total joint arthroplasty: An analysis of risk factors for transfusion. *J Bone Joint Surg*, in press.

The authors reviewed the charts of 489 total joint arthroplasty patients. Primary knee or hip arthroplasty patients with an initial hemoglobin value of 15.0 g/dL (n=67) and primary knee or hip arthroplasty patients with an initial hemoglobin level between 13.0 and 15.0 g/dL who were younger than 65 years old (n=63) had a minimal risk of transfusion. This transfusion risk was unaffected by the donation of autologous blood.

Nuttall GA, Santrach PJ, Oliver WC Jr, et al: The predictors of red cell transfusions in total hip arthroplasties. *Transfusion* 1996; 36:144–149.

The authors reviewed the charts of 299 primary and revision hip arthroplasty patients, calculated their average drop in Hgb, and discovered that the significant indicators for allogeneic transfusion were preoperative Hgb concentration, weight, age, estimated blood loss, and aspirin use.

Erythropoietin

Faris PM, Ritter MA, Abels RI: The American Erythropoietin Study Group: The effects of recombinant human erythropoietin of perioperative transfusion requirements in patients having a major orthopaedic operation. *J Bone Joint Surg* 1996;78A:62–72.

The investigators randomized 166 TJA patients to 3 groups: control, erythropoietin administration 300 international units/kg per day, and 600 international units/kg per day times 15 doses. There were significant increases in hemoglobin and decreases in transfusion rate for patients with a hemoglobin level between 10 and 13 g/dl in the latter 2 groups.

Acute Normovolemic Hemodilution

Oishi CS, D'Lima DD, Morris BA, Hardwick ME, Berkowitz SD, Colwell CW Jr: Hemodilution with other blood reinfusion techniques in total hip arthroplasty. *Clin Orthop* 1997;339: 132–139.

In a prospective randomized study of primary total hip arthroplasty, 17 patients who used ANH, PAD, and intraoperative cell salvage had an autologous transfusion rate of 41%, compared to 75% of patients who underwent PAD and intraoperative salvage alone.

Intraoperative Cell Salvage

Lemos MJ, Healy WL: Blood transfusion in orthopaedic operations. *J Bone Joint Surg* 1996;78A:1260–1270.

This current concepts review is an overview of transfusion risks and alternatives to allogeneic transfusion. The authors discuss the efficacy of intraoperative cell salvage.

Postoperative Cell Salvage

Ayers DC, Murray DG, Duerr DM: Blood salvage after total hip arthroplasty. *J Bone Joint Surg* 1995;77A:1347–1351.

In this prospective trial using PAD for primary and revision total hip arthroplasty, one group was randomized to receive postoperative cell salvage. Patients with postoperative cell salvage exhibited decreased exposure to allogeneic blood only if autologous units were unavailable.

Informed Consent

Goldman EB: Legal considerations for allogeneic blood transfusion. *Am J Surg* 1995;170(6A suppl):27S–31S.

The author discusses current legal standards for informed consent and strategies alternative to allogeneic transfusion.

Classic Bibliography

Consensus conference: Perioperative red blood cell transfusion. *JAMA* 1988;260:2700–2703.

Linden JV, Paul B, Dressler KA: A report of 104 transfusion errors in New York State. *Transfusion* 1992;32:601–606.

Nelson CL, Bowen WS: Total hip arthroplasty in Jehovah's Witnesses without blood transfusion. *J Bone Joint Surg* 1986; 68A:350–353.

Ritter MA, Keating EM, Faris PM: Closed wound drainage in total hip or total knee replacement: A prospective, randomized study. *J Bone Joint Surg* 1994;76A:35–38.

Woolson ST, Marsh JS, Tanner JB: Transfusion of previously deposited autologous blood for patients undergoing hip-replacement surgery. *J Bone Joint Surg* 1987;69A:325–328.

Chapter 8
Anesthesia for Hip and Knee Reconstructive Surgery

Introduction

The number of patients undergoing hip and knee reconstructive surgery has vastly increased over the past several years. This increase is the result of an aging population that remains active into their seventh and eighth decades of life. The ability to safely perform this type of surgery on older patients is the result, in large part, of advances in anesthetic techniques.

The administration and management of anesthesia are critical to the ultimate success of hip and knee reconstructive procedures. The anesthesiologist has many responsibilities in this process. These responsibilities include patient selection and preoperative medical optimization. Intraoperative responsibilities include maintaining the stability of physiologic parameters and ensuring appropriate surgical conditions. Postoperatively, pain management is an integral component in the rehabilitation and mobilization of patients. Furthermore, anesthesiologists play a vital role in treating acute medical conditions that may often arise in the perioperative period, especially following procedures such as bilateral joint reconstruction or complex revisions. Anesthetic management may affect both the acute medical care of the patient and the long-term outcome of a patient after joint reconstruction.

Preanesthetic Evaluation

The preanesthetic evaluation is an integral component in the care of any patient planning knee or hip reconstruction. As the population ages, patients with complex medical histories quite often come in for elective procedures. Concurrent medical conditions, such as coronary artery disease, hypertension, cerebrovascular disease, chronic obstructive pulmonary disease, and diabetes, are exceedingly common in this population of patients. The preanesthetic evaluation is a means of ensuring that the patient is in optimal medical condition to undergo the surgical procedure. Although the final decision to supply anesthesia rests with the anesthesiologist, if and when to proceed must truly be a multidisciplinary determination. This decision should ideally involve the anesthesiologist, orthopaedic surgeon, internist, and any subspecialist involved in the patient's care. This group must work together to determine if the patient is in optimum condition to tolerate invasive elective surgery.

The preanesthetic evaluation begins with a complete history and physical examination. A description of prior anesthetic experiences is essential, especially any issues regarding problems with the patient's airway. A list of current medications should be obtained. With the exception of diuretics, most medications should be continued in the perioperative period either by an oral or parenteral route. This is particularly true for beta blockers, because withdrawal has been associated with an increase in perioperative ischemic events. Patients who require hip or knee reconstruction are often taking nonsteroidal anti-inflammatory drugs as part of their analgesic regimen. Although these medications may inhibit platelet function, their use is not a contraindication to regional anesthesia.

Particular attention should be directed toward the preoperative cardiac, respiratory, and neurologic status of the patient. Coronary artery disease (CAD) affects approximately 10 million adult Americans. A significant percentage of patients for hip or knee reconstruction will have either overt or occult CAD. Risk factors associated with CAD include male gender, increasing age, hypertension, hypercholesterolemia, cigarette smoking, and diabetes mellitus. Furthermore, given the limited mobility of patients for hip and knee reconstruction, one of the best methods of determining myocardial oxygen reserve, exercise tolerance, is not particularly useful in this population. In patients who have known CAD (history of prior myocardial infarction, congestive heart failure, or angina) or who have multiple risk factors for CAD, it is prudent to consult a specialist. In this population of patients, further diagnostic testing may be warranted.

Chronic obstructive pulmonary disease (COPD) affects approximately 10 million Americans and is most often caused by cigarette smoking. Patients with COPD are extremely sensitive to the respiratory effects of anesthetics and analgesics, particularly following major surgery. Pulmonary function testing, measuring lung volumes both before and after bronchodilator therapy, is helpful in assessing patient readiness for surgery. Again, if patients have particularly severe COPD, consultation with a specialist is warranted.

Preanesthetic evaluation of neurologic status should include determination of both central and peripheral nervous system function. Preoperative documentation of neurologic deficits is essential. Although the incidence of peripheral nerve injury during hip and knee reconstruction is rare, it is important to distinguish between a preexisting neuropathy and one attributable to surgery or anesthesia. Confusion or mental status changes, as well as long-term cognitive dysfunction after hip and knee reconstruction, are not uncommon. It is therefore important to evaluate the patient's preoperative cognitive function (using a brief mental status examination) so that subtle postoperative changes can be seen. Furthermore, carotid disease should be evaluated either by history or physical examination. The presence of moderate or severe cerebrovascular disease may be a contraindication to hypotensive techniques often used in hip reconstruction.

Laboratory testing in patients undergoing hip and knee reconstruction should ideally be individualized to the patient's medical condition and the extent of procedure. Current guidelines for minimum preoperative testing are outlined in Table 1.

In summary, hip and knee reconstruction, being elective procedures, require that the patient be in optimal medical condition before proceeding. Good communication between the anesthesiologist, orthopaedic surgeon, and internist can insure appropriate patient selection and preparation, as well as the best possible outcome.

Table 1
Summary of preoperative test recommendations

Age	Men	Women
6 months to 40 years	None	Hematocrit ? pregnancy test*
40 to 50 years	Electrocardiogram	Hematocrit ? pregnancy test*
50 to 64 years	Electrocardiogram	Hematocrit ? pregnancy test* Electrocardiogram
65 to 74 years	Hemoglobin or hematocrit Electrocardiogram Blood urea nitrogen Glucose	Hemoglobin or hematocrit Electrocardiogram Blood urea nitrogen Glucose
Older than 74 years	Hemoglobin or hematocrit Electrocardiogram Blood urea nitrogen Glucose ? chest x-ray*	Hemoglobin or hematocrit Electrocardiogram Blood urea nitrogen Glucose ? chest x-ray*

* Debate exists as to whether these tests are essential as minimal standards
(Reproduced with permission from Roizen MF: Preoperative evaluation. *Anesthesia Analgesia*1994;78(suppl):78-85.)

Anesthetic Techniques

Hip and knee reconstruction can be safely performed with a variety of techniques including both regional and general anesthesia. The decision of which anesthetic to choose is based on many factors, including the patient's current medical condition, prior experiences and preferences and, finally, the anesthesiologist's abilities.

The most common regional techniques used for hip and knee reconstruction are spinal and epidural anesthesia. Spinal anesthesia involves placing a small (22 to 27 gauge) needle through the dura below the level of the spinal cord (below L2) and injecting a small dose and volume of local anesthetic into the cerebrospinal fluid. This produces a rapid (2 to 5 minute) onset of profound sensory and motor blockade. The duration of surgical blockade can vary from 30 minutes to 5 hours depending on the choice and amount of local anesthetic. Common drugs used for spinal anesthesia include bupivacaine, lidocaine, tetracaine, and mepivacaine. Narcotics, such as preservative-free morphine, may also be added to provide longer lasting analgesia. The advantages of spinal anesthesia include technical ease, a dense sensory and motor block, and a fast onset. The primary disadvantage of spinal anesthesia is its limited duration of action; on resolution of the block, there is no opportunity to use the anesthetic for postoperative analgesia. The incidence of the most widely publicized complication of spinal anesthesia, the "spinal headache," has decreased significantly in recent years (to less than 1%) due to the use of small gauge, pencil point needles.

Epidural anesthesia involves placing a larger needle (17 to 18 gauge) into the epidural space, usually at a low thoracic or lumbar level, and injecting a high volume (15 to 25 ml) of local anesthetic over several minutes. A catheter is threaded into the epidural space and secured for postoperative use. Similar local anesthetics and narcotics are used for spinal and epidural anesthesia. The disadvantages of epidural anesthesia include the occurrence of a patchy or incomplete block in a small percentage of patients, especially those with prior spinal surgery. The main advantage of epidural anesthesia is the ability to use the catheter for postoperative analgesic techniques. Important recent modifications of these methods include the combined spinal epidural (CSE) and the continuous spinal anesthetic techniques. These procedures offer both the advantages and complications of both spinal and epidural anesthesia.

A wide variety of general anesthetic techniques has been used successfully for hip and knee reconstructive surgery, including nitrous-narcotic, potent inhalational, and balanced methods. An ongoing debate exists as to whether there are any significant benefits of regional versus general anesthesia. Spinal and epidural anesthesia have been associated with less blood loss and a lower incidence of deep vein thromboses when compared with general anesthesia in patients undergoing hip and knee reconstruction. Studies have been divided as to whether regional anesthesia is associated with a lower morbidity and mortality when compared to general anesthesia. In a study in which spinal anesthesia was compared with general anesthesia in patients undergoing peripheral vascular surgery, no differences were noted with regard to perioperative morbidity; however, 1 population was identified as having a higher incidence of morbidity. That population was given a general anesthetic after a failed regional block. The authors concluded that anesthesiologists should perform those techniques with which they are most comfortable.

An area of current interest is the concept of preemptive analgesia. Proponents of this theory believe that by blocking painful stimuli before initiating the stimulus, dynamic pain pathways will be modified, and result in less postoperative discomfort. Spinal or epidural anesthesia would be advantageous with regard to this hypothesis.

Anesthesia for Hip Reconstruction

There are 2 primary objectives in the intraoperative anesthetic management of hip reconstruction. The first is meticulous cardiorespiratory monitoring and control during the operation. The second is maintenance of optimal intraoperative conditions. These conditions include appropriate and safe patient positioning, adequate muscular relaxation, and minimization of intraoperative bleeding. Maintaining these conditions allows the surgeon to operate expeditiously. Indeed, one of the primary determinants of deep venous thrombosis formation during total hip arthroplasty is duration of surgery. A dry surgical field may aid in reducing the duration of surgery. Limited bleeding facilitates optimal penetration of cement into cancellous bone, thereby providing an excellent bone-cement interface. Profound muscular relaxation allows unconstrained manipulation of the hip to achieve appropriate positioning and visualization of neurovascular structures.

The technique of hypotensive epidural anesthesia fulfills these criteria. An epidural injection is performed at a lumbar vertebral interspace with approximately 20 ml of a potent local anesthetic (0.75% bupivacaine or 2% lidocaine). This ensures a dense sensory and motor blockade that extends to the upper thoracic dermatomes. Consequently, an extensive sympathetic blockade ensues. Immediately after the local anesthetic is injected, an infusion of epinephrine is begun at a rate of 1 to 5 mcg/min to maintain cardiac output, filling pressures, and heart rate. This infusion is adjusted to provide a mean arterial pressure in the 50 to 60 mm Hg range. This technique has proven to be safe in a large population of patients; however, relative contraindications to this technique include moderate to severe aortic stenosis, hypertrophic obstructive cardiomyopathy, cerebrovascular disease, and moderate to severe renal insufficiency.

Controlled hypotension may also be instituted in conjunction with general anesthesia. Vasodilators, usually sodium nitroprusside or nitroglycerine, are used to lower the blood pressure. Negative inotropes, such as beta blockers or calcium channel blockers, may also be used to augment the hypotension and prevent reflex tachycardia.

Monitoring for hip reconstructive surgery should include continuous electrocardiography, pulse oximetry, and noninvasive blood pressure measurement. Also, with the use of hypotensive techniques and the potential for hemodynamic volatility, an arterial line is essential. Central venous or pulmonary artery monitoring is indicated based on the patient's preexisting medical status or for complex revisions and bilateral joint replacements. Patients who undergo hip revision surgery with long-stem cemented implants or bilateral hip or knee reconstruction are at a greater risk of developing bone-cement implantation reactions, and the ensuing cardiopulmonary and systemic complications. Central vascular access and monitoring may assist in the management of these reactions.

Reconstruction of the hip is a fairly uniform and predictable operation. The anesthesiologist should be familiar enough with the procedure to anticipate and treat the patient's responses and surgical needs during each particular phase. The operation begins with the dissection and exposure of the hip joint. The role of the anesthesiologist is to provide adequate conditions including profound relaxation and minimal bleeding. If controlled hypotension is being used, the blood pressure should be in the desired range by this time. After excision of the femoral head, the hip is dislocated. The resulting flexion and external rotation causes a "kinking" of the femoral artery and vein that may, to varying degrees, cause obstruction to both arterial and venous blood flow. Next, the acetabulum is prepared and the acetabular component is inserted. Excellent surgical conditions are again essential because sciatic nerve injury is possible. Hemodynamically, there are minimal effects on the cardiorespiratory system during insertion of the acetabular component. Preparation of the femoral shaft and cementing the femoral component carry the highest risk of hemodynamic and respiratory disruption. Debris, such as residual thrombus, bone fragments, and marrow components, may be forced under pressurization through bony sinuses into the circulation. A rise in pulmonary artery pressures, a fall in systemic blood pressure, and a fall in oxygen saturation may occur at this time. The anesthesiologist should be prepared for these events and resuscitate the patient, using epinephrine, fluids, and increased inspired oxygen. Furthermore, as previously noted, limited bleeding at this point may result in an improved bone-cement interface, with the potential for increased longevity of the implant. After the cement hardens, the hip is relocated. At this time, the femoral vessels are "unkinked" and, in a significant number of patients, the above-mentioned cardiorespiratory events may again occur as the debris is released into the central circulation. The effects of cementing and relocation on pulmonary artery pressures are shown in Figure 1. These events have been confirmed using transesophageal echocardiography as well. Once the hip is relocated, closure begins.

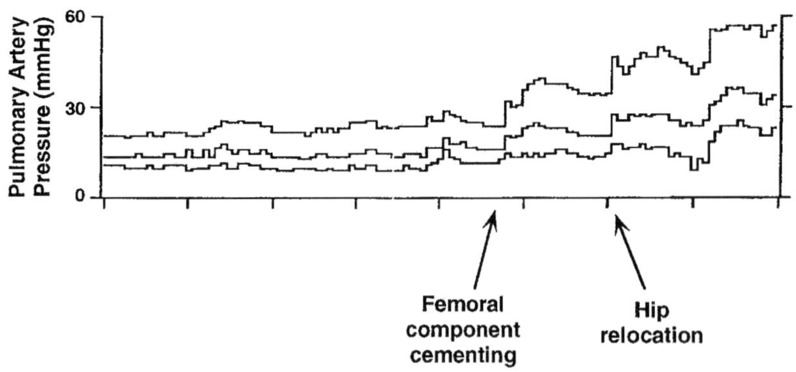

Figure 1

A trend of pulmonary artery pressure versus time during hip reconstruction, highlighting sudden elevations in pressure during femoral component cementing and hip relocation.

Anesthesia for Knee Reconstruction

Monitoring for patients undergoing knee reconstruction is similar to that for hip reconstruction; however, because hypotensive techniques are not required, the use of an arterial line may not always be indicated. However, if a patient's condition warrants the use of invasive monitors, then an arterial or central line may be indicated.

Knee reconstruction is often performed using a thigh tourniquet, resulting in minimal intraoperative blood loss. Despite this advantage, tourniquet use offers several challenges to the anesthesiologist. Tourniquet pain is an ill-defined phenomenon associated with tourniquet inflation. This pain is thought to be mediated by unmyelinated c-fibers and may be a response to localized ischemia under and adjacent to the tourniquet. It often occurs after approximately 60 minutes of inflation time and manifests as progressive hypertension and tachycardia. This phenomenon occurs during both regional and general anesthesia. However, certain local anesthetics may be more effective than others in preventing tourniquet pain during regional anesthesia.

On deflation of the tourniquet, significant hemodynamic and respiratory changes may ensue. The most common hemodynamic alterations are hypotension and tachycardia. However, in a significant percentage of patients, bradycardia may occur, and bradycardia and asystole have been reported following tourniquet deflation. A heightened awareness of these changes is imperative if resuscitation is to be successful. The anesthesiologist must be prepared to treat these events immediately. Metabolic changes associated with tourniquet release include an elevation in $Pa{CO_2}$ and a decrease in temperature. Finally, pulmonary thromboemboli and fat emboli, potentially leading to cardiovascular collapse and death, also have been reported with tourniquet release.

Following tourniquet release during knee reconstruction, bleeding may be significant. Patients should be adequately hydrated intraoperatively as well as during the postoperative period as significant blood loss also may be noted from the drains.

Although knee reconstruction can be performed successfully with general anesthesia, epidural anesthesia or CSE anesthesia offers many advantages for this procedure. One of the most important advantages is the presence of an epidural catheter, which allows for optimal postoperative pain management. Postoperative pain following knee reconstruction is quite often intense and more severe in comparison to hip arthroplasty. If a spinal or general anesthetic is used, appropriate arrangements must be made for adequate analgesia. Alternatives to epidural analgesia in these situations include parenteral narcotics or femoral and sciatic nerve blockade with long-acting local anesthetics, such as bupivacaine or ropivacaine.

Postoperative Care

Postoperative care of the patient following hip or knee reconstruction is often uneventful. However, before transferring a patient to an unmonitored setting, the patient's condition, including the residual effects of the anesthetic, should be determined. In addition, if a regional technique is used, it is imperative that the patient be kept in a monitored setting until complete resolution of the spinal or epidural anesthetic. Severe hypotension and bradycardia have been described following near-complete resolution of central blockade in the postanesthetic care unit. These events usually occur in the setting of hypovolemia, secondary to postoperative bleeding. Bradydisrhythmias are easily treated if acted upon immediately; any delay, however, may lead to a poor outcome.

Occasionally, patients may develop acute complications, such as hypoxemia, pulmonary hypertension, and right heart failure following hip or knee reconstruction. These complications occur more often after extensive procedures, such as complex revisions involving long-stem cemented femoral components or one-stage bilateral operations, but may occur after any joint replacement procedure.

Perioperative ischemia is a common event in the population of patients undergoing hip and knee reconstruction. It has now become apparent that the most important predictor of both long- and short-term cardiac outcome is the early recognition and treatment of ischemic events in the postoperative period. Recent studies have advocated the use of beta blockade as an effective method to reduce perioperative cardiac ischemic events.

Fat emboli syndrome is a potentially serious complication of both hip and knee reconstructive surgery. Echocardiographic studies have confirmed that embolic material is seen quite frequently during cemented hip arthroplasty. The spectrum of this event extends from mild postoperative hypoxemia to complete cardiovascular and respiratory collapse. The etiology seems to be related to the embolization of marrow fat cells into the pulmonary circulation. This embolization leads to a diphasic response, initially characterized by hypoxia. The lungs are subsequently affected by the metabolism of the fat, leading to endothelial damage, pulmonary edema, and alveolar collapse. As the fat migrates through the pulmonary circulation into the systemic circulation, alterations in consciousness and petechial hemorrhages are noted. Acute respiratory distress syndrome and disseminated intravascular coagulation may become evident in severe cases of this syndrome. Treatment is primarily supportive care. Although this syndrome may occur after any total hip or total knee arthroplasty, it is more commonly seen after long-stem cemented hip arthroplasties and bilateral joint replacements.

Postoperative Pain Management

Postoperative pain management plays an extremely important role in both the short-term and long-term outcomes following hip and knee reconstruction. Blunting the intensity of the pain and the neurohumeral stress response not only improves patient satisfaction but also may be associated with shorter hospitalizations and lower pulmonary, cardiac, and central nervous system morbidity.

The goal of postoperative pain management following hip and knee reconstruction is to allow for aggressive physical therapy while minimizing both pain and stress. Therefore, a delicate balance must be achieved in terms of providing adequate analgesia without causing oversedation or motor weakness that may inhibit mobilization. The conventional routine of "on demand" parenteral narcotic administration causes a cyclical pattern of pain and analgesia that may lead to wide swings in patient comfort, sedation, and stress responses.

If general or spinal anesthesia is used, intravenous patient-controlled anesthesia (PCA) may be used postoperatively. PCA is a process by which an analgesic medication (typically a narcotic) is delivered to the patient with a device that allows the patient to control the administration, with some preset limitations programmed by the clinician.

The intraoperative use of epidural or CSE anesthesia allows the clinician to use the epidural catheter for postoperative pain management. Patient-controlled epidural anesthesia (PCEA) is the process by which a combination of dilute local anesthetic and narcotic is infused into the epidural space under the patient's control, with some preset limiting parameters. Using a combination of these 2 drug classes allows the anesthesiologist to titrate a dilute concentration of each, thereby minimizing the side effects associated with both the narcotic (respiratory depression, sedation) and the local anesthetic (motor weakness). This, in turn, will allow the patient to proceed effectively with postoperative rehabilitation.

In either case, recent studies have confirmed that a dedicated acute pain service provides superior care in terms of patient satisfaction and minimizing side effects when compared with the patient's primary service physicians. PCA and PCEA, with the addition of acetaminophen or nonsteroidal anti-inflammatory drugs, form the basis of "balanced analgesia," which is highly effective following hip and knee reconstruction.

A large percentage of patients undergoing hip and knee reconstruction require postoperative anticoagulation. Epidural hematomas have been reported following placement and removal of epidural catheters in patients receiving anticoagulants. Extreme vigilance is required while using epidural analgesia in this population. With the recent introduction of low molecular weight heparin, there have been several reports of epidural hematomas, with an incidence greater than that observed with traditional anticoagulation regimens.

Annotated Bibliography

Preanesthetic Evaluation

Williams-Russo P, Sharrock NE, Mattis S, Szatrowski TP, Charlson ME: Cognitive effects after epidural vs general anesthesia in older adults: A randomized trial. *JAMA* 1995;274: 44–50.

This is the report of a randomized trial evaluating long-term cognitive dysfunction in patients after total knee arthroplasty under epidural or general anesthesia. The authors concluded that the incidence of long-term deterioration in cognitive function was 5%, but the choice of anesthetic did not affect the outcome.

Anesthetic Techniques

Bode RH Jr, Lewis KP, Zarich SW, et al: Cardiac outcome after peripheral vascular surgery: Comparison of general and regional anesthesia. *Anesthesiology* 1996;84:3–13.

This randomized, prospective trial compared morbidity and mortality in patients undergoing peripheral vascular surgery under either regional or general anesthesia. Whereas they found no significant increase in bad outcome in either group, the authors did note a significantly higher death rate in patients who had inadequate regional anesthesia.

Anesthesia for Hip Reconstruction

Sharrock NE, Salvati EA: Hypotensive epidural anethesia for total hip arthroplasty: A review. *Acta Orthop Scand* 1996;67: 91–107.

The authors provide a comprehensive review of this anesthetic technique including practical clinical applications, as well as its effects on both patient and surgical outcome.

Anesthesia for Knee Reconstruction

Liguori GA, Sharrock NE: Asystole and severe bradycardia during epidural anesthesia in orthopedic patients. *Anesthesiology* 1997;86:250–257.

This case series highlights the patterns of onset and settings in which sudden severe bradycardia and asystole occur during and after hip and knee surgery. Several cases of severe bradycardia occur in the postanesthesia care unit setting.

Postoperative Care

Mangano DT, Layug EL, Wallace A, Tateo I: Effect of atenolol on mortality and cardiovascular morbidity after noncardiac surgery: Multicenter Study of Perioperative Ischemia Research Group. *N Engl J Med* 1996;335:1713–1720.

The authors of this landmark prospective study conclude that perioperative treatment with beta blockers in patients who have or are at risk for coronary artery disease and who must undergo major noncardiac surgery can reduce the incidence of postoperative cardiac events.

Postoperative Pain Management

Horlocker TT, Heit JA: Low molecular weight heparin: Biochemistry, pharmacology, perioperative prophylaxis regimens, and guidelines for regional anesthetic management. *Anesth Analg* 1997;85:874–885.

This is a comprehensive review of low molecular weight heparin, concentrating on specific guidelines for the management of neuraxial blockade in patients receiving this medication in the perioperative period.

Stacey BR, Rudy TE, Nelhaus D: Management of patient-controlled analgesia: A comparison of primary surgeons and a dedicated pain service. *Anesth Analg* 1997;85:130–134.

This prospective study compared practice patterns of primary service physicians and a dedicated pain service in the management of patients receiving PCA, and demonstrated important management differences between the groups.

Classic Bibliography

Caplan RA, Ward RJ, Posner K, Cheney FW: Unexpected cardiac arrest during spinal anesthesia: A closed claims analysis of predisposing factors. *Anesthesiology* 1988;68:5–11.

Covino BG, Lambert DH: Epidural and spinal anesthesia, in Barash PG, Cullen BF, Stoelting RK (eds): *Clinical Anesthesia.* Philadelphia, PA, JB Lippincott, 1989, pp 755–786.

Ereth MH, Weber JG, Abel MD, et al: Cemented versus noncemented total hip arthroplasty: Embolism, hemodynamics, and intrapulmonary shunting. *Mayo Clin Proc* 1992;67:1066–1074.

Kahn RL, Marino V, Urquhart B, Sharrock NE: Hemodynamic changes associated with tourniquet use under epidural anesthesia for total knee arthroplasty. *Reg Anesth* 1992;17:228–232.

Mangano DT: Perioperative cardiac morbidity. *Anesthesiology* 1990;72:153–184.

Patterson BM, Healey JH, Cornell CN, Sharrock NE: Cardiac arrest during hip arthroplasty with a cemented long-stem component: A report of seven cases. *J Bone Joint Surg* 1991;73A: 271–277.

Roizen MF: Preoperative evaluation. *Anesth Analg* 1994; 78(suppl):78–85.

Valli H, Rosenberg PH: Effects of three anaesthesia methods on haemodynamic responses connected with the use of thigh tourniquet in orthopaedic patients. *Acta Anaesthesiol Scand* 1985;29:142–147.

Yeager MP, Glass DD, Neff RK, Brinck-Johnsen T: Epidural anesthesia and analgesia in high-risk surgical patients. *Anesthesiology* 1987;66:729–736.

Chapter 9
Imaging

Plain Radiographs

Plain radiographs should be the first type of imaging chosen in the setting of postoperative pain, which may herald component malalignment, osteolysis or aseptic loosening, or arthroplasty infection. Although certain adjuvant studies may be obtained to confirm a clinical and/or conventional radiographic suspicion of aseptic loosening or infection, technically advanced studies do not obviate properly performed routine radiographs.

Total Knee Arthroplasty: Radiographic Appearance

The optimally placed total knee arthroplasty (TKA) should be in 7° of anatomic valgus, as measured between the mechanical axis, which is defined by a line drawn from the middle of the femoral head to the middle of the ankle joint, and the anatomic axis, which is drawn along the shaft of the femur to the middle of the knee joint and then from the middle of the knee joint to the ankle joint. The femoral component should be approximately parallel to the long axis of the femur on lateral radiographs, such that the posterior aspect of the anterior flange of the prosthesis is parallel to and confluent with the native anterior femoral cortex. The tibial component should be perpendicular to the tibial shaft on an anteroposterior radiograph, and central or slightly posterior relative to the central line of the tibial shaft on the lateral view.

It has been noted that optimal TKA results are achieved in a posterior stabilized condylar knee when the height of the patella is 10 to 30 mm, as defined by the distance of a line drawn from the tibial component articular surface to the inferior edge of the patellar resurfacing.

Conventional radiographic criteria for aseptic loosening include progressive enlargement of lucencies at the bone-cement interface, component migration or subsidence, cement fractures, and in an uncemented TKA, increasing numbers of displaced porous-coating beads. Vigilant attention to imaging technique is important in detecting lucency; the X-ray beam should be as perpendicular as possible to the bone-cement interface to increase the conspicuity of thin radiolucent lines. Comparison with previous radiographs is essential for detection of interval change in component alignment and widening of the interface. Massive lucency typically is associated with particle osteolysis.

Polyethylene wear is suspected with progressive joint space narrowing on weightbearing plain radiographs. The so-called "synovial metal line" associated with joint metallosis is indicative of abnormal metallic contact resulting from progressive wear or displacement of modular polyethylene components of the TKA.

Although no plain radiographic findings are diagnostic of infection, aggressive patterns of laminated periosteal bone formation, rapid progression of osteolysis and progressive lucency at the bone-cement interface, and scalloped endosteal resorption, in combination with clinical parameters heralding joint infection, suggest infection.

Total Hip Arthroplasty: Radiographic Appearance

The optimally placed total hip arthroplasty (THA) has cup anteversion of 15° ± 10° as measured on a lateral radiograph of the groin. Given the effect of pelvic or thigh rotation on perceived angulation, groin lateral views are helpful only in assessing for either retroversion or excessive anteversion. Similarly, groin lateral views may be helpful in determining alignment of the femoral component.

The degree of femoral anteversion can be assessed accurately with computed tomographic (CT) examination, provided an image is obtained at the level of the femoral condyles to determine rotation of the femur. However, some authors believe that the degree of version of the acetabular component is determined optimally with fluoroscopic tilting of the X-ray beam, such that with proper attention to technique and maintenance of neutral rotation of the femur, reproducible measurements of the degree of anteversion of the acetabular component may be obtained.

A thin (less than 2 mm wide) lucency at the cement-bone interface reflects the fibrous layer that forms following cement placement. This becomes stable by 2 years after surgery and is delineated from the adjacent bone by a thin line of sclerosis. As noted in evaluation of TKA, optimal plain radiographic evaluation of THA is performed using review of serial radiographs. Progressive widening of the lucent line along the cement-bone interface generally heralds formation of a granulomatous membrane associated with component loosening and/or reaction to particulate debris. Rapid progression in the change of this lucency, combined with endosteal scalloping and periosteal response, often indicates joint infection.

Radiographic signs of loosening for cemented components include progression beyond the normal thin (1 to 2 mm) radiolucent zone at the cement interface and contiguous lucency around the components, particularly with progression over time. Minimal (less than 1 cm) subsidence of the femoral component without progression over time does not necessarily imply loosening. Reported signs of greater reliability for cementless component loosening include progressive subsidence or migration of the component, particularly when accompanied by pain.

Digital acquisition of plain radiographs has led to methods for obtaining more reproducible measurements of the degree of polyethylene wear than are available with conventional radiographic techniques using circular templates. There also is a significant reduction in observer subjectivity. These techniques incorporate the filtering of digitally acquired radiographic images and the selection of coordinate points to define sampling rays emanating from the center of the femoral head. Subsequent gray scale intensity profiling along the sampling rays and postprocessing through a computer algorithm identifies the edge of the backing of the acetabular component.

Arthrography

Total Knee Arthroplasty

Sensitivity of arthrographic techniques to detect loosening following TKA is enhanced with careful attention to technique, including adequate distention of the joint with contrast and obtaining additional films following exercise. Although identification of contrast at the periprosthetic interface is suggestive of loosening, negative arthrograms do not exclude loosening as a cause of pain. Serial plain radiographs, as opposed to a single contrast arthrogram, remain the best assessment for component lucency. Some studies suggest that a concurrent radionuclide arthrogram enhances sensitivity for detecting component loosening.

Total Hip Replacement

With cemented hip components, contrast material in the bone-cement interface extending past the intertrochanteric line of the femoral component or halfway down the stem for long-stem interfaces reflected loosening of the femoral component in 98% of surgically examined prostheses. Arthrography is less sensitive, however, in detecting component loosening on the acetabular side, particularly with uncemented acetabular components. Approximately one fourth of cemented acetabular components may show contrast material at the interface in asymptomatic subjects. False positive arthrograms are more common on the acetabular side than with femoral components. The most sensitive criteria for detecting acetabular loosening include contrast material around the entire acetabular component and more than 2 mm of contrast in any zone. Conspicuity of contrast at the bone-cement interface may be enhanced using digital subtraction radiographic techniques. Arthrographic technique may be limited by seepage of contrast into outpouchings of the pseudocapsule and by accessory bursae communicating with the joints. These accessory bursae may impair adequate capsular distention and limit forced elevation of intracapsular pressure.

Aspiration arthrography, whereby fluid may be obtained from the joint and cultured, remains an important imaging test in detecting infection. Recent studies suggest that routine hip aspiration performed before revision surgery is indicated only if there is a clinical suggestion of infection, based on comprehensive history, laboratory data, and/or radiographic findings.

Computed Tomography

With the advent of more rapid data acquisition with the use of helical (spiral) CT scanning techniques, CT has proved efficacious in detection of the degree of bone loss in cases of massive osteolysis (Fig. 1). Spiral scanning techniques also permit superior reformations from direct axial acquisitions, including coronal and sagittal images as well as 3-dimensional data sets. Such techniques are helpful in detecting the degree of bone loss when potential bone grafting is necessary before revision arthroplasty.

Bone Scintigraphy

Conventional radionuclide bone scanning using technetium phosphate complexes, particularly when performed with 3-phase techniques, provides a sensitive but nonspecific measurement of increased bone turnover surrounding sites of TKA. Radionuclide angiography, performed by acquiring sequential images every 3 to 5 seconds for a period of 1 to 2 minutes after intravenous injection of the technetium phosphate complex, allows for assessment of increased blood flow to the arthroplasty. A blood pool scan obtained immediately after the angiogram allows for assessment of regional soft-tissue hyperemia. Delayed static images should be obtained at least 3 hours after injection to maximize incorporation of the

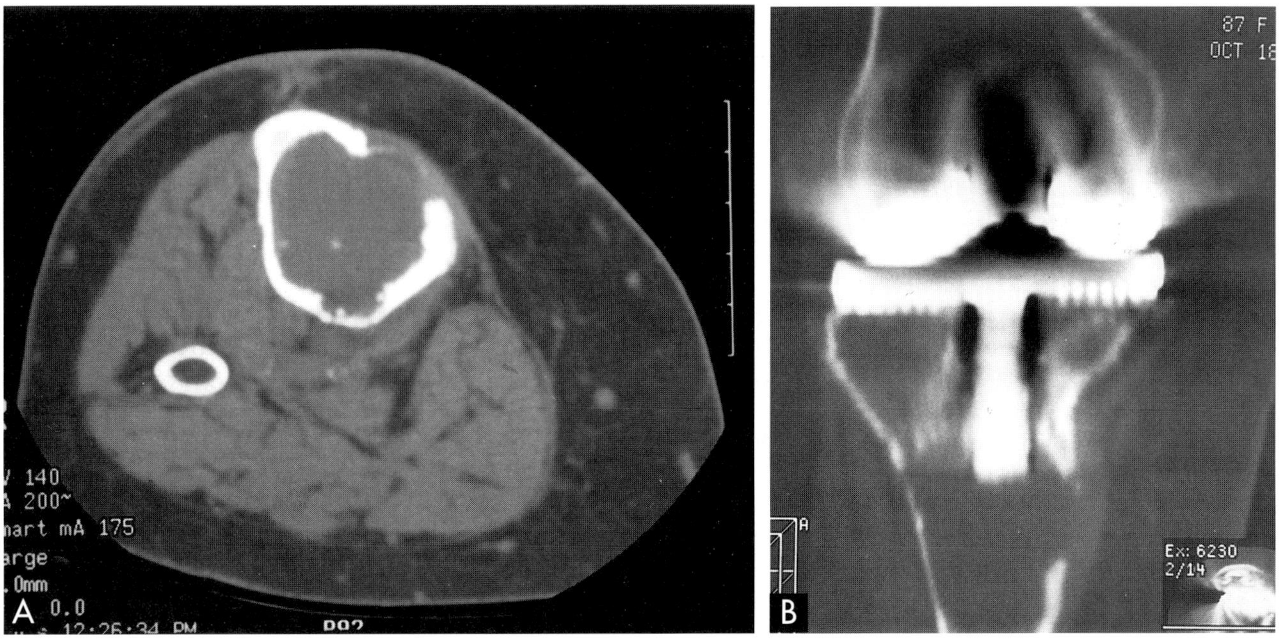

Figure 1

A, Axial computed tomography image in a patient with massive osteolysis related to particle debris. **B**, Subsequent coronal reformation demonstrates massive bone loss requiring bone grafting techniques before revision arthroplasty.

radionuclide into the hydroxyapatite matrix of bone. Although such techniques are sensitive in most series, false negative conventional bone scans have been reported in the settings of both infection and component loosening. No specific pattern of radionuclide uptake is characteristic of infection as opposed to aseptic loosening; however, a more diffuse pattern of increased radiotracer localization around the prosthesis typically is associated with infection, rather than the focal uptake associated with component loosening. Prosthetic loosening on radionuclide bone scan generally is denoted by mild to moderate increased radiotracer uptake in more than 2 radiographic zones. Serial plain radiographs remain the most effective method of detecting component loosening, but radionuclide bone scanning may be useful in cases where plain radiographs are inconclusive. There are no highly specific radiographic criteria, and the bone scan may show increased radiotracer activity around the tip of the femoral stem of uncomplicated THA for up to 2 years after surgery. As with plain radiographs, any progressive increase in the degree of radiotracer activity obtained with serial radionuclide bone scans suggests a pathologic state, either loosening or infection. Increased uptake has also been noted about uncemented acetabular components up to 2 years after surgery, with more than 75% of uncomplicated cases demonstrating increased radiotracer uptake. Similarly, TKA may show increased radiotracer activity for a variable period after uncomplicated surgery.

Infection on a radionuclide bone scan is denoted by a more diffuse pattern of uptake; however, positive cultures have been obtained from arthroplasties that demonstrated a more focal pattern. Slightly increased specificity is achieved with use of the 3 phases of radionuclide scan; however, sensitivities of only 33% have been reported. False positives include increased radiotracer activity in the presence of aseptic loosening, heterotopic bone formation, and stress fracture. In general, infection is deemed unlikely with a normal third phase bone scan and negative plain radiographs.

Gallium Scanning

Gallium-67 citrate accumulates both in infectious and noninfectious inflammatory processes because its action is largely via neutrophils. Although increased gallium localization is seen with increased bone turnover caused by infection, significant false positives exist with fracture and aseptic loosening. The combination of gallium with technetium bone scans has slightly increased accuracy for detecting infection. Combined scans are considered positive if uptake is spatially incongruent (increased gallium uptake where no significant increased technetium activity is noted) or the gallium uptake is more intense than the technetium uptake on spatially congruent scans. It has been reported, however, that less than one third of patients demonstrate either of these 2 patterns, limiting the predictive value of the combined gallium-technetium bone scan.

White Blood Cell Scanning

White blood cell scanning combined with technetium bone scans is more specific than sequential technetium bone and gallium scans for the diagnosis of infection. However, as seen with gallium, there are significant false positives, because indium may localize in uninfected reticuloendothelial tissue, such as the marrow of heterotopic ossification. In addition, white cell scans are most efficacious when the cellular response is primarily granulocytic, as in the setting of an acute or severe infection. In a low-grade infection, as is typical of delayed arthroplasty infection, the inflammatory response is primary lymphocytic, leading to potential false negatives. In addition, indium may localize in periprosthetic fracture, as well as in uncomplicated in-growth hip prostheses for up to 2 years. Again, the hallmark of an infected arthroplasty is either spatial incongruency between the technetium bone scan and the white cell scan, or more intense activity on the white cell scan. Postoperative alterations in bone marrow may lead to misinterpretation of indium localization, because indium may localize in marrow that is not infected. Redistribution of the cellular marrow after arthroplasty may be determined using concomitant radiolabelled colloid scan.

Experimental radionuclide agents include indium-labeled human polyclonal immunoglobulin (Ig), which has a reported sensitivity similar to that of radiolabeled white cell scans, but has the slight disadvantage of a decrease in target-to-background activity. Because preparation is easier and less time consuming than for white cell scans, Ig scans have some promise but are not yet approved by the Food and Drug Administration for routine clinical use in the United States, and the potential for induction of anti IgG antibodies may preclude serial scanning techniques. Additional experimental agents include streptavidin and indium-111-biotin, which demonstrate more rapid target-to-background accumulation. However, no large series has been reported showing superior accuracy in detecting soft-tissue infection. Clearly, the most specific technique by which to detect prosthetic infection remains joint aspiration with positive joint culture.

Ultrasound

The development of high-frequency transducers and digitized ultrasound images has enabled the expansion of ultrasound beyond conventional vascular imaging techniques. Ultrasound has been used extensively outside the United States to assess tendinous attachments, including the extensor mechanism and patellar tendon following arthroplasty. Ultrasound scanning techniques are made more appealing by applying dynamic contraction of muscle groups during image acquisition.

Cortical bone is echogenic and fluid is echolucent, yielding transmission of the ultrasound beam through the fluid collection. This permits reliable differentiation between the margins of cortical bone and adjacent fluid collections. In the setting of an infected arthroplasty, ultrasound is effective in detecting small loculated fluid collections and in tracking abscess collections beyond the confines of the joint into the pelvis or thigh. In addition, ultrasound has been used in THA to detect normal and abnormal pseudocapsules. In a small population, an increased distance between the anterior cortex of the femur and the pseudocapsule correlated with infection, as opposed to aseptic loosening. Although these results are preliminary, ultrasound shows promise in serving as an additional noninvasive test to evaluate the painful arthroplasty.

An ultrasound method also has been devised to detect polyethylene component wear in TKA patients. A characteristic bone-metal-polyethylene interface permits recognition of the polyethylene spacer and measurement of its dimensions. Consecutive measurements may be obtained to assess the degree of polyethylene wear more accurately than by measurement of progressive joint space narrowing on plain radiographs. These results also are preliminary; however, ultrasound may serve as a useful noninvasive technique to detect progressive liner wear.

Magnetic Resonance Imaging

Evaluation of TKA and THA with magnetic resonance imaging (MRI) has largely been limited by the susceptibility artifact created by the implants, which causes marked disturbance of the local magnetic field. More recently designed phased array coils, which inherently provide superior signal to noise, as well as software modifications that refocus the local field inhomogeneities induced by the arthroplasty allow for reproducible depiction of surrounding soft tissues. Additional techniques by which artifact reduction is achieved include the use of a wider receiver bandwidth, minimizing echo time, keeping the long axis of the frequency encoding gradient parallel to the long axis of the prosthesis, longer echo train length, and other techniques that diminish interecho spacing and subsequent signal decay.

The relative ferromagnetism of the components is less of a factor in the degree of artifact encountered than the orientation of the component relative to the long axis of the magnetic field (running parallel to the patient on a high magnetic field system). For this reason, complex revision THA cases generally encounter more imaging artifact than primary THA, and greater artifact is seen surrounding acetabular (as opposed to femoral) components of THA. Although susceptibility artifact is minimized on an open, lower magnetic field system, concurrent reduction of inherent signal to noise on the lower field strength system tends to minimize the lower field advantage.

When appropriate imaging techniques are used, adjacent soft tissues may be made apparent. Given the inherent superior soft-tissue contrast and direct multiplanar capabilities of MRI, it is superior to CT or ultrasound in characterizing soft-tissue masses surrounding knee or hip arthroplasty (Fig. 2). The characteristic paramagnetic effect of hemosiderin debris creates focal field disturbance, making MRI a suitable tool in detecting recurrent synovitis in cases of TKA performed for pigmented villonodular synovitis.

Patients with THA who have repeated posterior dislocations despite acceptable component alignment on plain radiographs pose a difficult problem for the hip surgeon. Using specialized MRI technique, the integrity of the posterior or soft-tissue envelope may be assessed, including the continuity of the pseudocapsule and integrity of the short external rotator muscles. Evaluation of these supporting structures may provide insight for the observed recurrent instability in this patient group.

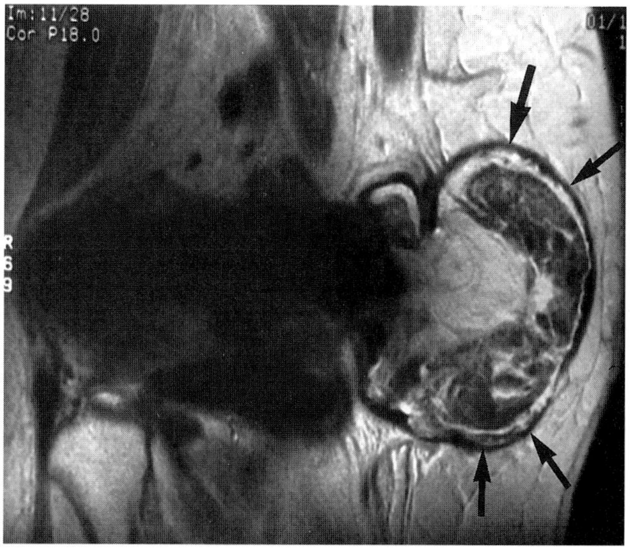

Figure 2

Coronal fast spin echo magnetic resonance image through posterior aspect of cemented total knee arthroplasty demonstrates a complex soft-tissue mass (arrows) at the medial joint space. The thick, hypointense rind with intermediate signal intensity debris as well as the central hyperintense debris is indicative of an organized granuloma. At surgical exploration, a polyethylene granuloma was removed.

MRI may also be used to assess the extent of the cement mantle in revision arthroplasty and to detect the proximity of extravasated intrapelvic cement to adjacent neurovascular structures without the characteristic beam hardening streak artifact seen on CT examinations. Similar to ultrasound, MRI may be used in the setting of fulminant or extra-articular spread of infection to detect small microabcesses and sinus tracks. MRI may also detect loculated collections or infected hematomas surrounding a joint arthroplasty that is refractory to conservative antibiotic management. Because of the increased cost of MRI when compared to conventional imaging techniques, routine MRI to detect arthroplasty infection is not currently warranted.

Magnetic Resonance Venography

The traditional imaging standard for detection of deep vein thrombosis (DVT) following TKA and THA is conventional contrast venography. However, conventional venography obtained by cannulation of the dorsal foot vein is limited in assessment of pelvic thrombosis, largely because of contrast dilution by unopacified pelvic veins. In addition, there is a potential risk of contrast allergy, regional soft-tissue damage created by potential extravasation of contrast at the site of venopuncture, and postvenographic thrombosis. Direct femoral venopuncture will provide superior depiction of pelvic veins; however, it is an invasive procedure that raises concerns about soft-tissue bleeding and/or infection over an area of recently performed THA. The importance of screening for DVT lies in the fact that patients will have clinically evident pulmonary emboli despite negative conventional screening techniques, including duplex color ultrasound and conventional contrast venography. It is apparent that the deep pelvic veins may serve as a source for occult thromboemboli.

Ultrasound is also a well established method for detecting DVT following joint arthroplasty. Although prior series comparing contrast venography to color Doppler indicate sensitivities of only 62%, improved scanning techniques and the addition of color flow as an imaging standard to traditional duplex Doppler ultrasound techniques significantly improve sensitivity in depicting proximal thrombi. Ultrasound, however, remains highly operator dependent, with accuracy varying widely depending on the expertise of the technician and on the equipment available. In addition, ultrasound is somewhat limited in detecting deep pelvic thrombosis given the limited compressibility of the pelvic veins, and in the immediate postoperative setting, the presence of associated ileus and bowel distention may cause reflection of the ultrasound beam.

Given these limitations, magnetic resonance venography (MRV) has recently been proposed as an additional noninvasive test by which to detect occult pelvic and thigh thrombi (Fig. 3). Whereas MRV has been studied in the trauma population, showing superior ability in detecting pelvic thrombi compared to conventional contrast venography, its application to the arthroplasty population has been limited. A recent study evaluating 191 patients following total joint arthroplasty with both MRV and standard contrast venography reported an initial limited (5/11 or 45%) sensitivity of MRV in detecting proximal thrombi; however, subsequent retrospective review of the MR venograms by a dedicated MR radiologist improved sensitivity to 91% (10/11). Clearly, detection of thrombi using MR venographic techniques requires an experienced MR radiologist with knowledge of potential vascular artifacts, which impair accurate image interpretation. Despite these limitations, MRV remains a promising technique to depict pelvic DVT. Artifactual reduction of signal surrounding the metallic acetabular component of THA has initially been reported as a potential pitfall for evaluating these patients. The advent of MRV with gadolinium contrast agents that have minimized echo times bypasses many of the velocity-dependent phase shifts and flow artifacts encountered in traditional MRV techniques and reduces magnetic susceptibility artifact, which may preclude visualization of the external iliac veins adjacent to the acetabular component. These techniques have been used in a small cohort of patients with success, achieving superior detection of pelvic veins adjacent to the acetabular components. Further study is warranted using these techniques, in order to assess their efficacy as well as to determine the true prevalence of pelvic thrombi following total joint arthroplasty.

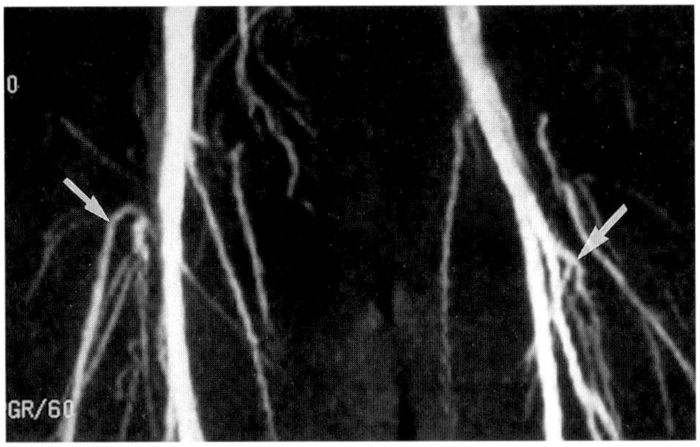

Figure 3

Maximum intensity projection magnetic resonance venographic image in a patient with bilateral THAs demonstrates superior visualization of the profunda femoris vessels (arrows), compared with conventional contrast venographic techniques obtained via dorsal foot vein cannulation. A venogram of both thighs may be obtained simultaneously with magnetic resonance venography.

Summary

With advances in imaging technology, new imaging tests have become available for evaluating the painful joint arthroplasty. Refinement in transducers has permitted superior resolution of surrounding soft-tissue structures using noninvasive ultrasound, and refinements in surface coil development and software reduction in susceptibility artifact from metallic components has allowed for MRI of total joints. However, the increased availability of sophisticated imaging tests does not preclude properly performed serial plain radiographs, which often have the best predictive value in evaluating for potential joint infection and aseptic loosening. Specialized MRI should be reserved for select cases, including evaluation for spread of infection beyond the joint space, assessing the soft-tissue envelope in cases of recurrent dislocation, or tissue characterization of soft-tissue masses surrounding joint arthroplasty. MRV techniques show superior sensitivity in detecting occult pelvic thrombi, but a larger series needs to be reported, with evaluation by experienced MR angiographers to assess the true prevalence of pelvic thrombosis in the immediate postarthroplasty setting.

Annotated Bibliography

Chik KK, Magee MA, Bruce WJ, et al: Tc-99m stannous colloid-labeled leukocyte scintigraphy in the evaluation of the painful arthroplasty. *Clin Nucl Med* 1996;21:838–843.

The authors evaluate the utility of leukocytes labeled with technetium 99m stannous colloid in the assessment of painful hip and knee arthroplasty. These techniques yielded a sensitivity of 70%, specificity of 100%, and diagnostic accuracy of 93%, which was improved compared to conventional bone scintigraphy.

Larcom PG, Lotke PA, Steinberg ME, Holland G, Foster S: Magnetic resonance venography versus contrast venography to diagnose thrombosis after joint surgery. *Clin Orthop* 1996;331: 209–215.

The authors evaluated 207 extremities (191 patients) with both conventional contrast and magnetic resonance venography. Initial prospective evaluation of magnetic resonance venograms yielded relative poor sensitivity (5/11, 45%) in detecting thrombi; subsequent retrospective review by experienced magnetic resonance angiographers detected 10/11 DVTs (91%). This report underscores the necessity for an experienced magnetic resonance radiologist to evaluate magnetic resonance venographic images.

Potter HG, Montgomery KD, Padgett DE, Salvati EA, Helfet DL: Magnetic resonance imaging of the pelvis: New orthopaedic applications. *Clin Orthop* 1995;319:223–231.

The authors report a preliminary study of the use of magnetic resonance venography in a small patient population, showing superior ability of magnetic resonance venography to detect pelvic thrombi compared to conventional techniques, including contrast venography and color Doppler ultrasound. In addition, the authors report new magnetic resonance techniques that permit visualization of the soft-tissue envelope surrounding total hip arthroplasty in patients having recurrent dislocations despite acceptable component alignment.

Schneider R, Gruen D, Brause B: Diagnosis of infected joint prostheses. *Semin Arthroplasty* 1995;6:167–175.

The authors provide a review of radiographic diagnosis of infected arthroplasty, with an emphasis on scintigraphic techniques, and caution that no single imaging test is consistently diagnostic of arthroplasty infection.

Shaver SM, Brown TD, Hillis SL, Callaghan JJ: Digital edge-detection measurement of polyethylene wear after total hip arthroplasty. *J Bone Joint Surg* 1997;79A:690–700.

A unique digital edge-detecting computer technique is described to measure polyethylene wear following total hip arthroplasty. Gradients of gray scale intensity on digitized radiographs are used. Digital edge detection proved more reproducible than manual measurement with conventional circular techniques, providing more accuracy in measurement of polyethylene wear.

Weissman BN: Imaging of total hip replacement. *Radiology* 1997;202:611–623.

The author provides a comprehensive review of plain radiographic, arthrographic and scintigraphic assessment of total hip arthroplasty, with a comprehensive review of current literature.

Yashar AA, Adler RS, Grady-Benson JC, Matthews LS, Freiberg AA: An ultrasound method to evaluate polyethylene component wear in total knee replacement arthroplasty. *Am J Orthop* 1996;25:702–704.

The authors report the use of ultrasound in a cadaveric model to detect polyethylene wear following total knee arthroplasty. High correlation was obtained between ultrasound derived measurements and direct measurements made by electronic caliper.

Classic Bibliography

Ghelman B: Three methods for determining anteversion and retroversion of a total hip prosthesis. *Am J Roentgenol* 1979;133:1127–1134.

Oyen WJ, Claessens RA, van Horn JR, vander Meer JW, Corstens FH: Scintigraphic detection of bone and joint infections with indium-111-labeled nonspecific polyclonal human immunoglobulin G. *J Nucl Med* 1990;31:403–412.

Seabold JE, Nepola JV, Marsh JL, et al: Postoperative bone marrow alterations: Potential pitfalls in the diagnosis of osteomyelitis with In-111-labeled leukocyte scintigraphy. *Radiology* 1991;180:741–747.

van Holsbeeck MT, Eyler WR, Sherman LS, et al: Detection of infection in loosened hip prostheses: Efficacy of sonography. *Am J Roentgenol* 1994;163:381–384.

Chapter 10 Outcomes Assessment in Hip and Knee Replacement

Introduction

The term "outcome" has become a buzzword to somehow connote more inherent significance or scientific reliability than the more traditional term "result". Orthopaedic surgeons have a long tradition of measuring and recording the results of their treatment as evidenced by the wide variety of hip and knee scales and scores. What new understanding can be gained using the term outcome? The study of outcomes is characterized by a broadening of the definitions of the surgical results from a strictly clinical context to the economic, social, and political consequences. This chapter deals with aspects of the growth and development of the outcomes movement as it relates to the practice of hip and knee arthroplasty, with the objective being to show that total hip and knee replacement is an excellent example of how the investigation of practice variations manifested in the differing rates for surgical procedures, the measurement of outcome, and the consideration of cost can help demonstrate the actual value of a particular technology and guide future efforts to continuously improve the quality of care.

Geographic Variation

A major event in the modern outcomes movement was when the significant variation in rates of certain surgical procedures performed within the context of relatively small geographic areas, referred to as Hospital Service Areas, were analyzed and reported. In 1982, total knee replacement was 1.75 times more likely and total hip replacement was 1.5 times more likely to be performed in Boston, MA. Demonstrating this variation called attention to the fact that there appears to be either uncertainty or disagreement regarding actual surgical indications. Surgeons confronted with these findings may be annoyed by outsiders who know little about the particulars of clinical care or the technical features of surgery. It may seem unlikely that by analyzing an administrative database that it could be concluded that the indications for a surgical procedure are actually poorly understood, and further, that a procedure may be overutilized in some areas. The question is, "Which rate is right?"

Defining precisely the correct indications for surgical procedures has not been an easy task. For total hip replacement alone there have been 2 National Institutes of Health Consensus Conferences in the last 20 years that have focused on the issues such as indications, technical solutions, complications, and outcomes. At each conference it was noted that the outcomes of surgery are not well understood because the measurements of the patients' health and functional status have been highly variable and imprecise. A conclusion shared at both conferences was that the reasons for the inability to define surgical indications more precisely are linked to a nonuniform and undefined system of outcomes measurement. It is important to know how a given surgical procedure will benefit the patient compared to an array of alternative treatments, or to no treatment at all. This benefit can only be accurately calculated by application of valid clinical measurement before and after treatment. Large-scale outcomes data of this sort are essential to compare with geographic variation data because of the importance of the issues involved here. For example, if, in an area of unusually high rates of total hip or knee replacement such as several of the western states, preoperative patient symptoms and function are better than the norm, and the outcomes are the same, a case could be made that surgery was being performed too early in the course of arthritis. Alternatively, patients in high rate areas have easier access to surgery and are influenced by good outcomes and patient satisfaction, and are more likely to seek treatment earlier. On the other hand, a comparatively low rate area may comprise patients who are significantly worse preoperatively, but whose results are also worse. Therefore, the benefit obtained from surgery is the same, but in one area more patients are being operated on early, and in the other the outcomes are worse and because of poor outcomes, limited access, or both, patients may wait longer for surgery. These hypothetical situations demonstrate the importance of obtaining clinical outcomes data to correlate with purely administrative data. There are many potential reasons for a variation of observed clinical outcomes. As the allocation of health care resources becomes more restricted and therefore more political, the importance of having rational explanations for phenomena such as geographic variations increases exponentially. Unlike many surgical procedures, total hip and knee replacement may very likely be underutilized in certain areas such as the inner city where the rates are lowest. Unfortunately, the most expedient assumption among health policy makers is that all high rates reflect inappropriate surgery. Orthopaedic surgeons as patient advocates, and as deliverers of these two highly cost effective procedures, need to find ways to aggregate valid outcomes data into databases that are powerful enough to match the global magnitude of currently used administrative databases that focus primarily on utilization and cost of health services.

Modern Outcomes Assessment

Instrument Validation and Data Aggregation

The fundamental principle guiding the development of modern outcomes assessment is that uniform and valid instruments should be used to collect outcomes data. Orthopaedic surgeons have been leaders in the systematic collection of data that documents the patient's preoperative and postoperative level of pain and functional impairment. The proliferation of hip and knee scales and scores attests to the widespread interest in this type of outcomes assessment. Several validated instruments are available that are patient-administered questionnaires and therefore capable of being used reliably in large populations without the problem of interobserver variability, which compromises the value of traditional hip and knee scores. The questionnaires are used to measure comorbidity, general health status, functional impairment, and levels of pain that may be general body pain, or referred to specific areas such as the hip or knee. A major issue of laterality (left or right), which is missing from large administrative databases such as Medicare, may also be addressed in modern clinical outcomes assessment for the purposes of documentation and tracking of individual joints in the same patient. Surgeon-generated information regarding procedures performed and complications are also essential. In older Medicare data, a total knee replacement 3 months after a contralateral primary replacement cannot be distinguished from a reoperation for early failure without significant work to examine hospital-specific data.

General Health Status Assessment

The SF-36 has become widely accepted in medicine as the "industry standard" in measuring patients' general health status. It was validated as part of the Medical Outcomes Study, an observational study conducted between 1986 and 1990 on adult patients in Boston, Chicago, and Los Angeles. Over 2,500 patients were surveyed at 6-month intervals over a 2-year period to provide normative age-adjusted health status data that can be used in outcomes assessment. The short form, containing 36 questions, emerged from this process. It contains 8 scales that measure physical function, role limitations caused by physical impairment, body pain, general health, vitality, social function, role limitations caused by emotional problems, and mental health. These scales can be consolidated into the physical component summary (PCS) and mental health component summary (MCS) scales. In 2 separate studies, Ritter and associates and McGuigan and associates have demonstrated statistically significant improvement in most SF-36 subscales. The PCS has been shown to be the most sensitive to patient improvement with either hip or knee replacement, but the MCS has also been shown to improve, and it may have some predictive value for the ultimate outcome of surgery.

Disease- and Region-Specific Questionnaires

Although the SF-36 is useful in demonstrating the benefit of total hip and knee replacement, especially when compared with other high volume or high profile surgery such as coronary artery bypass and transplantation, it does not specifically address the hip or knee status with the specificity of traditional hip and knee scores. The Western Ontario and McMaster University Osteoarthritis Index (WOMAC) is a disease- and region-specific questionnaire that was developed and validated in patients who have osteoarthritis of the hip or knee. The WOMAC contains 3 domains: pain (5 questions), stiffness (2 questions), and physical function (17 questions). The questions in the WOMAC refer to the same issues that are addressed by many of the traditionally used hip and knee scales, and therefore it has gained wide acceptance among orthopaedic surgeons. Laupacis and associates have shown that total hip replacement resulted in improvement in all 3 WOMAC domains. Ninety of these patients were followed for 2 years, at which time improvement was also noted in general health status and global health-related quality of life. The major problem with the WOMAC is that when used with the SF-36 there is significant overlap in content of questions dealing with functional impairment (in performing activities such as stairs, walking, housework, bending or kneeling, bathing, and shopping). A critical issue with patient-administered questionnaires is the so-called "respondent burden", or number of questions, that may limit the patient's willingness to fill out the form. There must be an effort to limit the length of questionnaires and the time required to complete them if the collection of outcomes data is to have widespread application.

In 1994, the American Academy of Orthopaedic Surgeons™ (AAOS), in conjunction with the Council on Musculoskeletal Subspecialty Societies, convened a meeting in Tarpon Springs, Florida, to form task forces that would develop questionnaire-based outcome assessment instruments for the spine, upper extremity, lower extremity, and pediatrics. The Lower Extremity Instrument was tested for reproducibility in 1995, and sensitivity in 1996 and 1997. Its original length has been significantly reduced during the validation process. It now contains a core of 7 questions (3 pain, 1 swelling, 1 stiffness, 2 function) that can be attributed either to the lower extremity in general, or to specific joints such as the foot and ankle, knee, or hip. Sports and foot and ankle modules containing additional questions were developed to supplement the core questions and enhance its sensitivity to change after treatment. The hip and knee module is capable of tracking the 3 pain questions for each individual hip and knee. The significant benefit of the AAOS Lower Extremity Instrument is that there is no overlap with the SF-36; therefore, respondent burden has been minimized without compromising the content or face validity of the data set.

Large Scale Databases

The explosion of powerful computer technology and data transmission capability has changed the face of medical record-keeping and clinical research. Whereas computerized health care data was predominantly administrative, and seemed far removed from the examining room or the patient's bedside, newer concepts in care, such as clinical pathways, practice guidelines, and electronic medical records designed to maximize and standardize clinical data capture, offer the prospect of merging large amounts of clinical data. One important goal of outcomes research is to match the supply of health care resources with the national and local need, and to continuously educate the public in a way that will modulate demand. This goal does not necessarily conflict professionally or ethically with what clinicians want to do for their patients. It is likely that better data on hip and knee replacement would strengthen the case for wider access to the procedures.

The Hip and Knee Registry

The problems with constructing high-quality, large-scale clinical outcomes databases are numerous. The legal and ethical dilemmas, and the issue of confidentiality, inherent in collecting sensitive patient data for national or international quality improvement are only beginning to be publicly debated. Despite these issues, the Hip and Knee Registry, initiated in 1995, has collected outcomes data on over 13,000 patients who underwent hip or knee replacement surgery performed by over 350 surgeons in North America. The core outcome instruments used in this database are the SF-36 and the WOMAC. Demographic, comorbidity, and technical data are also collected. At 1-year follow-up, patients with both hip and knee replacements have shown substantial improvements in the SF-36 (PCS) and the WOMAC. The Hip and Knee Registry has demonstrated the feasibility of building large-scale physician-controlled databases for joint replacement. Because the cost is high, long-term funding for these databases needs to be secured. In addition, accurate and comprehensive physician profiling as to the type of practice, overall surgical volume, and other issues is necessary to confirm the ability to generalize the data. The profiling data is necessary to confirm the ability to generalize the data, is not included in the Hip and Knee Registry, and is a controversial topic for many medical professionals. Without accurate information about doctors and hospitals to stratify and adjust the case mix, interpretations of administrative data may be misleading. The data for 8,774 hip replacements performed between 1988 and 1991 that were contained in a statewide hospital discharge registry in Washington were studied. There was a significant increase in the mortality and complication rate among low volume surgeons and hospitals (volumes of hip replacement below the 40th percentile). An implied conclusion to this study was that regionalization of hip and knee replacement should be considered. The findings of the study need to be confirmed by other studies using data from other states, hopefully with more information regarding the profiles of the surgeons and hospitals.

AAOS MODEMS Project

The AAOS has initiated a musculoskeletal database that includes the outcome assessment instruments already mentioned and including demographic patient data, comorbidity, and a physician and practice profile. As part of version 2.0 released in 1998, MODEMS-HK was introduced. This package was developed jointly by the AAOS and American Association of Hip and Knee Surgeons specifically for outcomes assessment of hip and knee replacement. It contains the Lower Extremity Instrument with attribution of pain to either left or right, hip or knee. In addition, a physical examination form, hip and knee surgical forms, and discharge and postdischarge complication forms are included. Future developments may add important modules such as a validated radiographic severity analysis for stratification of the technical difficulty of surgical cases. In contrast to the paper and pencil-based Hip and Knee Registry, MODEMS has contracted with computer software vendors who have adopted

MODEMS specifications and who offer a variety of office-based options that facilitate the integration of outcomes assessment into daily practice. Because of the additional time and work involved with implementing office-based outcomes assessment, it is widely believed that full integration is necessary for success. The integration of clinical outcomes data with utilization and billing will assist in a better local understanding of a practice's costs and effectiveness. This will become significant as total joint surgeons become more closely affiliated with hospitals that are accepting global payments from third parties such as the federal government. The recent initiative of the Health Care Financing Administration to establish "Centers of Excellence" for total hip and knee replacement is an example of a global approach to a definable episode of care. So far the emphasis has been on discounted rates that could possibly be offset by the increased volume that would occur as a result of being called a center of excellence. A glaring deficiency in this plan is that excellence in total hip and knee replacement has yet to be defined well enough to allow such an attribution to any center. Valid outcomes data collection, amalgamation, and dissemination is essential for this process to include quality as the important variable that it needs to be. MODEMS is a system of data collection that potentially could address this problem.

Conclusion

The current era of health care has been deemed one of assessment and accountability. During the last decade managed care has dictated the terms of assessment and has held physicians and hospitals accountable for carrying out an agenda that for the most part has removed the "capital" from the health care system and placed it in the open arms of outside investors. Now the pressure is mounting for the managed care industry to be more responsive to the rights of the patient. As beneficial as this development may be, the fundamental issue of quality, particularly in total hip and knee replacement, has yet to be seriously addressed. The cost of outcomes assessment in terms of time and money has been a major impediment. No one is eager to pay the price. But the price of not using available technology to implement a rational system of quality improvement is also high, and ultimately may be shouldered by the patient. As advocates for quality patient care, orthopaedic surgeons should make this issue the top priority.

Annotated Bibliography

American Academy of Orthopaedic Surgeons™, American Association of Hip and Knee Surgeons: MODEMS-HK Outcomes data collection module Version 2.0, 1997.

This module contains essential data elements for assessing outcomes of total hip and knee replacement. Included in the package are demographics, comorbidity, satisfaction, Lower Limb core questionnaire with attribution of pain to left, right, hip, and knee; SF-36, physical examination, hip surgical form, knee surgical form, discharge summary, and postdischarge complications. This data can be transmitted to a central site as part of the MODEMS program.

Johanson NA: Outcomes assessment, in Callaghan JJ, Rosenberg AG, Rubash HE (eds): *The Adult Hip.* Philadelphia, PA, Lippincott-Raven, 1998, vol 2, pp 853–863.

Outcomes movement as it relates to total hip replacement is reviewed. Issues addressed include expansion and variation of health care services, cost containment, managed care, guideline development, outcomes assessment instrument development, and amalgamation of clinical data into large-scale outcomes databases.

Kreder HJ, Deyo RA, Koepsell T, Swiontkowski MF, Kreuter W: Relationship between the volume of total hip replacements performed by providers and the rates of postoperative complications in the state of Washington. *J Bone Joint Surg* 1997;79A:485–494.

This important study documents the relationship between volume of total hip replacement of both hospitals and surgeons, and complications. However, the study is cross-sectional and does not track the complication rate over time and relate it to a rising or falling volume. This study is more difficult to perform, but essential to complete the analysis.

Lieberman JR, Dorey F, Shekelle P, et al: Differences between patients' and physicians' evaluations of outcome after total hip arthroplasty. *J Bone Joint Surg* 1996;78A:835–838.

This article reports on the discrepancy between physician- and patient-generated evaluations of the results of total hip replacement. When the result was good and the patient was experiencing little or no pain, patient and the physician evaluations were similar. In patients whose own evaluations were fair or poor and there was significant pain, the discrepancy between the patients' and the physicians' rating increased. This landmark article calls into question the validity of traditional methods of scoring for measuring the outcomes of hip replacement. It tends to complement the findings for the knee in McGrory and associates.

Mancuso CA, Ranawat CS, Esdaile JM, Johanson NA, Charlson ME: Indications for total hip and total knee arthroplasties: Results of orthopaedic surveys. *J Arthroplasty* 1996;11:34–46.

This article uses a survey technique to demonstrate the range of indications for total hip and knee replacement that are used among orthopaedic surgeons in New York City and in Canada. A striking finding was that Canadian surgeons tended to require more frequent pain and use of assistive devices for walking before considering surgery. Although a clear consensus for indications using precise criteria was not found, it was concluded that an integration of factors such as symptoms and functional impairment with the patient's desire to proceed with surgery was most likely an important driving force.

Mancuso CA, Salvati EA, Johanson NA, Peterson MG, Charlson ME: Patients' expectations and satisfaction with total hip arthroplasty. *J Arthroplasty* 1997;12:387–396.

This study reports on the results of 180 patient surveys 2 to 3 years after total hip replacement. Eighty-nine percent of patients were satisfied with the results. Lower levels of satisfaction were found among those patients who had better preoperative hip rating scores, and who had expected improvement in nonessential activities. It was concluded that patient satisfaction is a complex phenomenon, affected by expectations, actual outcome, and what patients know about the procedure from their community network.

MacWilliam CH, Yood MU, Verner JJ, McCarthy BD, Ward RE: Patient-related risk factors that predict poor outcome after total hip replacement. *Health Serv Res* 1996;31:623–638.

Factors that were found to be associated with a poor outcome in this report from the American Medical Group Association were race, education, and number of comorbid conditions. This finding underscores the necessity of collecting sufficient demographic and comorbidity data to adequately stratify the population under study. In addition, when the preoperative scores on the Health Status Questionnaire were high, there was less likelihood of achieving a sufficient benefit from surgery. For each increment of 10 points preoperatively there was an average of 6 points less benefit obtained.

McGrory BJ, Morrey BF, Rand JA, Ilstrup DM: Correlation of patient questionnaire responses and physician history in grading clinical outcome following hip and knee arthroplasty: A prospective study of 201 joint arthroplasties. *J Arthroplasty* 1996;11: 47–57.

This study compares the results of physician-generated hip and knee scores with those of a patient-administered questionnaire. Patient responses were more closely correlated with physician evaluations on hip evaluation than in the knee, where physicians gave significantly higher knee scores than patients.

McGuigan FX, Hozack WJ, Moriarty L, Eng K, Rothman RH: Predicting quality-of-life outcomes following total joint arthroplasty: Limitations of the SF-36 Health Status Questionnaire. *J Arthroplasty* 1995;10:742–747.

The SF-36 was administered to 114 hip and knee replacement patients preoperatively and 2 years postoperatively. Significant improvement in physical function, social function, physical role function, emotional role function, mental health, energy, and pain were noted. A predictive relationship between any of the health concepts measured preoperatively and the 2-year outcome was not found, and therefore it was concluded that the SF-36 would not be helpful in determining specific indications for surgery.

Ritter MA, Albohm MJ, Keating EM, Faris PM, Meding JB: Comparative outcomes of total joint arthroplasty. *J Arthroplasty* 1995;10:737–741.

The SF-36 was administered preoperatively, 6 months, 1 year, and 2 years postoperatively to 85 hip replacement patients and 158 knee replacement patients. Significant improvements occurred in all 8 health concepts, with no difference noted between hip and knee replacements.

Classic Bibliography

Johanson NA, Charlson ME, Szatrowski TP, Ranawat CS: A self-administered hip-rating questionnaire for the assessment of outcome after total hip replacement. *J Bone Joint Surg* 1992;74A: 587–597.

Keller RB: Outcomes research in orthopaedics. *J Am Acad Orthop Surg* 1993;1:122–129.

Laupacis A, Bourne R, Rorabeck C, et al: The effect of elective total hip replacement on health-related quality of life. *J Bone Joint Surg* 1993;75A:1619–1626.

Peterson MG, Hollenberg JP, Szatrowski TP, Johanson NA, Mancuso CA, Charlson ME: Geographic variations in the rates of elective total hip and knee arthroplasties among Medicare beneficiaries in the United States. *J Bone Joint Surg* 1992; 74A:1530–1539.

Wennberg J: Which rate is right? *N Engl J Med* 1986;314: 310–311.

Wright JG, Rudicel S, Feinstein AR: Ask patients what they want: Evaluation of individual complaints before total hip replacement. *J Bone Joint Surg* 1994;76B:229–234.

Section 2
The Hip

Chapter 11
Surgical Approaches and Anatomic Considerations

Chapter 12
Biomechanics of the Hip and Hip Reconstruction

Chapter 13
Osteotomy

Chapter 14
Design Evolution—Cemented Total Hip Replacement

Chapter 15
Evolution of Uncemented Femoral Component Design

Chapter 16
Osteonecrosis—Etiology, Pathophysiology and Treatment

Chapter 17
Deep Infection Complicating Total Hip Arthroplasty

Chapter 18
Dislocation

Chapter 19
Complications in Total Hip Arthroplasty

Chapter 20
Mechanical Failure—Loosening and Wear

Chapter 21
Osteolysis

Chapter 22
Results of Cemented Total Hip Replacement

Chapter 23
Cementless Primary Total Hip Arthroplasty

Chapter 24
Hybrid Total Hip Replacement

Chapter 25
Revision Total Hip Replacement

Chapter 11 Surgical Approaches and Anatomic Considerations

When considering hip surgery, the type of approach depends on factors such as extent of exposure required (iliac, acetabular, femoral), presence of scars from prior incisions, quality of tissue and skin, range of motion, leg length discrepancy, comorbid neuromuscular conditions, and the surgeon's goals and experience. Basic surgical approaches commonly used in North America include the direct lateral (Hardinge), anterior (Smith-Petersen), anterolateral (Watson-Jones), and posterior (Langenbeck/Moore). Extensive exposures, such as the trochanteric slide, vastus slide, and extended trochanteric osteotomy, may be required in revision arthroplasty.

General Principles

All exposures require positioning of the patient to ensure that potential pressure points are padded, the pelvis is immobilized, and the hip can move freely during surgery. The surgical pathology may show that conversion to a more extensive exposure may be necessary. Skin and soft-tissue problems can be minimized by incorporating scars from previous incisions or observing wide skin bridges, using internervous planes where possible, and using surgical drains to minimize hematoma formation in the postoperative period.

Anterior (Iliofemoral/Smith-Petersen) Approach

This exposure dissects the interval between the sartorius and rectus femoris muscles (femoral nerve innervation) and the tensor fascia lata and gluteus minimus and medius muscles (superior gluteal innervation). The anterior approach remains lateral to the sensory lateral femoral cutaneous nerve, which penetrates the sartorial fascia approximately 2 to 5 cm below the anterior-superior iliac spine (ASIS). Visualization of the superior portion of the hip and acetabulum has made this exposure useful for open reduction of developmental hip dysplasia, hip arthrotomy, hip arthrodesis, and reduction and fixation of hip fractures. The superior extension of this exposure allows for excellent visualization of anterior acetabular column and wall pathology. Disadvantages include poor access to posterior acetabular column and wall pathology. Positioning is supine with a sandbag under the ipsilateral buttock for slight elevation of the hemipelvis. The incision can be centered along a line running from slightly lateral to the ASIS to the lateral border of the patella. The plane between the tensor fascia lata and sartorius is identified. Once the lateral femoral cutaneous nerve is identified, the incision can be deepened to divide the plane between the rectus femoris and abductors (gluteus medius and minimus). The hip capsule can then be opened to access the anterior aspect of the hip.

Anterolateral (Watson-Jones) Approach

This exposure dissects the interval between the gluteus medius and tensor fascia muscles (superior gluteal innervation). It is described for biopsy, fracture reduction, and arthrotomy and in such cases may minimize dissection between muscle groups. The patient is usually positioned supine with a sandbag under the ipsilateral buttock. The incision is curvilinear apex posterior over the greater trochanter. After incising the fascia, the anterior edge of the gluteus medius is identified and a plane is developed between the tensor fascia lata and the gluteus medius. A portion of the gluteus medius may be reflected anteriorly with the tensor. Care must be taken to avoid injury or ligation of the superior gluteal neurovascular bundle, which runs from gluteus medius to tensor approximately 5 cm above the trochanter, because function of the tensor could be seriously compromised. Gentle release of the anterior portion of the gluteus medius and minimus tendons, with or without a wafer of bone, and reflection of the rectus femoris will facilitate exposure of the anterior hip.

Direct Lateral (Modified Hardinge) Approach

This approach (Fig. 1) dissects a plane between the anterior hip abductors and can provide excellent exposure to both the

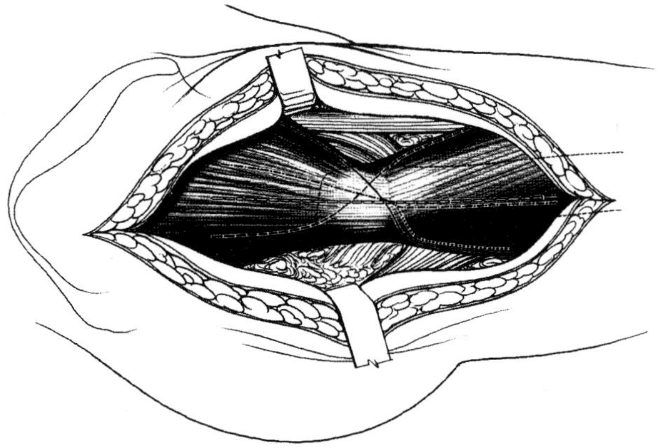

Figure 1

Modified lateral approaches to the hip, as seen from posterior proximal: 1) Hardinge, 2) Stracathro, 3) Bauer and 4) Frndak/Mallory. (Reproduced with permission from McGann WA: Surgical approaches, in Callaghan JJ, Rosenberg AG, Rubash HE (eds): *The Adult Hip.* Philadelphia, PA, Lippincott-Raven, 1998, pp 678–681.)

anterior hip and proximal femur with the ability to be extended distally for extensive femoral reconstruction. This approach provides excellent visualization for arthrotomy, arthrodesis, hip arthroplasty, and limited revision hip procedures. Decreased rates of sciatic nerve palsy and prosthetic dislocation with preservation of posterior hip tissues have been reported with this approach. In a recent review of 640 patients on whom total hip arthroplasty was performed using this approach, the dislocation rate was 0.3%. Disadvantages include limited proximal acetabular exposure, increased risk of heterotopic ossification, and possible slower abductor rehabilitation as a result of dissection through the anterior abductors. In the same series, a moderate or severe limp was reported in 10% of all patients at 2-year follow-up. Positioning is usually lateral; however, the supine position is preferred by some surgeons. After a direct linear incision is made centered over the greater trochanter, the fascia is incised for the length of the incision. The anterior third of the gluteus medius and minimus are then reflected together with the anterior vastus lateralis to allow exposure of the anterior hip capsule. A trochanteric wafer can be taken with the abductor tissues to facilitate healing of the abductor flap. Capsulectomy may be performed or the hip capsule may be reflected anteriorly with the anterior myofascial flap as a single flap. The drawback to this approach is the risk of injury to the superior gluteal neurovascular bundle when the gluteus medius division is extended more than 5 cm above the greater trochanter. For this reason, proximal dissection usually is limited to 3 cm above the trochanteric insertion of the abductors. Extension of the approach distally, with release of more of the vastus lateralis, may prevent undue tension on the superior gluteal bundle. When reflecting the myofascial flap anteriorly, blood loss can be minimized by cauterizing the ascending branch of the medial circumflex artery as it courses behind the greater trochanter and the transverse branch of the lateral circumflex artery in the proximal vastus lateralis. At closure, to minimize abductor weakness and limp, a careful reapproximation of the anterior abductors is required. Disruptions of abductor tendinous attachment of more than 2.5 cm correlate with a significant postoperative limp. Heavy nonabsorbable suture is used to reattach the anterior flap to the greater trochanter. Passing the suture through a generous cuff of peritrochanteric tissue or through drill holes in the greater trochanter can minimize dehiscence of the abductor repair.

Posterior Approach (Langenbeck/Moore)

This approach (Fig. 2) provides good visualization of the posterior capsule, posterior column, and entire acetabulum via splitting of the gluteus maximus, release of the short

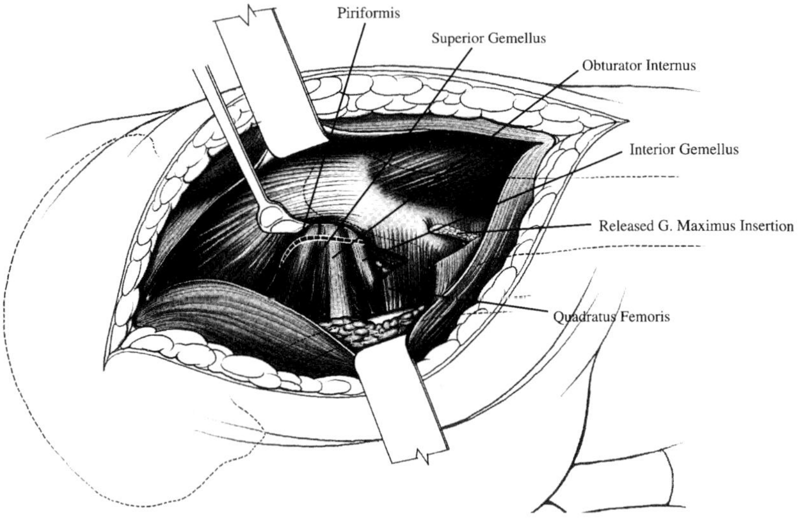

Figure 2

Posterior approach to the hip. The gluteus maximus is split and the short external rotators are reflected off their insertion into the greater trochanter. (Reproduced with permission from McGann WA: Surgical approaches, in Callaghan JJ, Rosenberg AG, Rubash HE (eds): *The Adult Hip.* Philadelphia, PA, Lippincott-Raven, 1998, pp 678–681.)

external rotators, and posterior capsulotomy. A complete posterior capsulectomy without reattachment of the rotators is sometimes performed, but it is preferable to detach the rotators and the posterior capsule in a single layer and to reattach them at the end of the procedure. The gluteus medius and minimus are retracted anteriorly to offer a better exposure superiorly. Further exposure is obtained by releasing the quadratus femoris in a subperiosteal fashion while carefully cauterizing the circumflex vessels. In addition, the gluteus maximus can be released near its insertion and reattached at the end of the procedure. An anterior capsulotomy is often required for soft-tissue balancing and can offer further exposure of the anterior wall and column.

The obvious advantage of this exposure is the preservation of the abductor mechanism. Easy exposure, quick rehabilitation, diminished operating time and a lower heterotopic ossification rate are factors that make this approach preferable over the Hardinge approach for primary arthroplasty. Although the postoperative rate of dislocation is high, this problem is effectively negated if the capsule is repaired and the patient is cooperative and neurologically intact. The tendency to place a component in an inadequate anteversion with this approach decreases with surgeon experience and familiarity with the approach.

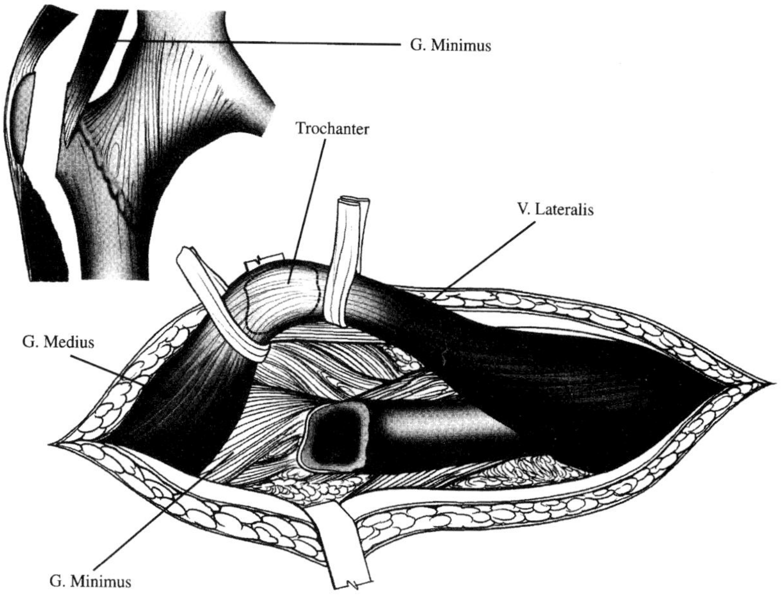

Figure 3

The trochanteric slide. The soft tissue is retracted anteriorly and may be held with retractors. The anterior capsule can then be dissected for exposure of the hip joint. (Reproduced with permission from McGann WA: Surgical approaches, in Callaghan JJ, Rosenberg AG, Rubash HE (eds): *The Adult Hip.* Philadelphia, PA, Lippincott-Raven, 1998, pp 678–681.)

Trochanteric Slide

Transtrochanteric approaches (Fig. 3) provide excellent visualization of the proximal femur and acetabulum. However, the traditional approach as popularized by Charnley is not widely used because of concerns regarding reattachment and possible nonunion of the trochanteric fragment. As a modification of the lateral approach, the trochanteric slide involves osteotomy of anterior trochanteric bone and reflecting it in continuity with the gluteus medius and vastus lateralis. The osteotomy is made just lateral to the gluteus minimus insertion or it can be made thicker to also include the gluteus minimus with the fragment. Reattachment of the osteotomy is performed by passing cerclage wire around the lesser trochanter and through the bony fragment. Stability is usually excellent following reattachment because of the opposing pull of the gluteus medius and vastus lateralis. This modification can improve visualization in the difficult primary arthroplasty case as well as in revision arthroplasty. In addition, proximal acetabular reconstruction can be performed without the increased risk of damage to the superior gluteal neurovascular bundle as described with the modified Hardinge approach. Dynamization of the trochanteric fragment can reestablish appropriate abductor tension and can facilitate fixation to proximal femoral allograft in cases of extensive femoral reconstruction.

Vastus Slide

As an extensile modification of the modified lateral approach (Fig. 4), the vastus slide allows wide exposure of the hip joint and femur. The superficial exposure is the same as for the modified lateral approach. The deep exposure is different in that the vastus lateralis is reflected off of the proximal femur from its posterior attachment to the lateral intermuscular septum. The vastus slide involves maintaining continuity between a proximal flap of the anterior gluteus medius and minimus and a large distal flap of the entire vastus lateralis as reflected off of the lateral intermuscular septum. Care must be taken to leave a cuff of vastus lateralis proximally on the

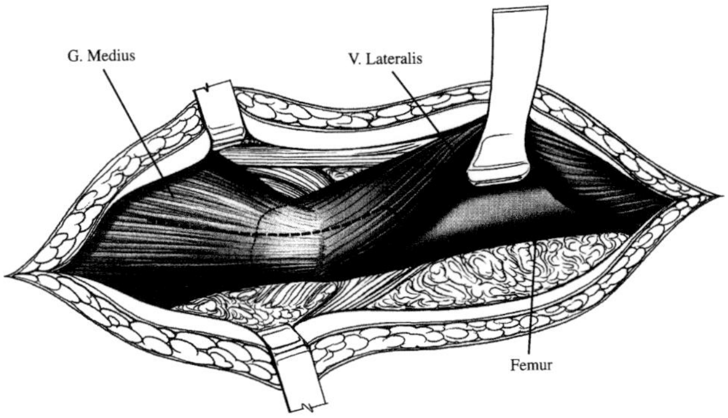

Figure 4

Extensile modification of the direct lateral approach. The gluteus medius and minimus are reflected anteriorly as is the vastus lateralis. (Reproduced with permission from McGann WA: Surgical approaches, in Callaghan JJ, Rosenberg AG, Rubash HE (eds): *The Adult Hip.* Philadelphia, PA, Lippincott-Raven, 1998, pp 678–681.)

greater trochanter to facilitate anatomic closure and repair of the soft-tissue sleeve. Blood loss can be minimized by careful ligation of vascular perforators as they course through the intermuscular septum. This approach provides excellent access and visualization of the hip joint and proximal femur. Although it provides excellent exposure of the proximal femur for femoral revision surgery, visualization and access to the acetabulum for extensive acetabular reconstruction are limited. The trochanteric slide or extended trochanteric osteotomy are better suited for complicated acetabular reconstruction.

Extended Trochanteric Osteotomy

This approach (Fig. 5) is a very useful approach in the revision of both cemented and noncemented femoral stems. It allows for controlled access to the femoral stem without compromising bone stock or significantly devitalizing the osteotomized segment. The varus bowing present in many failed total hip femurs is also addressed. Without the use of this approach, femoral bowing does not allow adequate seating of a revision implant and makes removal of the existing implant difficult, with an increased likelihood of fracture.

Preoperative planning for the extended trochanteric osteotomy is imperative. The length of the osteotomy should allow for easy removal of the porous-coated stem or retained cement while ensuring that adequate diaphysis is retained for subsequent fixation.

To perform this procedure, the posterior approach is extended distally along the posterior border of the gluteus medius and the posterior border of the vastus. The gluteus maximus muscle is detached and the interval between the posterior vastus and gluteus maximus is developed. The lateral third of the proximal femur is then osteotomized using an oscillating saw or a burr. The distal aspect of the cut should be rounded to prevent extension of a possible frac-

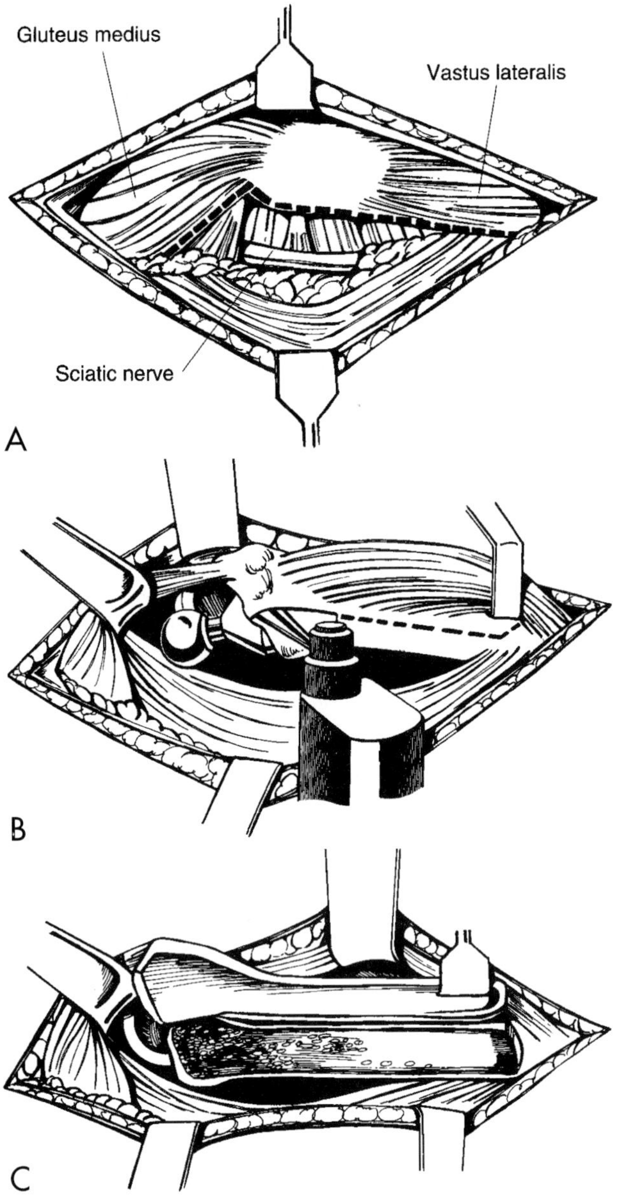

Figure 5

The extended trochanteric osteotomy. **A**, The posterior borders of the gluteus medius and vastus musculature are identified. **B**, The proximal lateral third of the femur is detached using an oscillating saw or a high-speed burr. **C**, The proximal fragment is then hinged forward to visualize the canal. (Reproduced with permission from Masterson EL, Masri BA, Duncan CP: Surgical approaches in revision hip replacement. *J Am Acad Orthop Surg* 1998;6:84–92.)

ture, and the distal cut should be rounded anteriorly and the anterior proximal portion cut to initiate the remainder of the osteotomy. Osteotomes can be passed into the osteotomized segment to spread and possibly allow removal of the implant; if this does not occur, an oscillating saw can be passed through the posterior osteotomy site and used to complete the anterior cut. If the latter maneuver is not possible, the osteotomy can be completed with the careful leverage of the osteotomized segments with the use of multiple osteotomes. Once the osteotomy is completed, care should be taken to preserve the muscular attachment on the proximal segment while freeing the soft tissue at the proximal and distal osteotomy sites to allow for adequate motion of the segment for subsequent reattachment. Once the implant is removed and the revision implant is placed, the osteotomized segment is reflected back into position and reattached using 2 tensioned cables.

The success rate with this technique has been very high. The advantages of the osteotomy include easier access to the distal bone-cement interface, predictable healing of the osteotomized fragment, proper tensioning of the abductors with distal advancement, neutral reaming of the femoral canal, decreased surgery time, and enhanced exposure of the acetabulum. Complications such as eccentric reaming, femoral perforations, and fractures have been less frequent in femoral revisions performed with an osteotomy.

Annotated Bibliography

General Principles

McGann WA: Surgical Approaches, in Callaghan JJ, Rosenberg AG, Rubash HE (ed): *The Adult Hip*. Philadelphia, PA, Lippincott-Raven, 1998, pp 663–718.

Surgical exposures for primary and revision arthroplasty are described and discussed.

Surgical Approaches

Aribindi R, Barba M, Solomon MI, Arp P, Paprosky W: Bypass fixation. *Orthop Clin North Am* 1998;29:319–29.

A review of 122 consecutive extended proximal femoral osteotomies with a minimum of 2 years follow-up is presented. There were no nonunions and no migration of the greater trochanteric fragment greater than 2 mm.

Masri BA, Campbell DG, Garbuz DS, Duncan CP: Seven specialized exposures for revision hip and knee replacement. *Orthop Clin North Am* 1998;29:229–240.

The authors describe the extended trochanteric osteotomy, the trochanteric slide, and the vastus slide for revision hip and knee replacement.

Mulliken BD, Rorabeck CH, Bourne RB, Nayak N: A modified direct lateral approach in total hip arthroplasty: A comprehensive review. *J Arthroplasty* 1998;13:737–747.

This is a retrospective review of 770 consecutive primary total hip arthroplasties. The direct lateral technique is described in detail. The complications are minimal (the dislocation rate is 0.3%, and 10% of patients have a limp).

Younger TI, Bradford MS, Magnus RE, Paprosky WG: Extended proximal femoral osteotomy: A new technique for femoral revision arthroplasty. *J Arthroplasty* 1995;10:329–338.

The authors describe the extended proximal femoral osteotomy.

Classic Bibliography

Baker AS, Bitounis VC: Abductor function after total hip replacement: An electromyographic and clinical review. *J Bone Joint Surg* 1989;71B:47–50.

Carlson DC, Robinson HJ Jr: Surgical approaches for primary total hip arthroplasty: A prospective comparison of the Marcy modification of the Gibson and Watson-Jones approaches. *Clin Orthop* 1987;222:161–166.

Crenshaw AH Jr: Surgical Approaches, in Crenshaw AH, Daugherty K (eds): *Campbell's Operative Orthopaedics*, ed 8. St. Louis, MO, Mosby-Year Book, 1992, pp 23–116.

Cuckler JM: Surgical Approaches, in Steinberg ME (ed): *The Hip and Its Disorders*. Philadelphia, PA, WB Saunders, 1991, pp 88–105.

Dall D: Exposure of the hip by anterior osteotomy of the greater trochanter: A modified anterolateral approach. *J Bone Joint Surg* 1986;68B:382–386.

Glassman AH, Engh CA, Bobyn JD: A technique of extensile exposure for total hip arthroplasty. *J Arthroplasty* 1987;2:11–21.

Hardinge K: The direct lateral approach to the hip. *J Bone Joint Surg* 1982;64B:17–19.

Head WC, Mallory TH, Berklacich FM, Dennis DA, Emerson RH Jr, Wapner KL: Extensile exposure of the hip for revision arthroplasty. *J Arthroplasty* 1987;2:265–273.

Turner RH, Mattingly DA, Scheller A: Femoral revision total hip arthroplasty using a long-stem femoral component: Clinical and radiographic analysis. *J Arthroplasty* 1987;2:247–258.

Chapter 12 Biomechanics of the Hip and Hip Reconstruction

Introduction

As a critical element of the human locomotor apparatus, the hip functions as a mechanical unit, and its behavior in health and disease may accordingly be explained by the principles of mechanics. Effective treatment of hip injuries or disease often depends on an understanding of hip mechanics. Critical elements include the motion (ie, kinematics), the forces (ie, kinetics), and the distribution of those forces (ie, the articular contact stresses and stresses through the bone).

Hip Kinematics

The anatomy of the hip provides considerable rotation in the 3 anatomic planes (sagittal, coronal, transverse). Although neither the acetabulum nor the femur are strictly spherical (the sagittal plane and coronal plane diameters are "out-of-round" by 1 to 3 mm) or congruent, they normally function as an effective ball-in-socket joint, a teleologically appropriate design for a proximal joint. Most normal subjects have a 120° to 140° arc of flexion-extension, a 60° to 80° arc of abduction-adduction, and a 60° to 90° arc of internal-external rotation. The "total" motion (sum of that in each of the 3 anatomic planar arcs) reaches 240° to 300°. These arcs are limited by capsular constraints and bony anatomy. Normal subjects achieve full extension (0 defined as the thigh axis being coincident with the flattened lumbar spine as the reference axis). Proximal femora that have greater anteversion will impinge (trochanter against the pelvis) posteriorly in extension with lesser external rotation, while proximal femora with lesser anteversion will tend to impinge anteriorly in flexion with lesser internal rotation.

The normally available arcs of hip motion substantially exceed those required for most activities of daily living, although obviously the limits are reached in some recreational or athletic activities. Level walking requires approximately 50° to 60° of flexion-extension, with relatively small amounts of internal-external rotation or abduction-adduction. However, putting on shoes and socks, perhaps the most motion-demanding activity of daily living, requires a total motion of 160° to 170° without using some unusual strategy (as would a patient with a hip fusion).

Hip Kinetics

The forces across the hip are considerable during activities of daily living, exceeding body weight (BW) by a factor of 2 or more. Until the advent of technology to manufacture implantable transducers (instrumented hip implants), investigators used various mathematical models to compute hip forces. All models before 20 to 25 years ago were static, 2-dimensional, and incorporated only 1 or several muscles. With the advent of laboratory-based digital computers, more sophisticated 3-dimensional dynamic models included many muscles. However, such models incorporated many assumptions, which often resulted in misleading absolute force magnitude estimates and, sometimes, even relative magnitudes from geometric changes produced by injury or disease. Typically, these models reported resultant hip joint loads in the range of 3 to 8 BW for most activities of daily living. Recent instrumented implants, however, demonstrate lower loads in the range of 2 to 4 BW for most activities. More recent modeling efforts have eliminated some of the assumptions resulting in the errors, but the results of modeling studies should be interpreted with some caution.

Quite obviously, forces in excess of BW cannot be generated by the body above the hip (approximately five sixths the total) and instead are generated by muscle forces. Muscle forces required for (static or dynamic) equilibrium are sensitive to their moment arms, and these are altered in conditions resulting in geometric distortion of the normal hip anatomy. In interpreting the literature, however, simple models cannot be relied on even to understand trends in reducing or increasing a single moment arm. Around the hip when 1 moment arm is changed as a result of some deformity (eg, healing of an intertrochanteric fracture in varus), others are also changed. The net effect on the hip forces depends on the changes in moment arms to all muscles as well as on muscle activation patterns. Because the net (resultant) hip force at a given instant is a vector sum of all muscle, ligament (capsule, scar), and articular contact forces, scarred or constrained capsules can also contribute to hip forces, although a normal mobile hip capsule likely contributes negligibly except at the end of the range of motion. Thus, although simple models suggest considerable change in the hip forces with geometric distortions such as proximal osteotomies, the net effects predicted by more plausible (and inclusive) models are often rather trivial. Osteotomies, then, do not likely achieve their effects by substantially altering the hip forces.

Because muscle contraction across the hip contributes the majority of the load, it is perhaps not surprising that the resultant force on the femoral head does not substantially change direction, regardless of hip position, because muscle directions follow the femur and are more or less in line with it. On the other hand, muscle directions change considerably relative to the pelvis during various activities, and accordingly, the resultant forces on the acetabulum (always equal and opposite in direction to those on the femoral head) change direction substantially. The forces acting posteriorly on the acetabulum are considerable (several times BW) during rising from a chair or bending, and may exceed the strength of an internal fixation construct for posterior wall fractures.

Falling directly on the hip causes considerable impact force to the bone and soft tissues about the hip. Only about 15% of the impact forces are distributed to the soft tissues, however, and muscle contraction does not significantly reduce those forces. Although young healthy bone has a margin of safety of 2 to 4 times, it is not surprising that the impact forces (essentially unaffected by soft tissue) cause substantial numbers of fractures in the elderly with markedly weakened bone.

The use of canes or other walking assists reduces the requirement for muscle activation and provides support for some of the BW. A properly used cane can reduce the total force up to 40%, and crutches at least 30% to 50%. However, the degree of force relief depends on the type of cane use, instructions to the patient, and muscle activation patterns. Because swinging of the leg is associated with substantial muscle activation, even nonweightbearing produces load across the hip.

According to output from an instrumented implant, ascending and descending stairs increases hip loads by 10% to 20% compared to level walking (mathematical models have predicted higher forces, but may not be reliable for reasons related to modeling assumptions). The resulting torsional moments are not substantially increased, but are at the high end of normal. However, the torsional moments generated are close to the moments shown experimentally to cause implant-interface failure, and they thus may be more critical than the axial loading.

Hip Articular Contact Stresses

As noted, neither the cartilaginous nor subchondral bone geometries are perfect spheres, and in no position are the unloaded acetabulum and femoral head completely congruent. Congruence is achieved under loads and with resulting deformation of the articular cartilage. In vitro studies of hip articular contact suggest normal activities result in stresses ranging from 1 to 8 MPa. In vivo studies of metal against articular cartilage from an instrumented hemiprosthesis demonstrate stresses as high as 18 to 20 MPa; however, it must be emphasized that these values are undoubtedly higher than those for cartilage-on-cartilage. Contact stresses are distributed on the femoral head in a "horseshoe" fashion reflecting those on the acetabulum. The higher contact stresses are found superiorly on the femoral head and the superior "dome" of the acetabulum, as would be intuitively expected.

Although acetabular and femoral osteotomies do not substantially alter the resultant loads across the hip, they do alter the locations and patterns of contact stresses and may well alter the magnitudes of peak or spatially averaged contact stresses. If osteotomies have a direct effect on the articular cartilage (in addition to underlying bone) it is likely because of alterations either in contact stress or stress gradient distributions. Observations over many years suggest that osteotomies induce remodeling in cartilage and subchondral and adjacent bone. Most likely, the stress redistribution in the bone, which would follow alteration of articular contact stresses, after osteotomy induces at least some of the long-term effects, although reduction of intramedullary hypertension may relate more to immediate pain relief. Osteotomies have long been advocated for treatment of established, symptomatic arthrosis, but in the past few decades they have been advocated to prevent (eg, the Salter innominate osteotomy in childhood) or retard (eg, the Ganz osteotomy in early adulthood) the development of hip arthrosis. Evidence suggests both periacetabular and femoral osteotomies relieve symptoms in a high percentage of patients, and appropriately selected patients do well in the short to medium term. Whether these osteotomies actually prevent or retard progression of arthrosis is unknown.

Whereas many conditions (eg, dysplasia, inadequately reduced intra-articular fractures) alter the contact stresses, the tolerance of the articular cartilage to load over time is not known. Cartilage is so compliant that small defects or malreductions do not lead to large increases of contact stress because the surrounding areas "recruit" a portion of the load. Furthermore, cartilage remodels to some extent over time, so that initially malreduced articular fracture margins do not cause sharp changes in contact pressure over long periods. There is little evidence that greatly elevated contact pressures per se relate to long-term arthrosis, although a stronger case might be made for elevated contact pressure gradients, which would be related to fluid and nutrition flow in cartilage, over many years.

Bone Stresses Around the Hip

All loads across the hip are distributed first to the articular surfaces, then to the underlying bone. Bone obviously undergoes deformation during loading, with resulting stresses and strains. While genetics plays a major role in the shapes of bones, these stresses and/or strains contribute to bone density, strength, and ultimate shape of the bone and the internal trabecular arrangement (ie, Wolff's law). Bone strains typically range from 100 to 1,000 με during the usual activities of daily living, and up to 4,000 με in vigorous activities. The trabecular patterns in the periacetabular region and in the femoral head and neck reflect the loading in some general way. Thickening of the subchondral plates suggests increase in local loading, and even density of the plates suggests normally distributed loads. After proximal femoral osteotomy, unevenly distributed subchondral density will sometimes become more evenly distributed, suggesting beneficial load distribution.

The ability of bone to adapt to the new mechanical environment created by a fracture, implant, or osteotomy depends on its ability to perceive and respond to its mechanical environment. This general notion, known as Wolff's law after Julius Wolff who popularized the notion that bone responds to principal and compressive stress, has never been formulated in such a way that all adaptation could be accurately predicted. It is possible to envision a number of limitations with such formulations: (1) Stresses and strains are concepts of continuum mechanics (eg, beam theory, finite element analysis) in which a solid (continuous), typically (but not always) homogeneous material is assumed. Bone is neither solid nor homogeneous. Local stresses or strains might be substantially higher or lower than the averages over some region computed by continuum mechanics. (2) Strain or stress calculations are very sensitive to modeling assumptions. (3) The levels of strain to which bone cells respond are not known. (The presumption is that they respond to strain or deformation resulting from gross tissue strain or fluid flow, rather than to stress.) Evidence suggests bone cells respond to strain well below the peaks most investigators have assumed. (4) Bone cells respond to some accumulation of strain events, but not merely sums of peak magnitudes times numbers of cycles. Frequently used simplifying assumptions (eg, using only 1 or a few muscle forces) may result in errors not only in magnitude, but trends. (5) Strain is not the only stimulus for bone adaptation; genetics, vitamins, hormones, and other systemic and local factors (eg, cytokines, growth factors) strongly influence responses. Nonetheless, substantial evidence supports a strong mechanical influence on the adaptation of bone to periprosthetic bone and on the short- and long-term success of arthroplasty.

Periacetabular cortical bone, being less "thick" than that on the femur, is structurally less stiff and consequently undergoes greater deformation. The deformations during level walking at various locations typically range from 15 to 60 mm; these are levels that could significantly contribute to micromotion between bone and a much more rigid implant. The initial stability of the implant and micromotion undoubtedly influences the nature of the developing bone-implant interface.

Bone Stresses in Osteonecrosis

Osteonecrosis compromises the strength of the femoral head bone in at least 2 ways. First, dead bone (in contrast to living bone) is subject to fatigue failure at physiologic magnitudes of loading and with relatively few (eg, 5,000 to 50,000) loading cycles. Second, the repair process resorbs dead bone and further compromises the structural integrity of the trabecular and subchondral bone. The structural compromise is intimately dependent on the size, location, and configuration of the femoral head. Smaller lesions or lesions in less critical locations are less likely to collapse and may repair without long-term consequences. Coring and/or grafting, often advocated for treatment, may improve or worsen the stress distribution and peak stresses, depending not only on the size, location, and configuration of the lesion, but also on the location, orientation, and depth of the core or graft. The best position for a core or graft is not always intuitively obvious, although a graft should abut the subchondral plate if substantial initial support is to be obtained.

Kinematics After Total Hip Reconstruction

Most patients with total hip reconstruction achieve adequate arcs of motion for activities of daily living without risk of dislocation. Although dislocation is often multifactorial, malpositioning of the components is among the more common causes. Placement of a femoral component in excess anteversion will increase the risk of anterior dislocation from posterior impingement in extension, and placement in excess retroversion will increase the risk of posterior dislocation from anterior impingement in flexion.

Kinetics After Total Hip Reconstruction

Implantation of a total hip replacement does not necessarily alter hip forces, presuming the hip center remains near the anatomic hip center, the motion is normal, and the muscle activation strategies remain the same (eg, no limp). However, within surgically achievable hip center locations, the hip forces can vary by a factor of 2. Quite naturally, such differences can be expected to affect loosening rates, and some evidence in long-term clinical follow-up suggests this is indeed the case. The lowest forces occur near the anatomic position and increase as the hip center is moved laterally, superiorly, and posteriorly, with lateral position causing the greatest increases.

Bone Stresses Around a Total Hip Reconstruction

Implantation of a total hip replacement considerably alters the normal distributions and magnitudes of bone stress and strain. These changes are substantial enough to result in long-term alterations in bone density (ie, remodeling). Quite obviously, the change in strains varies enormously from one design to another and with differing sizes of a given design. However, some areas of bone (eg, the proximal femur) always experience lower strains than normal, while others (eg, the region of the tip of the prosthesis) always experience increased strains. Strains may be reduced in the "calcar" region proximally as much as 90%. These changes suggest the joint load is transferred from the implant articular surfaces down the implant to the adjacent bone, in part bypassing ("stress shielding") the proximal bone. This phenomenon is associated with loss of proximal bone density. In most cases the changes are more or less subtle and not associated with any long-term clinical consequences. Theoretically and experimentally, femoral component stems of greater thickness increase proximal stress shielding. However, in only a small percentage of cases is bone loss considerable, thus raising concerns about fracture or difficulties revising the hip should that become necessary.

The long-term survival of a joint implant depends on the adaptation of periprosthetic bone to the new stress/strain situation. Bone normally exhibits a turnover of roughly 5% of the skeleton per year, with individual lamellae typically lasting a decade or more. Because bone scans are normal 6 to 12 months after total hip reconstruction, it may be presumed that the presence of an implant does not substantially alter bone turnover long term. The high rates of 10-year prosthesis survival (roughly 90% to 95%) suggest adequate adaptation to stresses within that time frame. However, whether longer-term (ie, after 10 to 20 years) failures reflect subsequent inappropriate adaptation to stress or reactions to particulate debris or other causes is not known. Given the usually slow rate of bone turnover, it is conceivable that markedly abnormal stresses around a prosthesis merely take a long time to make their effects obvious (perhaps in a fashion analogous to a "slow virus") because of slow bone turnover times. Thus, some long-term failures merely reflect the slow time required for complete adaptation.

Total Hip Component Migration

Migration or "settling" (subsidence) of femoral components is common if not nearly universal to some degree. Roentgenstereophotogrammetry (determination of relative position changes of 2 rigid bodies over time using at least 3 landmarks in each rigid body) affords assessment of settling with an accuracy of 0.5 mm and 2°. This is in contrast to plane radiographic interpretation, which likely is no more accurate (or reliable) than 3 to 5 mm and 3° to 5°. "Well-fixed" total hip components will migrate no more than 1 to 2 mm in the first year. However, components exceeding this amount of settling are associated with a higher risk of long-term radiographic and clinical loosening. Thus, the method has the potential to detect at a relatively early time a high risk of loosening in new devices.

Annotated Bibliography

Bergmann G, Graichen F, Rohlmann A: Hip joint loading during walking and running, measured in 2 patients. *J Biomech* 1993; 26:969–990.

The authors used an instrumented implant to ascertain the forces crossing the hip in 2 total hip reconstruction patients. In 1 patient, walking resulted in forces approximately 280% BW, while jogging increased forces to 480% BW. In the second patient, walking generated forces approximately 480% BW, while stumbling caused forces as high as 870% BW.

Bergmann G, Graichen F, Rohlmann A, Linke H: Hip joint forces during load carrying. *Clin Orthop* 1997;335:190–201.

Carrying loads of up to 25% BW has little effect on the ipsilateral hip, but causes the hip forces on the opposite side to increase by about two thirds. If a load of 25% BW is evenly distributed between 2 hands, the forces on both hips are increased by about 25%. Patients with total hip replacements should be aware it is best to carry loads on the affected sides.

Bergmann G, Graichen F, Rohlmann A: Is staircase walking a risk for the fixation of hip Implants? *J Biomech* 1995; 28:535–553.

Walking down stairs increases hip forces by about 20% compared to level walking at 3 km/hr, while walking up stairs increases the forces by about 10%. Torsional loads are at the high end of those for level walking, but are also near the tolerance limits for implants torsionally loaded in the laboratory. Thus, although not greatly elevated compared to level walking, torsional loading during stair ascending and descending appears to be high and with a lower margin of safety than axial loading.

Brand RA: Hip osteotomies: A biomechanical consideration. *J Am Acad Orthop Surg* 1997;5:282–291.

Osteotomies of the proximal femur do not substantially change hip joint forces, although they undoubtedly alter the manner in which those forces are distributed (ie, the articular contact stresses). The distribution of forces probably can be optimized through contemporary imaging and mathematical modeling.

Brand RA, Brown TD: The biomechanics of femoral head osteonecrosis, in Urbaniak JR, Jones JP Jr (eds): *Osteonecrosis: Etiology, Diagnosis, and Treatment.* Rosemont, IL, American Academy of Orthopaedic Surgeons, 1997, pp 315–321.

The distribution of stresses (and the propensity for collapse) in the femoral head intimately depends on the size, location, and configuration of the osteonecrotic lesion. The variable results of coring and grafting reported in the literature may relate to an improvement in stresses in some cases and a worsening of stresses in others. Patient-specific modeling might substantially improve the results of these procedures.

Brand RA, Pedersen DR, Davy DT, Kotzar GM, Heiple KG, Goldberg VM: Comparison of hip force calculations and measurements in the same patient. *J Arthroplasty* 1994;9:45–51.

To achieve comparable force magnitudes and patterns in a 3-dimensional, dynamic 47-element muscle model and output of an instrumented hip implant, considerable modification (greater anatomic realism) of the muscle model was required. Initial mathematical computations were quite high compared to forces recorded with the implant. The sort of changes required in the model had not previously been used, and the data suggest all previous models likely contain erroneously high estimates of hip forces.

Karrholm J, Herberts P, Hultmark P, Malchau H, Nivbrant B, Thanner J: Radiostereometry of hip prostheses: Review of methodology and clinical results. *Clin Orthop* 1997;344: 94–110.

Radiostereotometry (roentgenstereophotogrammetry) uses triangulation principles to compute relative positions of 2 rigid bodies and requires biplanar radiographs and at least 3 accurately definable landmarks in each rigid body. A number of studies have reported these techniques in total joint replacements by embedding at least 3 small tantalum beads in the bone, and then using beads or other landmarks on the prostheses to ascertain the relative changes in position of the implant relative to the bone. These studies have clearly identified the "normal" amount of settling that occurs but is neither symptomatic nor associated with long-term loosening. Perhaps more importantly, they define a level of settling (1 to 2 mm) associated with an increased risk of loosening in the longer term.

Kotzar GM, Davy DT, Goldberg VM, et al: Telemeterized in vivo hip joint force data: A report on two patients after total hip surgery. *J Orthop Res* 1991;9:621–633.

Two patients with instrumented total hip implants exhibited peak loads during walking of 2.1 to 2.8 times BW. The highest forces were seen with "instability" when the patient was standing on the affected leg and holding the hand of an attendant. With crutches, 1 patient at 23 days postoperatively exhibited forces ranging from 0.8 to 1.4 BW, while free (unassisted) walking resulted in forces of 1.8 to 2.4 BW. Cane use at 58 days resulted in 2.2 to 3.3 BW, whereas free (no assistive device) level walking at the same time resulted in similar forces of 2.3 to 3.3 BW. The levels of loading appeared more dependent on the time after surgery than the presence of a walking assist.

McNamara BP, Taylor D, Prendergast PJ: Computer prediction of adaptive bone remodelling around noncemented femoral prostheses: The relationship between damage-based and strain-based algorithms. *Med Eng Phys* 1997;19:454–463.

Although total hip femoral components are associated with substantial alterations in bone stresses or strains and with alterations in bone density, the direct link between stresses and density are not known. These authors explored 2 distinct theories (accumulated damage-based and strain-based) linking bone strain and long-term density changes. Flexible stems reduced stress shielding, but increased interface stresses. The study illustrates the practical aspects of implementation and differences in outcomes using 2 theories. This must be kept in mind when interpreting any study based on a given theory.

Millis MB, Murphy SB, Poss R: Osteotomies about the hip for the prevention and treatment of osteoarthrosis, in Pritchard DJ (ed): *Instructional Course Lectures 45.* Rosemont, IL, American Academy of Orthopaedic Surgeons, 1996, pp 209–226.

Osteotomies of both the periacetabular and intertrochanteric regions are used to treat or retard early hip osteoarthrosis. The notion of performing an "early" osteotomy to retard or prevent the development of later severe arthrosis is more recent than the purely therapeutic use. At short- to medium-term follow-up, early adulthood osteotomies relieve early symptoms in a large percentage of appropriately selected patients. Long-term follow-up should provide some indication as to whether the development of arthrosis is retarded, although a definitive study (ie, an adequately large controlled trial) is unlikely to be performed.

Neumann DA: Hip abductor muscle activity as subjects with hip prostheses walk with different methods of using a cane. *Phys Ther* 1998;78:490–501.

The amount of muscle activation around the hip (and thus the loads) is determined by the method of cane use. There are substantial variations from patient to patient, and while in most patients canes substantially reduce hip forces, this is not always the case. Because muscle activation is the primary source of hip loading, cane use may not always achieve its intended aims despite the patient using the device as instructed.

Noble PC, Paul JP: The deformation of the acetabulum during walking. *Trans Orthop Res Soc* 1995;20:709.

Deformation of periacetabular bone ranged from 3 to 58 mm during simulated single limb stance. The largest value was associated with "the width of the acetabulum," suggesting the anteroposterior diameter decreases during normal loading. Presuming the deformations are linear with load, these values might range from 2 to 4 times those in other activities of daily living. The deformations are in the range that could be associated with significant micromotion with implications for failure of initial stability.

Olson SA, Bay BK, Chapman MW, Sharkey NA: Biomechanical consequences of fracture and repair of the posterior wall of the acetabulum. *J Bone Joint Surg* 1995;77A:1184–1192.

Fracture and fixation of the posterior wall of the acetabulum leads to high contact stresses in the superior dome of the acetabulum. The explanation may be the relative flexibility of the construct with the result that the articular surfaces even when reduced cannot bear the weight, which is then shifted superiorly to the intact bone. The increases in stress may predispose to increased risk of long-term osteoarthrosis.

Robinovitch SN, Hayes WC, McMahon TA: Distribution of contact force during impact to the hip. *Ann Biomed Eng* 1997;25:499–508.

Despite the common and intuitive belief that soft tissues around the hip absorb impact forces during falls, the soft tissues in fact absorb only about 15% of that force and muscle contraction makes little difference.

Classic Bibliography

Bobyn JD, Mortimer ES, Glassman AH, Engh CA, Miller JE, Brooks CE: Producing and avoiding stress shielding: Laboratory and clinical observations of noncemented total hip arthroplasty. *Clin Orthop* 1992;274:79–96.

Brand RA, Crowninshield RD: The effect of cane use on hip contact force. *Clin Orthop* 1980;147:181–184.

Brand RA, Pedersen DR: Computer modeling of surgery and a consideration of the mechanical effects of proximal femoral osteotomies, in Welch RB (ed): *The Hip: Proceedings of the Twelfth Open Scientific Meeting of the Hip Society.* St Louis, MO, CV Mosby, 1984, pp 193–210.

Huiskes R, Weinans H, van Rietbergen B: The relationship between stress shielding and bone resorption around total hip stems and the effects of flexible materials. *Clin Orthop* 1992;274:124–134.

Johnston RC, Brand RA, Crowninshield RD: Reconstruction of the hip: A mathematical approach to determine optimum geometric relationships. *J Bone Joint Surg* 1979;61A:639–652.

Johnston RC, Smidt GL: Measurement of hip-joint motion during walking: Evaluation of an electrogoniometric method. *J Bone Joint Surg* 1969;51A:1082–1094.

Johnston RC, Smidt GL: Hip motion measurements for selected activities of daily living. *Clin Orthop* 1970;72:205–215.

Otani T, Whiteside LA, White SE: The effect of axial and torsional loading on strain distribution in the proximal femur as related to cementless total hip arthroplasty. *Clin Orthop* 1993;292:376–383.

Chapter 13
Osteotomy

Osteotomy may offer a satisfactory outcome in the treatment of several types of hip dysfunction. Intertrochanteric osteotomy should be considered when the predominant deformity is in the proximal femur. Classic indications for intertrochanteric osteotomy include malunions of fractures in the trochanteric region; pseudarthrosis of a fracture of the femoral neck in the presence of a viable femoral head; congenital coxa vara; osteonecrosis of the femoral head with a lesion of suitable size and location; and shortening, lengthening, and/or derotation osteotomies to realign the extremity. Additional indications include correction of deformity secondary to slipped capital femoral epiphysis, and coxa valga in some patients with mild dysplasia. Periacetabular osteotomy has recently emerged as the method of choice for young adults with significant hip dysplasia and minimal arthrotic changes. A particularly valuable procedure is isolated greater trochanteric advancement in a patient with an otherwise congruous hip but greater trochanteric overgrowth, the result of a previous capital femoral physeal arrest.

Principles of Contemporary Osteotomy

Normal activities, such as walking 1 km per hour, create forces across the hip of almost 3 times body weight. Jogging or stumbling increases those forces to between 5 to 8 times body weight. These forces are even greater if the hip is incongruous, because the loads are concentrated in a smaller surface area. If the hip dysfunction is secondary to a mechanical problem (malalignment), then theoretically it may be amenable to correction by osteotomy. Mechanical failure occurs when the unit load exceeds the adaptive capacity of articular cartilage and subchondral bone. In contrast, in inflammatory arthritis, normal loads become excessive for cartilage that is undergoing degradation by inflammatory processes. Patients with inflammatory arthritis are not candidates for osteotomy.

The first principle of osteotomy is to improve congruency by restoring proper biomechanics, that is, to increase the surface area available to transfer load, decrease the muscle forces across the joint, and reorient the weightbearing surfaces to transfer load in compression rather than shear.

The second principle is timely intervention. The prognosis is adversely affected by the presence of arthrosis, therefore, the ideal candidates for osteotomy are those with minimal radiographic changes of arthrosis in whom a realignment osteotomy of either the pelvis or proximal femur restores congruity, a maximum surface for load transfer, and a proper orientation of the load transfer surfaces. Ideal candidates for so-called reconstructive osteotomy tend to have minimal but progressive symptoms, presently satisfactory motion and function, radiographs that show no irreversible changes of arthrosis, but a poor prognosis without surgical intervention. In contrast, so-called salvage osteotomy may be indicated for patients with loss of motion, fair to poor function, and irreversible changes of arthrosis. Patients in the salvage category must understand that improvement in function is likely to deteriorate with time and that subsequent total hip arthroplasty is likely.

Technical Goals of Osteotomy

The technical goals of osteotomy include elimination of impingement, correction of deformity, and restoration of a pain-free functional range of motion. The surgeon must maintain the mechanical axis of the extremity in both the coronal and sagittal planes, maintain or restore equal leg lengths, and restore proper rotational alignment. With osteotomy, motion is neither gained nor lost, but its range can be altered. The patient must have sufficient preoperative motion so that correction leaves a functional range of motion. For example, a varus osteotomy decreases residual abduction by the amount of correction. Therefore, 20° of varus correction in a patient with a preoperative abduction range of only 10° will result in an adduction deformity of the extremity. With intertrochanteric osteotomy, technical complications can be minimized by making certain that: (1) the osteotomy is performed at the level of the proximal border of the lesser trochanter to ensure sufficient cancellous bone surfaces for uncomplicated union; (2) placement of the blade plate or other fixation device into the femoral neck leaves a cortical bridge of at least 1.5 cm between the entrance site of the fixation blade and the site of osteotomy; and (3) placement of the blade must be midneck and not midtrochanter in the sagittal plane to avoid injury to the retinacular vessels. The availability of blade plates of different fixed angles allows for exact preoperative planning to achieve the desired correction and to minimize complications.

Contemporary proximal femoral osteotomy combines elements of displacement and angulation. Correction is often in 3 planes: varus or valgus correction in the coronal plane, flexion or extension correction in the sagittal plane, and rotational realignment. In the frontal plane, varus correction without wedge resection minimizes leg length discrepancy. Medial displacement with varus osteotomy (afforded by the fixed 90° blade plate) maintains the proper mechanical axis of the lower extremity. In valgus osteotomy, wedge resection can be used to maintain length or shorten the extremity; with no wedge, the extremity can be lengthened. Wedge resection should not be performed in flexion or extension osteotomy; the fragments should be impacted in order to maintain a normal mechanical axis in the sagittal plane.

Dysplasia

In dysplasia, the primary developmental abnormality is usually a maloriented acetabulum that is considered globally deficient. Even if the acetabulum is restored to proper alignment, the volume of the joint available for load transfer is less than normal. The most common malalignment in dysplasia is an acetabulum that is anterolaterally deficient. Therefore, an anteroposterior (AP) radiograph will show an oblique rather than a horizontal acetabular subchondral plate and incomplete coverage of the femoral head. A common index by which to measure acetabular deficiency in the coronal plane is the center edge (CE) angle of Wiberg. The literature from Europe and North America suggests that in a patient whose AP radiograph shows a CE angle of less than approximately 15°, a periacetabular osteotomy is the procedure of choice; in contrast, the Japanese literature suggests that intertrochanteric osteotomy can be performed in patients whose CE angles are greater than zero. In a recent study from Japan, a group of patients whose average preoperative CE angle was less than 10° (-1.8° ± 12.2°) experienced good results following intertrochanteric osteotomy at a follow-up of 20 years as long as there were only minimal degenerative changes at the time of index surgery. In another Japanese study, in 13 severely dysplastic hips with subluxation in patients who had undergone periacetabular osteotomy, clinical and radiographic results were excellent in patients who had a preoperative CE angle of less than zero. The follow-up period was 10 to 19 years. It was concluded that periacetabular osteotomy prevented the onset of osteoarthrosis.

Acetabular deficiency in the sagittal plane is best seen by the false profile view where CE angles of approximately zero are common. The radiographic evaluation of a patient with hip dysplasia should include a standing AP pelvis view (which will show subluxation that might not be appreciated in a recumbent view), a false profile view, and an AP view of the hip in abduction. The latter view should show improved congruity rather than hinge abduction, suggesting improved congruity should acetabular redirection and/or intertrochanteric varus osteotomy be performed. It is generally agreed that the role of isolated intertrochanteric osteotomy for dysplasia is limited, but recent studies report that in appropriate patients in whom the major deficiency is on the femoral side, good intermediate term results can be achieved.

In dysplastic hips where there are abnormalities of both the proximal femur and the acetabulum, combined or staged realignment of both acetabulum and proximal femur are indicated. Varus osteotomy is usually performed in prearthrotic hips where the femoral head is spherical; in arthrotic hips where the head is elliptical, congruity may be better achieved with a valgus intertrochanteric osteotomy. In general, first consideration should be given to the acetabulum with or without concomitant intertrochanteric realignment.

Three studies point to the adverse prognostic influence of concomitant arthrosis and dysplasia. At a mean of 6.1 years postoperatively, clinical outcomes were better for patients who had isolated proximal femoral osteotomy for congenital dysplasia if they had minimal or no osteoarthrosis at the time of the index osteotomy. These same findings were reported in an early follow-up of the Bernese periacetabular osteotomy, discussed below. Patients who had osteoarthrosis were more likely to have had a major reoperation at 5 years postoperatively than those who had minimal or no preoperative osteoarthrosis. These studies emphasize the importance of early intervention in dysplasia to ensure favorable and enduring outcomes. Another recent study reports 20 years' follow-up of intertrochanteric osteotomy for treatment of dysplasia. Patients with prearthrosis, that is, more congruous hips, had much better survival at 20 years than patients with established arthrosis. More than 80% of the prearthrotic patients had good results at 20 years, whereas only approximately one third of the patients who had preexisting arthrosis had satisfactory results at 20 years.

The Bernese periacetabular osteotomy has emerged as a versatile and powerful technique to reorient the acetabulum. It has several advantages over other periacetabular osteotomies:

it is performed through a single incision; the acetabulum can be reoriented and medialized without disrupting the posterior column, and then securely fixed to allow the patient early mobilization; intra-articular pathology such as a torn acetabular labrum can be addressed; and the osteotomies are sufficiently distant from the articular surface so as to preserve acetabular vascularity.

In the experience of the developers of the Bernese osteotomy, a reoriented acetabulum, improved congruency, and coverage of the femoral head are goals that are usually achieved by periacetabular osteotomy alone. In some patients, the addition of concomitant or subsequent intertrochanteric osteotomy improves the congruency of the joint. In a recent review of more than 500 periacetabular osteotomies performed for dysplasia, 46 patients required subsequent supplementary intertrochanteric osteotomy to improve congruency, and/or to correct an excessive proximal valgus neck shaft angle.

Acetabular rim syndrome is often the cause of recurrent episodes of sharp groin pain and painful impingement in patients with hip dysplasia. In a recent study, patients reported a history of intermittent groin pain, usually with rotational movement, for up to 15 years; some had pain at night. Presenting symptoms included locking of the hip, a "dead leg" sensation, and a sensation of giving way. On physical examination virtually all had discomfort and apprehension when an impingement provocation test of flexion, adduction, and internal rotation was performed for lesions of the anterior superior acetabular rim. In 37 patients with dysplasia who were undergoing periacetabular osteotomy with these symptoms, 95% were found to have a labral tear. The most common site of the tear was the anterolateral quadrant. The labrum was excised in 21, repaired in 12, and not treated in 4 patients whose condition was considered not severe enough to require repair. At a mean follow-up of 4.5 years, pain was absent in 18 patients, mild in 3, and severe in 1.

Osteotomy in Osteonecrosis

Osteotomy may be considered when the size of the lesion encompasses less than 50% of the weightbearing surface of the femoral head. On plain radiographs, improved prognosis is seen with a combined necrotic angle of less than 200° on AP and lateral radiographs. There seems almost universal agreement that the size of the lesion and the ability to deliver it from the weightbearing sector determine the prognosis. For lesions of discrete size, particularly those in the anterolateral sector of the femoral head, valgus flexion or the flexion osteotomy of Imhauser have been used. Factors associated with failure include inability (usually because of a lesion that is too large) to rotate the necrotic fragment out of the weightbearing area.

In a recent study, 37 corrective osteotomies (Ficat stage II or stage III) were performed for osteonecrosis of the femoral head. At a mean follow-up of 11.5 years, results were good to excellent in patients whose hips had combined necrotic angles of less than 200°, and in patients who were not receiving continuing high doses of corticosteroids. Patients with more than 200° of combined femoral head involvement had poor results, leading to head collapse. The technical goal was to deliver the osteonecrotic area away from the zone of maximum load transmission during weightbearing. Varus osteotomy was performed in all patients, and flexion or extension components were added in an attempt to deliver the lesion from the weightbearing sector. The authors' current criteria for patient selection is an age of 45 years or younger, a painful hip with stage II or stage III involvement, no joint narrowing, a 20° arc of intact lateral femoral head to act as weightbearing support following varus osteotomy, a small to medium lesion of less than 200° on AP and lateral radiographs, and no continued use of high-dose corticosteroids.

In another study, 48 hips in 43 patients were treated with Sugiuka transtrochanteric rotational osteotomy. Results were poor when the preoperative area of necrosis was large. It was recommended that the surgical indications for rotational osteotomy be limited to hips in which the intact area is more than one third of the entire articular surface on the lateral radiograph. In 30 hips, Kaplan-Meier survivorship at 5 years was 60%, but in 6 hips in which the fraction of the intact area of the articular surface was decreased to less than 30%, the results were poor.

Retrieval of a Femoral Head After Osteotomy

The hip joint of a patient who had undergone intertrochanteric osteotomy for osteoarthrosis was retrieved at autopsy, 24 years after surgery. Radiographs 21 years after osteotomy showed improved congruence of the joint and maintenance of articular cartilage circumferentially. Histologic examination of articular cartilage on the superior portion of the femoral head showed 3 zones of articular cartilage, including a deep zone of proliferative hyaline cartilage. These findings support the theoretical foundations of osteotomy: timely intervention and reversal of an adverse mechanical environment can arrest degeneration of articular cartilage and even contribute to its regeneration.

Total Hip Arthroplasty After Previous Osteotomy of the Proximal Femur

Two studies report the results of total hip arthroplasty after proximal femoral osteotomy. In one study, there was no higher rate of complications in the group that had undergone osteotomy, although there was a trend suggesting improved survival of the implant in the group without previous surgery. Previous osteotomies may render subsequent conversion to total hip arthroplasty to be technically demanding because of distortion of the proximal femur. After varus osteotomy the greater trochanter may be prominent and obstruct access to the medullary canal. A trochanteric osteotomy is then indicated. Varus and valgus osteotomies may distort the neck shaft angle, and be rotationally malaligned; the latter problem can affect proper estimation of the anteversion of the femoral component. In general, as long as osteotomies are performed at the intertrochanteric rather than the subtrochanteric level, repeat osteotomy can generally be avoided. It is recommended that methods of intertrochanteric osteotomy that avoid major distortion are desirable. Contemporary methods that do not use wedge resection, particularly in flexion and extension osteotomies, should make subsequent conversion hip replacement less difficult.

In another study, 22 consecutive primary total hip arthroplasties were performed after proximal femoral osteotomies had failed. Of 19 hips studied, the osteotomies were subtrochanteric in 11 and intertrochanteric in 8. The osteotomies deformed the femur in 4 different ways: displacement and angulation of the osteotomy site, deformity in the intertrochanteric region, and canal narrowing because of endosteal new bone formation. These conditions often required novel solutions regarding the type and placement of the stem. There was an association between subtrochanteric osteotomy and its consequent deformities and loosening of the femoral component. Well-performed intertrochanteric osteotomy without excessive displacement or angulation is compatible with satisfactory long-term conversion of total hip arthroplasty.

Patient Selection

Each patient who has arthrosis or who is at risk of developing the condition must understand their prognosis if untreated, and the advantages and disadvantages of a variety of surgical interventions. The patient's age, occupation, level of activity, and functional goals must weigh prominently in the decision to perform osteotomy. The ideal candidate for a reconstructive osteotomy is a young adult (30 years of age or younger) in whom a reconstructive procedure is likely to delay hip replacement for at least 20 years. A salvage osteotomy may provide improved function for shorter periods of time. When restoration of a full range of motion is a chief reason why the patient seeks help, osteotomy is less likely to be deemed successful. Osteotomy neither increases nor decreases overall motion, but may restore a limited functional range of motion. In this context, total hip arthroplasty and osteotomy should be viewed as complementary rather than competitive procedures.

Annotated Bibliography

Dysplasia

Hersche O, Casillas M, Ganz R: Indications for intertrochanteric osteotomy after periacetabular osteotomy for adult hip dysplasia. *Clin Orthop* 1998;347:19–26.

In a minority of periacetabular osteotomies (46 patients in a group of more than 500 periacetabular osteotomies), concomitant intertrochanteric osteotomy was performed. After completing the periacetabular osteotomy the degree of restoration of hip joint space, congruency, and containment was assessed. If these factors are not optimal, either varus or valgus intertrochanteric osteotomy will be performed.

Iwase T, Hasegawa Y, Kawamoto K, Iwasada S, Yamada K, Iwata H: Twenty years' follow-up of intertrochanteric osteotomy for treatment of the dysplastic hip. *Clin Orthop* 1996;331:245–255.

Varus intertrochanteric osteotomy was performed on 52 hips with prearthrotic or early degenerative changes; in 53 patients, valgus intertrochanteric osteotomy was performed for established degenerative arthrosis. Kaplan-Meier survivorship at 10 and 15 years was 89% and 87%, respectively, for the prearthrotic or early arthrotic group; in contrast, the survival for the established osteoarthrotic group (valgus osteotomy) was 66% at 10 years and 38% at 15 years.

Leunig M, Werlen S, Ungersbock A, Ito K, Ganz R: Evaluation of the acetabular labrum by MR arthrography. *J Bone Joint Surg* 1997;79B:230–234.

In 23 patients undergoing periacetabular osteotomy for dysplasia, preoperative magnetic resonance arthrography showed a high sensitivity and good specificity identifying labral tears. Only 3 patients who had a positive arthrogram were found to have a normal labrum at arthroplasty.

Perlau R, Wilson MG, Poss R: Isolated proximal femoral osteotomy for treatment of residua of congenital dysplasia or idiopathic osteoarthrosis of the hip: Five to ten-year results. *J Bone Joint Surg* 1996;78A:1462–1467.

Intertrochanteric osteotomy was performed on a cohort of 18 hips for dysplasia and on a cohort of 16 hips with idiopathic osteoarthrosis. In both groups, patients who reported the most enduring improvement at 5 to 10 years were those who had the least arthrotic changes at the time of index surgery. Additionally, in the group with dysplasia, those with a predominant proximal femoral abnormality (rather than a predominant acetabular abnormality) reported the best improvements in function and pain relief.

Trousdale RT, Ekkernkamp A, Ganz R, Wallrichs SL: Periacetabular and intertrochanteric osteotomy for the treatment of osteoarthrosis in dysplastic hips. *J Bone Joint Surg* 1995; 77A:73–85.

Forty-two patients who underwent the Bernese periacetabular osteotomy were evaluated on an average of 4 years postoperatively. The likelihood of a patient requiring further surgery, that is, conversion to total hip arthroplasty or another osteotomy was increased if they had established osteoarthritic changes preoperatively.

Osteotomy in Osteonecrosis

Langlais F, Fourastier J: Rotation osteotomies for osteonecrosis of the femoral head. *Clin Orthop* 1997;343:110–123.

The authors performed either a Sugiuka anterior rotation osteotomy (16 patients) or a Kempf posterior rotation osteotomy (4 patients). Rotation osteotomy for osteonecrosis is recommended when the necrotic lesion can be delivered from the weightbearing zone of the acetabulum when the hip is in extension. In addition, if the necrotic lesion is deeper than the proximal third of the femoral head, rotational osteotomy is not recommended.

Mont MA, Fairbank AC, Krackow KA, Hungerford DS: Corrective osteotomy for osteonecrosis of the femoral head: The results of a long-term follow-up study. *J Bone Joint Surg* 1996; 78A:1032–1038.

Thirty-two patients (37 osteotomies) were evaluated at a mean of 11.5 years postoperatively. All underwent varus intertrochanteric osteotomy with additional flexion or extension sagittal plane correction, and all were either Ficat and Arlet class II or class III preoperatively. The best results were in patients who had not received corticosteroids and in those with an area of sector involvement of less than a sum of 200° on AP and lateral radiographs.

Total Hip Arthroplasty After Previous Osteotomy of the Proximal Femur

Boos N, Krushell R, Ganz R, Muller ME: Total hip arthroplasty after previous proximal femoral osteotomy. *J Bone Joint Surg* 1997;79B:247–253.

Seventy-four total hip arthroplasties (THAs) were performed following intertrochanteric osteotomy and compared to a control group of primary THAs. There were no significant differences in the rate of perioperative complications, or the incidence of sepsis or aseptic loosening. There was a frequent need to perform greater trochanteric osteotomy in the group with previous osteotomy to gain adequate access to the medullary canal.

Classic Bibliography

Ganz R, Klaue K, Vinh TS, Mast JW: A new periacetabular osteotomy for the treatment of hip dysplasias: Technique and preliminary results. *Clin Orthop* 1988;232:26–36.

Klaue K, Durnin CW, Ganz R: The acetabular rim syndrome: A clinical presentation of dysplasia of the hip. *J Bone Joint Surg* 1991;73B:423–429.

Marti RK, Schuller HM, Raaymakers EL: Intertrochanteric osteotomy for non-union of the femoral neck. *J Bone Joint Surg* 1989; 71B:782–787.

Millis MB, Murphy SB, Poss R: Osteotomies about the hip for the prevention and treatment of osteoarthrosis. *J Bone Joint Surg* 1995;77A:626–647.

Müller ME: Intertrochanteric osteotomy: Indication, preoperative planning, technique, in Schatzker J (ed): *The Intertrochanteric Osteotomy.* Berlin, Germany, Springer-Verlag, 1984, pp 25–66.

Poss R: Current concepts review: The role of osteotomy in the treatment of osteoarthritis of the hip. *J Bone Joint Surg* 1984; 66A:144–151.

Chapter 14
Design Evolution: Cemented Total Hip Replacement

Introduction

Although John Charnley was not the first to perform the total hip arthroplasty procedure, he, along with Maurice Mueller and Ken McKee, pioneered the cemented total hip arthroplasty procedure into an operation that provided a predictable short-term outcome. In the 4 decades since the inception of the procedure many design concepts have evolved. This chapter will review the evolution of cemented component design, femoral and acetabular, that has occurred during that time.

Rationale for Design Evolution of Cemented Total Hip Arthroplasty Components

When it became apparent that the long-term problem associated with cemented total hip arthroplasty was aseptic failure, surgeons studying this procedure began considering changes in the design of implants that could provide more durable results. On the femoral side of the construct, the recognition of stem breakage as an early cause of aseptic failure resulted in the development and use of metals with better material strength. When aseptic loosening was recognized, investigators switched their attention to the cause or causes of loosening. Initially, there was debate as to whether the initial event in the loosening process occurred at the bone-cement interface, at the prosthesis-cement interface, or within the cement. Design considerations required knowing which of these interfaces was the weak link in the construct. From long-term observations of the radiographic changes that occur around well-performed, well-designed, and well-functioning femoral implants that loosen, as well as from investigation of retrievals of well-functioning cemented femoral implants, it appears that fatigue fracture of cement (Fig. 1), especially in areas of thin cement mantles (Fig. 2), leads to loss of the sta-

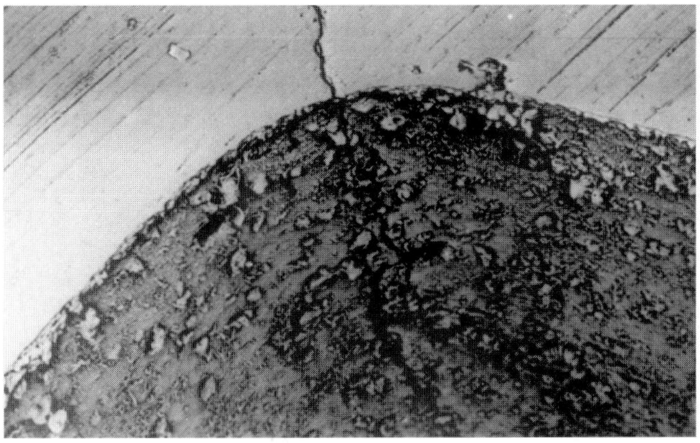

Figure 1

A fracture through the cement mantle in a specimen that had been implanted almost 10 years earlier. (Reproduced with permission from Jasty M, Maloney WJ, Bragdon CR, Haire T, Harris WH: Histomorphological studies of the long-term skeletal responses to well fixed cemented femoral components. *J Bone Joint Surg* 1990;72A:1228.)

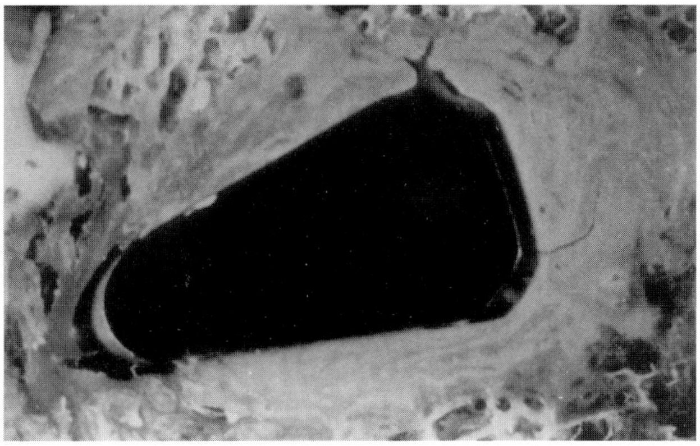

Figure 2

Proximal section of a Mueller prosthesis that had been inserted 13 years previously. The prosthesis has loosened from the cement mantle and has migrated medially. Despite this, there is excellent apposition between cement and bone, and the cement mantle is supported by the remodeled trabecular bone. (Reproduced with permission from Jasty M, Maloney WJ, Bragdon CR, Haire T, Harris WH: Histomorphological studies of the long-term skeletal responses to well fixed cemented femoral components. *J Bone Joint Surg* 1990;72A:1227.)

The author or the departments with which he is affiliated have received something of value from a commercial or other party related directly or indirectly to the subject of this chapter.

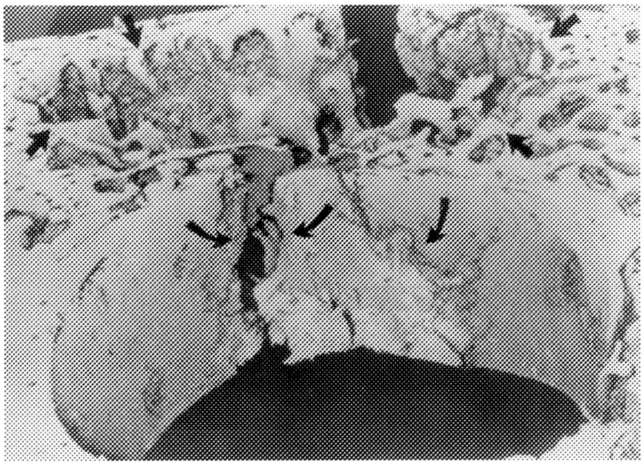

Figure 3

Scanning electron micrograph showing fracture in the thin cement mantle with fragmentation of the cement adjacent to a focal area of bone lysis (arrows). (Reproduced with permission from Maloney WJ, Jasty M, Rosenberg A, Harris WH: Bone lysis in well fixed cemented femoral components. *J Bone Joint Surg* 1990;72B:969.)

bility of the femoral component within the cement mantle (Fig. 3). This instability, represented by a radiolucency between prosthesis and cement, occurs initially in the proximal lateral aspect of the femur (Fig. 4), and is called debonding, although in the case of a polished implant the implant is never bonded to the cement. It is further demonstrated by cracks in the distal cement (a region of high stress in many cemented hip arthroplasty constructs) and subsidence of the femoral component within the cement mantle. Femoral component design and surgical instrumentation evolution have focused toward implants that minimize cement stresses and techniques and designs that accommodate adequate cement mantles. Controversy exists as to whether or not a prosthesis should be bonded to cement, and this issue will be addressed later in this chapter.

On the acetabular side of the cemented total hip arthroplasty construct, long-term radiographic analysis and autopsy retrieval studies have demonstrated that prosthesis-cement interface loosening and cracks in the cement mantle occur only rarely. Instead, loosening usually occurs at the bone-cement interface. It is hypothesized that a histiocytic cell membrane proliferation incited by particulate generation (mostly from wear at the bearing surface) proceeds from the periphery of the cement-bone interface to the dome of the acetabulum, with eventual loosening and superior migration of the construct (Fig. 5). Cemented acetabular design evolution was initially directed toward decreasing cement stresses; however, with better understanding of the loosening mechanism, it is now directed toward optimum bearing-surface mechanics and the peripheral bone-cement interface seal.

Femoral Design Evolution

Material

After recognizing the potential for femoral component fracture, manufacturers ceased using casted stainless steel and chromium cobalt implants and started using cold-worked, cold-forged micrograin implants made of chromium cobalt, titanium alloy, and stainless steel, which provided greater fatigue strength. As long as stress risers are not applied to these devices (especially on the anterolateral tension surface), these components should rarely break. When it appeared that bone-cement interface breakdown was the major cause of femoral component loosening, titanium (with one half the

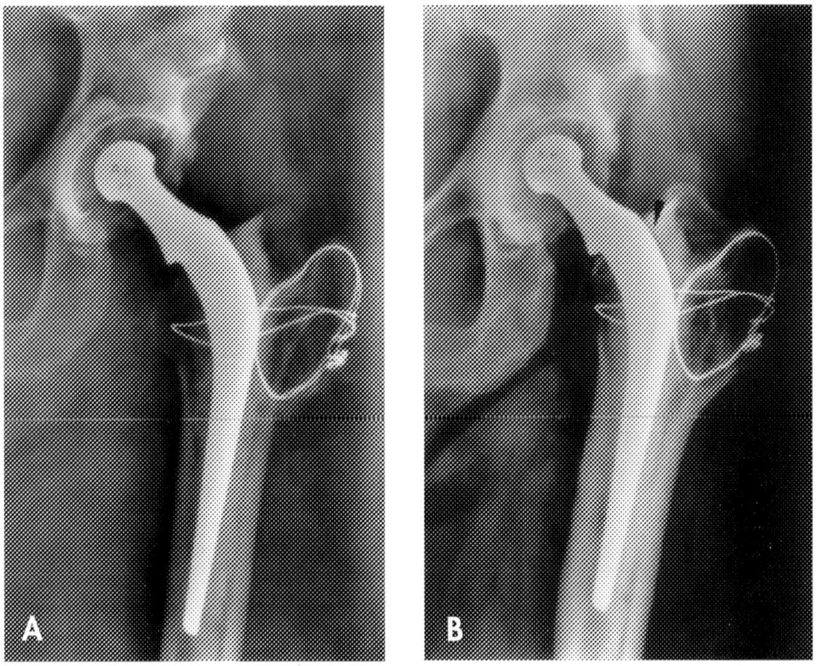

Figure 4

Postoperative (**A**) and follow-up (**B**) radiographs of a patient with a radiolucency between prosthesis and cement, so-called "debonding" (arrow), with maintenance of the bone cement interface.

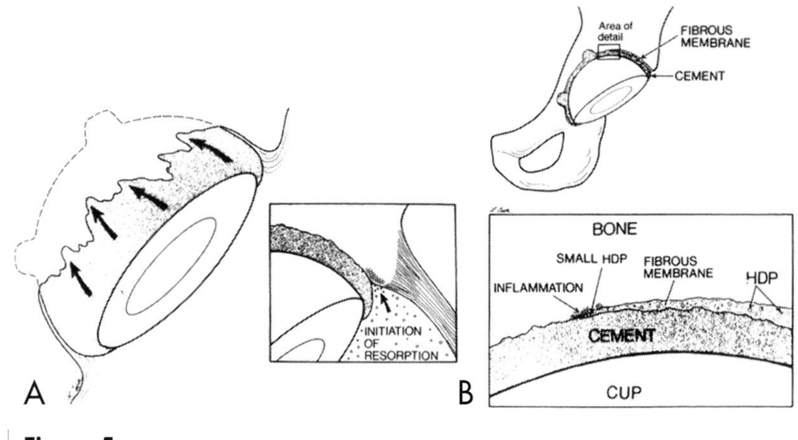

Figure 5

Mechanism of late aseptic loosening of cemented acetabular components. **A**, Bone resorption and membrane formation is initiated circumferentially at the intra-articular margin of the implant. Bone resorption and membrane formation then progresses in a 3-dimensional manner toward the dome of the implant. **B**, Microscopic evaluation of the transition zone from an area with membrane interposition between cement and bone to an area of intimate cement-bone contact was characterized by a cutting wedge of bone resorption. The hallmark of this region is extracellular and intracellular high density polyethylene (HDP) in macrophages with active bone resorption by macrophages. This process is fueled by small particles of HDP wear debris migrating along the cement-bone interface. (Reproduced with permission from Schmalzried TP, Kwong LM, Jasty M, et al: The mechanism of loosening of cemented acetabular components in total hip arthroplasty: Analysis of specimens retrieved at autopsy. *Clin Orthop* 1992;274:75.)

material modulus or stiffness of chromium cobalt or stainless steel) was introduced as a material for cemented femoral components, to potentially deliver more load to bone. However, with the realization that cement fatigue is the major initiator of cemented femoral component failure, stiffer materials (chromium cobalt and stainless steel), which decrease cement stresses and which are more abrasion resistant (harder), are usually used.

Implant Geometry

When it was recognized that fatigue of cement was a major cause of cemented femoral component loosening, designs that created high cement strains (such as the diamond-shaped Mueller prosthesis) were abandoned, and devices that provided broad medial borders with no sharp corners (to decrease cement strains) and broader lateral borders (to increase femoral component strength) were introduced (Fig. 6). The "cobra type" designs and other broad proximal geometries also decrease cement stresses at the tip of the prosthesis (a high stress area). Many contemporary designs incorporate this concept of reducing cement stresses both proximally and distally by altering stem geometry and by using stiffer materials (ie, chromium cobalt and stainless steel).

Because cement is stronger in compression than in tension, many stem designs have incorporated a taper to the mid and distal stem geometry. This design allows the stress transfer of load from the stem to the cement to occur mostly in compression. The Exeter femoral component is the most extreme example of this; however, many stem designs, including the original Charnley flatback design, were tapered distally.

When the transtrochanteric approach to the hip was abandoned for approaches that preserved the greater trochanter, optimization of joint mechanics and offset of the femur in relationship to the acetabulum was compromised. This led to the development of femoral components with greater offset (distance between a longitudinal line through the center of the stem and one through the center of the head of the implant on an anteroposterior projection) to restore the relationship of the greater trochanter and femoral shaft to the acetabulum to that of the normal hip. As large torsional loads are generated in the hip, especially in stair climbing, such offset in the prostheses could transfer high torsional loads to the cement. Although in vitro studies have demonstrated higher torsional loads with these high-offset implants, these loads have not exceeded the endurance limit of cement. However, due to the increasing offsets, designers now tend to use

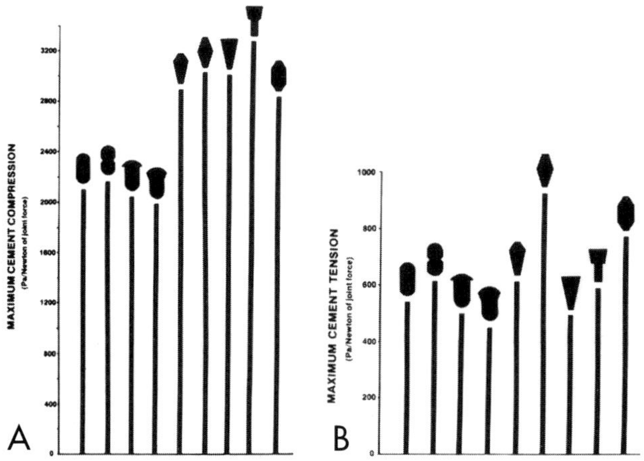

Figure 6

Maximum compression (**A**) and tension (**B**) stress resulting from various stem cross-sectional shapes. (Reproduced with permission from Crowninshield RD, Brand RA, Johnston RC, Milroy JC: The effect of femoral stem cross-sectional geometry on cement stresses in total hip reconstruction. *Clin Orthop* 1980;146:72–73.)

$$R_a = \frac{1}{l_m} \int_0^{l_m} |y|\, dx$$

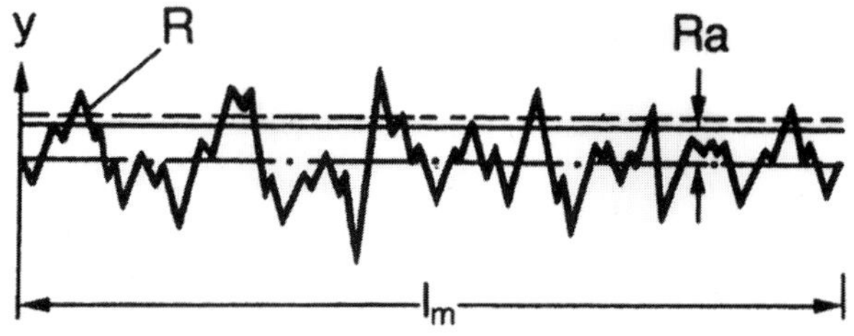

Figure 7

Definition of roughness profile characteristics of average roughness. (Reproduced with permission from Crowninshield RD, Jennings JD, Laurent ML, Maloney WJ: Cemented femoral component surface finish mechanics. *Clin Orthop* 1998;355:91.)

femoral implant geometries that optimize torsional stability so as to better accommodate these loads. Interestingly, the original Charnley flatback device incorporated many of the above design considerations (ie, cement protecting proximal geometry, tapered distal geometry, rotational stability with reasonable offset).

Collar

Most of the original femoral component designs included an internal collar (Charnley, Mueller, McKee prostheses). Charnley hypothesized that if the component subsided within the cement the internal collar would prevent excessive subsidence. Oh and Harris demonstrated that load could be transferred to bone and bypass cement if a large collar was applied to the prosthesis. However, some investigators have questioned the ability to obtain and/or maintain collar-calcar bone contact. In addition, some cemented designs, such as the Exeter stem, desire subsidence to better load the cement in compression and in such cases a collar would be undesirable. Practical issues concerning a collar include its ability to pressurize proximal medial cement, to stabilize the prosthesis while the cement hardens, and to provide a marker for how far to position the component down the femoral canal. Femoral components with and without collars have both functioned well long term.

Surface Finish

A number of variations in the surface finish of femoral implants have been tried over the 30 to 40 years experience with cemented total hip arthroplasty, and this remains one of the most controversial areas in cemented femoral component design today. The roughness of the surface finish of a femoral component is commonly measured using a profilometer. The average roughness (Ra), which is commonly reported by the manufacturer, is the arithmetical average of all departures from the center line of the roughness profile (Fig. 7). The center line is positioned such that the profile areas above and below the line are equal. Thus a surface with a higher Ra value has, on average, a greater distance between its peaks and valleys.

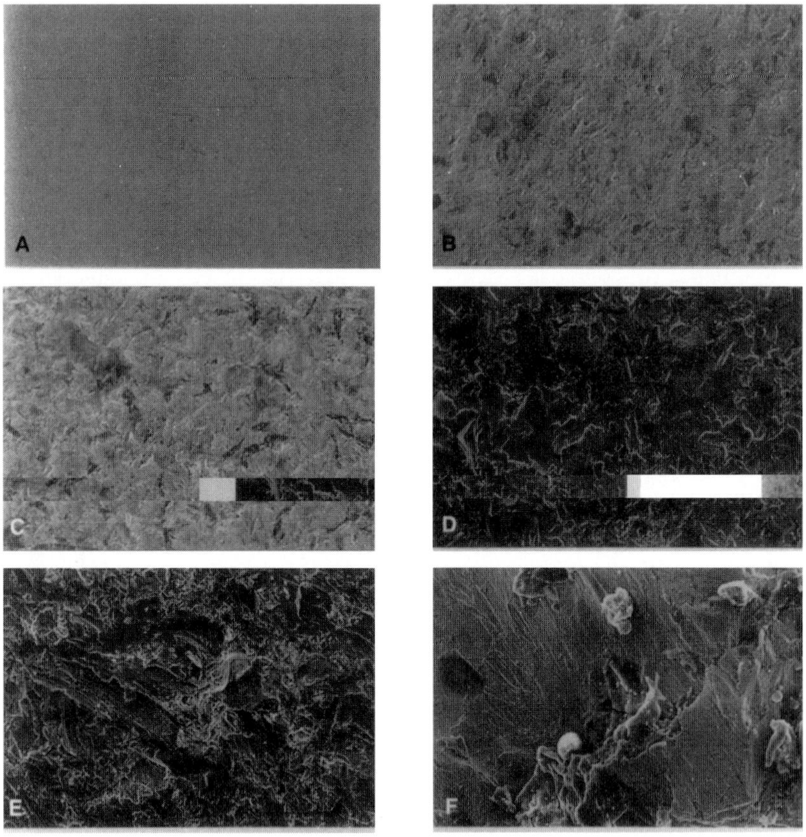

Figure 8

Scanning electron microscopic images of typical implant surfaces manufactured today: **A**, Ra = 0.05 micrometer, **B**, Ra = Ra = 0.64 micrometer, **C**, Ra = 0.08 micrometer, **D**, Ra = 1.22 micrometer, **E**, Ra = 2.2 micrometer, **F**, Ra = 14.2 micrometer. Ra=average roughness. (Reproduced with permission from Crowninshield RD, Jennings JD, Laurent ML, Maloney WJ: Cemented femoral component surface finish mechanics. *Clin Orthop* 1998;355:93.)

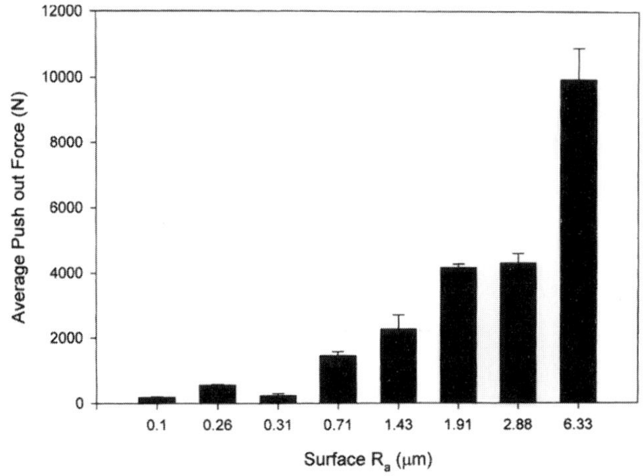

Figure 9

Average pushout force measured for various metal surface roughness. There is a general increase in cement metal attachment with increased metal surface roughness. (Reproduced with permission from Crowninshield RD, Jennings JD, Laurent ML, Maloney WJ: Cemented femoral component surface finish mechanics. *Clin Orthop* 1998;355:97.)

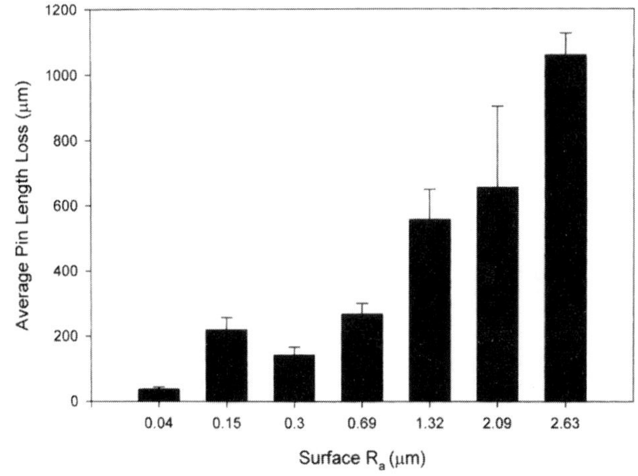

Figure 10

Average cement abrasion after 250,000 cycles for 0.5 mm cement metal displacement for various metal surface roughness. There is a general increase in cement abrasion with increased metal surface roughness. (Reproduced with permission from Crowninshield RD, Jennings JD, Laurent ML, Maloney WJ: Cemented femoral component surface finish mechanics. *Clin Orthop* 1998;355:98.)

The original Charnley flatback device was polished and had an Ra of less than 0.1 mm. The matte finishes commonly used by many manufacturers in the 1970s and 1980s were in the range of 0.6 to 0.75 μm Ra. The grit-blasted devices offered by many manufacturers in the 1990s had an Ra of 1.5 μm and above (Fig. 8). Devices with rougher surface finishes adhere better to cement (Fig. 9), because they use the cement as a glue. They transmit loads to the prosthesis-cement interface by a combination of tension, shear, and compression. Adherence of the prosthesis to cement decreases cement strains and lowers cement stresses. With cement-metal interface motion, these devices generate larger amounts of cement abrasion (Fig. 10). Implants with smoother surface finishes use cement as a grout and have weak bone-cement adhesion. They transmit load at the prosthesis-cement interface by compression, which results in higher cement stresses. However, with cement-metal interface motion, these devices create lower amounts of cement abrasion. Devices with smooth and rough surface finishes have performed relatively well over long periods of time. However, whenever a device has been used with both types of surface finishes, the results have been more durable when the component had a smoother surface finish. In addition, there is increasing evidence that failure can occur earlier, with more progressive and extensive osteolysis, when devices with a rougher surface finish demonstrate debonding from cement.

Centralization

Numerous finite element models of the cemented femoral component composite have demonstrated the beneficial load transfer of stresses from prostheses to cement when adequate circumferential cement mantles (at least 1 to 2 mm distally with as much as 3 to 7 mm recommended proximally) are obtained. In some series, especially in series of devices with rough surface finishes, failure has been attributed to cement mantle defects. Centralizers, both proximally and distally, have been developed and applied to cemented femoral components to avoid these defects and to provide more uniform cement mantles. Although laboratory models have demonstrated more uniform cement mantles when centralizers are used, no clinical studies have documented lower long-term loosening rates in series where these were applied. In addition, bony impingement (Fig. 11), cement voids around the centralizers (Fig. 12), and the potential for another interface failure are concerns.

Acetabular Component Design

Initially all-polyethylene acetabular components were used in the cemented total hip arthroplasty construct. Finite element modeling demonstrated the potential to decrease cement strains by backing the component with metal. Some studies have demonstrated less durable results in terms of loosening and component wear when these metal-backed components were used, although the literature is conflicting. The mechanism of loosening on the acetabular side of the construct is

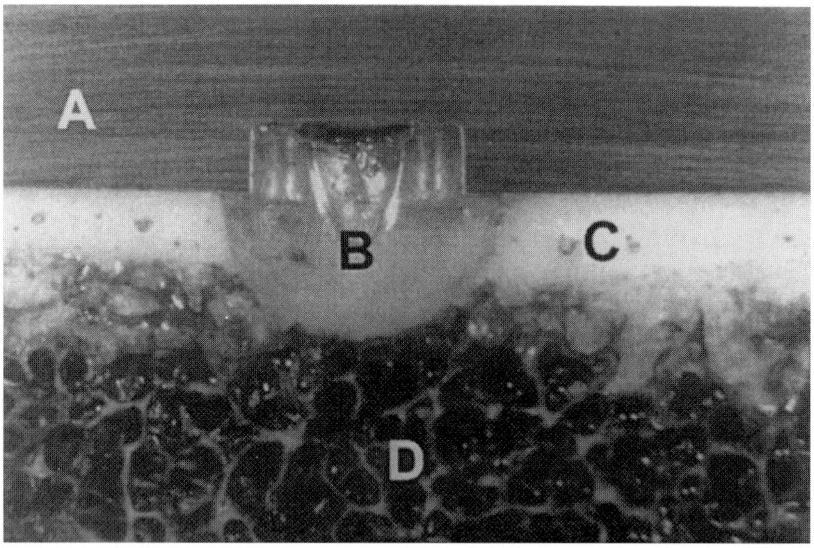

Figure 11

A magnified view (×12) of a section taken through a hemispheric centralizer (B) attached to the surface of a prototype prosthesis (A) and the cement mantle (C). This preparation illustrates the phenomenon of impingement of button-shaped centralizers in cancellous bone (D). (Reproduced with permission from Noble PC, Collie MB, Maltry JA, Kamaric E, Tullos HS: Pressurization and centralization enhance the quality and reproducibility of cement mantles. *Clin Orthop* 1998;355:84.)

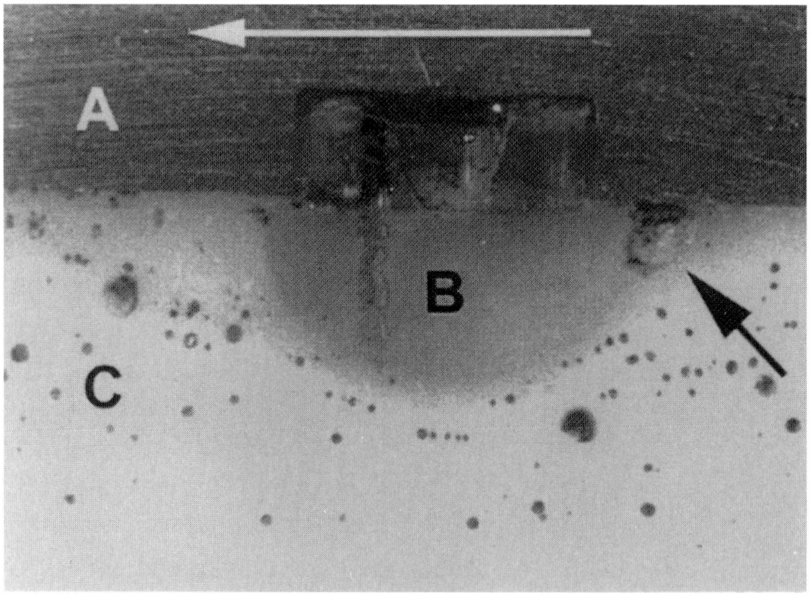

Figure 12

A photomicrograph (×14) of a section through a prototype prosthesis (A) implanted in cement (C), showing void entrapment. Motion of the implant (white arrow) during implantation has led to the accumulation of a void behind the button-shaped centralizer (B), as is indicated by the black arrow.

now thought to be biologic, with advancement of the histiocytic cell membrane (created by particulate debris) from periphery to dome. For this reason, acetabular cup design and preparation now focuses toward peripheral lips on the acetabular components (such as the Ogee injection cup design), to pressurize the peripheral cement, and toward techniques to reproducibly obtain cement-bone interfaces without peripheral bone-cement radiolucencies. All-polyethylene components are recommended because of their potential to use thicker polyethylene and because of the lower wear and loosening rates reported in some studies when compared to metal-backed components. Lower wear rates can potentially decrease the histiocytic cell response that contributes to loosening.

Annotated Bibliography

Mechanisms of Cemented Hip Replacement Loosening

Jasty M, Maloney WJ, Bragdon CR, Haire T, Harris WH: Histomorphological studies of the long-term skeletal responses to well fixed cemented femoral components. *J Bone Joint Surg* 1990;72A:1220–1229.

Autopsy retrieval of well-functioning femoral components demonstrated intact bone-cement interfaces, with cement mantle fractures and debonding of the prosthesis-cement interface in some specimens.

Maloney WJ, Jasty M, Rosenberg A, Harris WH: Bone lysis is well-fixed cemented femoral components. *J Bone Joint Surg* 1990;72B:966–970.

In 25 cases of focal femoral osteolysis, thin cement mantles or cement defects were associated with 60% of cases.

Schmalzried TP, Kwong LM, Jasty M, et al:

The mechanism of loosening of cemented acetabular components in total hip arthroplasty: Analysis of specimens retrieved at autopsy. *Clin Orthop* 1992;274:60–78.

An autopsy retrieval study of cemented, all-polyethylene acetabular components demonstrated that bone resorption was initiated circumferentially at the periphery of the component and progressed towards the dome, fueled by small particles of polyethylene that incited an inflammatory response. This study supports a biologic rather than mechanical mode of late aseptic loosening of cemented acetabular components.

Femoral Design

Material

Crowninshield RD, Brand RA, Johnston RC, Pedersen DR: An analysis of collar function and the use of titanium in femoral prostheses. *Clin Orthop* 1981;158:270–277.

This finite element study of femoral components demonstrates the high cement mantle stresses that can occur when components made of less stiff materials (ie, titanium) are used.

Woolson ST, Milbauer JP, Bobyn JD, Yue S, Maloney WJ: Fatigue fracture of a forged cobalt-chromium-molybdenum femoral component inserted with cement: A report of ten cases. *J Bone Joint Surg* 1997;79A:1842–1848.

This study reports on 10 fractures, of modern cemented femoral components, that initiated at the anterolateral aspect of the component where thermal changes to the microstructure of the alloy at that area probably caused a focal reduction in material strength.

Implant Geometry

Crowninshield RD, Brand RA, Johnston RC, Milroy JC: An analysis of femoral component stem design in total hip arthroplasty. *J Bone Joint Surg* 1980;62A:68–78.

This finite element study showed that femoral components made of stiffer metals (chromium cobalt instead of titanium), with broad proximal geometries and with longer stem length, provided the lowest cement stresses.

Crowninshield RD, Brand RA, Johnston RC, Milroy JC: The effect of femoral stem cross-sectional geometry on cement stresses in total hip reconstruction. *Clin Orthop* 1980;146:71–77.

In this finite element study, femoral components with broad medial borders, no sharp corners, and broader lateral borders proved optimal for minimizing femoral cement stresses.

Collar

Oh I, Harris WH: Proximal strain distribution in the loaded femur: An in vitro comparison of the distributions in the intact femur and after insertion of different hip-replacement femoral components. *J Bone Joint Surg* 1978;60A:75–85.

This study demonstrated that transfer of load directly to the calcar femorale through a larger collar in direct contact with the cortical bone restored 30% to 40% of the normal strain to the calcar femorale and shifted the strain pattern toward normal.

Markolf KL, Amstutz HC, Hirschowitz DL: The effect of calcar contact on femoral component micromovement: A mechanical study. *J Bone Joint Surg* 1980;62A:1315–1323.

This study demonstrated that it is difficult to obtain calcar-collar contact, even in the laboratory setting.

Ling RS: The use of a collar and precoating on cemented femoral stems is unnecessary and detrimental. *Clin Orthop* 1992;285:73–83.

This article reviews the benefits of using a tapered stem geometry and a polished femoral component, without a collar, so that loads are transferred from stem to cement in compression.

Harris WH: Is it advantageous to strengthen the cement-metal interface and use a collar for cemented femoral components of total hip replacements? *Clin Orthop* 1992;285:67–72.

This article reviews the benefits of using a grit-blasted, precoated, collared femoral prosthesis for cemented arthroplasty.

Surface Finish

Crowninshield RD, Jennings JD, Laurent ML, Maloney WJ: Cemented femoral component surface finish mechanics. *Clin Orthop* 1998;355:90–102.

This article reviews the definitions of surface finish and explains the choices and compromises associated with rough and smooth surface finishes on implants in relationship to adhesion and abrasion characteristics.

Schulte KR, Callaghan JJ, Kelley SS, Johnston RC: The outcome of Charnley total hip arthroplasty with cement after a minimum twenty-year follow-up: The results of one surgeon. *J Bone Joint Surg* 1993;75A:961–975.

This minimum 20-year follow-up of a polished Charnley femoral component demonstrated 2% revised for loosening at 20 years, and 7% radiographically loose (including the 2% revised).

Smith SW, Estok DM II, Harris WH: Total hip arthroplasty with use of second-generation cementing techniques: An eighteen-year-average follow-up study *J Bone Joint Surg* 1998;80A: 1632–1640.

This study demonstrates a 5% femoral revision prevalence at 18 years for aseptic loosening when a matte-finish femoral component with collar was used.

Middleton RG, Howie DW, Costi K, Sharpe P: Effects of design changes on cemented tapered femoral stem fixation. *Clin Orthop* 1998;355:47–56.

This study demonstrated more durable results when a tapered stem geometry with a polished finish, rather than a matte-finish stem, was used.

Collis DK, Mohler CG: Loosening rates and bone lysis with rough finished and polished stems. *Clin Orthop* 1998;355:113–122.

This study reviewed the loosening and osteolysis prevalence associated with 2 different femoral implant designs. Both rougher and smoother surface finishes had been used with both designs. Loosening and osteolysis was decreased by using a smoother surface finish.

Mohler CG, Callaghan JJ, Collis DK, Johnston RC: Early loosening of the femoral component at the cement-prosthesis interface after total hip replacement. *J Bone Joint Surg* 1995;77A: 1315–1322.

This study demonstrated rapid osteolysis and loosening after debonding occurred with a grit-blasted femoral component.

Centralization

Noble PC, Collier MB, Maltry JA, Kamaric E, Tullos HS: Pressurization and centralization enhance the quality and reproducibility of cement mantles. *Clin Orthop* 1998;355:77–89.

This article reviews the benefits of circumferential thick mantles in femoral cement fixation. It discusses the benefits and problems associated with centralizers.

Acetabular Component Design

Pederson DR, Crowninshield RD, Brand RA, Johnston RC: An axisymmetric model of acetabular components in total hip arthroplasty. *J Biomech* 1982;15:305–315.

This acetabular finite element model demonstrated a marked reduction in bone-cement strains when metal-backed components were compared to all-polyethylene components.

Ranawat CS, Peters LE, Umlas ME: Fixation of the acetabular component: The case for cement. *Clin Orthop* 1997;344: 207–215.

These authors demonstrate that achieving a cemented acetabular construct with no initial bone-cement radiolucencies is paramount for long-term survivorship of the component.

Bankston AB, Cates H, Ritter MA, Keating EM, Faris PM: Polyethylene wear in total hip arthroplasty. *Clin Orthop* 1995;317:7–13.

Comparing wear rates of cemented and cementless components, these authors demonstrated that the least wear occurred when cemented, all-polyethylene components that were compression-molded were used.

Chapter 15
Evolution of Uncemented Femoral Component Design

Introduction

Despite the widely acknowledged success of cemented femoral components of total hip arthroplasty, early and late failures due to loosening occur in a small number of patients. Uncemented femoral components were developed and have been refined over the last two decades in an effort to provide even better durability of femoral fixation, particularly in patients who, because of their age, activity, or size, place high demands on hip implants.

Failure caused by aseptic femoral loosening was common in some early cemented stems implanted with early cement techniques. These failures led to development of methods of fixing the femur without cement. When uncemented porous-coated implants were introduced in the 1980s, they were embraced enthusiastically in North America, but by the early 1990s problems with early loosening, thigh pain, and osteolysis led some surgeons to lose enthusiasm for their use. Simultaneously, long-term results demonstrated success of certain cemented femoral implant designs at more than 20 years, and favorable reports on femoral fixation with improved cementation techniques became available. This combination of factors led to a resurgence in cemented stem use in the 1990s. As the 1990s come to a close, the pendulum is perhaps swinging again toward enthusiasm for uncemented femoral implants. One factor responsible for this reassessment has been the premature failure of cemented femoral implants of certain designs—despite use of modern cement techniques. Perhaps even more importantly, over the last 15 years uncemented femoral implants have also continued to evolve, and several implants now have midterm results that rival those of the best cemented results at a similar time interval. Reported results of uncemented femoral components of a number of successful designs demonstrate very good clinical results, high rates of bone ingrowth, low rates of clinically troublesome thigh pain, and good midterm durability. This chapter discusses the evolution of uncemented femoral component designs and evaluates how increasing knowledge about uncemented implants has translated into design improvements that allow uncemented femoral implants to achieve a high level of success.

Implant Fixation

Satisfactory pain relief and good clinical function in hips with uncemented femoral implants are widely recognized to depend on stable initial and long-term prosthetic fixation to bone. Since the introduction of uncemented implants, much has been learned about how to achieve these goals. This section reviews what is known about the factors that lead to successful early and long-term implant fixation and how this information has affected uncemented femoral implant design.

Initial Stem Stability

Satisfactory initial stability of an uncemented stem is achieved when a stem has sufficient fixation on bone of sufficient strength to resist clinically applied loads. The initial fixation must provide stability until biologic fixation is achieved. The major advances in initial fixation have been in optimized implant geometries, expanded implant size options, and improved surgical techniques.

Implants must be able to resist translation in 3 planes: axial (subsidence), medial-lateral, and anterior-posterior. Implants must also resist rotation in the coronal plane (varus-valgus), rotation in the parasagittal plane (flexion and extension), and rotation in the transverse plane (ie, torsion around the long axis of the implant). Studies have shown that most uncemented implants, even successful ones, undergo a small amount of early subsidence after implantation, usually too small to measure with standard radiographs. Progressive subsidence, however, correlates with clinical failure. Resistance to torsional load (that is the resistance to rotation around the long axis of the implant) appears to be particularly important and is a key distinguishing feature of successful uncemented implants.

Obtaining initial implant stability requires not only proper implant design but also that the implant is placed in contact with bone of sufficient strength to support the implant rigidly. Bone strong enough to meet these demands is typically either cortical or hard, dense cancellous bone near the cortex. Different implant designs obtain fixation in different parts of the femur: the metaphysis, the metaphyseal-diaphyseal junction, and the diaphysis. Some implants are designed to obtain fixation in several of these areas simultaneously, and some obtain initial stability that resists certain forces (such as torsional loads) in one part of the femur, but obtain stability that resists other forces (such as axial loads) in another part of the femur.

Implant Geometry

Implant geometry is a key determinant of initial implant stability. Uncemented femoral implant geometries have evolved according to a number of different philosophies, and it now seems clear that several different varieties of implant geometry reliably can provide stable implant fixation.

Any classification system is arbitrary and grouping of some implants is difficult. Nevertheless, most common implant geometries fall into 4 categories: wedge-shaped metaphyseal-filling implants that obtain fixation in the metaphysis, single wedge-shaped implants that are relatively thin in an anterior to posterior direction, tapered stems that are designed to get most fixation at the metaphyseal-diaphyseal junction, and distally cylindrical or fluted stems designed to obtain initial fixation in the diaphysis (Fig. 1). The metaphysis provides most axial and torsional stability for most wedge-shaped proximally porous-coated metaphyseal-filling implants, the metaphyseal-diaphyseal junction provides axial stability in most tapered designs, and the diaphysis provides torsional stability in extensively porous-coated implants and fluted implants. Collared implants may also obtain axial stability in part from the femoral neck.

Midterm information suggests that each of the above categories of implant geometry can provide a high level of success. Each implant geometry has a unique set of advantages and disadvantages, and each also has a specific set of pitfalls associated with insertion.

Implant Sizes

Early in the development of uncemented implants most systems had only a few stem sizes. This limitation compromised the surgeon's ability to fit the stem to the patient's bone, and hence to provide reliable initial implant stability. An important part of the evolution of uncemented stems has been an expanded number of stem sizes, which now allow the surgeon a greater opportunity to match the implant to an individual patient's femur. The broader array of sizes allows surgeons to achieve implant stability more regularly, with less bone removal and less risk of fracture.

The size of the femoral metaphysis relative to the diaphyseal canal diameter varies markedly from patient to patient. Different approaches have been developed to deal with this discrepancy. Some implant systems allow the surgeon to choose different metaphyseal implant geometries or sizes for a given diaphyseal size or different diaphyseal sizes for a given metaphyseal size (Fig. 2). Modular femoral implants allow the surgeon to construct many combinations of proximal and distal prosthetic femoral geometry with an off-the-shelf implant.

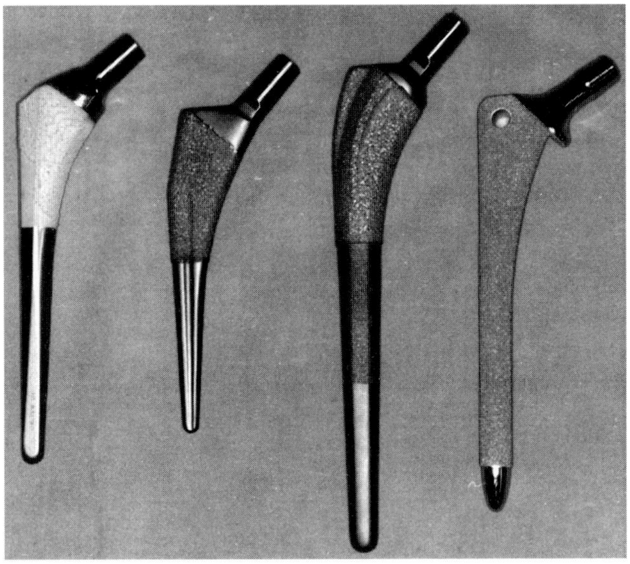

Figure 1
From left to right, examples of a metaphyseal-filling implant, a single wedge-shaped implant, a tapered implant, and an extensively porous-coated implant.

Surgical Technique and Instrumentation

A tight fit of the implant with bone correlates with the highest likelihood of good initial and long-term stability. For any implant, an important variable that affects initial stem stability is the surgeon's ability to obtain an intimate fit between the implant and strong bone. Implant-bone contact can be increased by using instruments to prepare the femoral canal that are sized smaller than the real implants, but the greater the size discrepancy the greater the risk of fracture.

Different methods to prepare the femur include broaching, reaming, milling by hand, and milling with computerized robotic techniques; each has its own set of trade-offs between simplicity and efficacy. Familiarity with the nuances of technique required for proper implant sizing, bone preparation, and implant insertion also makes a major difference in quality of initial fixation. Thus a learning curve is associated with implanting each specific design and as surgeons become more familiar with techniques better results can be expected.

Modularity

The value of modularity (exclusive of modular femoral heads) has been one of the most controversial of all aspects of

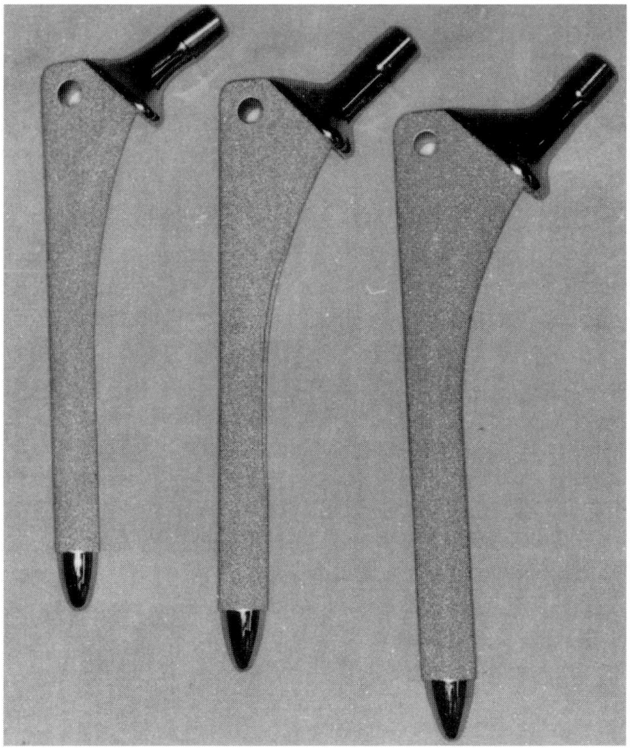

Figure 2

Implants of the same design with 3 different metaphyseal wedge sizes. These allow accommodation to different relative dimensions and shapes of the metaphysis and diaphysis.

uncemented implant design. Modularity allows more versatility in matching the proximal and distal aspects of femoral geometry and also allows the surgeon to manipulate implant anteversion relative to the patient's anatomic anteversion (Fig. 3). On the other hand, modular junctions have some theoretical disadvantages. They could fail catastrophically, leading to arthroplasty failure, or, more insidiously, they could produce particulate debris by fretting or corrosion. That particulate debris could lead to osteolysis directly or indirectly by acting as a third body at the bearing surface. To date, there are few reports of major clinical problems with modular junctions, although with longer follow-up times these problems may still develop. There presently is no consensus about the value of routine use of modular implants in uncemented total hip arthroplasty. However, modular implants are recognized to be useful for unusual femoral geometries or femoral deformities that cannot readily be managed with standard off-the-shelf implants. Concerns about the long-term risk of fretting, corrosion, or failure of modular junctions need to be considered along with the benefits these implants may provide.

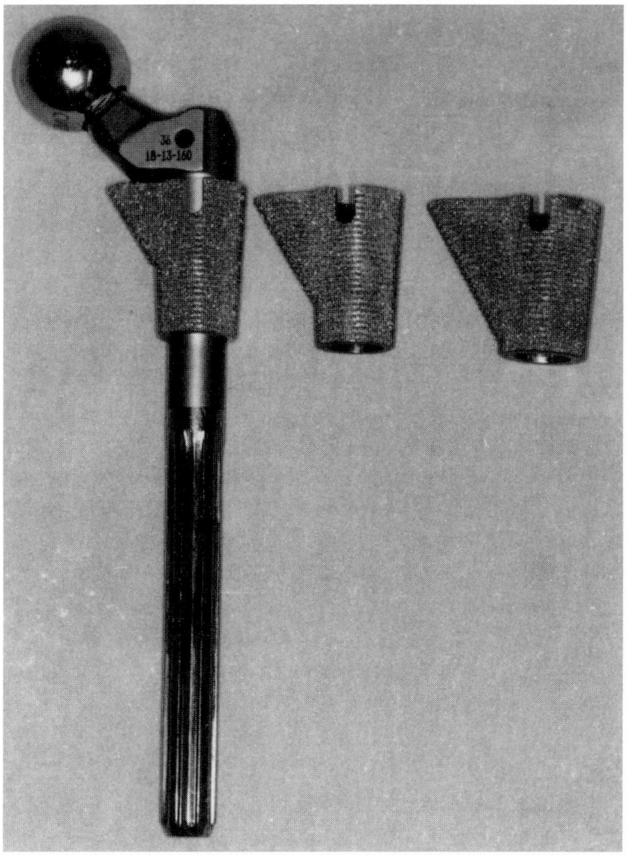

Figure 3

Example of a modular femoral stem with different metaphyseal sleeves. Many different stem and sleeve combinations are possible. The stem and sleeve are joined by a taper fit.

Long-Term Implant Stability

Long-term implant stability, which is bony fixation of an uncemented implant, occurs when bone grows onto or into the surface of the femoral implant. For bony fixation to occur, the implant must have sufficient initial stability. Studies have shown that implant micromotion of less than 50 mm of displacement is required for reliable bony fixation. For bone ingrowth or ongrowth to occur, the implant also must make sufficient contact with viable bone. Precise surgical preparation of the femoral envelope is necessary to provide an intimate fit between the biologically active portion of the implant and native bone. The difficulty of obtaining a perfect match between the implant and the prepared canal helps explain why retrieval studies typically show ingrowth in only a portion of the available implant surface area.

In addition to stable initial fixation and good contact with native bone, bony fixation also requires a prosthetic surface into or onto which bone can grow. Smooth metallic surfaces have not provided satisfactory results and mostly have been abandoned for porous-coated surfaces, roughened surfaces, or surface coatings of biologically active materials such as hydroxyapatite. A sufficient surface area of biologically active implant must also be available to provide for long-term biologic fixation.

Level of Implant Coating

The amount of stem covered with a biologically active surface varies from the proximal one third of the stem to coating of the entire stem. Press-fit designs with completely smooth metal surfaces have been abandoned by most surgeons except for treatment of elderly, inactive patients with hip fractures. Several early uncemented stem designs had porous bead coatings of the entire implant and achieved successful biologic fixation. However, concerns about difficulty of extraction and stress shielding led to efforts to limit the amount of biologically active surface to the upper portion of the stem. Some stem designs with limited porous coating have reliably achieved bone ingrowth, but others have not. Although adverse experience with a reduced area of surface coating in some designs proves that certain designs fare poorly with limited porous coating, this finding cannot necessarily be generalized to all uncemented stems. In general, better success is achieved when the porous or biologically active coating or finish extends to the level of the stem at which primary fixation is achieved. Several metaphyseal-filling stems have achieved good fixation with proximal coatings, most successful tapered stems have coatings that extend to the metaphyseal-diaphyseal junction, and most stems designed for primary fixation in the diaphysis have done best when coatings extend well into the diaphysis of the femur.

There is general agreement that porous coatings or surface enhancements should be applied circumferentially around porous implants rather than in patches. Early "patch porous coated" designs provided channels between patches that served as routes for distal egress of particulate debris from the bearing surface and led to diaphyseal osteolysis. Some implants with limited patches of porous surface have also developed late loosening, possibly as a consequence of stress fracture or traumatic fracture through the limited areas of bone ingrowth provided by small areas of porous coatings.

Types of Coatings

Early uncemented implants had smooth metal surfaces with or without macro texturing or macro geometric features such as fenestrations in the implant. Smooth metal surfaces have not provided reliable long-term bone fixation in the absence of a rough surface texture or porous coating. Macro features alone also have not provided reliable biologic fixation. Thus, most devices presently have some form of surface enhancement to promote bone ingrowth or bone ongrowth. Different surface enhancements include roughened titanium, porous coatings made of cobalt chromium or titanium beads, titanium wire mesh, plasma-sprayed titanium, and bioactive nonmetallic materials such as hydroxyapatite or tricalcium phosphate (Fig. 4).

Factors that affect the success of surface coatings are now better understood, and refinements in porous coatings have evolved accordingly. For porous implants, best bone ingrowth has been demonstrated for pore sizes of 100 to 400 µm. Presently there is not agreement on a single optimal pore size, nor is there agreement that a single type of metal or surface enhancement is most successful. Implant manufacturers have improved the bond between porous coatings and implants, which reduces the likelihood of separation of the coating from the substrate implant.

Hydroxyapatite and tricalcium phosphates are osteoconductive calcium phosphate ceramic compounds that may be applied to metal surfaces. Bone can heal directly to these compounds, thereby providing prosthetic fixation. These compounds may be used in different ways, either as the primary form of long-term implant fixation or to enhance bone ingrowth or ongrowth to an underlying roughened or porous metal surface. The needs in each case are different. Compounds that allow a strong initial bond with bone and resorb slowly are preferred for long-term fixation, while highly biologically active compounds that are more rapidly resorbed may be preferred as a surface enhancement over an underlying porous substrate. Several factors are known to influence the biologic activity and the rapidity of resorption or dissolution of these compounds. Tricalcium phosphate appears to dissolve more rapidly than hydroxyapatite. More crystalline hydroxyapatite is resorbed more slowly than less crystalline hydroxyapatite. Greater porosity of hydroxyapatite increases the resorption rate and reduces mechanical strength.

The thickness of hydroxyapatite coatings has evolved. Very thick coatings (200 µm or more) may be at risk for fracture or delamination, and very thin coatings might be resorbed too quickly. Most manufacturers now provide coatings of around 50 µm. Different methods are available to apply hydroxyapatite to the metal substitute; the method chosen is important because it determines the bond strength between the two. To date, most techniques involve spraying hydroxyapatite onto a rough surface. Because hydroxyapatite is deposited in a unidirectional manner, the ability to deposit

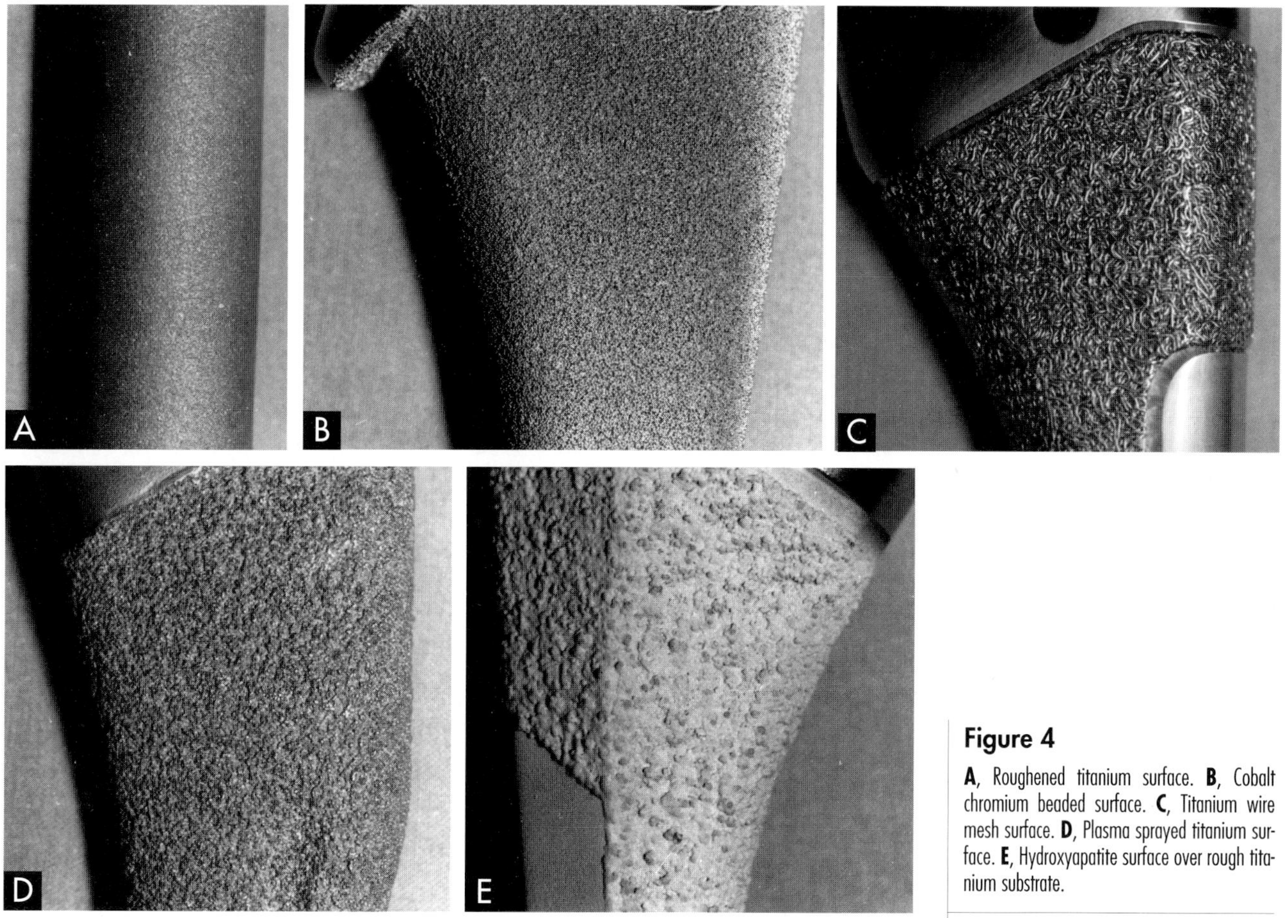

Figure 4

A, Roughened titanium surface. **B**, Cobalt chromium beaded surface. **C**, Titanium wire mesh surface. **D**, Plasma sprayed titanium surface. **E**, Hydroxyapatite surface over rough titanium substrate.

hydroxyapatite evenly onto porous surfaces has been limited. Efforts continue to improve methods of applying calcium phosphate ceramics to porous or rough metal surfaces.

Prevention of Periprosthetic Bone Loss

Bone loss around the femoral implant of a hip arthroplasty can occur by either of two main mechanisms: stress shielding or osteolysis. Stress shielding represents a diffuse loss of bone around an implant in accordance with Wolffs' law. If the presence of a prosthetic implant leads to less stress on the bone, over time bone loss occurs. In contrast, osteolysis is focal bone loss that occurs around an implant and is understood to be caused predominantly by particulate debris—from any part of the prosthesis—that gains access to bone around the implant. Finally, bone loss can occur when implants require extraction. This bone loss is mechanical in nature but has important consequences for a subsequent arthroplasty. This section reviews the factors that lead to periprosthetic bone loss of each type and how implants have evolved to address these issues.

Osteolysis

Osteolysis around uncemented implants occurs when particulate debris—usually from the bearing surface—gains access to the bone around the femoral implant. Proximal femoral osteolysis can occur with any implant design, but osteolysis extending to the diaphysis is mostly associated with loose implants and so-called patch porous-coated implants, both of which provide access channels by which particulate debris from the bearing surface can reach the diaphyseal bone (Fig. 5). Most well-fixed implants with circumferential coating around the upper femoral implant provide bone or soft-tissue ingrowth or ongrowth around the circumference of the upper femoral implant, thereby forming a so-called "gasket-seal". This process seems to restrict access of debris from the bearing surface to most of the femur.

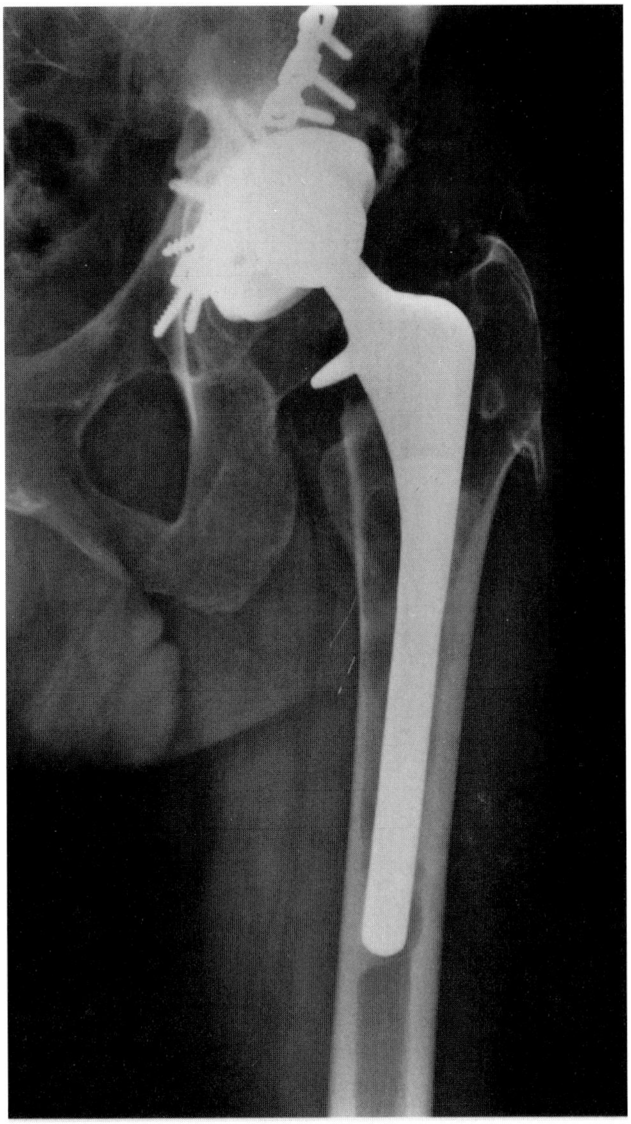

Figure 5

Diaphyseal osteolysis around a well-fixed patch porous-coated femoral component.

Stress Shielding

Stress shielding, related to changes in the physiologic loads experienced by the proximal femur, occurs to some degree around both cemented and uncemented femoral implants. The severity of stress shielding is a function of demographic and implant factors. Bone quality before implant placement is important; the more osteopenic the bone, the greater the chance of severe stress shielding. Stress shielding around uncemented implants also relates to the geometry of the implant, the stiffness of the implant, and the length of the implant covered with porous or biologically active coating. Stiffer, longer implants that allow more distal bone ingrowth appear to be at greater risk for marked proximal femoral stress shielding (Fig. 6).

Extractability and Ease of Revision

Design features that provide good early stability and long-term biologic fixation also create conditions that can make implant extraction difficult and are likely to be associated with significant bone loss. Proximally fixed shorter stems are easier to extract than distally fixed longer stems. However,

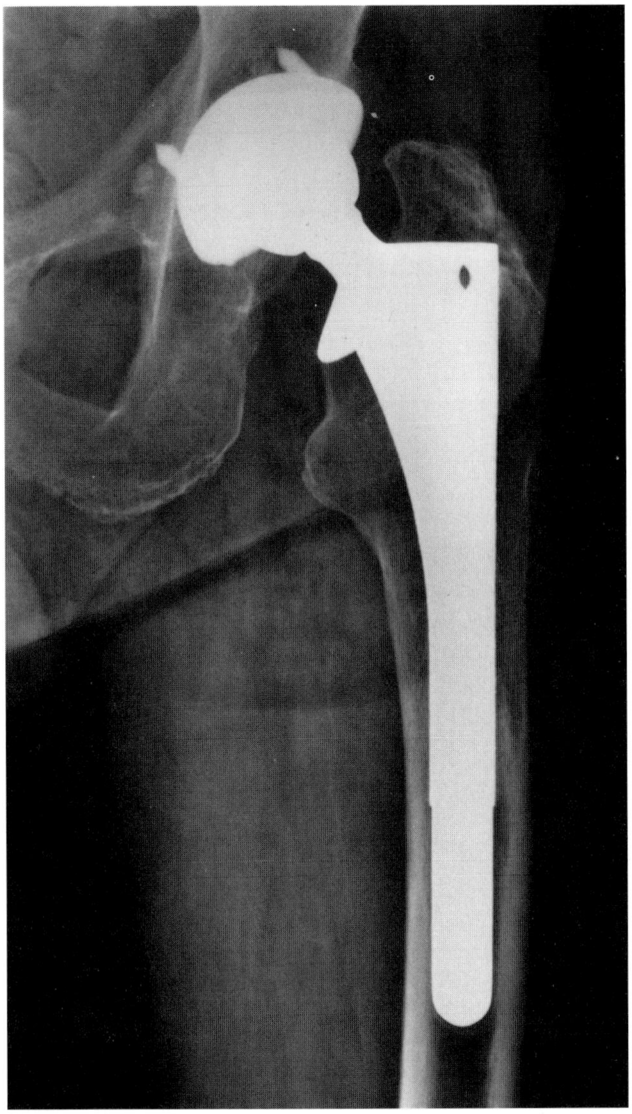

Figure 6

Proximal stress shielding around a bone ingrown extensively porous-coated femoral component.

after extraction, proximal canal-filling implants may leave less bone in the metaphyseal area than some distally fixed designs.

Optimizing Clinical Results

Good clinical results of uncemented hip implants depend on pain relief and restoration of hip mechanics. The most important factor providing pain relief is stable implant fixation. However, it is also recognized that especially for uncemented femoral implants, occasional thigh pain can occur even with well-fixed implants. This section discusses what has been learned about the causes of thigh pain in association with uncemented implants and what has been done to reduce the frequency of this problem. This section also discusses the advances in the proximal geometry of the implants that have improved the surgeon's ability to optimize the biomechanics of a hip reconstruction and, hence, the functional results.

Thigh Pain

Clinically problematic thigh pain around uncemented implants most frequently is a consequence of stem loosening or of fibrous rather than bony tissue stabilization of the implant. Occasionally, marked thigh pain also occurs around bone-ingrown uncemented implants; the etiology of thigh pain in these circumstances is not known with certainty. One hypothesis is that motion of the flexible femur bone occurs around a stiff, less flexible femoral implant, leading to micromotion between the two and pain. One strategy to reduce such micromotion between implant and stem is to extend porous coatings or surface roughening to the tip of the stem. Another is to reduce contact between the tip of the stem and cortical bone of the diaphysis by thinning or tapering stem tips distally. An alternative hypothesis to explain thigh pain is that stress concentration at the tip of a stiff, stable femoral implant causes pain. Several approaches have been used to reduce the modulus of elasticity of the distal stem: these include slots, cutouts, and slimming or boring out the center of the distal stem (Fig. 7). Entire femoral stems made of composite materials with a very low modulus of elasticity to date have not been clinically successful, primarily due to high implant loosening and implant fracture rates.

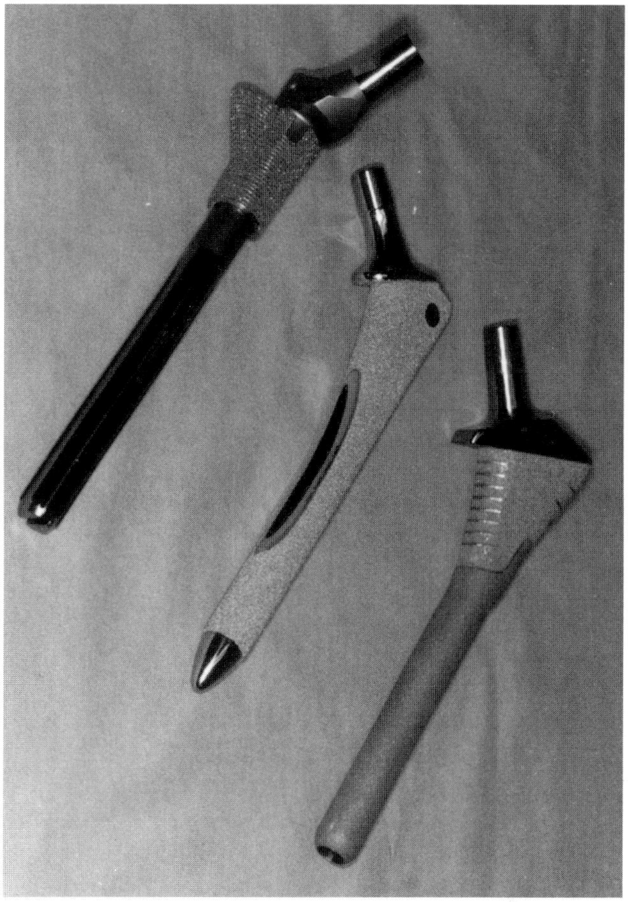

Figure 7
Three methods of reducing stem stiffness; From left to right: a stem with a slot, a stem with a diaphyseal cutout, and a stem that is hollow distally.

Biomechanics

The femoral component has two major functions. It anchors the prosthetic femoral head to the femur, and it substitutes for the femoral head and neck, thereby taking over the biomechanical functions of the proximal femur. For good hip function, the proximal features of femoral implant design that optimize hip biomechanics (neck length, neck angle, neck anteversion, femoral offset, trunion diameter) are as important as femoral stem body design. In recent years greater attention has been paid to these aspects of stem design and, consequently, surgeons are better able to optimize leg length, restore abductor power, optimize hip stability, reduce joint reaction forces, and perhaps reduce bearing surface wear.

By the mid 1980s most implants had modular heads that allowed the surgeon to adjust neck length even after implant insertion. Further refinements of the upper part of the implant allowed better reproduction of the wide range of proximal femoral geometries encountered. Some implant systems allow the surgeon to choose between implants with standard and extra femoral offset. These options are helpful for the patients with a large amount of femoral offset due either to a long femoral neck or a varus femoral neck. Some implants have anteversion built into the stem, which in some instances may improve posterior hip stability. Manufacturers have made an effort to reduce the femoral neck trunion diameter and optimize its shape, thereby improving range of motion before prosthetic neck-socket impingement. Improvements in the geometry of the proximal portion of uncemented hip implants help the surgeon optimize leg length and hip stability and optimize hip biomechanics, which can reduce postoperative limp. By reducing joint reactive forces and prosthetic impingement, these modifications may also reduce bearing surface wear, although this has yet to be proved.

Annotated Bibliography

Engh CA Jr, Culpepper WJ III, Engh CA: Long-term results of use of the anatomic medullary locking prosthesis in total hip arthroplasty. *J Bone Joint Surg* 1997;79A:177–184.

The authors report the results of using an extensively porous coated cobalt chromium stem in 174 hips followed 10 to 13 years. Stem survivorship free of revision was 97% at 12 years. Six patients had activity limiting thigh pain.

Havelin LI, Espehaug B, Vollset SE, Engesaeter LB: Early aseptic loosening of uncemented femoral components in primary total hip replacement: A review based on the Norwegian Arthroplasty Register. *J Bone Joint Surg* 1995;77B:11–17.

The likelihood of early femoral revision for aseptic loosening of multiple uncemented stems was strongly based on implant design.

Geesink RG, Hoefnagels NH: Six-year results of hydroxyapatite-coated total hip replacement. *J Bone Joint Surg* 1995;77B: 534–547.

The survival rate free of revision for loosening at 6 years for 118 hydroxyapatite-coated titanium stems was 100%. No femoral components were radiographically loose.

Jaffe WL, Scott DF: Total hip arthroplasty with hydroxyapatite-coated prostheses. *J Bone Joint Surg* 1996;78A:1918–1934.

This review article discusses the basic science and clinical results of hydroxyapatite-coated implants.

Kienapfel H, Sprey C, Wilke A, Griss P: Implant fixation by bone ingrowth. *J Arthroplasty* 1999;14:355–368.

This article presents a review of the basic requirements for bone ingrowth, including implant materials, surface geometry characteristics, implant stability, and interface distances.

Malchau H, Herberts P, Wang YX, Kärrholm J, Romanus B: Long-term clinical and radiological results of the Lord total hip prosthesis: A prospective study. *J Bone Joint Surg* 1996;78B: 884–891.

The 10-year survival rate free of femoral revision was 98% for an extensively porous coated femoral component.

Maloney WJ, Sychterz C, Bragdon C, et al: Skeletal response to well fixed femoral components inserted with and without cement. *Clin Orthop* 1996;333:15–26.

Autopsy retrievals from patients with unilateral cemented or uncemented femoral components were retrieved and bone loss around implants was evaluated. Patients with lower bone mineral density in the control femur experienced a greater percent decrease in bone mineral density around the hip prosthesis.

McLaughlin JR, Lee KR: Total hip arthroplasty with an uncemented femoral component: Excellent results at ten-year follow-up. *J Bone Joint Surg* 1997;79B:900–907.

One hundred forty-five hips treated with a titanium uncemented femoral component were followed 8 to 12.5 years. One stem was revised for aseptic loosening. Ninety-four percent of stems were bone ingrown, 3% had stable fibrous fixation, and 3% were loose.

Mont MA, Hungerford DS: Proximally coated ingrowth prostheses: A review. *Clin Orthop* 1997;344:139–149.

A review of the results of first-generation and second-generation proximally porous coated femoral implants. Second-generation devices followed at least 5 years demonstrated low aseptic loosening rates (1% to 3%) and less thigh pain.

Mulliken BD, Bourne RB, Rorabeck CH, Nayak N: A tapered titanium femoral stem inserted without cement in a total hip arthroplasty: Radiographic evaluation and stability. *J Bone Joint Surg* 1996;78A:1214–1225.

Four hundred sixteen total hip arthroplasties were performed with an uncemented tapered titanium stem and followed 2 to 6.5 years. There were no revisions for stem loosening or for thigh pain. Six percent of patients had thigh pain.

Rothman RH, Hozack WJ, Ranawat A, Moriarty L: Hydroxyapatite-coated femoral stems: A matched-pair analysis of coated and uncoated implants. *J Bone Joint Surg* 1996;78A: 319–324.

A matched pair analysis of the same femoral component implanted with porous coating or hydroxyapatite demonstrated no difference in clinical or radiographic results at a mean of 2.2 years.

Urban RM, Jacobs JJ, Sumner DR, Peters CL, Voss FR, Galante JO: The bone-implant interface of femoral stems with non-circumferential porous coating: A study of specimens retrieved at autopsy. *J Bone Joint Surg* 1996;78A:1068–1081.

Noncircumferential porous coating provides pathways for migration of particulate debris to the distal part of the stem, thus allowing distal osteolysis to occur.

Vresilovic EJ, Hozack WJ, Rothman RH: Incidence of thigh pain after uncemented total hip arthroplasty as a function of femoral stem size. *J Arthroplasty* 1996;11:304–311.

Two hundred ninety-seven total hip arthroplasties performed with wedge-shaped uncemented femoral components were evaluated at a minimum of 2 years. Thigh pain was directly correlated with increasing stem size and implant moment of inertia for bending in the medial-lateral plane.

Xenos JS, Callaghan JJ, Heekin RD, Hopkinson WJ, Savory CG, Moore MS: The porous-coated anatomic total hip prosthesis, inserted without cement: A prospective study with a minimum of ten years of follow-up. *J Bone Joint Surg* 1999;81A:74–82.

This article presents minimum 10-year follow-up results of 100 proximally porous coated first-generation metaphyseal filling cobalt-chrome femoral components. Five femoral components were revised, 2 for loosening and 3 for osteolysis. An additional 12% of patients had thigh pain.

Classic Bibliography

Bourne RB, Rorabeck CH, Ghazal ME, Lee MH: Pain in the thigh following total hip replacement with a porous-coated anatomic prosthesis for osteoarthrosis: A five-year follow-up study. *J Bone Joint Surg* 1994;76A:1464–1470.

Callaghan JJ: The clinical results and basic science of total hip arthroplasty with porous-coated prostheses. *J Bone Joint Surg* 1993;75A:299–310.

Engh CA, Bobyn JD: The influence of stem size and extent of porous coating on femoral bone resorption after primary cementless hip arthroplasty. *Clin Orthop* 1988;231:7–28.

Engh CA, Glassman AH, Suthers KE: The case for porous-coated hip implants: The femoral side. *Clin Orthop* 1990;261:63–81.

Heekin RD, Callaghan JJ, Hopkinson WJ, Savory CG, Xenos JS: The porous-coated anatomic total hip prosthesis, inserted without cement: Results after five to seven years in a prospective study. *J Bone Joint Surg* 1993;75A:77–91.

Kärrholm J, Malchau H, Snorrason F, Herberts P: Micromotion of femoral stems in total hip arthroplasty: A randomized study of cemented, hydroxyapatite-coated, and porous-coated stems with roentgen stereophotogrammetric analysis. *J Bone Joint Surg* 1994;6A:1692–1705.

Lombardi AV Jr, Mallory TH, Eberle RW, Mitchell MB, Lefkowitz MS, Williams JR: Failure of intraoperatively customized non-porous femoral components inserted without cement in total hip arthroplasty. *J Bone Joint Surg* 1995;77A:1836–1844.

Martell JM, Pierson RH I-II, Jacobs JJ, Rosenberg AG, Maley M, Galante JO: Primary total hip reconstruction with a titanium fiber-coated prosthesis inserted without cement. *J Bone Joint Surg* 1993;75A:554–571.

Rorabeck CH, Bourne RB, Laupacis A, et al: A double-blind study of 250 cases comparing cemented with cementless total hip arthroplasty: Cost-effectiveness and its impact on health-related quality of life. *Clin Orthop* 1994;298:156–164.

Sweetnam DI, Lavelle J, Allwood WM, Cohen B: Poor results of the Ribbed Hip System for cementless replacement. *J Bone Joint Surg* 1995;77B:366–368.

Chapter 16
Osteonecrosis–Etiology, Pathophysiology, and Treatment

Introduction

Although the most common cause of osteonecrosis (ON) of the femoral head is a displaced transcervical fracture, this is best covered in a section dealing with fractures of the hip. This chapter will therefore focus on nontraumatic ON of the adult hip and emphasize etiology, pathophysiology, and treatment.

Despite a growing interest in this condition, many gaps remain in the knowledge of ON, partly because no good animal model is currently available. It is estimated that approximately 10,000 to 20,000 new cases of ON are diagnosed annually and that ON accounts for approximately 10% of primary total hip replacements (THR) being performed. Young adults between the ages of 25 and 45 years are most frequently affected, and the condition is bilateral in over 50% of patients. If the hips are affected, then other joints are involved approximately 15% of the time. Without specific treatment, most clinically diagnosed cases will progress and eventually require hip arthroplasty. It is therefore important that the condition be diagnosed early and treatment instituted promptly. Although the term "osteonecrosis" is currently preferred, the condition frequently is referred to as avascular necrosis, ischemic necrosis, or aseptic necrosis.

Etiology

ON is not a single disease entity, but is rather the end point for a number of factors that cause an impairment of the circulation to a specific area of bone, resulting in its death. ON may be due to a single pathologic process, although it often is multifactorial. The more common mechanisms implicated in causing ON are listed in Outline 1. Of these, the most important is currently believed to be intravascular coagulation or thrombosis. A number of factors have been associated with the development of ON (Outline 2), although the pathologic mechanisms by which they act are not always clear. Of these factors, the 2 most frequently encountered are chronic steroid administration and excessive alcohol intake, which are associated with ON in over 65% of patients. It is presumed that these factors act in part through alterations in circulating lipids and coagulation mechanisms. A minimal dose and duration of both steroid and alcohol is necessary to cause ON; however, the specific amount has not been conclusively determined, and there is a marked difference in the sensitivity of patients to the effects of these factors. In many instances, some underlying abnormality is present that predisposes the patient to develop ON in response to a specific insult. For example, fewer than 5% of patients exposed to heavy alcohol consumption and between 5% and 10% of those receiving

Outline 1
Mechanisms that cause osteonecrosis

- Gross disruption of vessels
  - Displaced femoral neck fractures
  - Dislocation
- External vascular occlusion
  - Dislocation
  - Joint effusion
  - Increased intraosseous pressure
  - Marrow infiltration or replacement
  - Marrow hypertrophy
- Embolization
  - Lipid droplets
  - Blood clots
  - Nitrogen bubbles
  - Sickle cells
- Thrombosis
  - Coagulopathies
    - Thrombophilia
    - Hypofibrinolysis
  - Vascular disorders
- Cytotoxicity
- Idiopathic

Outline 2
Conditions and factors associated with osteonecrosis

Chronic systemic steroid administration
Excessive alcohol intake
Systemic lupus erythematosus and other connective tissue disorders
Chronic renal disease
Organ transplantation
Sickle-cell disease and other hemoglobinopathies
Coagulopathies
Caisson disease or dysbarism
Chronic liver disease
Inflammatory bowel disorders
Pancreatitis
Hyperlipidemias
Gaucher's disease
Gout
Pregnancy
Radiation
Arteriosclerosis and other occlusive vascular disorders
Smoking
Cushing's disease and endocrine disorders
Miscellaneous allergic conditions
Hypersensitivity reactions
Sarcoidosis
Chemotherapy and other toxic chemical agents
Tumors
Idiopathic

high doses of corticosteroid develop ON. The factors that distinguish those patients who develop ON from those who do not have not been completely determined. However, subtle coagulation defects have been found in approximately 70% of patients with ON. These include thrombophilia, an increased tendency to develop intravascular thrombosis, often caused by decreased levels of protein C, protein S, or antithrombin III, or resistance to activated protein C (RAP-C). Hypofibrinolysis, a relative inability to lyse intravascular thrombi, has also been found in association with ON. This problem may be caused by elevated levels of plasminogen activator inhibitor (PAI). Other factors that may lead to abnormal coagulation include altered levels of antiphospholipid antibodies (immunoglobulins G and M) and lupus anticoagulant.

Conditions associated with ON include such diverse entities as inflammatory bowel disease, various allergic states, organ transplantation, and systemic lupus erythematosus. Patients with these disorders are regularly treated for prolonged periods with high doses of corticosteroid. Although vascular pathology may be present in some cases, probably the steroid itself rather than the underlying disorder being treated is primarily responsible for the development of ON. Another significant factor is the regional vascular anatomy. There are obvious differences in the circulation to the femoral and humeral heads, for example, as compared with circulation to other long bones, which make these areas more prone to develop ON. The lateral epiphyseal vessels supply the superolateral aspect of the femoral head with little collateral circulation. Therefore, this region is sensitive to circulatory impairment and is, in fact, the most frequent site for ON. There may also be significant differences in the vascular supply between individuals, which predisposes them to ON.

External vascular occlusion may be caused by marrow infiltration or replacement. This is seen in Gaucher's disease, in dysbaric ON, and in conditions leading to hypertrophy of marrow cells. Increased intraosseous pressure is frequently found in the proximal femur of patients with ON and may contribute to the development of ON. Different types of emboli, including blood clots, clumps of sickle cells, lipid droplets, and nitrogen bubbles, can block smaller arteries and arterioles. This, in turn, often leads to intravascular coagulation or thrombosis.

In many series, the etiology is listed as "idiopathic" in 15% to 20% of patients. As knowledge concerning pathologic mechanisms improves and as efforts to identify these mechanisms increase, the number of cases listed as idiopathic will continue to diminish.

Pathophysiology

Whichever factor or factors may be responsible for the development of ON, the common mechanism of action is to decrease or obliterate the circulation to a specific area of bone. If the involved area is small and not adjacent to an articular surface, the infarct may remain asymptomatic and have little clinical effect. However, if the infarct is large and near a weightbearing surface, the clinical consequences often are significant. Within approximately 6 hours after the vascular insult, death of marrow and fat cells is noted. Osteocyte death occurs at the same time, but it may not be detected histologically until several days later when the disappearance of osteocytes from their lacunae is noted. There follows a sequence of reactions to the injury with attempts at repair. Local edema develops and may extend a considerable distance beyond the necrotic lesion as seen histologically and on magnetic resonance imaging (MRI). Areas completely devoid of circulation may remain stable for quite some time. However, with mechanical stresses transmitted to subchondral trabeculae, microfractures occur that now cannot be repaired. This lack of repair leads to progressive weakness of the subchondral bone.

At the same time, areas of the necrotic lesion that are adjacent to intact vessels and viable cells undergo a process involving resorption of dead bone and new bone formation (Figs. 1 and 2). Unfortunately, bone resorption usually outpaces bone formation, and further weakening of the bone structure usually occurs. Progressive collapse of the subchondral trabeculae takes place and may be associated with the appearance of a radiolucent "crescent sign" before flattening of the articular surface (Fig. 3). Eventually this process involves the cartilage and subchondral end plate, causing gross collapse of the articular surface of the femoral head. These changes have now become irreversible and will eventually lead to progressive joint damage and increasing symptoms.

The necrotic process initially affects only the bone of the

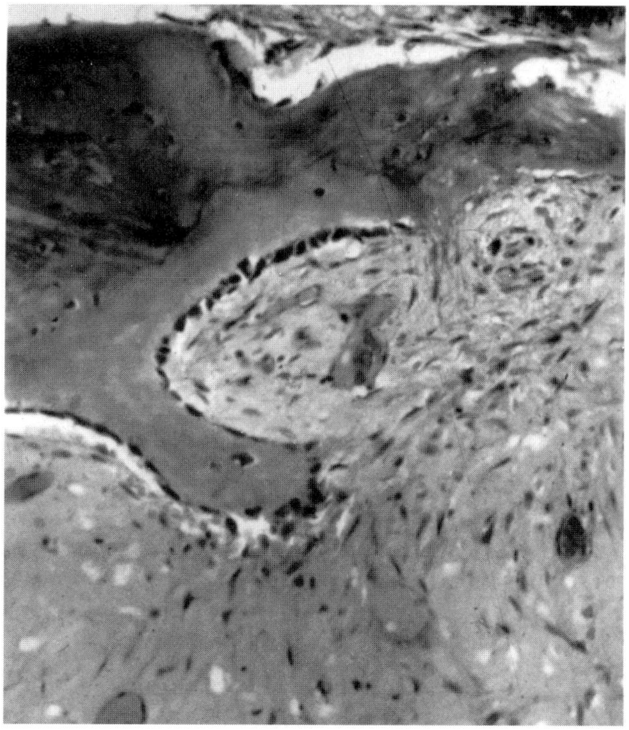

Figure 1

Photomicrograph showing the reparative process with new bone being laid down, on old dead trabeculae (hematoxylin and eosin, × 100). (Reproduced with permission from Steinberg ME, Steinberg DR: Avascular necrosis of the femoral head, in Steinberg ME (ed): *The Hip and Its Disorders.* Philadelphia, PA, WB Saunders, 1991, pp 623–647.)

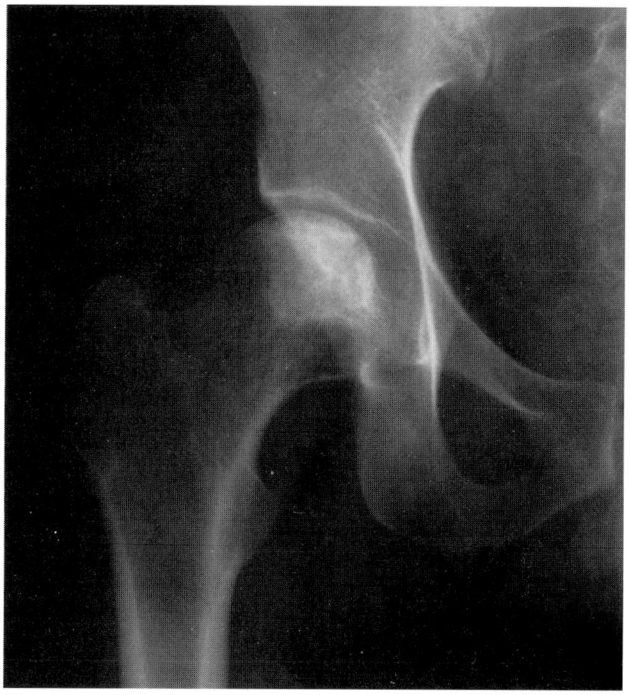

Figure 2

Characteristic radiograph of a hip with stage II osteonecrosis. The necrotic lesion is surrounded by a dense sclerotic border, formed by the apposition of new bone onto old dead trabeculae.

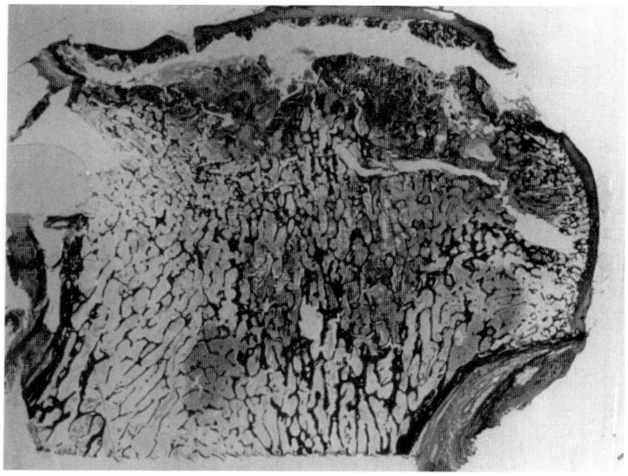

Figure 3

Low power photomicrograph of a stage IV femoral head showing flattening of the articular surface, collapse of subchondral trabeculae (giving a crescent sign on radiographs), and the presence of dead bone and marrow, necrotic debris, granulation tissue, and new bone formation scattered throughout the area of involvement (hematoxylin and eosin, × 2). (Reproduced with permission from Steinberg ME, Steinberg DR: Avascular necrosis of the femoral head, in Steinberg ME (ed): *The Hip and Its Disorders.* Philadelphia, PA, WB Saunders, 1991, pp 623–647.)

femoral head. Primary involvement of the acetabulum is uncommon. The articular cartilage of the femoral head remains intact and viable until after trabecular collapse occurs, because it receives its nutrition through the synovial fluid and is not dependent on circulation from within the femoral head (Fig. 4). After collapse of the femoral head, the articular cartilage is subjected to abnormal mechanical pressures that lead to progressive degeneration. The irregularity of the femoral articular surface, in turn, transmits abnormal stress to the acetabular cartilage and it, too, begins to undergo degenerative changes. At this point, radiographs of the hip reveal no acetabular abnormalities (Fig. 5), but these changes are readily seen on both gross and microscopic examination

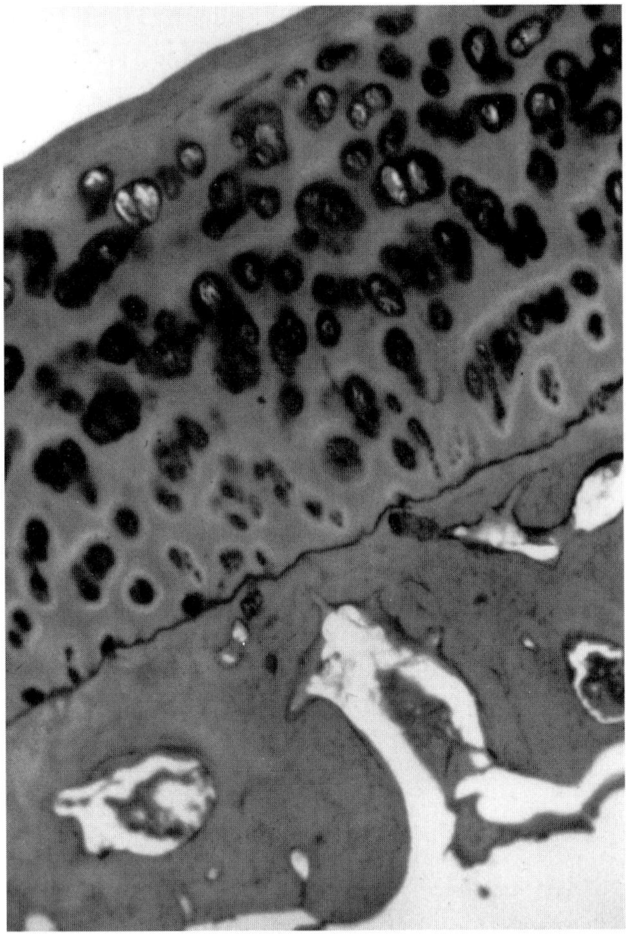

Figure 4

Photomicrograph of articular cartilage with attached subchondral bone. The articular surface is regular and chondrocytes are viable although not normal. The subchondral bone is dead (hematoxylin and eosin, × 50). (Reproduced with permission from Steinberg ME, Steinberg DR: Avascular necrosis of the femoral head, in Steinberg ME (ed): *The Hip and Its Disorders.* Philadelphia, PA, WB Saunders, 1991, pp 623–647.)

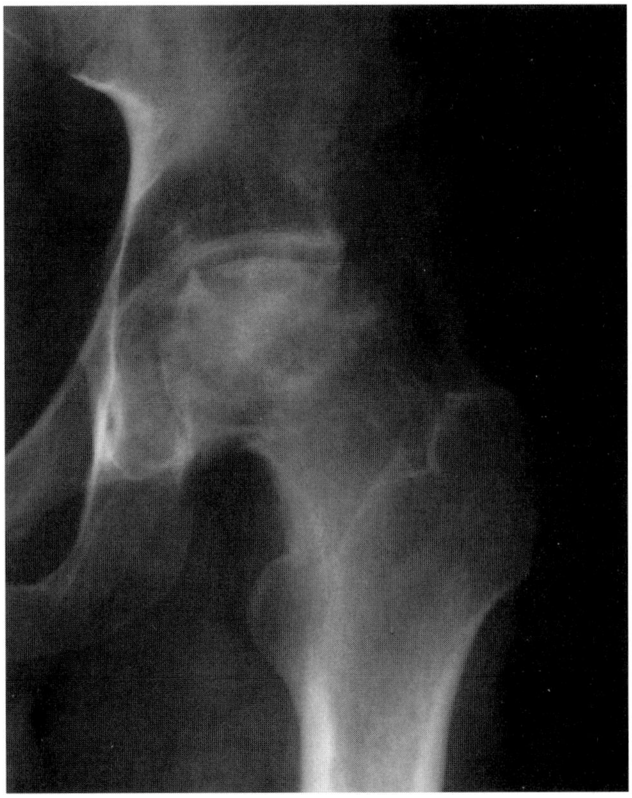

Figure 5

Radiograph of a stage IV hip showing lucent and sclerotic areas and flattening of the femoral head. The acetabulum appears radiographically normal.

of the acetabular cartilage at the time of arthroplasty. Progressive degeneration of the articular cartilage leads to a radiographic picture of joint line narrowing and eventually sclerosis and formation of cysts and marginal osteophytes. During the late stages of ON, the picture is that of advanced secondary degenerative joint disease.

Both the size and location of the necrotic lesion are important determinants of outcome. Small lesions that are not in an area of major weightbearing may remain asymptomatic, undergo spontaneous healing, and have no clinical consequences. Japanese investigators have identified a small group of patients in whom the necrosis affects a relatively small area in the medial aspect of the femoral head. These patients have a relatively good prognosis. If the necrotic segment is large and in an area of weightbearing, it will usually go on to collapse without specific treatment. Unfortunately, most lesions are located in the anterosuperior aspect of the femoral head, the area of major weightbearing. This location may be a result of thrombosis of the lateral epiphyseal vessels that supply this region.

Approximately 70% of hips diagnosed clinically with ON

go on to femoral head collapse. This may be a relatively rapid process and occur within a period of weeks to months. In some instances the collapse is slow and only partial. These patients may continue to function for several years during which progressive degenerative changes develop. The sequence of pathologic changes can be made apparent by modern imaging techniques and forms the basis for most systems of staging ON. Good quality anteroposterior and lateral radiographs are routinely required and should be supplemented by MRI if plain films of 1 or both hips are normal. If present, preradiographic changes can be detected by MRI in over 90% of cases. Bone scans, computed tomography, or single photon emission computed tomography are seldom required.

Treatment

Despite increased efforts during the past several years, the treatment of ON leaves much to be desired. Protected weightbearing does not affect the natural progression. The primary goal is to diagnose and treat ON early in order to retard or prevent progressive changes and preserve the femoral head. Several techniques have been described to accomplish this. Unfortunately, the published data are so variable and inconsistent that it is difficult to determine accurately the relative indications for and effectiveness of these different approaches.

Optimum treatment of ON requires a thorough evaluation of the whole patient as well as the involved joints. Several factors must be considered, including age, gender, general health, life expectancy, associated medical conditions, and etiologic factors. The hip itself must be evaluated clinically using an accepted hip evaluation protocol and radiographically with a modern and effective method of staging that includes a determination of both the type and extent of involvement.

Nonsurgical Treatment

Prevention

The best treatment for ON is prevention. Certain risk factors have been identified, and these should be eliminated or minimized to the extent possible. This applies to smoking and particularly to alcohol ingestion and steroid administration, the 2 leading causes of this condition. Established guidelines must be followed by divers and those working under hyperbaric conditions.

Medical Management

Certain systemic disorders, such as hyperlipidemias, coagulopathies, and the presence of certain antibodies, have been associated with an increased incidence of ON. Under ideal circumstances patients with ON should be screened for the presence of these disorders using a lipid profile, liver function tests, anticardiolipin antibodies, lupus anticoagulants, and coagulation studies. The coagulation studies should include a determination of prothrombin time, partial thromboplastin time, and levels of protein S, protein C, antithrombin III, PAI, and RAP-C. If definitive abnormalities are identified, the decision should be made as to whether or not to treat them and which agents to use. There has been some recent interest in the use of nifedipine (a vasodilator), stanozolol (an anabolic steroid that alters lipoproteins and suppresses certain clotting factors), other agents to lower circulating lipids, and long-term anticoagulation to treat coagulopathies. Neither the effectiveness nor safety of these agents has been determined nor are there appropriate guidelines for their use at this time.

Symptomatic Treatment

Symptomatic treatment, including protected weightbearing, has not been shown to alter the natural course of ON. However, small lesions, particularly those in the medial aspect of the femoral head, have a relatively good prognosis and often do well without surgical intervention. If this approach is elected, the patient should be followed carefully for signs of clinical or radiologic progression, in which case surgery should be considered. Nonsurgical or symptomatic treatment might also be elected in cases where the patient's age, overall prognosis, associated medical conditions, or wishes contraindicate surgical intervention. Symptomatic treatment is also used in the patient with advanced stages of ON that is no longer amenable to procedures designed to preserve the femoral head, yet has not reached the stage at which reconstructive surgery is indicated.

Electrical Stimulation

Because of its ability to enhance bone formation and fracture healing, there has been ongoing interest in the role of electrical stimulation for the treatment of ON. Three specific types of signal have been used: direct current (DC), capacitive coupling (CC), and pulsing electromagnetic fields (PEMF). All have been used as supplements to core decompression and CC and PEMF can also be used alone without surgical intervention. These 2 signals are transmitted to the bone by means of surface electrodes or coils placed on the skin over the hip. Despite indications of an early response to DC stimulation, long-term studies failed to show a lasting effect of either DC or CC. Results with PEMF, both in individual studies and in a multicenter study, were promising. PEMF was shown to be more effective than symptomatic management in precollapsed and early collapsed hips, as effective as core decompression in precollapsed lesions, and more effective in hips with early collapse, in regard to both radiographic progression and delaying the need for arthroplasty. However, a special signal, different from that used to treat fractures, was used to treat ON and to date this signal is not available for routine use. If further evaluation by other investigators confirms these earlier findings, use of PEMF may be added to the treatments of ON.

Surgical Procedures to Retard Progression

In most instances the goal is to diagnose and treat ON as early as possible, well before the onset of femoral head collapse. Several procedures have been proposed to accomplish this. Unfortunately, it is virtually impossible to compare the effectiveness of these procedures accurately. In some instances there have been only a few reports regarding a specific procedure, with limited numbers of patients and short follow-ups. In other instances several studies have been published, but they include so many variables that a comparison is difficult. These variables include criteria for performing surgery, surgical technique, patient demographics, method of clinical and radiographic evaluation, and the criteria for determining outcome.

Core Decompression

Core decompression (CD) is perhaps the most frequently used prophylactic procedure for the treatment of ON. It is technically a simple procedure, but it must be done carefully so as not to miss the necrotic lesion, perforate the femoral head, or lead to postoperative fracture. CD presumably acts through a number of mechanisms, including reducing the elevated intraosseous pressure usually found in association with ON, opening channels through sclerotic bone for vascular ingrowth, and stimulating the processes of repair. Published results have varied significantly, from those reporting no effectiveness and a high incidence of complications to those reporting 90% success. The authors of a recent extensive review of the literature studied 42 reports of 2,025 hips, of which 1,206 were treated by CD and the other 819 by nonsurgical means. Satisfactory clinical results were noted in 64% of hips in 24 studies of CD, but in only 23% of hips in 21 studies of nonsurgical management. In hips treated before collapse, good results were obtained in 71% treated with CD as compared with 35% treated nonsurgically. In addition, the best results are obtained in hips with smaller necrotic lesions. The incidence of fracture and other complications is quite low with careful technique.

CD can be performed as originally described, removing 1 or 2 relatively large cores of bone with diameters between 8 and 10 mm (Fig. 6). Some have advocated the use of multiple drill holes in the femoral head; however, it should be noted that this technique, originally referred to as "Forage", did not appear to be effective. CD can be supplemented with cancellous bone grafting, electrical stimulation, or the addition of material with osteoinductive properties, such as bone morphogenetic protein or demineralized bone matrix. Preliminary results with some of these adjunctive measures seem encouraging.

Grafting Procedures

Cortical Strut Grafts In 1949, the use of tibial strut grafts for posttraumatic ON was described. This technique was subsequently modified to include the use of fibular and tibial grafts, taken either from the ipsilateral limb of the patient or from the bone bank. Most studies reported between 70% and 80% satisfactory results. This procedure combines the effec-

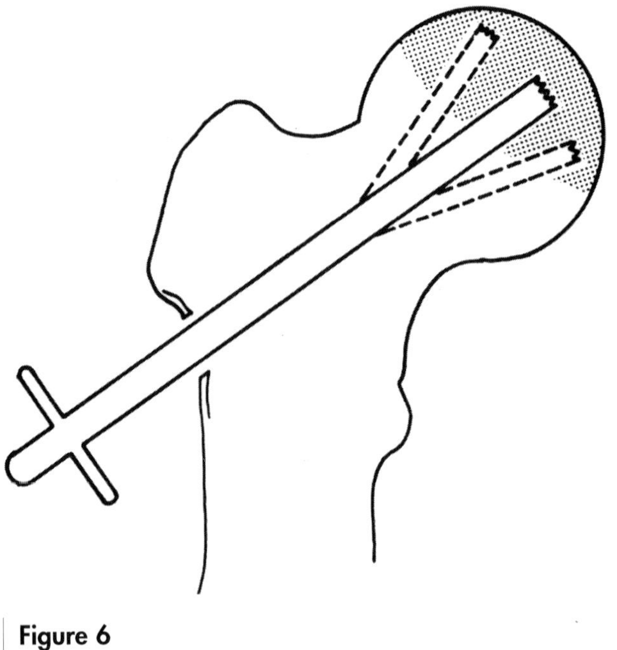

Figure 6

Schematic of a core decompression in which an 8-mm trephine is used to make a single channel into the necrotic segment and a 5- to 6-mm trephine is used to make 2 additional channels closer to the periphery. Viable bone removed from the intertrochanteric region can be used as a supplemental graft. (Reproduced with permission from Steinberg ME, Brighton CT, Hayken GD, Tooze SE, Steinberg DR: Early results in the treatment of avascular necrosis of the femoral head with electrical stimulation. *Orthop Clin North Am* 1984; 15:163–175.)

tiveness of core decompression with that of providing mechanical support to the femoral head, thus retarding its tendency to collapse.

Free Vascularized Fibular Grafts Since 1979, free vascularized fibular grafts (FVFG) have been used in a small number of centers to treat ON. The greatest experience in the United States is that of Urbaniak and associates who have done over 1,000 such surgeries during the past 20 years. Patients are operated on in the lateral decubitus position by 2 teams working simultaneously. Surgery is performed through the lateral femoral cortex. The joint is not opened, nor is the hip dislocated. As much of the necrotic bone as possible is removed by the use of burrs. The periphery of this area is then packed with cancellous bone. (Alternatively, the graft can be inserted without further excision of necrotic bone.) A section of fibula from the ipsilateral limb is then inserted into the center of the femoral head, and a microvascular anastomosis to local vessels is completed (Fig. 7). Patients are maintained on protected weightbearing for 6 months in unilateral cases and up to 1 year if both hips are operated on.

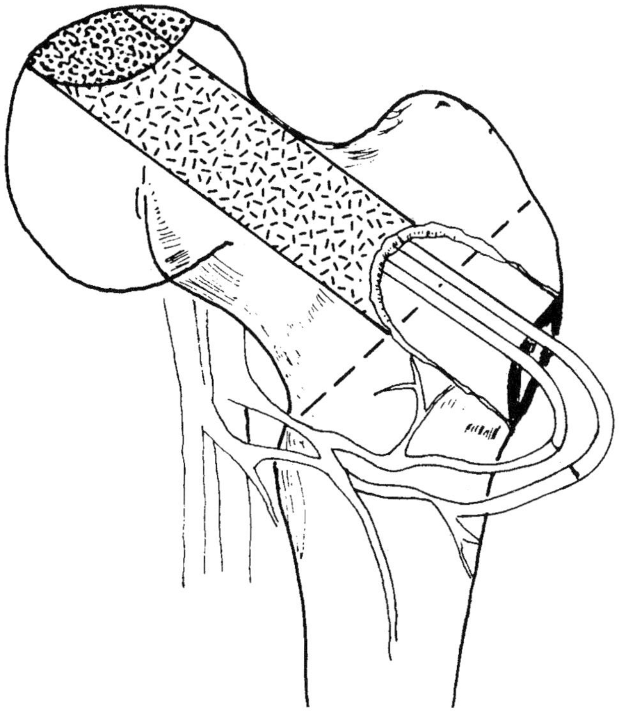

Figure 7

Schematic of a free vascularized fibular graft extending from the lateral femoral cortex into the necrotic lesion. Anastomosis of the fibular vein and artery to local vessels has been completed. (Reproduced with permission from Richards RR: Bone grafting with microvascular anastomosis in osteonecrosis of the femoral head. *Semin Arthroplasty* 1991;2:198–207.)

Complications have been reported in approximately 15% of cases. Successful results, that is, delaying THR by more than 5 years, were achieved in 70% of hips that already had some degree of femoral head collapse and in more than 80% of hips treated before collapse. This procedure is technically difficult and time-consuming and requires special equipment and trained microvascular surgeons. Several questions remain to be answered, however. Is it clearly superior to less complicated methods of grafting, such as those using nonvascularized cortical struts or cancellous bone? Will bank bone give equal results, thus significantly decreasing the incidence of complications? Should it be used for virtually all cases of ON or only for advanced cases with femoral head collapse, which are less responsive to simpler techniques?

Muscle Pedicle Bone Grafts In an effort to preserve the viability of the bone graft, techniques have been developed using muscle pedicle bone grafts. Donor sites have included the iliac crest and the insertion of the quadratus femoris as well as other areas. This technique requires that the joint be opened either anteriorly or posteriorly and that a window be made in the femoral neck. Relatively few cases in which this technique was used have been reported, and the results have been variable.

Cancellous Grafts There are several techniques by which cancellous bone is used to replace the necrotic tissue removed from the femoral head. The simplest, perhaps, is to use the cancellous bone removed with a trephine from the intertrochanteric region as a supplement to a classic core decompression. Other techniques involve a more aggressive attempt to remove the majority of necrotic material from the femoral head and to replace it with cancellous graft taken from the host. This can be done through the lateral femoral cortex, without opening the joint, or through the femoral neck, entering the joint either anteriorly or posteriorly. Necrotic material can also be removed through a flap or "trap door" of articular cartilage and subchondral bone after dislocating the hip. A combination of cancellous and cortical bone can be used, thus restoring the normal configuration of a collapsed femoral head. This technique was first described in 1965 but has experienced renewed interest recently. More cases and longer follow-up will be required to determine the effectiveness of and the indications for these procedures.

Osteochondral Allografts If the articular cartilage over the collapsed segment of femoral head is badly degenerated, the entire segment can be removed and replaced with an osteochondral allograft after replacing the necrotic material with bone graft. There are many technical problems to be overcome when using this approach and experience with it to date is very limited.

Osteotomies

Several authors have used proximal femoral osteotomies to shift the necrotic and often collapsed segment of the femoral head out of the major weightbearing region, replacing it with normal cartilage and bone. This can be done by a combination of varus and valgus, flexion and extension, and rotation, either anteriorly or posteriorly. It has been shown repeatedly that the best results are obtained if the lesion is relatively small and located in an area that can be replaced with normal cartilage and bone by the osteotomy. These procedures are technically demanding, have a significant complication rate, are frequently ineffective, and make later arthroplasty difficult. As a result they are infrequently used in the United States today, although they are still used in selected centers in Asia and Europe.

Hip Reconstruction

Once significant femoral collapse has taken place, results with most of the prophylactic procedures described decline rapidly. The surgeon must then decide what type of reconstructive procedure to select and when to perform the surgery.

Endoprosthetic Replacement In the past, femoral endoprostheses were often used to treat the hip with a collapsed head but radiographically "normal" acetabulum. Results were frequently poor even with modern techniques of achieving stable femoral fixation and carefully sizing the head to the acetabulum. Results did not improve with the use of bipolar rather than unipolar prostheses. The poor results often were caused by degeneration of the acetabular cartilage and protrusio of the femoral head. Examination of acetabular cartilage removed at the time of THR done for ON in hips with radiographically "normal" acetabuli revealed that in virtually all instances the cartilage had already undergone degenerative changes. At the present time the use of femoral endoprostheses in ON is not routinely advocated.

Total Hip Replacement Although results with THR in young patients with ON are generally inferior to results in older patients with degenerative arthritis, recent studies have shown definite improvement with modern techniques and devices. When compared with endoprostheses, results with THR are clearly superior. In studies involving the use of endoprostheses for ON, the incidence of good to excellent results generally varies from 48% to 59% with a follow-up ranging from 5 to 9 years. Although early results with THR in ON were poor, more recent reports indicate that good to excellent results can be achieved in 80% to 94% of patients with a follow-up of 5 to 7 years. In 1 study the probability of survival was estimated at 85% at 10 years. Results in patients with sickle-cell disease and those on chronic renal dialysis were, however, disappointing.

Currently, THR is usually the procedure of choice in the patient with advanced stage ON who is in need of an arthroplasty, especially if significant acetabular involvement has already taken place. With continued improvement in components and surgical techniques, it is anticipated that the useful life of THR, even in the young patient with ON, can be increased significantly.

Modified Cup Arthroplasty and Hemisurface Replacement Arthroplasty Conventional cup arthroplasties did not work well and were essentially abandoned with the advent of THR. A limited interest remained in the use of a modified cup arthroplasty in patients with ON. In these procedures, a metallic or ceramic cup was placed over the femoral head after reaming and held in place either by a press-fit or by cement. Accurate sizing of the acetabulum was important. A number of authors reported satisfactory results in 80% to 85% of hips in an average follow-up of 5 to 9 years. This procedure was used to "buy time" before resorting to conventional THR.

Results with older surface replacement arthroplasty (SRA), using metallic femoral cups to articulate with thin polyethylene acetabular liners, were generally poor and this technique was abandoned by most surgeons. Recently, however, there has been renewed interest in using this technique to resurface only the femoral head in cases of ON, allowing the metallic cup to articulate with the intact acetabulum. Components are now available in 1-mm increments, because careful acetabular sizing is now known to be essential. The techniques and devices have been refined since the early days of SRA. Relatively few cases of hemisurface replacement arthroplasty have been reported to date and the follow-up is generally short. However, the results so far seem encouraging. This approach should not be used if significant acetabular degeneration is already present. Advocates of hemi-SRA believe that it is a worthwhile, conservative procedure used to postpone, perhaps for several years, the need to perform the more extensive procedure of THR. More cases and longer follow-up are required to determine the role of hemi-SRA as compared to conventional THR.

Surface Replacement Arthroplasty A limited number of investigators have expressed renewed interest in the role of SRA in ON, using metal-on-metal articulations. Only a small number have been performed, and the follow-up is relatively short. It therefore has yet to be determined whether these components have overcome the problems with older SRAs.

Miscellaneous Procedures

Fusion Hip fusion is rarely resorted to in patients with ON. In a small number of cases with selected indications, this may be an alternative. For example, in the young active male with unilateral ON in whom THR may be clearly contraindicated for a variety of reasons, fusion may be considered.

Resection Arthroplasty Resection arthroplasty is another alternative for treatment of a patient with ON in whom THR is contraindicated. It can be used in patients with bilateral disease and is particularly useful when motion rather than stability is required.

Summary

This chapter has given a brief overview of the etiology, pathophysiology, and treatment of ON of the hip. Advances have been made during the past several years in understanding and treating this condition. Much more has yet to be learned. Further knowledge regarding the etiology and pathogenesis may help decrease the incidence and improve the medical treatment of ON. Earlier diagnosis and better methods of prophylaxis will help save a number of hips from collapse. Improvements in arthroplasty components and techniques will enable treatment of patients with advanced stages of involvement and may lead to devices that will not only function well, but that will last a lifetime, even in the younger patient with ON of the hip.

Annotated Bibliography

Aaron RK, Ciomber DM: Electrical stimulation, demineralized bone matrix, and bone morphogenic protein. *Semin Arthroplasty* 1998;9:221–230.

This is a timely discussion on the role of electrical stimulation in the treatment of ON and on the use of demineralized bone matrix and bone morphogenetic protein as supplements to core decompression.

Amstutz HC, Sparling EA, Grigoris P: Surface and hemi-surface replacement arthroplasty. *Semin Arthroplasty* 1998;9:261–271.

The authors describe recent modifications in components and techniques for surface replacement and hemisurface replacement arthroplasty specifically for the treatment of ON.

Bauer TW, Plenk H Jr: The pathology of early osteonecrosis of the femoral head. *Semin Arthroplasty* 1998;9:192–202.

This is a practical and theoretical review of the earliest changes seen in the pathogenesis of ON.

Cabanela ME: Femoral endoprostheses and total hip replacement for avascular necrosis. *Semin Arthroplasty* 1998;9: 253–260.

The author reviews early and more recent results with femoral endoprostheses and THR in the treatment of ON.

Jones JP Jr: Etiology and pathogenesis of osteonecrosis. *Semin Arthroplasty* 1998;9:184–191.

This article contains some of the latest information available on current theories regarding etiology and pathogenesis of ON.

Santore RF: Intertrochanteric osteotomies for femoral head necrosis. *Semin Arthroplasty* 1998;9:242–252.

This is a practical evaluation of the role of intertrochanteric osteotomy in the treatment of ON of the femoral head.

Steinberg ME: Core decompression. *Semin Arthroplasty* 1998;9: 213–220.

This is an overview of the status of core decompression, which includes both a review of the literature and the author's own experience with this technique and its modifications.

Sutker BD, Urbaniak JR: Grafting procedures for osteonecrosis. *Semin Arthroplasty* 1998;9:231–241.

This is a comprehensive review of the various grafting procedures used for the treatment of ON with emphasis on the author's own experience using free vascularized fibular grafts.

Urbaniak JR, Jones JP Jr (eds): *Osteonecrosis: Etiology, Diagnosis, and Treatment.* Rosemont, IL, American Academy of Orthopaedic Surgeons, 1997.

This book contains the published proceedings of an International Symposium on ON, which included participants from several countries and contains the latest information concerning etiology, pathogenesis, and treatment. It is perhaps the most comprehensive compendium on this topic currently available.

Classic Bibliography

Aaron RK: Osteonecrosis: Etiology, pathophysiology, and diagnosis, in Callaghan JJ, Rosenberg AG, Rubash HE (eds): *The Adult Hip*. Philadelphia, PA, Lippincott-Raven, 1998, pp 451–466.

Ficat RP: Idiopathic bone necrosis of the femoral head: Early diagnosis and treatment. *J Bone Joint Surg* 1985;67B:3–9.

Glueck CJ, Freiberg R, Tracy T, Stroop D, Wang P: Thrombophilia and hypofibrinolysis: Pathophysiologies of osteonecrosis. *Clin Orthop* 1997;334:43–56.

Mont MA, Hungerford DS: Non-traumatic avascular necrosis of the femoral head. *J Bone Joint Surg* 1995;77A:459–474.

Mont MA, Carbone JJ, Fairbank AC: Core decompression versus nonoperative management for osteonecrosis of the hip. *Clin Orthop* 1996;324:169–178.

Petty W: Osteonecrosis: Strategies for treatment, in Callaghan JJ, Rosenberg AG, Rubash HE (eds): *The Adult Hip*. Philadelphia, PA, Lippincott-Raven, 1998, pp 467–491.

Steinberg ME, Hayken GD, Steinberg DR: A quantitative system for staging avascular necrosis. *J Bone Joint Surg* 1995;77B: 34–41.

Steinberg ME, Mont MA: Osteonecrosis, in Chapman MW (ed): *Operative Orthopaedics*, ed 3. Philadelphia, PA, Lippincott-Williams & Wilkins, in press.

Urbaniak JR, Coogan PG, Gunneson EB, Nunley JA: Treatment of osteonecrosis of the femoral head with free vascularized fibular grafting: A long-term follow-up study of one hundred and three hips. *J Bone Joint Surg* 1995;77A:681–694.

Chapter 17
Deep Infection Complicating Total Hip Arthroplasty

Incidence

The rate of infection after total hip arthroplasty (THA) has been relatively stable since the introduction of prophylactic antibiotics, various means of maintaining ultraclean operating rooms, and refinement of surgical technique. The incidence remains approximately 1% after primary and 3% to 4% after revision hip surgery. Currently, approximately 200,000 THAs per year are done in the United States, accounting for between 4,000 and 5,000 new cases per year of infected hips that require treatment. Deep sepsis represents a devastating complication for the patient and costs $250 million per year. Most important, there is increasing evidence that the ability to combat these new infections is lagging behind the evolution of bacterial defense mechanisms.

Etiology

Evolution of Microbial Flora

The most important factor in understanding periprosthetic infections in the late 1990s is the emergence of resistant bacterial flora. Bacteria develop resistance to antimicrobials via the use of genetic carriers called plasmids or transposons, which enable these organisms to alter the drug target, inactivate the drug, or inhibit drug access to the target. These carriers provide bacteria with the genetic information needed to alter the microbial phenotype.

Historically, it has taken bacteria between 1 and 10 years to develop resistance in the form of a genetic response to newly introduced antibiotics. This evolution has been noted with many first-generation antibiotics such as penicillin, but is now being seen regularly with new antimicrobials synthesized to treat such resistance. Recently, an institution reported 5% of their *Staphylococcus aureus* and 30% of their *S epidermidis*, which cause 50% to 75% of all arthroplasty infections, were oxacillin resistant. In a Scottish study of the incidence of cephalosporin resistance in 740 infected THAs, 30 had positive cultures at the time of surgery. Of these, 18 were identified as *S epidermidis*, and two thirds of these were methicillin resistant. In fact, the incidence of methicillin resistant *S aureus* (MRSA) strains in the United States has jumped from 2% in 1975 to 35% in 1996. Aminoglycoside resistance also is becoming increasingly common among the *Staphylococcus* and *Streptococcus* species.

Gram Positive Organisms and Vancomycin Resistance

Resistance to vancomycin has been reported in the United States for 2 strains of *S aureus*. In vitro bacterial transfer of Van A, a phenotype capable of imparting this resistance, has already been accomplished. At a university hospital in Japan, 20% of *S aureus* isolates were vancomycin resistant secondary to a transfer of another potential phenotype, the Mu3. Overuse of vancomycin for perioperative, revision cement-antibiotic mixture, and other nonorthopaedic applications renders this problem imminently larger and potentially untreatable.

Organisms other than *Staphylococcus* species are also rapidly developing resistance to vancomycin. *Enterococcus feacalis* is capable of preventing vancomycin and other glycopeptides from binding, prohibiting cell wall synthesis. Vancomycin resistant *Enterococcus* (VRE) has become increasingly common, possibly evolving from chronic intestinal exposure to antibiotics eluted from bone cement used in revision THA. The data support vancomycin's role as a risk factor for infection or colonization by VRE. This virulent organism has demonstrated the ability to transfer vancomycin resistance to other organisms such as staphylococci (in vitro). The Hospital Infection Control Practice Advisory Committee has identified certain risk factors for developing an outbreak of VRE. These include proximity to another patient with VRE, and sharing a nurse with a VRE-positive patient.

Gram-Negative Organisms

Gram-negative bacilli are also developing resistance to antibiotic therapy faster than effective antimicrobials can be developed. Their presence has been associated with a worse prognosis after hip replacement, and is at times a contraindication to further surgery. These findings stress the importance of establishing preoperative protocols for obtaining antibiograms for every organism cultured, before instituting any form of therapy.

The Glycocalyx

There is increasing interest in organisms capable of forming a glycocalyx, the polysaccharide biofilm that permits increased adherence and survival of bacteria on biosynthetic surfaces, thereby conferring resistance to the hosts' humoral and cellular defenses. Currently, 90% of existing bacteria produce some form of a slime layer. Although one study suggests that resistance to antibiotics can increase up to 500 times under these circumstances, there is in vitro evidence that antibiotics can be effective before these slime layers develop (during the planktonic phase of microbial development). Although there are laboratory tests capable of characterizing glycocalyx producers, their value remains incompletely defined.

Biomaterial Hypersensitivity and Infection Risk

The presence of rapid osteolysis or early radiographic loosening after THA can signify deep infection. It has also been suggested that these findings can reflect an allergic hypersensitivity reaction to the metal alloys used or the accelerators such as N,N-dimethylparatoluidine contained in bone cement. Hypersensitivity should be considered extremely rare. Skin patch testing can be effective in the event that all other laboratory and clinical data are equivocal. However, additional biomaterials research suggests that both material and structural properties of the implants used may affect the ability to eradicate infection.

Recent animal studies using *S aureus* inoculums have found that different indwelling metals seem to increase susceptibility to infection at differing rates. One group noted a 40% higher rate of infection using titanium versus steel plates, while another noted a 15-fold lower concentration of bacteria required for infection using cobalt chrome versus titanium. These differences are likely multifactorial in nature, related to each metal's relative biocompatibility, available surface area or geometry, and time to bony ingrowth. This competition between host and bacteria for binding to newly introduced synthetic interfaces has been coined "the race" for colonization of the biomaterial surface. The concept may be particularly relevant in the setting of chronic, indolent periprosthetic infections, which are thought to occur from very small inoculums of less virulent bacteria at the time of surgery.

Microbial Adherence

Patterns of microbial adherence are evolving and recently have been found to transpire through 3 independent mechanisms: van der Waals and hydrophobic interactions, covalent or hydrogen bonding, or receptor-ligand recognition. In fact, certain microorganisms have demonstrated affinity both in vivo and in vitro toward different biomaterials such as polymers or metals. Host defense mechanisms are further impaired by the presence of any particulate foreign debris that might be generated after THA. This debris elicits an inflammatory response that releases multiple mediators, such as free oxygen radicals, interleukin-1 (IL-1), tumor necrosis factor-α and γ-interferon, which result in tissue and cellular destruction that increases the host's susceptibility to infection.

As a consequence, ongoing tissue engineering research is aimed at biochemical and microstructural alteration of biomaterials to promote the host's control of the interface. Creation of surface receptors for host cells such as osteoblasts and white blood cells would, if successful, support more rapid development of osseointegration and surface coating with host cellular defenses. This could improve immunoresponse around the indwelling foreign body and significantly thwart microbial resistance to present treatments.

Mycobacterial and Fungal Infection

The resurgence of mycobacterial and fungal infections is also of concern. Despite the recent increase in tuberculous disease in the United States, tuberculous and fungal periprosthetic infection remain rare, with only isolated cases being reported. Therefore, there is little experience to fall back on in deciding how best to manage these patients.

Recent anecdotal evidence has suggested that traditional staged reimplantation may not be required for revision if the components are stably fixed, because antitubercular chemotherapy alone can be effective. This evidence should be interpreted very cautiously given the recent emergence of multidrug-resistant mycobacteria and the fact that such data are inadequately validated. Other recent data indicate that the majority of such cases represent mycobacterial reactivation, supporting that successful outcomes may still depend on both medical and surgical intervention.

Fungal organisms, especially the various *Candida* species, are another potential periprosthetic threat because of the host toxicity often inflicted in treating these infections with the appropriate antibiotics. Positive candidal cultures should not be considered a contaminant in otherwise healthy hosts, because most patients with fungal infections have no identifiable premorbid risk factors. All of these pathogens should also be considered in patients with otherwise unexplainable prosthetic failure.

Prophylaxis

It remains difficult to draw accurate conclusions when assessing the literature dealing with infection because of the varying scientific methodology, the heterogeneous patient mix included in the various studies, the lack of unified outcome measures, and the lack of prospective studies with the necessary number of subjects (study power) and control groups.

Some researchers advocate against prophylaxis for deep infection. They note that most periprosthetic infections are nonhematogenous in origin, and that most do not occur as a result of medical interventions. Many argue that antibiosis implemented on such a broad scale carries a high risk of host toxicity, bacterial resistance, cost, and medicolegal issues that may outweigh its benefits. The majority of clinicians, however, strongly support the continued use of antibiotic prophylaxis.

Which Antibiotic is Best?

Currently, the most widely advocated and used prophylactic antibiosis for THA is first generation cephalosporins. Although many centers administer this antibiotic regimen for 48 hours, increased effectiveness beyond 24 hours of administration has not been demonstrated, and recent reports suggest that only 1 to 2 postoperative doses might be equally effective. However, these recommendations are being increasingly challenged as a result of the rapid evolution of bacterial resistance among common skin commensals. For example, the report of a recent prospective study indicated that on skin swabs taken from 100 preoperative THA patients, 25% of the staphylococcal organisms were methicillin-resistant *S epidermidis* (MRSE), one of the most common proven causes of THA infections. Such data indicate that current antibiotic usage and prophylaxis must be adjusted to avoid catastrophic infection risks. The United States Center for Disease Control and Prevention (CDC) is currently making this issue one of its premier epidemiologic research focuses.

Under CDC supervision, many states are carrying out surveillance for the presence of VRE and community-acquired MRSA. Although how long to provide prophylaxis remains unclear, deciding which antibiotic to use has become even more uncertain. It is clear that judicious prophylactic use of vancomycin is vital to its preservation as an effective drug. Although this problem is to some degree imminent, its acceleration can be minimized with preventative measures. CDC guidelines to help control the spread of resistance must be followed. These guidelines include prudent use of antimicrobials, education of hospital personnel, rapid laboratory detection and communication of VRE, prompt isolation of infected patients, and detection and reporting of both vancomycin-resistant *S aureus* (VRSA) and vancomycin-resistant *S epidermidis* (VRSE).

Antibiotics in Cement

Another controversial issue in prophylaxis is the use of antibiotics in cement during both primary and revision THA. A revision risk study of 148,359 primary THAs by the Swedish Registry found the lowest risk of revision in their patients with Palacos-gentamicin cement. In analyzing how best to prevent septic complications, these researchers identified a positive correlation between prevention and the use of gentamicin-impregnated Palacos cement in combination with either intravenous penicillin or cephalosporin prophylaxis. They found no significant effect with ventilated suits or use of laminar flow, and noted an improved durability of bone cement with the use of gentamicin. The infection rate was 7.2% in all revisions. These findings are in agreement with a recent report evaluating survival of 10,905 primary cemented THAs in the Norwegian Registry. In this study, the lowest incidence of infection occurred in patients receiving both systemic antibiotics and antibiotic-impregnated cement, as compared with either alone or nothing at all. The revision rate was 4.3 times higher using only systemic antibiotics, 6.3 times higher using antibiotic-impregnated cement, and 11.5 times higher using no prophylaxis.

The United States Food and Drug Administration is currently evaluating routine use of gentamicin-impregnated cement during primary THA. Their concern is the evolution of resistant organisms. Resistance may occur because although high antibiotic levels leach out of cement in the first 1 to 2 weeks after implantation to potentially wipe out surrounding organisms, any bacteria that subsequently invade would be exposed to low levels of the antibiotic. This exposure could increase predisposition to the development of resistance. Some infectious disease experts dismiss this argument as irrelevant. They believe that gentamicin is too cytotoxic to ever be considered the intravenous agent of choice, and that its incorporation in cement results in minimal systemic doses.

Many human and animal studies have corroborated that using antibiotic-loaded acrylic cement during treatment of infected joint replacements does not result in antibiotic serum levels higher than 3 mg/l, rendering this a very safe option. The literature suggests a safe concentration limit of about 2 g of antibiotic powder per 40 g of bone cement, an amount that does not significantly alter the cement biomechanically.

Recent Guidelines

Orthopaedic surgeons should be aware of the 1997 Advisory Statement issued by the American Academy of Orthopaedic Surgeons® (AAOS) in conjunction with the American Dental Association, which refers to antibiotic prophylaxis for the prevention of hematogenous spread in dental patients with total joint replacement. Prophylaxis is not routinely indicated for most dental patients with total joint replacements, based on the analysis of risk-benefit and cost-effectiveness ratios. However, antibiotic prophylaxis is indicated 1 hour before dental procedures with high bacteremic risks and during the first 2 years after surgery. About 50% of hematogenously spread infections occur within 2 years of surgery. Immunocompromised or suppressed patients and those with rheumatoid arthritis, lupus erythematosus, diabetes, previous history of periprosthetic infection, malnourishment, and hemophilia are at increased risk and are candidates for prophylaxis. Benefits must be weighed against the risks of antibiotic toxicity and allergy, as well as the development and transmission of microbial resistance. The suggested regimen for patients not allergic to penicillin includes cephalexin, cephradine, or amoxicillin, 2 g orally. If patients are unable to take oral medication, cefaxolin (1 g) or ampicillin (2 g) given intramuscularly or intravenously are recommended. If the patient is allergic to penicillin, 600 mg of clindamycin should be given orally. If the patient is allergic to penicillin and is unable to take oral medication, the same dose of clindamycin can be given intramuscularly or intravenously. No recommendation for a second dose of the drug is suggested. The recommendations include maintenance of effective daily oral hygiene and aggressive treatment of any acute orofacial infection.

The AAOS also issued an Advisory Statement in 1998 regarding the use of prophylactic antibiotics in orthopaedic medicine related to the emergence of vancomycin-resistant bacteria. The AAOS recommends that vancomycin be reserved for the treatment of serious infections with beta-lactam resistant organisms or for treatment of infections in patients with life-threatening allergies to beta-lactam antimicrobials. The advisory statement also recommends hand washing with antibacterial soap, to prevent nosocomial spread, and isolation of patients infected with VRE, VRSE, or VRSA who demonstrate intermediate resistance to vancomycin. One preoperative and one postoperative dose should be sufficient prophylaxis in institutions that have a high rate of MRSA or MRSE infections.

Future Trends in Prophylaxis

Recently, scientists have also been working on means of preoperatively augmenting a host's cell-mediated immune response to combat potential infection. Host macrophages are primed via introduction of recognizable, phagocytosable remnants that serve to accelerate their function and activate the cellular immune response of T lymphocytes and natural killer cells.

IL-12 and γ-interferon, 2 cytokines that mediate these interactions, are also upregulated. Such augmentation has already been demonstrated in animal models, with peak antimicrobial resistance noted to be around 3 days after introduction. This has enormous clinical potential in THA, because any organisms present in the host after introduction of an implant would encounter an activated immunodefense system, theoretically decreasing the chances of successful postoperative bacterial colonization and infection. It has already been successful in thwarting infection in animals introduced to both *S aureus* and *Pseudomonas aeruginosa.*

Diagnosis

The consequences of misdiagnosis of a chronically infected hip replacement are significant, and efforts to improve the accuracy of diagnosis are therefore extremely important. Incorrect diagnosis as aseptic loosening leads to inappropriate surgical procedures and high failure rates that are disappointing to both surgeon and patient. Infection after THA presents a diagnostic challenge for which no single test can be considered the standard. Diagnosis relies on the judgment and experience of the surgeon in assembling the various pieces of the diagnostic puzzle. It begins with a careful history and physical examination and review of radiographs. Although there has been no drastic change in the ability of many diagnostic tests to document the presence of infection, certain improvements in the classification of infection and refinement of some diagnostic modalities has perhaps made it easier to rapidly identify and properly treat infected THAs.

Classification

Infected THAs are not homogenous. Roughly half of these infections are either introduced at the time of surgery or spread from a contiguous source, and about a third are hematogenous. The remainder are considered cryptogenic. Such broad variability makes classification necessary. Although a staging classification of types I through III has been used to guide the treatment of infection, a recent system has been introduced that may be more inclusive and treatment-oriented. This system includes early postoperative infection (EPOI), which occurs 0 to 4 weeks after index procedure, late chronic infection (LCI), which occurs later than 4 weeks postprocedure, usually with insidious loss of function or increase in pain, and acute hematogenous infection (AHI), which is a late, sudden decrease in a previously well-functioning joint replacement. A fourth subgroup recently has been suggested, to include patients presumed to be aseptically loose but who are found to have positive intraoperative cultures (PIOC) after a prosthesis has been implanted. Of 106 treated infections, 31 were in this latter category, defined as having at least 2 of 5 positive intraoperative cultures. Follow-up averaged almost 4 years, with 71% (25 of 35) of the EPOI group, 85% (29 of 34) of the LCI group, 50% (3 of 6) of the AHI group, and 90% (28 of 31) of the PIOC group having a good result when this classification was used to guide treatment. Success was defined as retention of a functional prosthesis (either primary or staged) at last follow-up without evidence of infection for at least 2 years after cessation of antibiotic therapy.

Although this new classification system has some merit, results should be interpreted carefully. For example, 9 of the patients treated successfully later developed loosening of their implants. Additionally, it is still unclear what the false positive rate is in this classification scheme, particularly in patients with PIOC who have no other clinical indicators of infection. This system seems to be a step forward in the understanding of periprosthetic infections; however, further advances in understanding the pathophysiology will lead to more sophisticated classification schemes. Ideally, these systems would account for the presence or absence of particular organisms, biomaterials, and glycocalyx, as well as the timing and source of infection. A universally adaptable, consensual system will be mandatory in the future to properly compare data and to help revolutionize treatment.

Erythrocyte Sedimentation Rate (ESR)

This indirect indicator of acute phase reactant activity is a very specific but not very sensitive indicator of infection. Based on multiple reports, a level of 30 to 35 mm/h is considered to be a good cutoff for guiding an index of suspicion for infection. With these values, sensitivities have been reported from 0.60 to 0.96, and specificities from 0.65 to 1.00. In a recent prospective study of 202 revision THAs, sensitivity was 82%, specificity 85%, predictive value of positive test (PVPT) 58%, and predictive value of negative test (PVNT) 95%. In a consecutive series of 105 revision THAs, sensitivity was 75%, specificity 90%. Thus, a normal ESR can safely rule out infection but an elevated ESR requires further investigation. The ESR takes over 1 year to return to normal after an operation.

C-Reactive Protein (CRP)

This acute phase reactant peaks 48 hours postoperatively and should rapidly decline to normal in only 2 to 3 weeks without persistent infection or inflammation. Thus, its value may be better suited for postoperative monitoring of the success of treatment rather than for the diagnosis of infection. Based on multiple studies, CRP values are most useful in ruling out infection when the value is less than 10 mg/1. This test is considered most meaningful when interpreted in conjunction with the ESR. Recent papers cite a sensitivity and a specificity of around 0.90 to 0.93, and in the prospective series with 202 patients, the PVPT was 74% and the PVNT was 99%.

White Blood Cell Count (WBC)

This is rarely abnormal in patients with infected THA, and, although it is an additional piece of information, WBC carries little weight in deciding the absence of infection if it is not elevated.

Plain Radiographs

Plain radiography remains of limited use in the diagnosis of infection. Most patients with infection initially have few or no radiographic changes unless they have chronic, protracted infections. There are a few findings, however, that should alert the physician to the possibility of infection, especially in the absence of other obvious causes of bony change, such as polyethylene wear, endosteal scalloping, early loosening, rapidly progressive radiolucent lines, periosteal new bone formation, or lacy periostitis.

Magnetic Resonance Imaging (MRI)

MRI is valuable not for the diagnosis of infection, but for identification of radiolucent cement after infection is diagnosed. This cement shows up as a signal void within the femoral medullary canal. MRI can also be valuable in delineating the extent of the periprosthetic abscesses, particularly if there is an intrapelvic extension.

Ultrasound

Ultrasound also has a limited role in the diagnosis of infection. It may be helpful in identifying thickened joint capsules or abscesses that could be associated with an underlying septic process. In the event of a negative joint aspirate, it can also guide needle position to aspirate a surrounding abscess. In 1 series, ultrasound was especially effective in identifying effusions in infected patients. No hip evaluated by ultrasound was infected if the distance between the anterior hip capsule and proximal femur measured less than 3.2 mm (the mean distance for infected hips was 10.2 mm). All patients with an abnormal combination of intra- and extra-articular fluid were found to be infected. These data, however, need to be validated in a larger, more carefully designed investigation.

Radionuclide Scans

The various radionuclide scans (RS) that are available to help diagnose infection are costly, time consuming, and frequently inconsistent when used individually. There has been a paucity of new studies documenting any improved accuracy of these tests in diagnosing periprosthetic infections.

However, RS power should not be underestimated in equivocal clinical situations. Sensitivities and specificities of technetium-99 (^{99}Tc), gallium, and various indium-111 white blood cell (^{111}I) scans range from about 0.40 to 1.00. The combination of various RS or the use of immunoglobulin-G scans have sensitivities and specificities in excess of 90%. A negative scan can be considered fairly reliable in ruling out the presence of infection or mechanical failure after hip implantation.

Technetium Tc-99 scans have been reported to possess a sensitivity of 33% and specificity of 86%, with a positive predictive value of 88%. Indium-111 labeled WBC RS have a sensitivity of 83% and a specificity of 85%, with an accuracy of 84%. When combined, Tc-99 and sulfur colloid I-111 can produce a sensitivity of 100%, specificity of 97%, and accuracy to 98%. I-111 polyclonal antibodies possess 100% sensitivity, specificity, and accuracy, but need to be studied in the context of infected joint replacements.

Aspiration/Arthrogram

Although hip aspiration might be the most direct and predictable preoperative diagnostic test for hip infection, it has a false positive rate between 0 and 15%, and most authors have warned against its routine use before revision. Opinions on preoperative aspiration vary from it being a valuable test necessary for every revision to it having little intrinsic value. Part of this difference may relate to the technique of aspiration and subsequent sample handling. Transport should be rapid to allow immediate incubation and minimize the risk of a false negative aspiration, particularly when the organism might be of poor vitality. Requests for an immediate Gram stain speed processing of the specimen. The use of blood culture bottles for synovial fluid aspiration seems to increase the risk of false positive (FP) cultures, as demonstrated by a 58% FP rate in a recent study.

Results should be interpreted broadly using all available data, such as culture results, WBC count, differential WBC, protein, and glucose levels. Overall, aspiration successfully identifies an organism about 90% of the time. In a recent prospective study, the use of preoperative aspiration was reevaluated in 150 consecutive revision THAs, of which 142 were successfully aspirated for fluid. Using positive intraoperative cultures as the definitive diagnostic test and defining a positive aspiration as either frank pus or growth on solid medium, the authors found a 92% sensitivity, 97% specificity, and 96% accuracy. One negative aspiration was identified PVNT (0.7%). They identified an increased likelihood of infection when the ESR was concomitantly high or if the prosthesis was less than 5 years indwelling. They reaffirmed the selective use of preoperative hip aspiration, and suggested that ESR and in situ prosthesis time be codeterminants of its use.

Another recent report of a similar number of patients cited lower sensitivity (50%) and specificity (88%). These data are corroborated by a spectrum of sensitivity (0.50 to 0.91) and specificity (0.82 to 0.97) values reported in the literature, and signify the difficulty in interpreting such results. The literature suggests the PVNT to be in the mid 90th percentile, while the PVPT is roughly one third lower. Thus, routine preoperative aspiration cannot be recommended, although selective aspiration remains an invaluable diagnostic tool.

Although arthrography itself is rarely useful for the diagnosis of infection, it has recently been reported that the accumulation of dye in pockets may suggest abscess formation. As with ultrasound, arthrography may aid needle sampling of an associated extra-articular abscess when the joint aspirate is negative. Aspiration or arthrogram is probably most indicated when the ESR and CRP are elevated in a painful, symptomatic, failed THA performed initially for noninflammatory hip disease.

Molecular Biology and Genetic Engineering

Molecular diagnostic tools such as polymerase chain reaction (PCR) testing have the potential advantage of sensitive and rapid microbial identification when a cause for infection cannot be identified on culture. Assays being developed for more specific identification of both bacterial DNA and ribonucleic acid (RNA) targets will improve diagnostic accuracy. Bacterial species causing arthroplasty infections have a highly conserved genomic sequence encoding the 16S RNA of the small ribosomal subunit, and sometimes the 23S ribosomal RNA (rRNA) subunit. Researchers can use bacterial primers or probes to amplify these sequences and analyze them, using hybridization techniques to facilitate bacterial detection. Synovial fluid aspirates of 50 patients with total knee arthroplasty (TKA) and symptoms suggestive of infection were analyzed for the presence of bacterial DNA using a PCR protocol. The investigators noted 32 positive culture and PCR specimens. There were no false positive PCRs in 21 negative control specimens obtained from aseptic joints. These results highlight the sensitivity, utility, and reliability of PCR analysis on synovial fluid. However, because a small amount of bacterial genomic material is necessary to produce a positive test and most wounds are colonized, PCR has been associated with a high incidence of false positives and low specificity.

Ribotyping has also increased understanding of the complexity of periprosthetic infection. It now is known that multiple isolates of the same bacterial species can be present within a given infection despite identification of one species on culture. Another promising approach is immunoglobulin labeling using antigranulocyte monoclonal antibodies to detect septic loosening.

Surgical Opinion

Although finding overt pus in an inflamed joint usually leads to a proper diagnosis of infection, the numerous possible etiologies of more common intraoperative scenarios of either synovitis, turbid joint fluid, fibrinous exudate, soft-tissue edema, or normal appearing tissue often confound an accurate surgical diagnosis. Surgical experience probably has an increased role under these equivocal circumstances, and it is best to assume infection and treat accordingly. One group recently correlated the intraoperative surgical opinion with the pathologic diagnosis for a sensitivity of 70% and a specificity of 87%.

Intraoperative Gram Stain

The Gram stain remains a very specific but terribly insensitive test for infection; sensitivity ranges from 0 to 23%. Gram stains have been associated with a very high false negative rate. In less virulent infections, the bacterial load is not enough to allow reliable determination on Gram stain. In a series of 194 revision THAs and TKAs, in which intraoperative Gram stains were obtained in all patients, there were no positive Gram stains despite the presence of infection in 32 cases, as confirmed by culture.

Intraoperative Frozen Section

Intraoperative frozen section is a useful procedure, the reliability of which can be increased by attention to detail and elimination of sampling error. Specimens should be taken from the most inflamed tissue at the time of surgery. There are no conclusive criteria for a positive result on histology. Recent reports range from using 1 to 10 polymorphonuclear cells per high power field (PMN/HPF). Sensitivity of frozen section has ranged from 0.18 to 1.00, and specificity from 0.90 to 0.99.

In a recent prospective study of 33 consecutive revision THAs and TKAs, sensitivity was 100% and specificity was 96% using the criterion of at least 5 PMN/HPF. There was a 100% correlation between frozen and permanent sections in this study. In a follow-up prospective study of 175 consecutive revisions (142 THAs, 33 TKAs), the reliability was evaluated of intraoperative frozen section in identifying active infection as confirmed by intraoperative culture. Based on the final cultures, 3 of 152 joints with negative intraoperative frozen sections and only 16 of 23 with positive intraoperative frozen sections were found to be infected. Of the 23 positive frozen sections, 18 had >10 PMN/HPF, including all 16 of those found to be infected. Thus, when comparing 5 versus 10 PMN/HPF, the sensitivity is 84% for both, the specificity is 96% versus 99%, respectively, with a negative predictive value of 98% for both, and a positive predictive value of 70% versus 89%, respectively (a statistically significant difference). To minimize false positives, the authors suggested considering >10 PMNs as predictive of infection, 5 to 9 PMNs as a grey zone requiring further clinical assessment, and < 5 PMNs as inconsistent with infection. The test is most helpful when experienced pathologists study the samples.

Intraoperative Culture

This procedure is most often used as the "gold standard" in the confirmation of periprosthetic joint infection. At least 3 tissue samples from the most inflamed areas should be sent for culture to improve yield and minimize diagnostic error. All cultures should be incubated for 5 days. Recent studies have confirmed the rate of false positives to be around 6% to 13% for patients immediately after revision THA. This incidence probably is related directly to a break in sterility while obtaining, transferring, and plating these specimens. In a recent prospective study of revision THAs, at least 3 tissue samples were obtained in each, and the removed implants were swabbed for culture and sensitivity 3 times. At least 2 out of 3 samples had to be positive for the culture to be considered a true positive. Tissue culture had a sensitivity of 94%, specificity of 97%, PVPT of 77%, and PVNT of 99%, while swab culture had a sensitivity of 76%, specificity of 99%, PVPT of 93%, and PVNT of 97%. Because the swab cultures were less sensitive than the tissue cultures, the authors recommended sampling of inflamed tissue only during revision.

Treatment

Adequate treatment of infected THAs is based on the time and symptoms of the infection, the virulence and antibiotic sensitivity of the pathogen, the clinical status of the patient, and the condition of the wound and intraoperative findings. The duration and type of treatment should mirror the clinical picture.

General Treatment

Treatment of infected THAs and TKAs is best dictated by the timing of diagnosis, medical presentation, and patient expectations. Patients whose infection is diagnosed only by PIOC can be adequately treated with subsequent meticulous surgical debridement and soft-tissue management followed by 6 weeks of intravenous antibiotics and no further surgery. Any patient failing this treatment should undergo revision with delayed exchange arthroplasty. Patients who have an EPOI can be treated with appropriate surgical debridement, exchange of any easily removable foreign bodies such as polyethylene liners, and component retention if it is well-fixed, followed by 6 weeks of intravenous antibiotics.

Patients who have LCI should be treated with debridement and removal of all foreign bodies including components. Thereafter, the patients are mobilized with or without a spacer in place and receive specific intravenous antibiotics, based on either postpeak serum bactericidal titers or minimum inhibitory concentrations against the particular offending organism. An infectious disease specialist should be involved. Either 1-, 2-, or 3-stage reimplantation is considered thereafter, depending on wound healing, effectiveness of the antibiotic therapy, quality of the soft tissues and bone, clinical status of the patient, and potential for rehabilitation. Seventy percent of periprosthetic infections are reimplanted, with a recurrence rate of approximately 5%. The appropriate period of antibiotic treatment, role of antibiotic beads and spacers, time between removal and reimplantation, definition and role of virulent organisms in deciding treatment, use of allografts, and use of antibiotic bone cement remain controversial in these situations. It has so far been impossible to effectively isolate such issues for adequate comparison. Systemic antibiotics should be used in this situation because the literature indicates an average success rate of only 58% in 1-stage exchange without antibiotics.

Antibiotic Suppression

Before institution of antibiotic suppression, 1 of the following conditions must be met: the patient is either too sick for a surgical procedure or refuses surgery, the organism is identifiable and sensitive, the prosthesis is well-fixed, there are no signs of systemic sepsis, and an appropriate oral antibiotic is available and is tolerated. Compliance is an issue, because incomplete treatment can lead to subtherapeutic antibiotic levels and, hence, to resistant strains of bacteria. The ability to eradicate infection with suppressive antibiotics is becoming increasingly more difficult because exposure to foreign material (ie, implants, cement) lends itself to the formation of biofilms. Coagulase negative staphylococci are an example of bacteria that have capitalized on this, presumably because of a slowed growth rate.

Most antibiotics have been found to be effective only on rapidly growing bacteria. In fact, a recent study suggested rifampin, which affects messenger RNA (mRNA) synthesis, to be the only drug capable of inducing strong enough pharmacodynamic effects to inhibit both growing and nongrowing *S epidermidis*. Amikacin, ofloxacin, imipenem, and vancomycin were effective only against growing bacteria. Recent research suggests that the combination of a low electrical current with current antibiotics may act synergistically in eradicating slime-producing bacteria. As yet, the actual therapeutic value of electricity remains undefined.

New methods of local antibiotic delivery have also been introduced in an effort to enhance delivery and minimize toxicity in the host. The efficacy of experimental antibiotic-impregnated implants made of polylactide and polyglycolide has been investigated using a canine model. In this study, concomitant intravenous antibiotics were not required for successful eradication of infection. Potential clinical advantages of this technique include obviating the need for peripheral venous access, improvement of 1-stage exchange results, and shorter hospital stays.

Certain antibiotics have been found to be helpful in reversing the tissue destruction produced by local matrix metalloproteinases released in the presence of loose or inflamed hip replacements. In an evaluation of cephalothin, doxycycline, tetracycline, and gentamicin, only cephalothin was capable of inhibiting this enzymatic activity in periprosthetic tissues. Although the mechanism of action was found to be unrelated to any antimicrobial activity, such antibiotics could have additional clinical applications in the setting of a destructive infectious process.

Oral antibiotic therapy can also be indicated for therapeutic as opposed to suppressive means. Some authors suggest that 6 weeks of intravenous antibiotics alone without further surgery are acceptable in treating patients exhibiting only PIOC. Oral suppressive antibiotics are valuable in treating EPOI that involve only the surrounding soft tissue when they are used in conjunction with debridement, polyethylene liner change, and component retention. Duration of antibiotic therapy remains controversial, but should be between 4 and 6 weeks, with some combination of intravenous and oral coverage.

Long-term suppression is reported to have about a 30% success rate, with the outcome being retained implants. This number is misleading, because it does not take function into account. If caught very early, many of these infections are potentially curable without having to remove the prosthesis because the septic process has not yet invaded the periprosthetic interface. The chance of salvage depends heavily on the sensitivity of the organism. However, it still is difficult to identify this small subpopulation of organisms that remain only in the soft tissue and thus are potentially curable. If there is any question as to whether the interface is infected or if the bacteria are resistant, then all foreign material should be removed, deferring reimplantation to a second stage. Very selected cases of acute hematogenous infection caused by sensitive bacteria in healthy patients who have sought immediate medical attention have been treated using arthroscopic debridement and copious lavage, followed by 2 to 4 weeks of intravenous antibiotic therapy and oral suppression thereafter. After a mean follow-up of 5 years (4 to 9), none of the 7 patients have required further procedures.

Surgical Debridement and Component Retention

Debridement and retention of an infected THA has limited success and should be reserved for patients who cannot tolerate further surgery or have limited life expectancy. Studies indicate that the results of this treatment improve with the urgency of treatment. A recent investigation of 33 *S aureus* joint infections identified failure of treatment in 21, as defined by relapse of infection. The 1-year cumulative probability of failure was 54% (36% to 71%, confidence interval [CI]), which went up to 69% (52% to 86%, CI) at 2 years. A median of 4 (range, 1 to 9) additional surgical procedures were required to control infection in these 21 cases. Those patients debrided more than 2 days after onset of symptoms had a higher probability of failure, 82% (62% to 100%, CI) versus 30% (8% to 52%, CI), p value < 0.01.

The optimal number of cultures to be sent during debridement has not been determined. Specimens taken from the most involved areas of the joint on both sides should be sent for aerobic, anaerobic, fungal, and other special cultures. All antibiotics should be held until these are obtained. The most important issue in determining the extent of debridement necessary is the overall burden of anything left behind. The more foreign or devitalized tissue remaining, the worse the expected result. This includes the implant if it is not well-fixed. An extended proximal femoral osteotomy has been described to efficiently remove difficult cement mantles during revision surgery. Union rates are apparently good as long as the vascularity of the flap is maintained.

One-Stage Exchange Arthroplasty

Better understanding and treatment of periprosthetic infection and the increased pressure of cost-containment have stimulated revisiting the role of 1-stage reimplantation. Results are encouraging if adherence to strict guidelines regarding patient selection and type of infecting organism are followed. This method was considered to have a higher reinfection risk and carried the possibility of nonspecific antibiosis in the form of either systemic therapy or impregnated cement. It is considered inappropriate when massive bone loss requiring grafting is anticipated or when microbial identification is elusive or involves glycocalyx producers. One-stage reimplantation has been indicated for elderly patients who could not tolerate multiple operations or prolonged bed rest. It also is indicated in healthy hosts devoid of reinfection risk who have adequate bone and soft tissue for reconstruction and a known susceptible or low-virulence pathogen.

In a recent study, there was an 86% success rate with 1-stage exchange in the face of discharging sinuses; the authors concluded that the presence of a discharging sinus should not be considered a contraindication. In a prospective review of 20 consecutive infected THAs treated by one surgeon with an average follow-up of 10 years, the most common infecting organism was *S epidermidis*. After 1-stage exchange infection did not recur in any of these cases. This was attributed to careful surgical debridement, sensitivity-directed intravenous antibiotics, and the use of antibiotic-loaded cement. There were 2 revisions for aseptic loosening, one at 9 years and the other at 17 years after surgery. Patient selection criteria excluded any patient who was immunocompromised, infected with MRSA or Gram negative resistant organisms, or had any significant soft-tissue or bony defect that could compromise wound treatment or implant stability. In another study, 18 patients with infected megaprostheses placed after malignant tumor resection had 1-stage. At a mean follow-up of 52 months, 14 were infection-free. All treated patients had sensitive organisms, and in all cases the components were left unchanged. Thus, this technique may also be advantageous for salvage operations requiring endoprosthetic replacement.

Through careful patient selection and refined treatment, the results of 1-stage exchange seem to be approaching those of a 2-stage procedure. Thus, in the future, acceptable and effective treatment could consist of 1 hospitalization, with associated lower cost, morbidity, and disability for the patient. One-stage exchange procedures may avoid any interim instability, loss of bone density, disuse atrophy, limb shortening, and soft-tissue scarring associated with a second procedure. There appears to be no statistical difference when comparing the incidence of mechanical failure in 1- versus 2-stage procedures using survival analysis.

Two-Stage Exchange Arthroplasty

Two-stage exchange with the use of antibiotic-loaded cement has traditionally been the standard for treating patients with LCI, AHI, or patients having failed radical debridement and antibiotics in EPOI. This combination has had the lowest overall reinfection risk of any procedure under these circumstances. In 1 study, the 2-stage exchange had success rates of 83% without and 87% with antibiotic-loaded cement, whereas the 1-stage procedure had success rates of only 52% and 79%, respectively. This difference is particularly noticeable when evaluating results of more severe infections or virulent pathogens. Staged exchange has the added advantage of treating an organism immediately with specific antibiotics, and it allows clinical assessment of treatment prior to reimplantation. It does, however, require a great deal more effort on the part of the patient, physician, and health care resources.

Research is continuing to define the limitations of 2-stage exchange arthroplasty. Using uncemented porous implants during 2-stage exchange instead of an implant with antibiotic-loaded cement was studied in 34 patients with infected cemented THAs. After a 4-year follow-up, the authors noted an 18% recurrent infection rate and a 68% complication rate; they recommended the use of cemented implants for staged exchange arthroplasty. In another study with similar follow-up, there were 5 recurrences (13%) out of 40 arthroplasties using cementless revisions.

Three-Stage Exchange Arthroplasty

A new technique of 3-stage revision has been reported for infected THAs with concomitant severe bone loss. It is similar to the traditional 2-stage procedure except that in the second stage, bone grafting of any femoral or acetabular defects is performed 3 to 12 months after the initial stage using autograft and/or allograft. During the third stage, which is carried out 9 months from the initial resection, reconstruction is performed with cementless components. So far, this technique has been adopted by only a few surgeons and is based on retrospective studies with small sample sizes. It may have value for young patients whose successful outcome demands restitution of bone stock.

Resection Arthroplasty

Resection arthroplasty is an uncommon but occasionally necessary salvage procedure after a failed THA secondary to infection. This procedure is dissatisfying to both patient and physician. Resection arthroplasty is most indicated in patients who, for whatever surgical or medical reason, are not candidates for a staged reimplantation or are unable to comply with a postoperative rehabilitation protocol. Recent resection arthroplasty reports suggest that there is a decrease in function and ambulation as a result of a shortened limb. Nevertheless, many still consider this operation to be the ultimate salvage procedure because of its excellent success rate in eliminating infection and relieving pain.

Arthrodesis

Arthrodesis is a technically demanding procedure to undertake after infected THA, primarily because infection often leaves behind incompetent bone and soft tissue. It may have a limited indication in the younger, more active patient, but should really be considered anecdotal, as relatively few cases have been reported in the hip literature.

Amputation

This procedure is mentioned for the sake of completion. It is a rare operation performed only on patients who have a life- or limb-threatening infection or have massive tissue loss or vascular injury.

Use of Antibiotics During Exchange Arthroplasty

Review of the current literature makes it evident that antibiotic-impregnated bone cement improves outcome of periprosthetic infection regardless of the mode of treatment. There is clearly an increased elution of antibiotic when more than 1 antibiotic is used in the cement spacer. In the event of anaerobic infection, clindamycin-cement admixture may become the future thermostable drug of choice to be placed in cement or spacers. Some in vitro studies support the alternative use of antibiotic-impregnated bioresorbable beads made of polydilactide or polycoglycolide. They appear to have better elution properties than polymethylmethacrylate and have the added advantage of being biodegradable. They also appear to release sustained high concentrations of all contained antibiotics long enough to combat infection; this is in contradistinction to cement spacers, which elute different antibiotics at differing rates. Further study is required for this promising alternative.

Duration of antibiotic therapy and timing between stages remains controversial. It appears best to delay the second stage (implantation) for 6 weeks after the initial debridement, pending good clinical progression with antibiotics, and wound healing. Based on their results, some authors have recently recommended at least 3 months for less virulent organisms and 1 year for more virulent organisms. There are no studies adequate to reasonably compare the efficacy of delay periods shorter than 6 weeks.

Intervening Spacers During Exchange Arthroplasty

The use of PROSTALAC (prosthesis of antibiotic loaded acrylic cement) implants during the interim period between staged exchange continues to be evaluated for its efficacy and cost effectiveness as compared to traditional cement spacers. Its proposed advantages of better mobilization, control over limb-length discrepancy, earlier outpatient discharge, and antibiotic delivery remain inadequately proven. In a recent study with a 4-year follow-up, its use was investigated in 30 infected THAs with proximal segmental bone loss, for which the first 15 had a cement-on-cement articulation and the latter 15 had a custom metal-on-poly articulation. The average duration of hospitalization was 38 days. Most patients were considered mobile with the use of various assistive devices, although none bore weight on their affected limbs. Twenty-six reported no to moderate pain between stages and 96% were without evidence of infection at last follow-up. The ability of this spacer to mobilize patients to be discharged between stages might be advantageous in the setting of segmental bone loss; the large reconstruction needed to address this defect should probably not be performed in the presence of a contaminated bed. This technique was reported to be successful in eradicating infection in 94% of patients (45 of 48) after a minimum follow-up of 2 years. Review of 60 PROSTALAC staged exchanges revealed 5 patients sustained dislocations and 2 had periprosthetic fracture after the latter stage. The mean length of stay in the hospital was 12 days after the first stage and 9 after the second, with a mean interim delay of 91 days. The cure rate was 93%. Other similar techniques also have been reported recently. A spacer shaped like the femoral component of a hemiarthroplasty has been described, as well as autoclaving and reuse of the infected implant itself. What is most cost-effective and patient-friendly during this interim period of two-stage exchange remains debatable.

Allografts and Infection

The use of allografts for reconstruction after an infected THA remains controversial. The reinfection rate after the use of fresh frozen morcellized or bulk sterilized allografts during 2-stage revisions is reported to be between 5% and 11%. This does not differ significantly from the rate of reinfection after revision for septic failure without the use of allografts (9%). In addition, recent reports of marginally greater patient numbers using allograft in a nonseptic revision setting identify the infection risk to be around 2% to 4%, which is identical to recently reported infection rates for similar revision cases without the use of allograft. In most of the cases, allografts united to host bone after a medium-term follow-up. These results are interesting but must be interpreted cautiously in light of the small patient populations studied.

Future Developments

The most promising new technology in the ongoing effort to avert the potential threat of untreatable periprosthetic infection is immunization research. In a recent US study, investigators have for the first time capitalized on bacterial phenotypic expression to develop a broadly protective vaccine against many strains of *S aureus*, including some multidrug-resistant ones. They are using antibodies against poly-N-succinyl β-1-6 glucosamine (PNSG), an in vivo expressed surface polysaccharide produced principally during active human and animal infection and presumed vital to disease progression. Promising preliminary results in laboratory animals show effective conferral of immunity to infection in many cases. If successful in humans, such vaccines directed against expressed bacteria-specific factors such as staphylococcal PNSG could have a major impact on the preventive treatment of prosthetic and other infections, significantly improving patient care and providing enormous economic relief to the health care system.

Annotated Bibliography

General

Garvin KL, Hanssen AD: Infection after total hip arthroplasty: Past, present, and future. *J Bone Joint Surg* 1995;77A: 1576–1588.

This is an excellent and well-referenced overview of the evolution of infection and its management in total hip arthroplasty over the past 20 years.

Incidence and Etiology

Brause BD: Sepsis: The rational use of antimicrobials, in Callaghan JJ, Rosenberg AG, Rubash HE (eds): *The Adult Hip*. Philadelphia, PA, Lippincott-Raven, 1998, vol 2, pp 1343–1349.

A very up-to-date reference on the causes of periprosthetic infection, this chapter summarizes the types and prevalence of current pathogens and outlines the patterns of emerging bacterial and fungal resistance that have been identified. Appropriate antibiotic use and prophylaxis for the future are described as well.

Mahoney CR, Schneider JA, Garvin KL: Abstract: The emergence of resistant bacteria associated with failure of total joint arthroplasty. Proceedings of the American Academy of Orthopaedic Surgeons 65th Annual Meeting, New Orleans, LA. Rosemont, IL, American Academy of Orthopaedic Surgeons, 1998, p 345.

This paper highlights the science behind evolving microbial resistance, particularly with respect to the Staphylococcal and Enterococcal species. It provides Centers for Disease Control and Prevention practice guidelines for preventing the spread of bacterial resistance, and has many references on this issue.

Prophylaxis

Deacon JM, Pagliaro AJ, Zelicof SB, Horowitz HW: Prophylactic use of antibiotics for procedures after total joint replacement. *J Bone Joint Surg* 1996;78A:1755–1770.

This article outlines the appropriate use of antibiosis following total joint replacement. Prophylaxis for medical, dental, and varying surgical procedures are summarized, identifying the common bacteria and necessary spectrum of coverage required in each situation based on a literature review and 180 reports of hematogenously induced infection.

Hanssen AD, Osmon DR, Nelson CL: Prevention of deep periprosthetic joint infection. *J Bone Joint Surg* 1996;78A: 458–471.

A complete summary of the many variables influencing prosthetic infection in the perioperative period, this report addresses means of optimizing the prevention of infection, with historic perspective. Risks and recommended measures are discussed regarding the patient, operating environment, surgical technique and materials, and common pathogens.

Diagnosis

Spangehl MJ, Younger AS, Masri BA, Duncan CP: Diagnosis of infection following total hip arthroplasty. *J Bone Joint Surg* 1997;79A:1578–1588.

This review encompasses most of the current literature recommendations regarding the various modalities used to diagnose an infected total hip replacement. It is most helpful for understanding the various preoperative and intraoperative diagnostic investigations available to the surgeon, although the usefulness of some of these remains controversial as a result of limited available data.

Treatment

Masterson EL, Masri BA, Duncan CP: Treatment of infection at the site of total hip replacement. *J Bone Joint Surg* 1997;79A: 1740–1749.

A thorough summary of modern surgical technique and principles for treating infected total hip arthroplasties, this article describes both a protocol and options list for management. It is a valuable review of current, albeit controversial, literature on treatment methods.

Tsukayama DT, Estrada R, Gustilo RB: Infection after total hip arthroplasty: A study of the treatment of one hundred and six infections. *J Bone Joint Surg* 1996;78A:512–523.

One hundred six infections were treated in 98 hips with a mean follow-up of 3.8 years. A very useful management protocol is presented based on an updated and more inclusive classification scheme that categorizes patients into those with either a positive intraoperative culture, an early postoperative infection, a late chronic infection, or an acute hematogenous infection.

Future Developments

McKenny D, Pouliot KL, Wang Y, et al: Broadly protective accine for staphylococcus aureus based on an in vivo expressed antigen. *Science* 1999;284:1523–1527.

This is the first article to present promising data on the ability to engineer antibacterial vaccines generated from microbial antigens phenotypically expressed during human infection. Antibodies to poly-N-succinyl β-1-6 glucosamine, a surface polysaccharide synthesized by *S aureus* during infection, are found to confer protective immunity against even some multidrug-resistant Staphylococcus species in certain animals.

Chapter 18
Dislocation

Dislocation, probably the most frequent and distressing early complication for the patient who has a total hip arthroplasty (THA), is sudden, very painful, and causes immediate disability. Dislocation is a source of great anxiety for both the patient and the surgeon and may be a cause for loss of patient confidence in the surgeon and lead to medical malpractice litigation.

Early dislocation occurs within the first 12 months after the THA. In 1 report, 81% of hip dislocations occurred within the first 3 months after surgery. Late dislocation is a distinct pathologic entity that can occur after several years of implantation. A classic report on late dislocations described 32 patients who had an initial dislocation of a Charnley prosthesis between 5 and 10 years postoperatively. The identified risk factors were a greater range of motion and acetabular loosening.

The direction of dislocation of a THA is usually posterior, with anterior dislocation occurring much less frequently. In 1 report, the direction was posterior in 77% and anterior in 23%. Superior or "lateral" dislocation has also been described, but, in these cases, it is unclear if a cross-table lateral radiograph had been obtained before reduction.

Prevalence

The prevalence of dislocation of primary THA has been reported to range from less than 1% to more than 9%, with the number of hips in each study ranging from 427 to 10,000 or more. The overall general prevalence is considered to be 2% to 3% for primary THA. However, over the past decade, the prevalence of dislocation may have increased because of multiple factors, including earlier discharge from the hospital, modular components, and different methods of fixation. Recent studies have reported dislocation rates of 3.5% (anterior approach), 4.6% (posterior approach), and 7.6% (transtrochanteric approach) between 1985 and 1991, as performed by a large number of surgeons using a wide variety of prostheses. In 2 series of hybrid THA performed by 1 surgeon through a posterior approach, the prevalence of dislocation was 4% and 5.6%, respectively. In a multisurgeon series using the same components through an anterior approach, the rate of dislocation was only 2.1%. In a multisurgeon series in which hydroxyapatite coated femoral components were used, the rate of dislocation was 4.7%. It is obvious that with these newer techniques, a wide range (2% to 6%) of prevalence of dislocation after primary THA exists.

The prevalence of dislocation is much higher after revision THA. The rate of dislocation was 9% in one report of 169 revisions and 10% in another report of 530 revisions using a standard acetabular liner. However, the prevalence of dislocation after a primary bipolar hemiarthroplasty is lower than after a THA. A rate of dislocation of 1.5% was reported in a group of over 1,900 bipolar procedures performed at 2 institutions. However, recurrent dislocation was much higher (52%) with this procedure.

Causes and Risk Factors

Early dislocation of THA is directly related to patient-related factors, factors under the surgeon's control (such as technique and implant design), and other miscellaneous causes.

Patient-Related Factors

Gender has been considered an important risk factor for dislocation. In several studies performed during the 1980s, dislocation was reported to occur twice as frequently in female than male patients. However, in a report of primary Charnley hip arthroplasty from the Swedish National Register, gender had no influence on the rate of dislocation. In another United States study, there was no relationship between gender and the rate of dislocation after either primary or revision arthroplasty. Prior studies, as well as the previous 2 reports, have shown that patient age, height, weight, obesity, and preoperative diagnosis were not related to the rate of dislocation. However, previous hip surgery-revision arthroplasty has the highest rate of dislocation, at least twice that of primary arthroplasty. Primary THA performed in elderly (≥ 80 years of age) patients and in patients with an acute femoral neck fracture have a rate of dislocation of 8% to 10%. Emotional and psychiatric problems (such as depression and presenile dementia) have not yet been statistically correlated with a higher rate of dislocation. Two reports suggest that a history of excessive intake of alcohol or a suspicion of alcohol abuse in men was more common in groups with a dislocation compared to groups without a dislocation.

Surgical Factors

Previous reports from several centers have shown that the rate of dislocation is higher with the posterior approach than with the anterior or transtrochanteric approach. However, 2 recent reports challenge this assertion. In a Swedish study of more than 3,000 Charnley THA performed in 2 centers between 1979 and 1991 in similar patient groups, the rate of dislocation was 3.4% for the transtrochanteric approach and 3.3% for the posterior approach. More recently, 2 surgeons have reported dislocation rates of zero (395 patients) and 0.8% (160 hips) doing a hybrid THA through the posterior approach with an enhanced posterior soft-tissue repair. The surgeon's experience is also related to the rate of dislocation. In another Swedish study (at 3 centers) of 4,230 primary THAs performed using the posterior approach, the rate of dislocation was 3%. The less experienced surgeons had twice the number of dislocations than the more experienced surgeons. The frequency of dislocation decreased with increasing numbers of operations and leveled off after 30. For every 10 primary THA performed annually, the risk of dislocation decreased by 50%.

The orientation or position of the acetabular component has been related to dislocation, and in 1 study, a third of recurrent dislocations were caused by cup malposition. A retroverted component predisposes to posterior dislocation, and excessive anteversion predisposes to anterior dislocation. Vertical orientation (> 55°) has also been considered a risk factor. However, recent studies question the relationship between cup orientation and dislocation. A computed tomography study of component alignment in 38 THAs that dislocated and 14 uncomplicated arthroplasties showed no difference between the alignment of the components in either group. It was concluded that muscular imbalance rather than malposition of components was the major factor determining dislocation. In another study of 97 primary THAs, the abduction angle and version angle measured on standardized anteroposterior and cross-table lateral radiographs were not significantly different between those hips with or without a dislocation. In a report on 391 primary and 169 revision hip arthroplasties, a matched-pair radiographic analysis of acetabular component position was performed. There was no association between either the version or the abduction angles of the acetabular component (within the ranges seen) and the risk of dislocation in either group. These 3 studies demonstrate that patient-related factors or noncompliance with precautions may be more important than acetabular position as a risk factor for dislocation.

Trochanteric avulsion, nonunion of a trochanteric osteotomy, or abductor muscle malfunction caused by superior gluteal nerve injury have all been associated with a higher rate of dislocation.

Several prior clinical studies have failed to confirm a theoretical concern that a smaller femoral head (22 mm) would have a higher rate of dislocation than larger (28 and 32 mm) femoral heads. A Swedish report found no difference in the rate of dislocation between the 22-mm Charnley prosthesis (2.5%) and the 32-mm Lubinus prosthesis (2.4%) at 1 year. However, there was a higher rate of recurrent dislocation (2.3 times the risk) when the smaller femoral head was used. In a small, prospective, randomized study of modular THA, hips with a 22-mm modular head had an increased rate of dislocation compared to those with a 28-mm modular head.

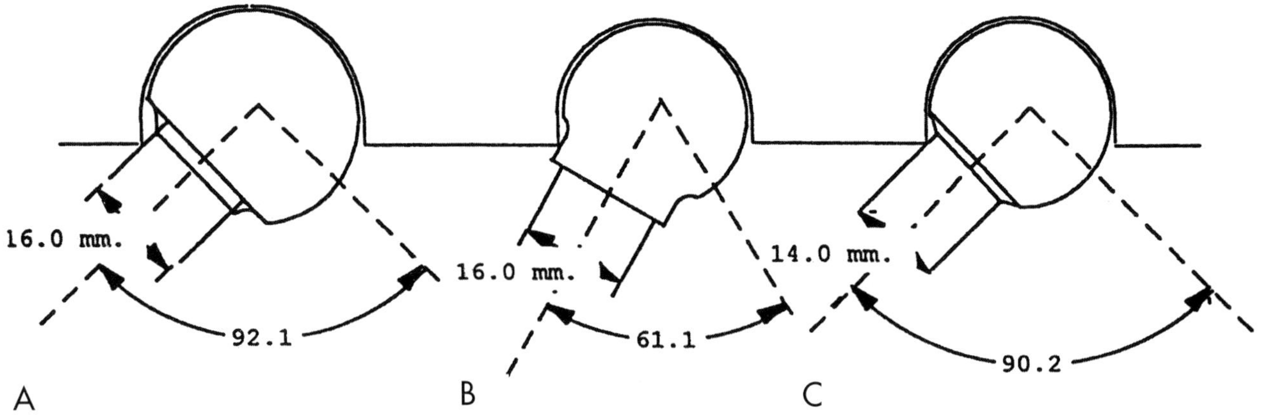

Figure 1

Estimated ranges of motion of a 32-mm Lubinus head on the 14/16 taper (**A**), collar-reinforced (skirt) 28-mm head on the 14/16 taper (**B**), and 28-mm head on the 12/14 taper (**C**). (Reproduced with permission from Hedlundh U, Carlsson AS: Increased risk of dislocation with collar reinforced modular heads of the Lubinus SP-2 hip prosthesis. *Acta Orthop Scand* 1996;67:204–210.)

There was also an important relationship between the outer size of a cementless acetabular component and the risk of dislocation. Using a 28-mm modular femoral head, the rate of dislocation for acetabular components 60 mm and larger was significantly increased compared to components 58 mm and smaller. The rate of dislocation for each head size was related to outer acetabular component size, with increased rates for component diameters 54 mm and larger with a 22-mm head, and 60 mm and larger with a 28-mm head.

Modularity and Dislocation

Modular prostheses have introduced both new problems and possibly new solutions for dislocations of THA. Modern femoral components have a separate modular femoral head that attaches to the femoral stem through a Morse taper impaction-attachment. There are several reports of dissociation of the femoral head from the stem with attempted closed reduction. Open reduction was required. Some modular femoral heads with long necks have a reinforcement at their base, commonly called a skirt, and these have been reported to have an increased risk of dislocation with a 28-mm head prosthesis. The range of motion of a total hip with a femoral head skirt is less than that of one without such a modification (Fig. 1). This femoral head skirt can impinge against an acetabular liner and cause the head to lever out as well as lead to premature loosening or wear of the acetabular component. There is a case report of dislodgement of a press-fit femoral stem with attempted reduction of a dislocation.

Modular acetabular component liner dissociation has also occurred following reduction of a dislocation. Elevated rim liners (10° and 20°) placed into a modular acetabular component may provide both increased prevention of a first-time dislocation and a possible treatment for recurrent dislocation in a hip with slight malposition of the acetabulum as the presumed etiology. In a report of over 5,000 THAs, the 2-year probability of dislocation was 2.19% for hips with a 10° elevated rim liner and 3.85% for those with a standard liner, a statistically significant difference. In revision THA, the risk of dislocation was also significantly lower with the elevated rim liner (5%) compared with the standard liner (10%). However, the range of motion of a hip with an elevated rim liner is decreased compared to one with a neutral liner (Fig. 2). There is also concern that the neck of a femoral component can impinge on an elevated rim and lever the head out of the acetabular component. The torsional forces of this impingement could increase the likelihood of loosening of the acetabular component (Fig. 3).

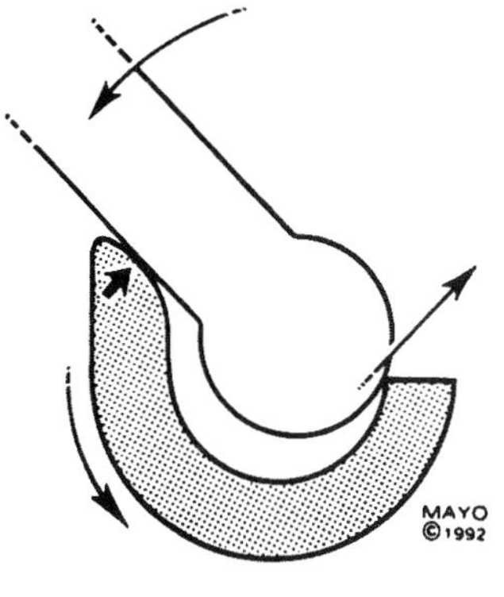

Figure 3

The neck of the femoral component can impinge on an elevated rim liner and lever the head out of the acetabulum. The curved arrows show the torsional forces that could increase the likelihood of acetabular component loosening. (Reproduced with permission from the Mayo Foundation, Rochester, MN.)

Miscellaneous Factors

Occult infection of a THA, with septic fluid accumulation and a stretched or failed capsule, can be an overlooked factor for a first or second dislocation. Trauma, such as a fall from a height or motor vehicle accident, can be a direct cause of dislocation. Profound weight loss, with its accompanying loss of muscle mass (as a result of cancer or chronic illness), may also be related to late dislocations.

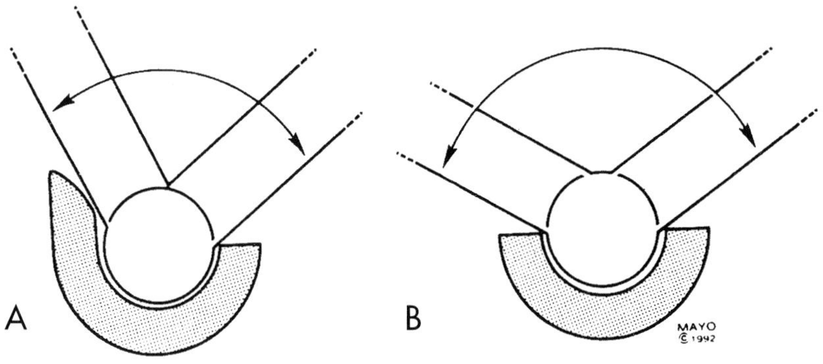

Figure 2

The influence of elevated rim (**A**) and neutral liners (**B**) on the range of motion. The elevated rim decreases the range of motion. (Reproduced with permission from the Mayo Foundation, Rochester, MN.)

Treatment

After confirmation of the diagnosis with biplane radiographs, the immediate treatment for a dislocated THA is closed reduction, either under heavy intravenous sedation in the emergency department or under general or regional anesthesia in the operating room. One report recommended the latter method because of the chance of disengagement of a modular prosthesis. The usual method of reduction is longitudinal traction with the hip in slight flexion. A recent report described a new technique for closed reduction in which the surgeon's upper arm serves as a fulcrum for a flexed hip. Traction is applied through the knee while the surgeon grasps the ankle to control rotation.

Following reduction, the hip should be placed through a range of motion maneuver to determine the overall stability. Although there is no study that confirms the efficacy of postoperative immobilization, it is generally wise to immobilize the hip with an above-knee orthosis, which limits flexion, adduction, and rotation, for 4 to 8 weeks after a dislocation.

Prognosis

It has been shown that approximately two thirds of patients with an initial dislocation of the hip will have no further problems; a third will have recurrent dislocations. However, recent studies have reported that hips may eventually stabilize after a second or third dislocation without further surgery. One report of 3,685 primary Charnley or Charnley hybrid THAs found that 121 hips had a dislocation. Only 35% of patients with a first dislocation remained stable, but a total of 65% stabilized without surgery after a second or third dislocation. Another study determined that approximately 70% of hips stabilized after the first or second dislocation. These reports suggest that counseling and/or immobilization is justified until a third dislocation occurs.

Reoperation for Recurrent Dislocation

In recent reports on a variety of prostheses, approximately 1% to 2% of primary THAs undergo revision for recurrent dislocation. Preoperative evaluation should be directed toward determining the cause of recurrent dislocation. Radiographic studies to determine the version of the acetabular and femoral components are still recommended. The status of the trochanter and the gluteal muscles should be determined. A careful history should determine if alcohol abuse or neurologic-psychiatric problems are present.

Reoperation for recurrent dislocation has been reported to be successful in 40% to 80% of hips. The prognosis has been shown to be worse for hips with a 22-mm femoral head. In one series, 45% of multiple revisions for recurrent dislocation failed. In another series of 121 Charnley hips, less than a third of revisions for recurrent dislocation were successful if the surgeon was unable to determine the cause of dislocation, but 70% were successful if a technical error was corrected.

Repositioning of a retroverted acetabular component was reported to be successful in 70% of revisions for recurrent dislocation. With the availability of modular components and elevated rim liners (10° and 20°), this option should be considered for components with minimal or no acetabular malposition. Presently, there are no reports on the results of liner exchange for recurrent dislocation. Repair of a trochanteric avulsion or trochanteric osteotomy nonunion should be attempted if this is the identifiable cause of recurrent dislocation. Distal advancement of the greater trochanter has a reported success rate of 80% when soft-tissue (capsule or abductor muscle) laxity is considered to be the cause of recurrent dislocation.

Salvage of a hip with recurrent dislocation by conversion to a bipolar hemiarthroplasty may be considered in elderly, low-demand patients with sufficient acetabular bone structure. Over the past several years, treatment of hips with recurrent dislocation has included the use of constrained or captive devices; with the S-ROM® constrained acetabular liner, recurrent dislocation occurred in 29% and 10%, respectively, in 2 series with short-term follow-up. Open reduction is usually required to correct this complication. Disassembly and loosening of this acetabular component have been reported. Recently, a study of the Omnifit® constrained acetabular insert reported only 4 recurrent dislocations of 77 hips in patients still alive at 2 to 8 years (mean, 5 years) of follow-up. However, judicious use of this component as a salvage procedure was recommended because of long-term concerns of increased polyethylene wear and acetabular loosening.

Prevention

Instruction in THA precautions both before and after surgery is important for the prevention of dislocation. In those patients with a history of alcohol abuse or an abnormal mental status (for example, confusion), a prophylactic hip orthosis should be in place soon after surgery and worn for 6 weeks. For those surgeons who use a posterior approach for THA, careful repair of the posterior capsule, short external rotator tendons, quadratus femoris, and gluteus maximus should be performed to decrease dead space and serve as a check-rein to internal rotation. This technique reduced dislocation in 1 surgeon's practice from 4% to 0% in 395 patients at 1-year follow-up. The routine use of an elevated rim (10°) liner in primary THA is controversial. At 2 years' follow-up in a retrospective, nonrandomized study of over 5,000 THAs, the 1% decrease in the rate of dislocation with the elevated rim liner was statistically significant. The difference was 5% in revision arthroplasty. A companion study reported that there was no difference in the probability of revision for loosening with an elevated rim liner at a mean follow-up of 5 years. However, routine use of elevated rim liners in primary THA was not recommended in this study. Elevated rim liners should be considered in revision arthroplasties performed for loosening.

Annotated Bibliography

Cobb TK, Morrey BF, Ilstrup DM: The elevated-rim acetabular liner in total hip arthroplasty: Relationship to postoperative dislocation. *J Bone Joint Surg* 1996;78A:80–86.

This is a retrospective, multisurgeon study of dislocation after 2,469 THAs using a 10° elevated rim liner and 2,698 using a standard liner. At 2 years, those hips with an elevated rim had a statistically significant lower probability of dislocation (2.19% versus 3.85%). This difference was significant for the anterior and transtrochanteric approaches, but not for the posterior approach.

Cobb TK, Morrey BF, Ilstrup DM: Effect of the elevated-rim acetabular liner on loosening after total hip arthroplasty. *J Bone Joint Surg* 1997;79A:1361–1364.

This is the companion study to the above to determine the effect of a 10° elevated rim liner on loosening and revision of the components. Five-year follow-up data were available for 1,237 hips (174 with an elevated rim and 1,063 with a standard liner). No significant differences were found in the survival of the acetabular or femoral components at this short follow-up time.

Goetz DD, Capello WN, Callaghan JJ, Brown TD, Johnston RC: Salvage of total hip instability with a constrained acetabular component. *Clin Orthop* 1998;355:171–181.

This is a retrospective review of 101 Omnifit® constrained acetabular inserts performed by 2 very experienced surgeons. Of the 77 hips in living patients, with a mean follow-up of 5 years, there were only 4 cases of recurrent dislocation. The authors recommended judicious use of this component as a salvage measure.

Hedlundh U, Ahnfelt L, Hybbinette CH, Wallinder L, Weckstrom J, Fredin H: Dislocations and the femoral head size in primary total hip arthroplasty. *Clin Orthop* 1996;333:226–233.

There was no difference at 1 year in the dislocation rate of the Charnley (22 mm) prosthesis and the Lubinus (32 mm) prosthesis. However, almost all late dislocations occurred with the Charnley, and the risk of recurrent dislocation was increased by 2.3 times with the 22-mm head.

Hedlundh U, Ahnfelt L, Hybbinette CH, Weckstrom J, Fredin H: Surgical experience related to dislocations after total hip arthroplasty. *J Bone Joint Surg* 1996;78B:206–209.

After 4,230 primary THAs, twice the number of dislocations occurred for inexperienced surgeons compared to experienced ones. The frequency of dislocation leveled off after approximately 30 surgeries.

Hedlundh U, Fredin H: Patient characteristics in dislocations after primary total hip arthroplasty: 60 patients compared with a control group. *Acta Orthop Scand* 1995;66:225–228.

Sixty patients with a primary Charnley arthroplasty and at least 1 dislocation were compared to a randomly selected group of 118 patients with no dislocation. There was an increased mortality rate in patients with a dislocation. Gender, height, weight, diagnosis, psychiatric disorder, or use of pharmaceuticals had no influence on dislocation. Half of the male patients in the dislocated group were alcoholics.

Kelley SS, Lachiewicz PF, Hickman JM, Paterno SM: Relationship of femoral head and acetabular size to the prevalence of dislocation. *Clin Orthop* 1998;355:163–170.

In a prospective, randomized study, a modular 22-mm head had a significantly higher rate of dislocation than a modular 28-mm head. In a retrospective group of 308 primary hips with a modular 28-mm head, the rate of dislocation was significantly higher in hips with acetabular components with an outer diameter of 60 mm and larger.

Paterno SA, Lachiewicz PF, Kelley SS: The influence of patient-related factors and the position of the acetabular component on the rate of dislocation after total hip replacement. *J Bone Joint Surg* 1997;79A:1202–1210.

There was no relationship between age, gender, obesity, or preoperative diagnosis and dislocation after primary or revision hip arthroplasty. There was a higher rate of dislocation in patients with a history of excessive alcohol intake. In a matched-pair analysis, there was no association between either acetabular version or abduction angle and the risk of dislocation.

Pellicci PM, Bostrom M, Poss R: Posterior approach to total hip replacement using enhanced posterior soft tissue repair. *Clin Orthop* 1998;355:224–228.

Using an enhanced posterior soft-tissue repair after hybrid THA through a posterior approach, a dislocation rate of 4% in 395 patients prior to using the repair was reduced to zero in 395 patients by 1 surgeon. A dislocation rate of 6.2% (160 hips) was reduced to 0.8% (124 hips) with the identical enhanced posterior repair.

Pollard JA, Daum WJ, Uchida T: Can simple radiographs be predictive of total hip dislocation? *J Arthroplasty* 1995;10:800–804.

The postoperative radiographs from a control group of 90 THAs was radiographically compared with those of a group of 7 known dislocating hips using a standardized protocol. Neither the abduction angle nor the version angle of the acetabular component was a predictor of dislocation.

Classic Bibliography

Hedlundh U, Hybbinette CH, Fredin H: Influence of surgical approach on dislocations after Charnley hip arthroplasty. *J Arthroplasty* 1995;10:609–614.

Hedlundh U, Sanzen L, Fredin H: The prognosis and treatment of dislocated total hip arthroplasties with a 22 mm head. *J Bone Joint Surg* 1997;79B:374–378.

Vosburgh CL, Vosburgh JB: Closed reduction for total hip arthroplasty dislocation: The Tulsa technique. *J Arthroplasty* 1995;10:693–694.

Barnes CL, Berry DJ, Sledge CB: Dislocation after bipolar hemiarthroplasty of the hip. *J Arthroplasty* 1995;10:667–669.

Hedlundh U, Carlsson AS: Increased risk of dislocation with collar reinforced modular heads of the Lubinus SP-2 hip prosthesis. *Acta Orthop Scand* 1996;67:204–205.

Fisher DA, Kiley K: Constrained acetabular cup disassembly. *J Arthroplasty* 1994;9:325–329.

Pierchon F, Pasquier G, Cotten A, Fontaine C, Clarisse J, Duquennoy A: Causes of dislocation of total hip arthroplasty: CT study of component alignment. *J Bone Joint Surg* 1994;76B: 45–48.

Morrey BF: Difficult complications after hip joint replacement: Dislocation. *Clin Orthop* 1997;344:179–187.

Chapter 19 Complications in Total Hip Arthroplasty

Introduction

The list of potential complications following total hip arthroplasty (THA) is endless. The greatest concerns of Charnley's era, wear and sepsis, were addressed by the introduction of high molecular weight polyethylene and antibiotic prophylaxis. Later, the mischaracterization of osteolysis as "cement disease" led nearly an entire generation of orthopaedic surgeons to embrace cementless fixation. The subsequent experience with intraoperative fracture, postoperative thigh pain, and failure of fixation resulted in further modification of technique and design, which will undoubtedly create unforeseen complications in the future.

Infection

Aside from the life-threatening complications of total hip replacement, no postoperative complication can be more devastating than infection. In the earliest cemented THAs the infection rate was noted to be as high as 11%. Charnley frequently reported on osteomyelitis from THA despite sterile cultures. In retrospect, this probably represented what we currently refer to as lysis and probably exaggerated the actual incidence of infection. Only through identification of the risk factors and development of prophylaxis has the incidence of infection decreased. Advances in treatment in the identification of infection have offered some hope in solving this devastating problem. It is important to realize that a THA should not be painful, and if it is, the possibility of infection must always be considered.

Deep infection has been shown to be related to the premorbid state of the patient. Increased risks of infection have been shown to occur with rheumatoid arthritis (1.2%), psoriatic arthritis (5.5%), diabetes mellitus (5.6%), and, in males, following postoperative urethral instrumentation (6.2%). Prophylaxis against infection begins with identifying which organisms are most prevalent. *Staphylococcus aureus*, coagulase-positive, is the most common cause of acute infection after surgery; *S epidermidis* and *S albus* are common causes of late infection. Any prophylactic regimen must be aimed at these common organisms.

Exposure to the staphylococcal organisms can occur at the time of the skin incision. Antibiotic prophylaxis must therefore be directed at having a high tissue concentration at the time of the skin incision. Most commonly, first-generation cephalosporins are used prophylactically. Other measures designed to reduce the incidence of infection include sealing off the skin edges, and the use of body exhaust suits, laminar flow, and ultraviolet lights, which destroy airborne bacteria. Small doses of antibiotic (tobramycin) within cement, which have been shown to produce high local diffusion rates without significantly altering the mechanical substrate of the cement, can be beneficial when cemented components are selected for postseptic reimplantation. Antibiotic-impregnated cement provides a low systemic concentration that, theoretically, is better tolerated by the patient. However, even at these low systemic concentration levels, irreversible toxic reactions can occur and should be identified.

Postoperative urinary tract infection occurs in approximately 7% to 14% of patients. However, no correlation has been shown between the bacteria isolated from urine and those isolated from deep septic infections. Late hematogenous infection has been reported following dental, gynecologic, urologic, or gastroenterologic procedures. As a result, various protocols for antibiotic prophylaxis have been proposed (Table 1).

The identification of a postoperative infection can be quite obvious or deceptively subtle. An infection must be suspected in the setting of unexplained postoperative pain or component loosening (Fig. 1). The diagnosis of infection relies on clinical examination, supported by radiologic and laboratory studies. The aspiration arthrogram is the final step in the work-up of a septic hip following total hip replacement. A negative aspirate, however, does not mean that infection does not exist. Radiologic findings suggestive of infection include irregular or scalloped endosteal borders, with a lacy pattern of new bone formation (Fig. 2). Infection may fall into 1 of 3 categories: acute, delayed, or late.

The acute postoperative infection is typically depicted as an erythematous, draining, painful hip in the febrile patient

Table 1
Suggestions for prophylactic antibiotic regimens for patients with prosthetic joints*

Procedures	Treatment
Dental Procedures (associated with gingival hemorrhage)	Amoxicillin–2 g, po, 1 hour before procedure or clindamycin–300 mg, po, 1 hour before procedure
Certain Genitourinary/ Gastrointestinal Procedures	Ampicillin 2 g, IV plus Gentamicin 1.5 mg/kg (not to exceed 80 mg), IV or IM plus Metronidazole 500 mg, po, 30 minutes before procedure followed by Amoxicillin 1.5 g, po plus Metronidazole 500 mg, po, 6 hours after initial doses For patients allergic to ampicillin, amoxicillin, or penicillin: Vancomycin 1 g, IV (1 hour infusion) plus Gentamicin 1.5 mg/kg (not to exceed 80 mg), IV or IM plus Metronidazole 500 mg, po, 1 hour before procedure followed by Metronidazole 500 mg, po, 6 hours after initial dose

*The use of prophylactic antibiotics in patients with prosthetic joints for events/procedures associated with anticipated bacteremias is controversial. The specific indications for their use have not been established. Schedules shown here are for consideration by those physicians who wish to employ prophylactic antibiotics in some settings for certain patients. po = by mouth; IV = intravenous; IM = intramuscular

with an associated leukocytosis. In a delayed infection, the findings may or may not be so obvious. The presence of a draining sinus accompanied by fever and leukocytosis is a standard presentation. Pain at rest should alert the surgeon to possible deep-seated infection. Elevation of the erythrocyte sedimentation rate and C-reactive protein has been correlated with postoperative infection. A variety of nuclear studies are available to help differentiate between septic and aseptic loosening. Although the technetium-99m scan will not differentiate between aseptic and septic loosening, indium scans have been shown to be increasingly accurate in diagnosing low-grade musculoskeletal sepsis. As previously mentioned, an aspiration arthrogram should be considered when the diagnosis of sepsis is a possibility.

Treatment of infection is predicated on identification of the organism and sensitivity patterns, host defenses, and fixation of the implant. A superficial infection must be drained completely at an early stage. Early salvage is related to the stability of the fixation and the sensitivity of the bacteria. If an attempt is made to retain the components, a closed-suction drainage system is used. Infections delayed longer than 6 months frequently require removal of components and all cement. An immediate exchange arthroplasty or a delayed two-stage reimplantation, following removal of implants and cement, may be considered. The principles of reimplantation are based on the condition and physiologic age of the patient, the sensitivity of the organism to antibiotics, and the absence of active infection. In many cases, resection arthroplasty provides a pain-free alternative and allows ambulation using external support and a shoe lift. In this situation, fusion is difficult to achieve because of the decrease in bone stock.

Thromboembolism

Thromboembolism, the most common complication following THA, is the leading cause of postoperative morbidity. The incidence of deep vein thrombosis (DVT) has been shown to be as high as 70% and as low as 8%. Fatal pulmonary embolus occurs in 1% to 2% of patients who are left untreated. The incidence of DVT is reported to be highest on postoperative

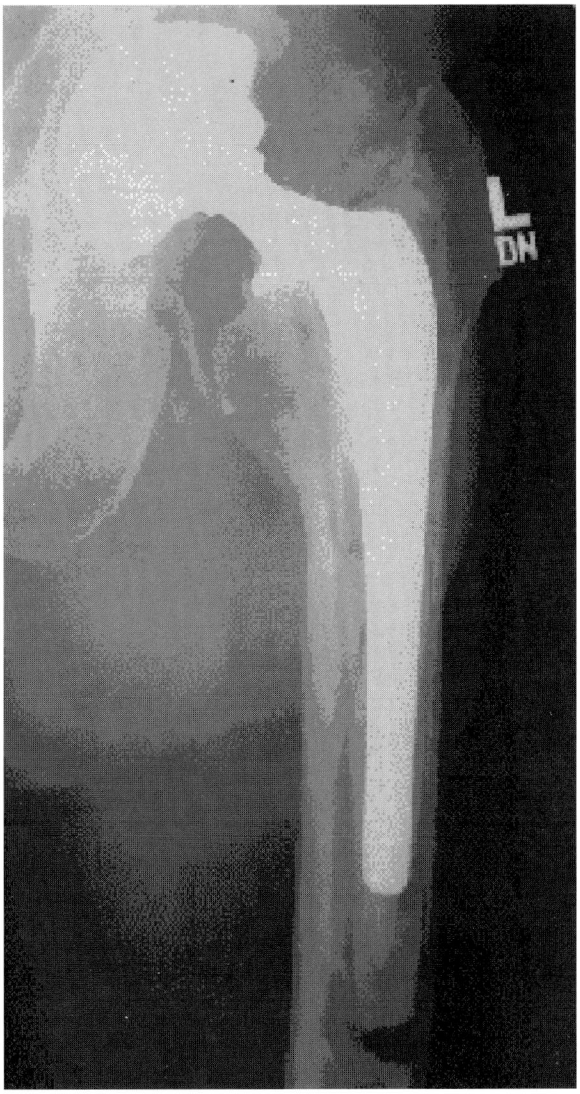

Figure 1

Unexplained loosening of a cemented femoral prosthesis 4 years postoperatively. Sepsis work-up, including aspiration, was negative. Review of the original operative note described femoral canal preparation for cementless fixation, which was abandoned in favor of cement when mechanical stability could not be achieved.

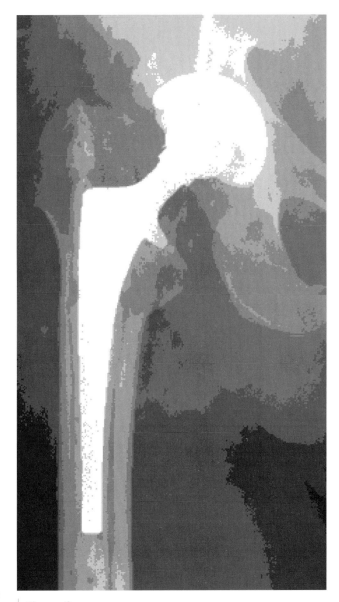

Figure 2

Deep sepsis 3 years following placement of a cemented femoral stem. A complete radiolucent line at the cement bone interface is shown with subsidence and distal endosteal scalloping.

day 4. Other authors have implicated the intraoperative period as a time frame in which DVT can develop, reporting that there is a strong systemic activation of the clotting cascade associated with local vessel injury and stasis in the femoral vein. Detection of thromboembolism may be clinically obvious or subtle. The classic presentation of a pulmonary embolus, consisting of shortness of breath, pleuritic chest pain, and mental status changes, is not always present. The presence of calf tenderness (Homan's sign), a low grade fever, fatigue, tachycardia, and diaphoresis may or may not be evident. Standard treatment for a suspected pulmonary embolus includes immediate administration of oxygen therapy.

A chest radiograph, followed by ventilation perfusion scanning (if the chest radiograph is negative), may screen a large majority of pulmonary emboli. An electrocardiogram may be helpful in ruling out cardiogenic causes for the patient's symptomatology. The "gold standard" for detecting a pul-

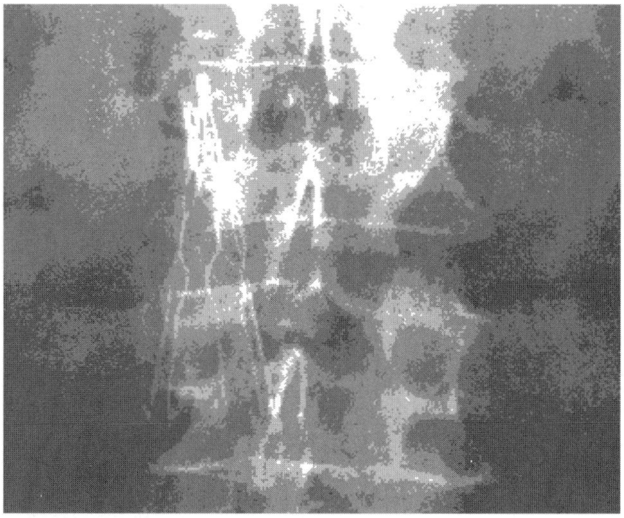

Figure 3
Greenfield vena caval filter in place.

monary embolus is still the pulmonary angiogram. Therapy is instituted immediately, with the goal of preventing a fatal pulmonary embolus from occurring. In addition to oxygen, hemodynamic support is initiated. Therapeutic (nonprophylactic) anticoagulation is instituted with the goal of preventing further propagation of DVT and the development of a fatal pulmonary embolism. The use of a Greenfield filter (Fig. 3) may be necessary if additional pulmonary emboli develop despite anticoagulation, or if anticoagulation is not tolerated. When used properly, the Greenfield filter has been shown to be a safe, easy, and effective method of preventing fatal pulmonary embolism in selected patients: those who are at exceptionally high risk for thromboembolism, as a method of preoperative prophylaxis; those who have a documented thromboembolism and in whom therapeutic anticoagulation is contraindicated; and those who have complications secondary to therapeutic anticoagulation.

The risk of bleeding complications resulting from therapeutic anticoagulation has been shown to be excessively high in the postoperative period. A 45% incidence of bleeding complications is attributed to the treatment of postoperative thromboembolic disease with heparin when it is administered intravenously within the first 6 days after THA. Antiembolic treatment is therefore directed at prophylaxis and prevention of potentially fatal thromboembolic events. A variety of drugs and therapeutic modalities, used individually or in combination, have attempted to decrease the incidence of postoperative thromboembolism. Coumadin, low

Table 2
New England Baptist Hospital guidelines for anticoagulation*

	Category I	**Category II**
Risk Factors	History of PE, DVT Varicosities, thrombophlebitis History of carcinoma Bilateral THR	Everyone else
INR	1.5–2.0	1.5–2.0
Ultrasound examination	No (unless clinically indicated)	Yes
Treatment	Coumadin for 6 weeks	Coumadin as inpatient until Doppler ultrasound. If negative, discharge on 1 ecotrin/day for 6 weeks. If positive and minor clot is present, continue Coumadin for 6 weeks. If positive and major clot is present (eg, common femoral vein and > 5 cm), consider heparin.

*PE = pulmonary embolism; DVT = deep vein thrombosis; THR = total hip replacement; INR = international normalized ratio

molecular-weight heparin, unfractionated heparin, low molecular-weight dextran, dihydroergotamine, phenylbutazone, aspirin, sulfinpyrazone, and hydroxychloroquine (plaquenil) have all been used as prophylactic agents. Antiembolic stockings, external sequential pneumatic compression boots, and early mobilization have also been used.

Only the number of diagnostic procedures used to detect thromboembolic phenomena has rivaled the variety of treatment modalities. Doppler ultrasonography, venography, impedance plethysmography, lung scans, and radioactive iodine fibrinogen scanning have all been used preoperatively and postoperatively to detect thromboemboli. The lengthy list of therapeutic and diagnostic modalities related to the treatment and detection of thromboembolic disease attests to the complexity of the problem and to our failure to eradicate it. The current anticoagulation protocol for THA used at The New England Baptist Hospital is outlined in Table 2.

Heterotopic Ossification

The incidence of heterotopic ossification following THA has been reported to be between 0.6% and 61.7%. Heterotopic ossification may vary from slight to complete bony ankylosis from the femur to the pelvis (Fig. 4). Its etiology and pathogenesis are still obscure and has been shown to be related to the duration of the surgical procedure and to the amount of soft-tissue dissection. Heterotopic ossification is associated with such conditions as ankylosing spondylitis, Forestier's disease, and posttraumatic arthritis. One particular group identified as being at high risk is males with considerable bilateral osteophytic osteoarthritis. Heterotopic ossification is usually painless and rarely requires removal. Ectopic bone formation does not seem to affect the functional result unless apparent bone ankylosis is present.

Various treatment modalities have been developed in an effort to reduce the incidence of heterotopic ossification following THA. Radiation has been shown to aid in the prevention of heterotopic ossification (2,000 rads given in 10 fractions) but was found to be of doubtful value, however, once the ectopic bone is visible on radiograph. A protocol of 1,000 rads has been shown to be as effective as treatment with 2,000 rads, and may be preferable because it reduces the risk of malignancy and length of hospitalization. Various reports of successful prevention of heterotopic ossification, with as little as 500 rads given as a single dose, are promising. In a canine model, the pullout strength of a titanium fiber implant was significantly reduced by a dose of radiation commonly used in the prevention of heterotopic ossification.

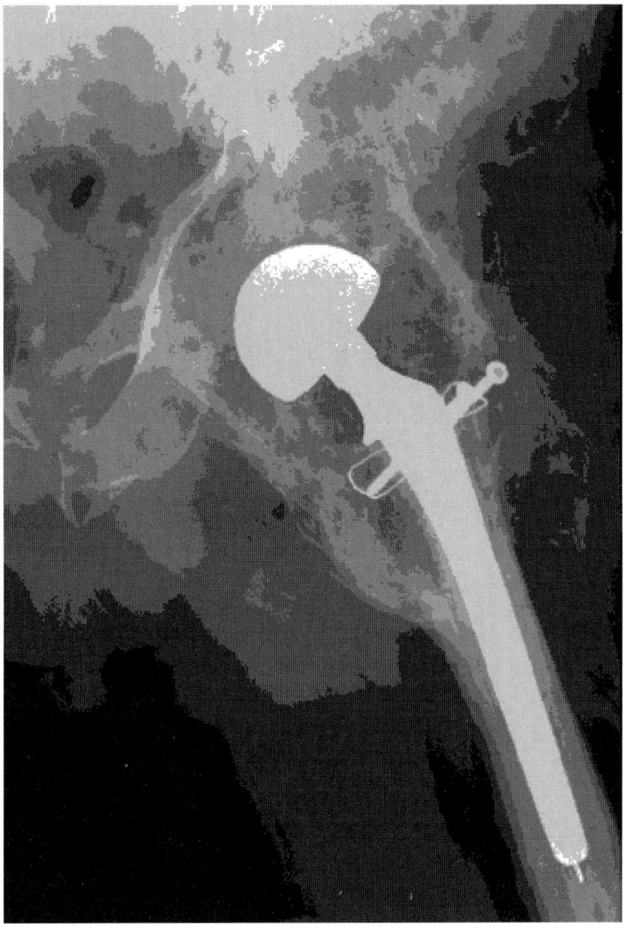

Figure 4

Extensive heterotopic ossification with bony ankylosis following bipolar hemiarthroplasty for femoral neck fracture.

If irradiation is chosen for prophylaxis, either the porous implant should be adequately shielded, or a cemented implant should be used. Indomethacin, ibuprofen, and diphosphonates have been used as prophylactic agents. Not surprisingly, porous-coated implants in laboratory animals treated with indomethacin, ibuprofen, and high-dose aspirin have demonstrated decreased bone ingrowth. Diphosphonates have been demonstrated experimentally to delay mineralization of osteoid rather than to prevent heterotopic bone formation. This delay, however, does not significantly improve the range of motion following THA. Heterotopic ossification, although a frequent occurrence following THA, is usually painless, rarely requires removal, and does not seem to affect the functional result unless it is severe.

Intraoperative Fracture

Intraoperative femoral fractures are most commonly seen in the revision situation. However, with "fit and fill" techniques, an effort is made to press fit the femoral component, if possible, into the proximal femur. This approach has raised the incidence of intraoperative femoral fractures to 3% in some series. Another situation in which fracture is likely is when a straight component is used in a bowed femur. When a femur is fractured during an uncemented procedure, the loosening rate has been shown to increase to 10% at 2 years. If an intraoperative femur fracture is detected, a longer stem component should be used, one that bypasses the defect by a distance measuring 1.5 diaphyseal diameters (Fig. 5). Intraoperative femoral perforations or fractures require protracted periods of restricted weightbearing postoperatively, and they usually heal without incident.

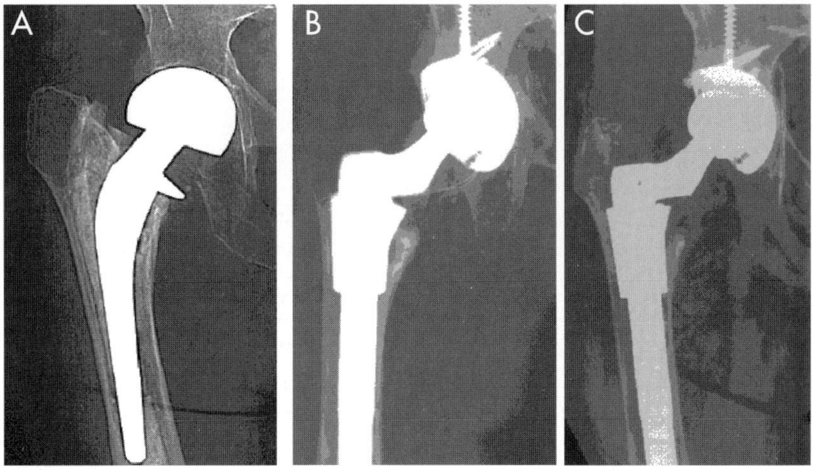

Figure 6

A 68-year-old woman presented with thigh pain 10 years following cemented bipolar hemiarthoplasty (**A**) implanted following hip fracture. At the time of femoral revision, the bipolar acetabular component was converted to a fixed hemispherical cup. The postoperative recovery room film (**B**) revealed a displaced fracture of the acetabulum exiting through the sciatic notch. Following 3 months of protected weightbearing, the fracture has healed (**C**).

Periprosthetic fractures of the acetabulum during and following THA have been reported. The use of press-fit techniques, in which the acetabulum is underreamed in relationship to the size of the acetabular component, is desirable to create immediate stability of the implant. The amount of underreaming is determined by the quantity and quality of the patient's bone, the geometry of the implant, and the force with which the implant is seated. Periprosthetic fracture of the acetabulum can potentially occur with impaction of the oversized component into the host bone (Fig. 6).

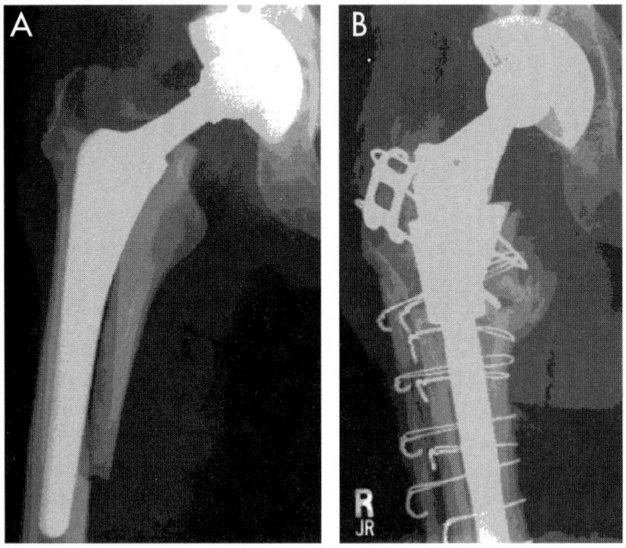

Figure 5

Periprosthetic femoral fracture (**A**) detected 1 week postoperatively. A 225-mm stem bypasses the fracture (**B**) sufficiently with supplemental onlay strut grafting.

Trochanteric Nonunion

The virtues of trochanteric osteotomy, including greater exposure and the ability to lateralize the abductor mechanism, seem to have been outweighed by the increased risk of complication when it is used in the primary setting. The increased intraoperative blood loss and operative time, coupled with slower rehabilitation, have decreased the number of trochanteric osteotomies that are performed. The bursitis associated with trochanteric wire breakage and the increased incidence of heterotopic ossification have encouraged many to abandon it in certain situations. The 5% incidence of trochanteric nonunion (Fig. 7), as with the other complications listed, have led to disenchantment with the trochanteric osteotomy, and many surgeons now reserve it for revision or dysplastic reconstruction. The overall decrease in the incidence of trochanteric nonunion is related to the decreasing incidence with which it is performed. Reattachment of the trochanter is technically demanding, and success is based on the size of the bone and contact area, appropriate tension on the abductor mechanism (10° to 15° of abduction), and stability of the fixation. The success of the reattachment is ulti-

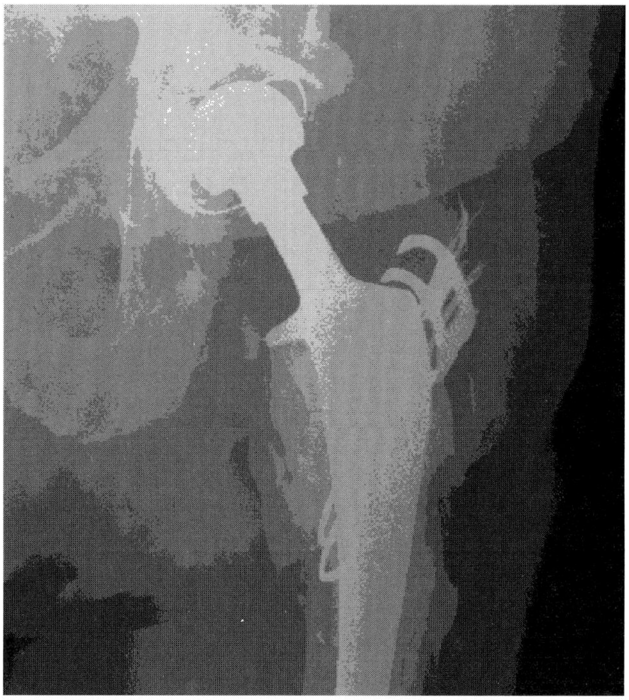

Figure 7

Chronic trochanteric nonunion following long stem cemented femoral revision surgery. The loss of host bone along the lateral aspect of the femur precludes bony union. Any type of fixation used can only serve to stabilize the hip temporarily until a pseudocapsule is formed.

mately related to the host response and the protection of the fixation. With displacement of the trochanteric nonunion greater than 2 cm, relaxation of soft-tissue structures has been implicated in an increased risk of dislocation, loosening, and stem failure.

Preoperative evaluation of proximal femoral geometry is essential. The anteroposterior (AP) radiograph must be scrutinized for trochanteric overhang. With the femoral stem template aligned within the canal, a line is drawn proximally to predict the path of femoral component insertion. If an excessive amount of trochanter is shown to overhang, one of several potential complications can occur. (1) If the trochanteric bone is not resected, the new femoral stem will be placed in varus, with or without lateral femoral perforation. (2) If too great a lateral force is placed on the trochanter during canal preparation or stem insertion, a trochanteric fracture can result. (3) The trochanteric bed may be thinned excessively in order to introduce the femoral stem, resulting in trochanteric fracture on abductor avulsion (Fig. 8).

A template of the selected implant should be placed over the AP radiograph. The presence of trochanteric overhang, as mentioned previously, should alert the surgeon to potential problems. The temptation to preserve the trochanter can result in excessive thinning of the bone or inadvertent detachment of the abductor tendon. A trochanteric slide, extended trochanteric osteotomy, or transverse femoral osteotomy should be considered in these situations. Although the concept of femoral osteotomy may seem somewhat radical, it avoids the potential pitfalls of trochanteric fracture or abductor injury and may actually be a more conservative option.

The heightened awareness of trochanteric complications has led to an increase in use of the extended (Fig. 9) and transverse (Fig. 10) femoral osteotomies, which reduce the risk of distal femoral perforation, decrease operating time, allow neutral positioning of the femoral component, and preserve trochanteric bone and abductor musculature. The incidence of nonunion is minimal, primarily as a result of the abundant soft-tissue coverage.

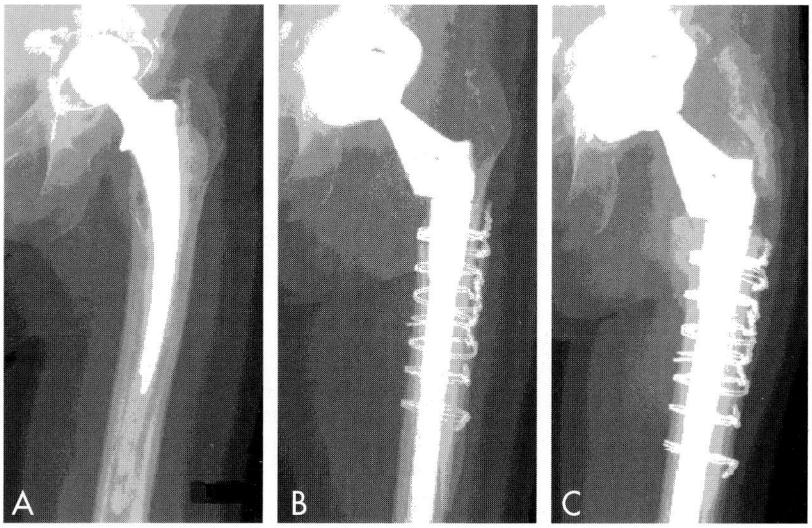

Figure 8

Femoral revision for a loose cemented prosthesis (**A** and **B**) required lateralization of the trochanter to access distal cement and to avoid varus positioning of the stem. Four months postoperatively the patient suffered a trochanteric fracture (**C**) as a result of minimal trauma.

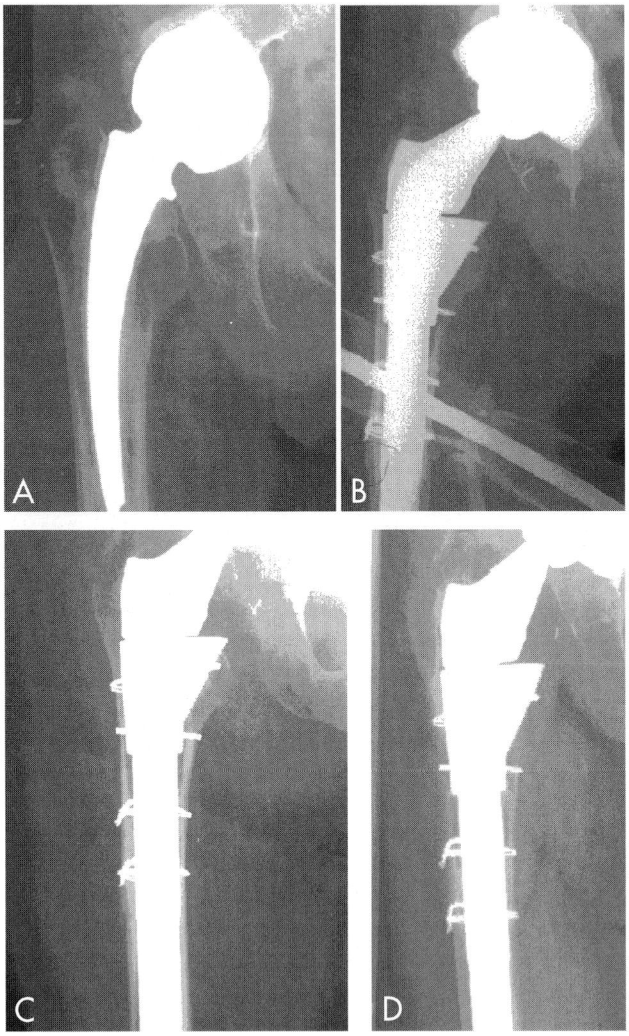

Figure 9

To facilitate cement removal (**A**), an extended trochanteric osteotomy (**B**) was performed at revision. The osteotomy did not preclude the use of a proximally modular femoral stem. The trochanter is shown at 6 weeks (**C**) and is completely healed by 3 months (**D**).

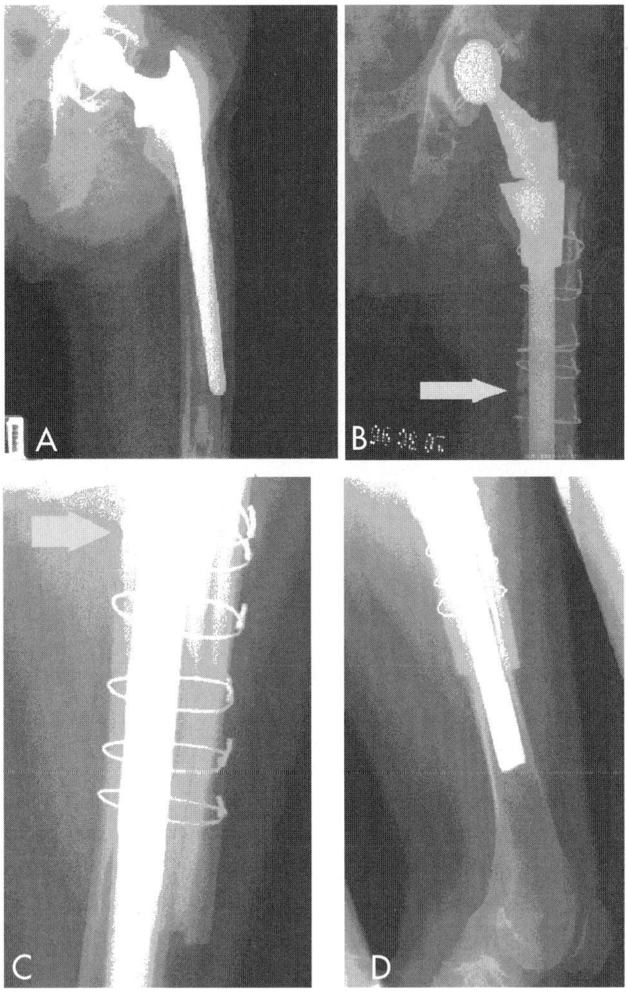

Figure 10

A varus deformity (**A**) of the femur required the use of a transverse femoral osteotomy (**B**), which is completely healed by 3 months (**C, D**).

Dislocation

The overall incidence of dislocation following THA is reported to be 3%. There is a slight predisposition to dislocation with the posterior approach versus the anterolateral and transtrochanteric approaches. The etiology of the dislocation must be identified to determine appropriate treatment. Many factors have been implicated as increasing the risk of postoperative dislocation. The presence of a shortened rotated limb postoperatively requires immediate attention (Fig. 11). Patients who have neuromuscular problems are at risk as a result of weakness and proprioceptive deficits (Fig. 12). A certain degree of patient compliance, in the absence of mental confusion, is important to ensure limb positioning. A history of previous surgery has been shown to double the incidence of postoperative dislocation. Trochanteric nonunion, as has been previously described, leads to shortening of the abductor mechanism, and relaxes the soft-tissue dynamic stabilizers about the hip (Fig. 13).

Many dislocations, however, result from technical errors at the time of surgery. Malposition (Fig. 14) of the components and impingement must be avoided. Placement of the acetabulum in greater than 25° of anteversion, any amount of retroversion, or greater than 60° of inclination in the vertical plane have been implicated in painful recurrent dislocations.

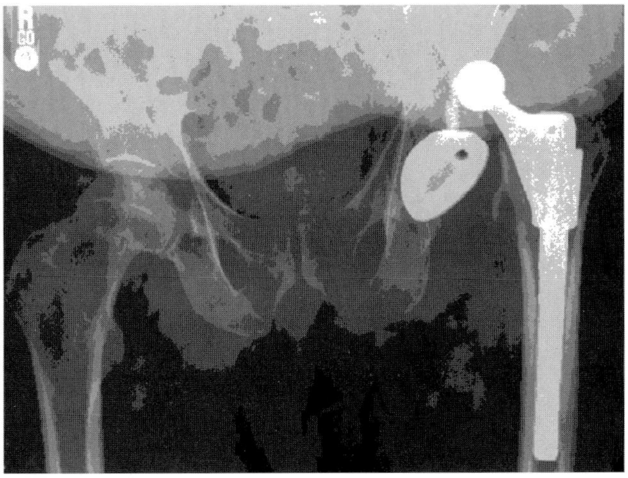

Figure 11

Dislocated hip. The profile of the lesser trochanter suggests that the hip has dislocated anteriorly.

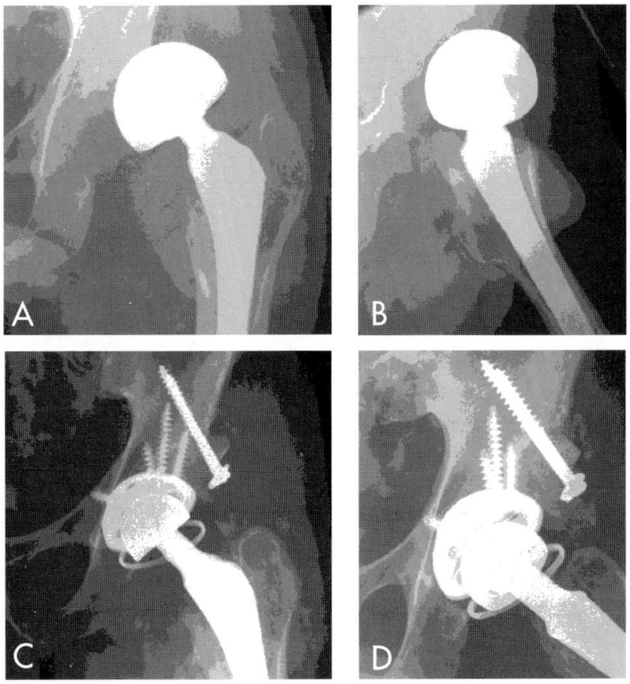

Figure 12

A 30-year-old man suffered an L3 vertebral injury with subsequent neuropathic arthropathy of the hip, for which a bipolar hemiarthroplasty was performed. The hip became unstable and remained dislocated for 6 months, allowing the bipolar component to erode the superior (**A**) and lateral (**B**) rim of the acetabulum. Reconstruction of this neuropathic hip required structural allografting with a constrained tripolar acetabular component (**C** and **D**). At the time of surgery, 70% of the acetabular component was in contact with the host bone. The patient was placed in a hip spica cast for 6 weeks following surgery and subsequently wore a brace for 3 months.

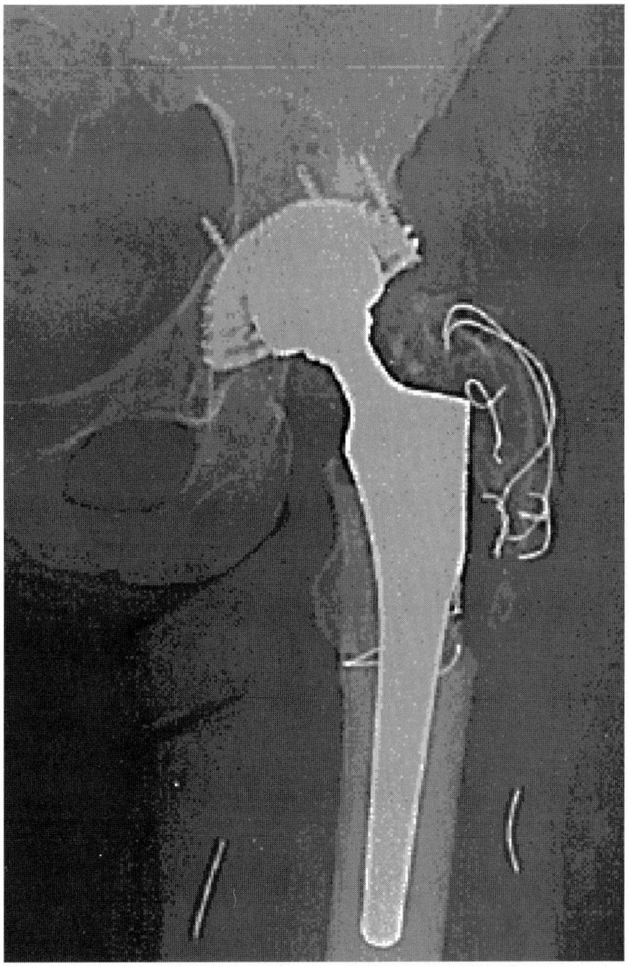

Figure 13

Chronic trochanteric nonunion in a 48-year-old woman with asymmetric polyethylene wear and zone II acetabular osteolysis.

Similarly, more than 15° of femoral anteversion can contribute to instability. A computed tomography scan may help delineate malposition of the components in the event of unexplained recurrent postoperative dislocation. Any form of impingement of the proximal femur on the pelvis, acetabular cup, or cement must be checked and corrected at the time of surgery. Osteophytes and cement masses may act as a fulcrum to lever the head out of the cup, stressing the importance of their removal to prevent impingement. Impingement of the trochanter on the pelvis must be relieved by trochanteric osteotomy and reattachment. Impingement of the femoral neck on the acetabular cup has been reduced by using chamfered cups and oval or trapezoidal necks with a larger head-to-neck diameter ratio (Fig. 15). Adherence to the postoperative regimen of restricted motion is mandatory.

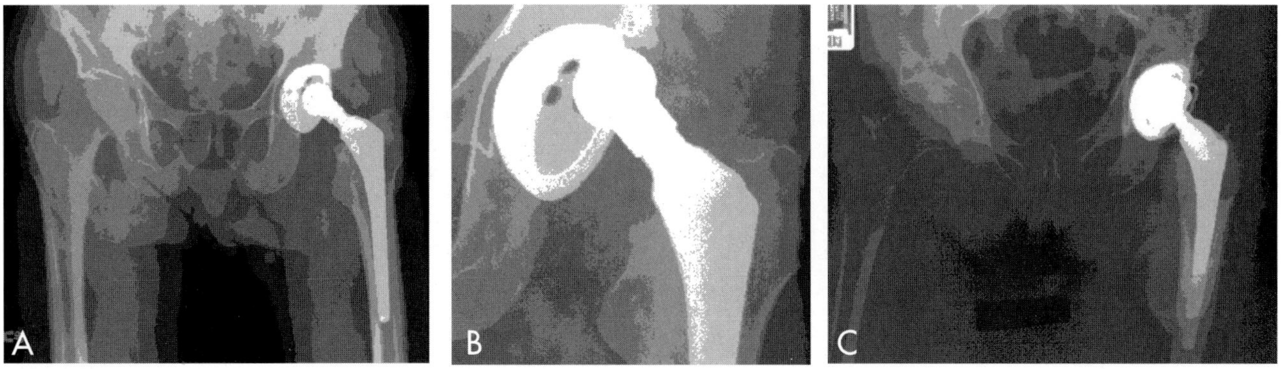

Figure 14

Excessive abuction of the acetabular component (**A**) contributed to anterior instability (**B**). Intraoperatively, a skirted 26-mm head was found to impinge on a 20° elevated liner that had been placed posteriorly. At revision (**C**), a constrained insert was used with the elevated portion of the liner positioned superiorly.

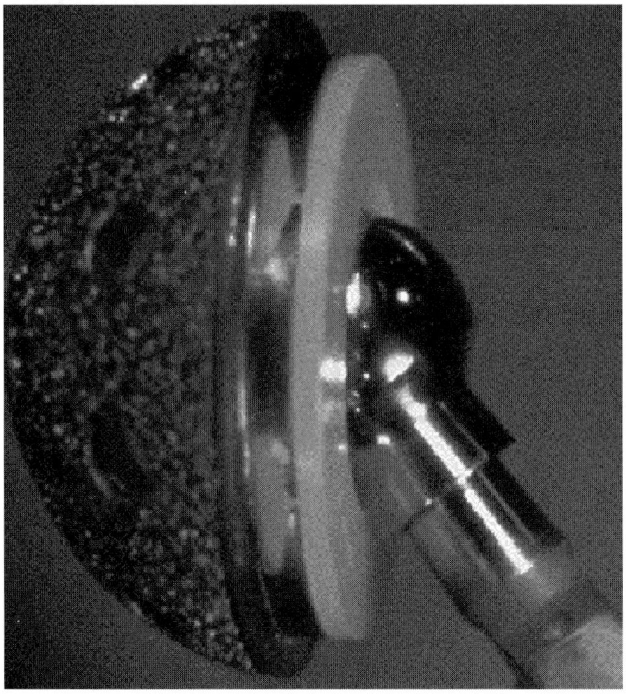

Figure 15

Impingement of the femoral head skirt upon the rim of the polyethylene liner.

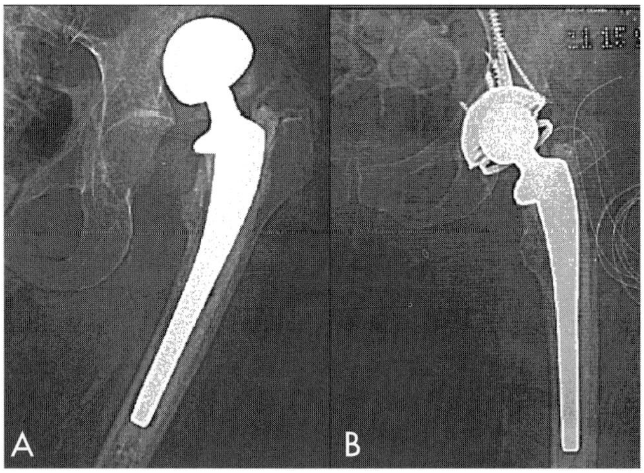

Figure 16

A 90-year-old woman sustained a femoral neck fracture treated with a cemented bipolar hemiarthroplasty which recurrently dislocated (**A**). A constrained acetabular component (**B**) was used at revision in conjunction with adductor tenotomy.

Restricted range of motion must be continued, based on the approach used, until a pseudocapsule has been allowed to form. An acute traumatic dislocation responds well to reduction followed by restriction of motion for several weeks. Recurrent painful dislocations, however, often require revision to be ultimately corrected (Fig. 16).

Stem Failure

Breakage of stems, which peaked in the 1970s, has been shown to be related to the size of the stem and the strength of the material. Deformation and fatigue fracture of the stem is a response to cyclic loading and occurs years after surgery. Modern stems made with super alloys now outlast patient life expectancy. Most early stem fractures were related to the use of stainless steel components that had inadequate cross sectional area and excessive head-stem offset (Fig. 17). In the early stainless steel femoral stems, an incomplete fatigue fracture would occur in the area of greatest tension (anterolater-

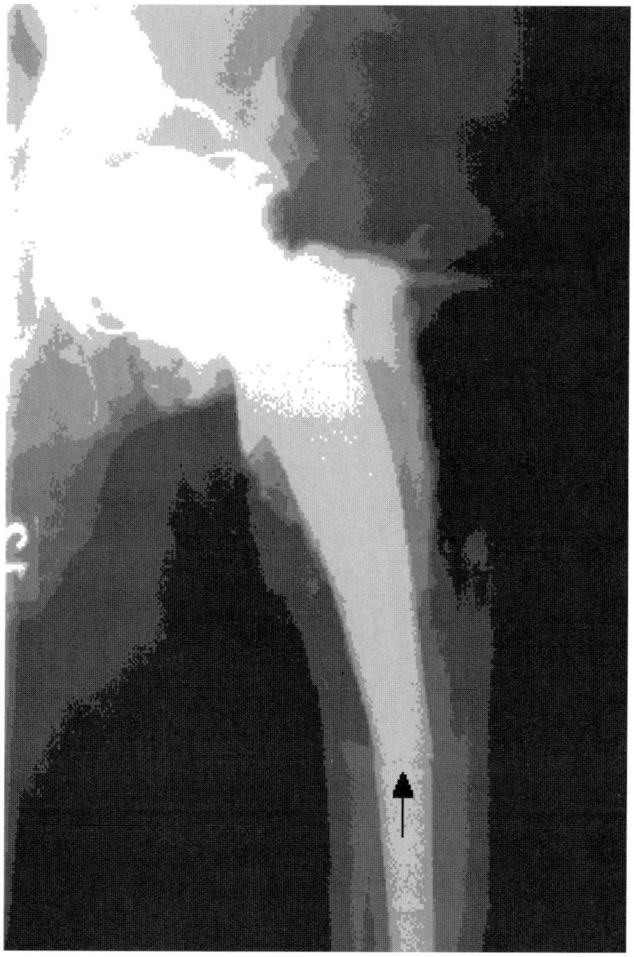

Figure 17
A fractured stainless steel femoral stem (arrow).

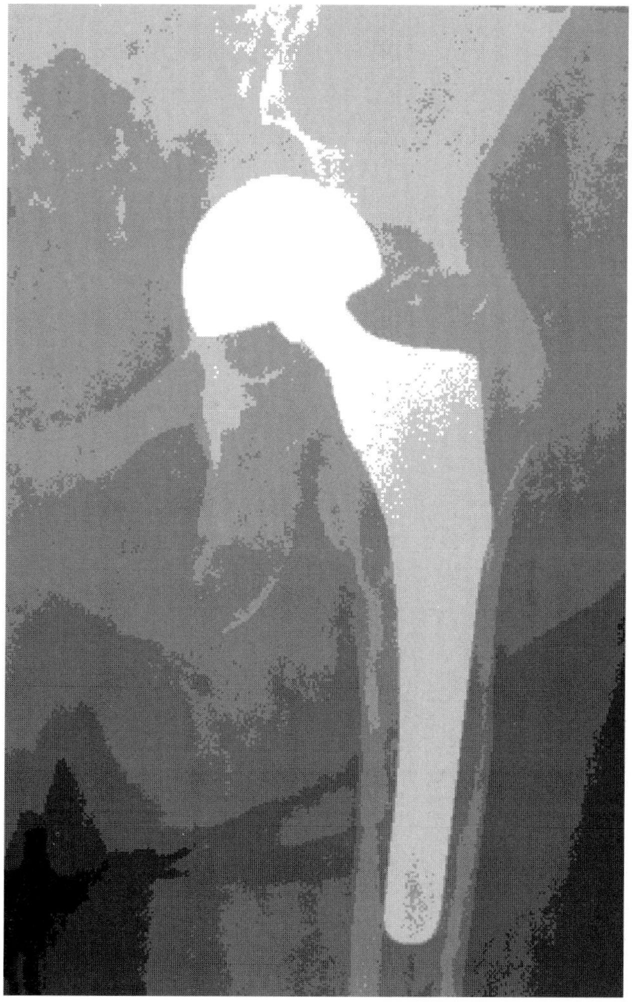

Figure 18
Intrapelvic protrusion of the acetabular component places the internal iliac artery and vein at risk for injury.

ally), and this would be followed by progression to a complete fracture. Factors that predisposed patients to femoral stem fracture in the Charnley era were inadequate strength of the metal, weight and activity of the patient, design and position of the stem, and quality of fixation. In the post-Charnley era, noncemented components in younger patients are expected to survive longer than their predecessors. The application of a porous coating, however, weakens the stem to a certain degree. With longer survival, an increased exposure to cyclic loading may challenge the strength of modern super alloys.

Nerve and Vascular Injury

Nerve palsy is certainly one of the most distressing complications of total hip replacement for both surgeon and patient. The prevalence of nerve palsy after total hip replacement has been reported to be from 0.6% to 3.7%. The incidence increases to 5.2% following the primary arthroplasty for congenital dislocation or dysplasia of the hip and 3.2% after revisions. The proposed causes for a neuropathy after total hip replacement include direct trauma, excessive tension caused by lengthening of the extremity, ischemia, intraneural hemorrhage, extrusion of methylmethacrylate or the heat of its polymerization, constriction by a trochanteric wire or suture, migration of a trochanteric wire, and dislocation of the femoral component. In most instances, neuropathy is not diagnosed until after the patient awakens. Often the cause of the neuropathy is never identified. The incidence of vascular injury is 0.2% to 0.3%. Injuries to the femoral artery and nerve have been reported, as have injuries to the obturator artery and nerve when the ligamentum teres and transverse acetabular ligament are removed from the inferior margin of the cup. In acetabular protrusio (Fig. 18), the risk of injury to the common iliac and superficial iliac vasculature may warrant a preoperative angiogram and/or venogram. The placement of acetabular screws into major intra-abdominal vascular cavities has been reported with catastrophic results. Anatomic studies have defined acetabular quadrants as being formed by drawing a line from the anterior superior iliac spine through the center of the acetabulum to the posterior fovea, forming halves. Safe and dangerous zones have been demonstrated to be adequately defined with respect to this line. The posterior-superior quadrant has been shown to be the safest area for placement of acetabular screws.

Summary

Modern hip replacement surgery has provided pain relief and improved function for many patients. These benefits must be weighed against the potential complications. Complications occur and must be identified and treated. Antiembolic and antibiotic prophylaxis has greatly reduced the incidence of thromboembolic and infectious complications. As total joint surgery enters the 21st century, the variety of complications and their management will continue to challenge surgeons.

Annotated Bibliography

Evaluation and prevention of postoperative complication, in Bono JV, McCarthy JC, Thornhill TS, Bierbaum BE, Turner RH (eds): *Revision Total Hip Arthroplasty*. New York, NY, Springer-Verlag, 1999, pp 359–464.

A comprehensive review of major postoperative complications including infection, thromboembolism, heterotopic ossification, fracture, trochanteric nonunion, dislocation, stem failure, and nerve and vascular injury.

Chapter 20
Mechanical Failure—Loosening and Wear

Loosening

Biomechanical and histologic analyses, performed postmortem on well-functioning hips with cemented femoral components, have demonstrated variable degrees of separation of the metal femoral stem from the surrounding cement mantle, so-called debonding. Debonding results from the peak torsional forces in retroversion, such as when arising from a chair and climbing stairs, with the stem shifting into a more retroverted position within the cement mantle. A component of axial subsidence may be present as well. Debonding is manifest radiographically as a lucency at the metal-cement interface, most commonly in zone 1.

The role of debonding in the clinical successes and failures of cemented femoral components involves an interplay of stem geometry, stem surface finish, and surgical technique. Debonding may not be progressive and does not necessarily lead to mechanical instability and clinical failure. Clinical and radiographic evaluation of the Charnley femoral prosthesis with a polished surface indicate nonprogressive debonding in over 30% of well-functioning hips with 20-year follow-up.

There continues to be controversy over the optimal conditions for the interface between the femoral stem and the cement mantle. Is it preferable for there to be no motion at this interface or is some limited motion preferable? How much motion can be tolerated and how is it limited? The answers to these questions involve consideration of the stem surface finish (the roughness of the metal surface) and the 3-dimensional (3-D) shape of the stem. There is experimental data indicating that a roughened metal surface can increase the strength of the bond between that surface and bone cement (polymethylmethacrylate [PMMA]). The addition of a thin layer of factory-applied PMMA (so-called precoat) to the metal surface can further increase the strength of the bond to the cement mantle.

Although there are intermediate-term reports of good results in hips reconstructed using femoral stems with a grit-blast roughened surface and precoated, such stems can still debond. Debonding can be rapidly progressive, resulting in stem-cement interface loosening and endosteal osteolysis in regions with a thin or absent cement mantle. With progressive debonding, relative motion between the roughened surface and the cement mantle fuels an abrasive wear mechanism that generates numerous small particles of metal and bone cement. Regardless of the stem surface finish, a defect in the cement mantle can allow access of joint fluid and small particles to endosteal bone with the subsequent development of osteolysis in that location. All other factors being equal, a stem with a smoother surface finish may have an advantage when there are imperfections in the cement mantle. Although there are few examples, whenever a cemented stem has been manufactured with more than 1 surface finish, in single-surgeon series better clinical results have always been associated with the smoother surface.

Wear Modes

It is important to distinguish among adhesion, abrasion, and fatigue, the fundamental wear mechanisms; the changes in the appearance (morphology) of the bearing surfaces, referred to as wear damage; and the conditions under which the prosthesis was functioning when the wear occurred, which have been termed the wear modes. Adhesion involves bonding of the surfaces when they are pressed together under load. Sufficient relative motion results in material being pulled away from one or more surfaces, usually from the weaker material. Abrasion is a mechanical process, wherein asperities on the harder surface cut and plough through the softer surface, resulting in removal of material. When local stresses exceed the fatigue strength of a material, that material then fails after a certain number of loading cycles, with release of material from the surface. One or more of the classic wear mechanisms may be operating on the prosthesis in a particular wear mode, and a prosthesis may function in several wear modes over its in vivo service life. The predominant type of wear occurring from one prosthetic joint to the next

The author or the departments with which he is affiliated have received something of value from a commercial or other party related directly or indirectly to the subject of this chapter.

can be different. Further, in a specific joint, there may be different types of wear occurring at different times during the service life. The damage on an implant is a result of all of the wear mechanisms that have acted over the service life, with the greatest influence from the most recent events.

Mode 1 wear results from the motion occurring between the 2 primary bearing surfaces, as intended, such as the prosthetic femoral head moving against the polyethylene acetabular bearing surface. Mode 2 refers to the condition of a primary bearing surface moving against a secondary surface which is not intended. An example of this wear mode would be when a femoral component penetrates through a modular polyethylene bearing and rubs against a secondary surface such as the metallic tibial base plate or acetabular shell. Mode 3 refers to the condition of the primary surfaces moving against each other, but with third-body particles interposed. In Mode 3, the contaminant particles directly abrade one or both of the primary bearing surfaces, which is known as three-body abrasion or three-body wear. The primary bearing surfaces may be transiently or permanently roughened by this interaction.

Mode 4 refers to 2 secondary (nonprimary) surfaces rubbing together. Examples of Mode 4 wear include impingement of the prosthetic femoral neck on the rim of the acetabular component; wear due to stem-cement or bone-cement interface motion or from relative motion of a porous coating, or other metallic surface, against bone; relative motion of the external surface of a modular polyethylene component against the metal support, so-called backside wear; fretting between a metallic substrate and a fixation screw; fretting and corrosion of modular taper connections as well as extra-articular sources. The particles produced may be composed of bone, PMMA, metal, metallic corrosion products, or hydroxyapatite. Wear particles produced by Mode 4 wear can induce an inflammatory reaction as well as be transported to the bearing surfaces and induce 3-body wear (Mode 3).

Mode 1 wear is a consequence of the intended motion of the joint prosthesis, whereas Modes 2, 3, and 4 are generally unintended. The operating conditions in vivo are variable and several types of wear can occur simultaneously. The clinical importance and interaction of wear modes may be clarified by a hypothetical example: (1) A well-fixed and well-functioning total hip or knee replacement prosthesis functions in Mode 1, with a low rate of wear of the polyethylene articular surface(s). (2) The gradual release of polyethylene particles to the periprosthetic tissues can result in a slow rate of interfacial bone resorption, which can result in an increase in the relative motion between the implant and the adjacent bone. Such relative motion causes Mode 4 wear that, depending on the type of joint prosthesis, can generate particles of bone, cement, metal, or hydroxyapatite. (3) These hard particles can affect the baseline Mode 1 wear by passing through the articulation, resulting in a transient 3-body wear mechanism, Mode 3. The femoral component can be scratched by this interaction. Additionally or independently, hard particles may become embedded in the polyethylene and act as an ongoing abrasive source. Increased roughness of the bearing surface of the femoral component can then increase the rate of polyethylene wear in Mode 1 as a result of increased 2-body abrasive wear. This can increase the rate of polyethylene particle production, which increases the rate of periprosthetic bone resorption leading to additional relative motion, and can eventually result in clinical failure of the implant. The time course for such a sequence of events is variable. From a practical perspective, if there is a problem with fixation, there will be a problem with wear, and vice-versa.

Friction and Frictional Torque

Friction is the resistance to movement between 2 surfaces in contact. The degree of resistance is proportional to the load. The ratio between frictional force and load (friction/load) is the coefficient of friction, μ. Frictional torque is the force created as a result of the friction of the bearing. Charnley initially selected a stainless steel on polytetrafluoroethylene bearing couple because of a low coefficient of friction. The small, 22.25-mm diameter head (subsequently referred to as simply a 22-mm head) was selected to minimize the moment arm of the frictional forces and, thus, minimize frictional torque (coefficient of friction [μ] $\times$ r^2). Thick walls of polyethylene increased the outer diameter of the Charnley socket, which distributed the frictional torque over a large fixation area.

Contrary to theoretical considerations, frictional torque has not been demonstrated to be important in the initiation of aseptic loosening of either femoral or acetabular components. Accumulating evidence indicates that wear particles have a far greater effect on the durability of implant fixation than frictional torque. From this perspective, the subsequent success of the Charnley low friction arthroplasty with a polyethylene acetabular component is primarily a function of the low volumetric wear of the 22-mm metal bearing, not low frictional torque. Larger diameter bearings can be successful if the wear rate is low. This is an important consideration because methods to substantially reduce polyethylene wear, such as extensive cross-linking of polyethylene, or the use of hard-on-hard bearings (such as ceramic-on-ceramic and metal-on-metal), are being investigated.

Countersurface Roughness

For joint prostheses with 1 polyethylene bearing surface, the other bearing surface is commonly referred to as the countersurface. The base material and the specifics of manufacturing, such as the method of polishing, determine the initial (as-manufactured) surface characteristics of a femoral head or femoral component of a total knee. The microtopography of the surface determines its roughness. A contact or noncontact (laser) stylus can be used to scan the surface and make an analog recording of the peaks and valleys over a specified length of the surface. As a result of Mode 3 wear, the original surface can be damaged in vivo, resulting in a rougher surface.

Increased femoral countersurface roughness may accelerate 2-body abrasive wear of polyethylene. Polyethylene wear is sensitive to the specific type of surface damage. Damage to the countersurface is found on the majority of retrieved femoral heads, resulting in a surface roughness that is substantially higher than the as-manufactured surface. The affected areas are usually discrete, measuring from 1 to 20 mm^2. Increased femoral head surface roughness has been associated with substantially higher in vivo polyethylene wear rates, with the magnitude of the increase dependent on the nature of the damage to the femoral countersurface. The combined effects of increased countersurface roughness and increased oxidation on wear may be synergistic rather than simply additive.

The mechanisms for generating an increased countersurface roughness in vivo apply to all materials but the susceptibility to scratching is a function of the hardness of the material. Compared to stainless steel and cobalt-based metal alloys, the decreased hardness of titanium alloy results in decreased abrasion resistance. Although the initial surface roughness of a titanium alloy femoral head may be equivalent to that of other bearing materials, there is greater potential for surface roughness to increase in vivo. In an environment with few or no hard third bodies, the wear performance of titanium alloy against polyethylene can be comparable to the other metals but the performance of titanium alloy against polyethylene is adversely affected to a greater degree by the presence of hard third bodies, such as particles of cement or metal.

Ceramics are harder than stainless steel and cobalt-based metal alloys and are therefore more resistant to damage by third-body particles than metal countersurfaces. For this reason, the increased hardness of ceramic materials is advantageous. Ceramic materials may not, however, demonstrate a significant advantage in a laboratory joint simulator where there are little or no third bodies. In clinical comparisons, however, where the operating environment of the articulation is more variable, ceramic heads have demonstrated wear rates that are lower than those of metallic heads.

Assessing Wear In Vivo

The clinical assessment of the wear of a polyethylene bearing has traditionally been based on radiographic studies. Using standard radiographs, the degree of penetration of the femoral component into the polyethylene component is considered the linear wear of the bearing. Linear wear rate is conventionally expressed as millimeters per year. A more accurate term for this measurement is linear penetration rate. With polyethylene bearings, linear wear has historically been used synonymously for linear penetration. However, linear penetration includes several factors in addition to wear, which is the removal of material from the femoral-acetabular articulation with the generation of wear particles. Linear penetration includes creep (plastic deformation) and wear. The contribution of creep to linear penetration is greatest early and decreases with time, becoming negligible by 12 to 18 months. Additionally, there is an initial running-in of the bearing that results in better conformity, lower contact stresses, and lower wear. In longer-term studies, decreasing patient activity over time will result in decreased wear, and there may also be a survival selection for the better functioning implants (those with lower wear rates). For these reasons, short-term linear penetration rates are higher than long-term rates. Modularity is another factor that can contribute to linear penetration. Because of issues related to creep, manufacturing tolerances, and the in vivo assembly of modular acetabular components, the acetabular liner may change position relative to the acetabular shell, resulting in a change in the position of the femoral head and an increase in the short-term linear penetration rate. So-called backside wear of the modular polyethylene liner could also contribute to higher linear penetration rates.

Volumetric wear is a measure of the amount of material removed from the bearing surface. The simple formula, $v = \pi r^2 w$, has commonly been used to calculate volumetric wear, in which v is the volume change in the polyethylene bearing, r is the radius of the femoral head, and w is the measured linear wear. This formula assumes a single, cylindrical wear track, but this assumption is not supported by some retrieval studies.

In this decade, computer-assisted wear measurement techniques have been developed. Standard radiographs can be digitized to create a computer model of the femoral head and acetabular component. Use of both anteroposterior and lat-

Table 1
Wear of total hips in vivo*

Study	Acetabular Bearing	Femoral Head	Diameter (mm)	Number of hips	Average linear wear rate (mm/yr)	Range linear wear rates (mm/yr)	Average volume wear rate† (range)	Comments
Charnley et al 1969	PTFE	SS	22	39	2.26		859	
Charnley and Cupic 1973	PE	SS	22	72	0.12		46	
Charnley and Halley 1975	PE	SS	22	72	0.15	0–0.6	57	
Griffith et al 1978	PE	SS	22	493	0.07	0–0.24	27	
Wroblewski 1985	PE	SS	22	21	0.21	0–0.41	80	Radiographic
				21	0.19	0–0.52	72	Direct
Wroblewski 1986	PE	SS	22	103	0.10	0–0.43	36	15 to 21-year follow-up
Ohashi et al 1989	PE	CoCr	32	13	0.04		35	
		SS	28	106	0.04		26	
		Alumina	28	187	0.03		15	
Okumura et al 1989	PE	SS	22		0.14		53	
		Alumina	28		0.08		49	
Livermore et al 1990	PE	SS	22	227	0.13	0–0.39	49	
		SS	28	98	0.08	0–0.30	49	
		CoCr	32	60	0.10	0–0.32	80	
Wroblewski et al 1992	PE	SS	22	57	0.07	0.01–0.2	27	19- to 25-year follow-up

eral projections allows construction of a 3-D model. Comparison of serial radiographs gives both the magnitude and the direction of the femoral head displacement. Such computer-assisted techniques can reduce measurement variability caused by difficulties related to single reference point identification, angle of the radiographic beam, and patient positioning. Edge-detection techniques have been developed, which infer the margins of the components by evaluating gray-scale intensity on digitized images of the radiographs. These techniques minimize the potential for intraobserver and interobserver variability and should enable accurate comparisons of results between institutions.

The amount of wear of hard-on-hard bearing surfaces, such as metal-on-metal or ceramic-on-ceramic, is typically so low that it cannot be measured on routine clinical radiographs. Computerized coordinate measuring machines have been used to quantify the amount of wear on retrieved specimens. These devices can be used to assess the sphericity of bearing surfaces by comparing the measured dimensions in multiple planes to the best-fit sphere. The volume of wear can be calculated by integrating the depth of multiple individual wear points on the worn surface.

Studies of Wear In Vivo

Several investigations that report polyethylene wear rates in total hip replacement have been summarized in Table 1. Many variables exist that influence polyethylene wear in vivo; consequently, polyethylene wear rates are highly variable. Looking not only at the average linear wear rates but also at the range of wear rates (when reported), these studies demonstrate substantial variability. Regardless of the length of follow-up, some hip replacements have no radiographical-

Table 1 *continued*
Wear of total hips in vivo*

Study	Acetabular Bearing	Femoral Head	Diameter (mm)	Number of hips	Average linear wear rate (mm/yr)	Range linear wear rates (mm/yr)	Average volume wear rate† (range)	Comments
Isaac et al 1992	PE	SS	22	87	0.21	< 0.005–0.6	80	Direct
Schmalzried et al 1992	PE	CoCr		12	0.12	0.04–0.30	36 (14–102)	Autospy
Kabo et al 1993	PE	SS	22	5	0.13		48	Direct
		CoCr	26	3	0.23		122	
			28	23	0.23		144	
		CoCr	32	9	0.21		172	
			36–54	20	0.38		314	
Cates et al 1993	PE	Ti alloy	28	99	0.08	0–0.37	49	all-poly MB
Hernandez et al 1994	PE	Ti alloy	28	97	0.14	0–0.92	86	Hybrid hips
		Ti alloy	28	134	0.22	0–1.41	135	Cementless hips
Bankston et al 1995	PE	SS	28	77	0.06		37	Patient matching
		CoCr	28	77	0.05		31	Patient matching
		Tr alloy	28	77	0.08		49	Patient matching
Callaghan et al 1995	PE	SS	22	23	0.12		46	5-year machined
		SS	22	61	0.11		42	5-year molded
		CoCr	28	20	0.14		86	5-year molded
		CoCr	28	43	0.11		68	5-year molded MB
		CoCr	28	63	0.07		43	5-year machined hybrid
		CoCr	28	43	0.11		68	7- to 8-year molded MB
		SS	22	23	0.12		46	10-year machined
		SS	22	61	0.08		30	10-year molded
		CoCr	28	20	0.12		74	10-year molded
		SS	22	23	0.11		42	15-year machined
		SS	22	61	0.09		34	15-year molded
		SS	22	23	0.10		38	20- to 22-year machined

ly measurable wear and others demonstrate wear that is several times the average for that study. These large patient-to-patient variations in wear rate have not been explained by differences in the wear resistance of the polyethylene. This is not surprising considering the number of variables that contribute to wear in vivo.

Patient-related variables include age, gender, weight, general health, and activity level as it relates to use of the hip prosthesis. Variables related to the hip reconstruction include the implanted materials (including but not limited to the polyethylene bearing material), design, and manufacturing, and variables related to the surgical implantation procedure including surgical techniques, biomechanical considerations, and the initial as well as the long-term fixation of the implants. These variables are important from a wear perspective because they can affect the loads and motions of the bearing, lubrication, and degree of 3-body wear mechanisms. Differences in the method of wear assessment and the limitations of the measurement techniques have an effect as well.

Based on theoretical models and retrieval analyses, volu-

Table 1 *continued*
Wear of total hips in vivo*

Study	Acetabular Bearing	Femoral Head	Diameter (mm)	Number of hips	Average linear wear rate (mm/yr)	Range linear wear rates (mm/yr)	Average volume wear rate† (range)	Comments
Nashed et al 1995	PE	Ti alloy		24	0.10			Cemented poly cup
		Ti alloy		62	0.13			Cememted MB cup
		Ti alloy		15	0.25			Cementless
		CoCr		74	0.17			Cementless
Bankston et al 1995	PE	CoCr	28	54	0.05		31	Compression molded
		CoCr	28	54	0.11		68	Machined bar stock
Devane et al 1995	PE	CoCr	26, 32	141	0.15			2-D computer
					0.26		79	3-D computer
Woolson and Murphy 1995	PE	CoCr	28	80	0.14	0–0.35	86	Cementless cups
Sychterz et al 1996	PE	CoCr or A1	32	26	0.07	0.02–0.18	245 (13–779)	Autopsy
Wroblewski et al 1996	XLP†	Alumina	22	19	0.06	0.024–0.32	22	Average 77-mo follow-up
				14	0.23		87	First 18 months
				14	0.04		13	Average 91 months follow-up
								> 8 years follow-up
							13	
				9	0.03			
Hop et al 1997	PE	SS, CoCr	22, 28	181	0.086		52	Cable reattachment
		SS, CoCr	22, 28	189	0.074		46	Wire reattachment
Jasty et al 1997	PE			22			35 (8–116)	Autopsy
				84			62 (8–256)	Cemented
				22			94 (12–284)	Cemented, MB

metric wear rates of polyethylene components increase with increasing head diameter. Volumetric wear increases with increasing head size because of an increase in the contact surface, and during the same gait cycle, sliding distance (the motion of the surface ball relative to the surface of the socket) increases with increasing bearing size. In clinical studies, the linear wear rates of polyethylene against 32-mm heads have been equivalent to or greater than those with smaller head diameters and have been associated with higher rates of bone resorption and component loosening. Strictly from a wear perspective, 32-mm heads have not compared favorably to smaller diameter heads. Because of their large diameters, surface replacement components have polyethylene volumetric wear rates that are 4 to 10 times higher than those of conventional total hips with 28-mm heads. It is important to recognize that if the wear rate of the bearing is sufficiently low (such as with hard-on-hard bearings and extensively cross-linked polyethylene), then larger diameter bearings may be clinically successful.

The association between volumetric wear and periprosthetic bone resorption is related to the number of polyethylene wear particles generated and released into the so-called effective joint space, which include all periprosthetic spaces and tissues in communication with joint fluid. Assuming a 28-mm diameter bearing with a conservative linear wear rate of 0.05 mm per year (a volumetric wear rate of about 30 mm^3) and wear particles equal in volume to a 0.5-μ sphere, this results in 500 billion particles. Assuming 1 million steps per

Table 1 *continued*
Wear of total hips in vivo*

Study	Acetabular Bearing	Femoral Head	Diameter (mm)	Number of hips	Average linear wear rate (mm/yr)	Range linear wear rates (mm/yr)	Average volume wear rate† (range)	Comments
Livingston et al 1997	PE	CoCr	28	50	0.12			Average age 67.2 years
	Hylamer	CoCr	28	26	0.13			Average age 66.5 years
	Hylamer	CoCr	28	138	0.29			Average age 62.8 years
	Hylamer	CoCr	28	20	0.29			Average age 47.7 years
	Hylamer	Alumina	28	7	0.33			Average age 42.6 years
Sychterz et al 1997	PE		28,32	84	0.22			Average age 54.2 years
	Hylamer		28,32	138	0.15			Average age 64.3 years
Devane et al 1997	PE	Ti alloy	28	69	0.15			2-D cemented
					0.23		99	3-D cemented
	PE	Ti alloy	28	70	0.25			2-D cementless
					0.36		155	3-D cementless
Shaver et al 1997	PE	CoCr	28	43	0.15		47	2-D short-term
					0.09		27	2-D steady state
Sychterz et al 1997	PE	CoCr	32	96	0.17	0.02–0.45	137(16–362)	2-D computer
		Alumina	32	9	0.16			

*PTFE = polytetrafluoroethylene; PE = polyethylene; XLP = cross-linked polyethylene; SS = stainless steel; CoCr = cobalt chromium alloy; Ti = titanium; Al = alumina; MB = metal backed; 2-D = 2-dimensional; 3-D = 3-dimensional.
†For radiographic studies, volumetric wear calculated from linear wear: v = pr2w

year, this translates to 500,000 particles per step. Such estimates are very sensitive to particle size. The number of particles produced by a given wear volume varies with the cube of the diameter of the particle. A single 10-μ spherical particle comprises the same volume as 8,000 0.5-μ particles. With larger particles, equal in volume to a 10-μ sphere, there would only be about 63 million particles with the same degree of volumetric wear (30 mm^3). At 1 million steps per year, this translates to only 63 wear particles per step.

Studies of wear particles retrieved from periprosthetic tissues and of worn polyethylene surfaces are consistent with an average particle size in the 0.5-μ range. Assuming constant wear particle size, increases in volumetric wear lead to increased numbers of polyethylene wear particles. From a combined mechanical and biologic perspective, optimization of in vivo wear requires not only a reduction of wear volume but a reduction in the generation of the most biologically active wear particles. A lower wear rate may not necessarily be preferred clinically if a higher number of biologically active wear particles are generated.

Clinical wear rates have traditionally been expressed using a denominator of time. This has been done as a matter of convenience, not accuracy. More appropriately, in vitro laboratory wear simulator studies have always used the number of loading cycles as a denominator. The wear of a prosthetic hip is a function of use or the number of cycles and not a function of time in situ. The assumption made in clinical studies is that the activity of joint replacement patients, the actual use or number of cycles on the bearing, is about the same from patient to patient, or that any differences will average out over a large sample size. The limitations of this assumption must be recognized.

The walking activity of 111 total joint replacement patients has been studied using an electronic digital pedometer. These patients were averaging about 0.9 million cycles for each lower extremity joint per year. The most important result, however, was not the average but the fact that there was a 45-fold difference in the range of gait cycles between the least active and the most active patient. The most active patient averaged 3.2 million cycles per year, about 3.6 times higher than average. These data indicate that individual differences in patient activity are a substantial source of variability in wear rates. A 45-fold range in wear rates and wear rates of more than 3.5 times the average wear rate can be accounted for by differences in patient activity. Age correlated with daily walking activity but with a high degree of variability (SD = 3,040 steps per day). Patients younger than age 60 years walked about 30% more on average than those 60 years or older ($p = 0.023$). Male patients walked 28% more on average than the female patients ($p = 0.037$) and males under 60 years of age walked 40% more on average than the other patients ($p = 0.011$). Thus, variation in patient activity contributes to the variability in wear rates consistently seen in in vivo studies. These data on patient activity should be considered when analyzing the results of in vivo wear studies based on time in situ.

Annotated Bibliography

Brand RA: The papers presented at the Hip Society Meeting 1998. *Clin Orthop* 1998;355:2–253.

At the open meeting of the Hip Society in 1998, 9 papers were presented that addressed various aspects of cemented fixation of femoral components. The variables discussed include the 3-dimensional geometry of the stem as well as the specific characteristics of the stem surface finish. The role of surgical technique was also recognized including variability in the preparation and insertion of bone cement and the characteristics of the resulting cement mantle, the implant-bone interface and the cement-bone interface.

Davies JP, Singer G, Harris WH: The effect of a thin coating of polymethylmethacrylate on the torsional fatigue strength of the cement-metal surface. *J Appl Biomater* 1992;3:45–49.

The interface between the femoral prosthesis and the bone cement in total hip arthroplasty is repetitively subjected to high torsional loads. This study evaluated the efficacy of a thin layer of polymethylmethacrylate (PMMA) precoating in increasing the torsional fatigue strength of the cement-metal interface. The PMMA precoating significantly and substantially increased the torsional fatigue strength of the cement-metal interface. Regardless of the presence or absence of precoat, however, failure always occurred at the metal-cement interface. Even in this laboratory test, there was extreme variability in the strength of the metal-cement interface. The performance of the specimen with the lowest fatigue strength compared to that with the highest differed by a factor of more than 3,000.

McKellop H, Campbell P, Park SH, et al: The origin of submicron polyethylene wear debris in total hip arthroplasty. *Clin Orthop* 1995;311:3–20.

In the absence of significant third-body abrasive damage, the articulation of the ball in the cup produced a visually polished surface on the polyethylene. Despite the grossly bland appearance, at high magnification the morphology of the worn polyethylene surfaces revealed features on a submicron scale that have a high morphologic and dimensional similarity to polyethylene wear particles retrieved from periprosthetic tissues.

Schmalzried TP, Callaghan JJ: Wear in total hip and knee replacements. *J Bone Joint Surg* 1999;81A:115–136.

This article addresses the multifactorial nature of wear in vivo addressing the complex interaction of the mechanical and biologic aspects of wear.

Schmalzried TP, Szuszczewicz ES, Northfield MR, et al: Quantitative assessment of walking activity after total hip or knee replacement. *J Bone Joint Surg* 1998;80A:54–59.

This article documents extreme variability in patient walking activity, which should be considered in radiographic and retrieval studies of wear.

Schulte KR, Callaghan JJ, Kelley SS, Johnston RC: The outcome of Charnley total hip arthroplasty with cement after a minimum 20 year follow-up: The results of one surgeon. *J Bone Joint Surg* 1993;75A:961–975.

At a minimum of 20 years after the implantation, 90% of 322 hips had retained the original implant until the patient died or until the most recent follow-up examination. Aseptic loosening of the acetabular component occurred in 13% of all hips and in 22% of the hips in patients who survived beyond 20 years. Aseptic loosening of the femoral component occurred in 6% of all hips and in 7% of the hips in patients who survived beyond 20 years. Radiographic evidence of a lucency at the stem-cement interface (so-called debonding) was present in 38% of well-functioning hips.

Chapter 21
Osteolysis

Periprosthetic osteolysis is the most common and important long-term complication associated with total hip replacement. The prevalence of this problem increases over time, and it can potentially limit the longevity of the reconstruction. Osteolysis was originally associated with cemented total hip arthroplasty and therefore was often referred to as "cement disease;" as a result, cementless technologies were developed. Eliminating bone cement, however, has not solved the problem of osteolysis, which has been reported both with cemented and cementless total hip arthroplasties and cobalt-chrome and titanium alloy implants. In addition, it has been reported in implant systems such as ceramic on ceramic-bearing surfaces in which there is no bone cement or polyethylene.

Although aseptic loosening and osteolysis historically have been thought of as separate processes, they are similar from a biologic standpoint. For example, the histology associated with aseptic loosening of a cemented socket appears radiographically as a linear pattern of osteolysis at the interface between cement and bone. This is similar to the histology of the expansile, focal type of osteolysis that has classically been associated with cementless implants. The differences in the radiographic patterns of bone resorption are not likely determined by the biologic response to wear debris but by issues related to access of joint fluid and wear debris to the implant bone interface and surrounding bone and particle load.

Periprosthetic bone resorption, whether linear or expansile in its radiographic appearance, is related to 3 major factors: generation of particulate debris, access of particle-laden joint fluid to the implant-bone interface or periprosthetic bone, and the biologic reaction to the implant that results in macrophage and osteoclast activation leading to bone resorption.

Production of Particulate Debris

Wear and production of particulate debris has emerged as the major problem that threatens the long-term survival of total hip replacements. There are several potential sources of wear particles in a hip reconstruction, the most common being the articulation between the femoral head and acetabular liner. Scanning electron microscopic studies have demonstrated that the majority of polyethylene wear particles in hip replacements are less than 1 mm in size. Based on the volume of polyethylene wear seen in some hip replacements and average particle size, it has been estimated that up to 500,000 particles of polyethylene can be generated with each gait cycle. Several factors are likely important in wear of polyethylene in total hip replacements. The first and perhaps most important overall is femoral head size. Laboratory and clinical studies have suggested that volumetric wear of polyethylene is proportional to the size of the femoral head. Larger femoral heads have a longer sliding distance that in turn results in greater wear. In primary surgery, 32-mm heads have been abandoned in preference for 28- or 26-mm heads, and in some cases 22-mm heads.

Finite element studies suggest that in a relatively constrained environment such as a hip articulation, polyethylene thickness is not a critical factor. However, clinical experience suggests that thin polyethylene liners have not performed well and therefore most surgeons avoid them. Implant design may also play an important role when evaluating the wear of polyethylene liners. Congruity and stability of the liner within the shell may be important and modern implant design addresses these issues to maximize both stability and congruency. Factors inherent to the polyethylene itself are also important for wear. The preparation and sterilization of polyethylene are likely critical. Oxidative degradation over time in implants that have been sterilized using gamma radiation in air is deleterious. Radiation produces free radicals that are chemically reactive sites that can react with oxygen to form ketone esters and carbolic acid groups. This chemical reaction prevents recombination and decreases the molecular weight of the material. It also decreases its tensile strength and fracture toughness. From an industrial standpoint, most if not all manufacturers have now eliminated gamma sterilization in air and have looked to other methods of sterilization. This includes the use of radiation in the absence of oxygen or alternative methods such as sterilization with ethylene oxide.

Recent efforts in terms of the manufacturing processes used to make polyethylene have focused on cross-linking the polyethylene using a variety of different techniques. Increasing the cross-linking of the polyethylene improves its wear characteristics in in vitro testing machines using hip simulators. Although promising, clinical studies will be necessary to demonstrate long-term efficacy in vivo.

The importance of counterface abrasions in terms of affecting wear is unclear. However, it makes sense to optimize the surface finish in order to minimize wear. Femoral heads are now polished to an ultrasmooth surface finish. Although it is possible for articulation surfaces to wear polish in vivo, roughening that occurs either in vivo or during implantation will likely have a deleterious effect on the performance of polyethylene. Thus, it is important for the surgeon to handle the femoral head carefully during implantation to avoid scratching.

Other factors specifically related to the patient are also likely to be important in polyethylene wear. The most relevant is likely to be the activity level of the patient. It has been demonstrated through studies using pedometers that there is a tremendous variation in the activity of patients who have had total hip replacement surgeries. Although the average number of gait cycles is approximately 1 million per year, the variation in activity in terms of gait cycles from patient to patient is 45-fold. Thus, when doing an analysis of polyethylene wear the activity of the patient must be taken into account.

Although the articulation is probably the most common source of particles, there are other potential particle generators. The second most important potential source of particles is modular junctions. Corrosion products from modular head-neck junctions have been demonstrated to occur relatively frequently. These particles can migrate into periprosthetic tissues and into the articulation itself. The most common corrosion product identified is chromium orthophosphate. This develops as a result of crevice corrosion and has been demonstrated at the head-neck junction of hip components. Histologic analysis of periprosthetic tissues have demonstrated that these particles appear to be biologically active in that they are present within macrophages and surrounded by foreign body giant cells. This material is relatively hard and if it migrates into the articulation can lead to accelerated polyethylene wear secondary to 3-body phenomenon. It is important to remember that any modular junction has the potential to be a source of particles and that potential complication must be compared with the benefits of using modularity.

Cables, which are braided wire, are another source of particles. These cables have been used to wire allografts in place and to wire trochanteric osteotomy fragments and have the potential to abrade and generate numerous metallic fragments. In general, these metal fragments are relatively large and may not be very important from a biologic standpoint. However, if they migrate into the articulation, they again may be an important source of 3-body wear accelerating the wear of the polyethylene.

The cement-bone interface is also a potential source of wear debris. When a femoral component debonds and micromotion develops between cement and metal, the cement itself may wear. Several studies have demonstrated that the fate of the debonded stem is in part likely related to the surface finish of the stem. Although smooth stems may debond at a higher rate, the potential exists for them to remain clinically asymptomatic for a longer period of time. This is likely due to the fact that a rougher stem, once debonded, will generate a higher particle load in terms of cement debris. This debris stimulates periprosthetic osteolysis, leading to clinical loosening. Once the stem is grossly debonded, studies have shown that regardless of surface finish the longevity of the implant decreases over that of nondebonded stems.

Clinical Presentation of Osteolysis

The clinical presentation of periprosthetic bone resorption is integrally related to the fixation of the components. With well-fixed components, osteolysis for the most part is an asymptomatic disease. There are exceptions to this rule. Patients who have high wear may develop synovitis and will present with groin pain. Aspiration with the injection of corticosteroids can alleviate symptoms at least in the short term in these patients. To avoid infection, a strict sterile technique must be used when introducing a needle into a hip replacement.

The patient may also present with pain related to spontaneous fracture through an osteolytic defect. This most commonly occurs in the greater or lesser trochanter. These fractures have been reported in up to 1% of patients who have had hip replacement with extensively porous-coated stems inserted without cement, with a minimum 10-year follow-up.

Access to the Implant Bone Interface and Periprosthetic Bone

The prevalence and location of osteolytic lesions following hip replacement surgery is in part dependent on the ability of particle-laden joint fluid to gain access to the implant bone interface and periprosthetic bone. The effective joint space has been defined as all periprosthetic regions that are accessible to joint fluid and wear debris. This concept is important when evaluating any given implant system. If the implant design and the typical bony remodeling pattern that occurs around a given implant are known, the effective joint space for that implant system, along with where osteolytic lesions are likely to occur, can be predicted.

During activities of daily living, fluid within the joint is subject to high pressures. This pressure distributes fluid along the path of least resistance, transporting particles from the articulation to the implant-bone interfaces and periprosthetic tissues. This concept helps in the evaluation of the radiographic patterns of osteolysis seen around total hip replacements. Examples of this concept are described below.

Cemented Versus Cementless Sockets

The difference in pattern of periprosthetic osteolysis most commonly seen with cemented and cementless sockets illustrates the concept of the effective joint space. Following cemented socket replacement, autopsy studies have shown that the subchondral plate usually reforms. This dense bone is a barrier for ingress of joint fluid and wear debris into the trabecular bone of the ilium. Thus, instead of developing expansile lysis in the ilium, a linear pattern of osteolysis develops at the cement-bone interface, leading to the radiolucency seen on clinical radiographs. Autopsy studies have also demonstrated that this radiolucency represents a soft-tissue membrane that contains macrophages with numerous intracellular polyethylene particles. In addition, there is evidence of osteoclastic bone resorption at the cement-bone interface. As bone resorption progresses around the implant, component fixation is compromised. When the radiolucency, and thus the soft-tissue membrane, is complete, the socket is loose. The prevalence of socket loosening has been directly correlated with polyethylene wear in several studies, supporting the theory that polyethylene wear debris drives this process.

In contrast, the pattern of bone remodeling after implantation of a porous-coated noncemented socket is quite different. Dense pods of ingrowth into the porous-coating are seen, rather than reformation of the entire subchondral plate. Access channels exist through noningrown areas and potentially through screw holes into the trabecular bone of the ilium. Therefore, in cementless sockets with bony ingrowth, the pattern of osteolysis is different. Instead of linear osteolysis, such as that noted with cemented sockets, expansile lytic lesions that extend into the ilium are more commonly seen with cementless porous-coated cups. These lesions, which can become large without compromising implant stability, remain asymptomatic. Loosening is late and results from acute catastrophic loss of support.

Although the radiographic appearance of these expansile lesions with cementless sockets is impressive, the amount of bone loss can be equally devastating with both patterns of osteolysis. Once the soft-tissue membrane around a cemented socket is complete and stability is compromised, the socket migrates into the radiolucency as the bone destruction progresses, usually superior and medially. Factors that must be considered when estimating the amount of bone loss that occurs with aseptic loosening of a cemented socket are the superior migration of the socket and the presence or absence of ischial lysis. When the socket has migrated more than 2 to 3 cm superiorly and ischial lysis is present, the posterior column is compromised and may be absent.

Patch Porous Coating Versus Circumferential Porous Coating

The effective joint space is also illustrated by the pattern of periprosthetic osteolysis in association with cementless femoral components that have either patch (incomplete) porous coating or circumferential porous coating. Clinical studies have clearly shown that diaphyseal osteolysis and patch porous-coated implants are linked. In contrast, with circumferential porous-coated implants, osteolysis is almost exclusively limited to the metaphyseal region of the femur. Autopsy studies have demonstrated that noncoated portions of the implants are conduits for polyethylene debris and joint fluid to gain access to the diaphyseal canal. In contrast, when bone ingrowth occurs, circumferential porous coating is a relative barrier to the ingress of wear particles. This has been further supported in animal studies.

Biology of Osteolysis

Periprosthetic tissue in osteolytic regions has been examined in detail. Wear debris is phagocytosed by macrophages. Larger particles that are nonphagocytosable are surrounded by foreign body giant cells. The normal cellular response to foreign material is to phagocytize the particles and wall them off, forming a granuloma through cell interactions between macrophages and fibroblasts. When the ability of this system to handle the particle load has reached capacity, aggressive osteolysis can occur. Activated macrophages and fibroblasts have the ability to produce significant amounts of bone-resorbing factors, including interleukin-1 (IL-1), interleukin-6 (IL-6), tumor necrosis factor-α (TNF-α), prostaglandin E_2 (PGE_2), and collagenases. In addition, wear debris may have a negative influence on osteoblast function, which in turn could lead to inhibition of bone repair. For example, titanium particles have been shown to suppress the expression of the gene that codes for collagen. In addition, the synthesis of both type I and type III collagen was decreased in cells that were exposed to titanium particles.

In general, there appears to be no significant difference in the levels of various bone resorbing factors comparing failed cemented and uncemented hip prostheses and between failed titanium and cobalt-chromium alloy components. One study did demonstrate that membranes around loosened bipolar components have been shown to produce larger amounts of PGE_2 than those around loose total hip arthroplasties. This may be related, in part, to the particle load. Bipolar hemiarthroplasties have been shown to produce large amounts of polyethylene wear debris. It is important to remember that these studies are retrospective analyses of membranes retrieved at revision surgery from failed total hip replacements. Several factors that have been shown to be critical in in vitro studies are not controlled in these retrospective histologic studies. These factors include particle load, particle size and surface area, and specific biomaterial present.

In vitro studies have shown that particle load as measured by particle concentration or number is a critical determinant of the biologic response. Important bone-resorbing factors have been shown to increase in concentration in macrophage studies when exposed to increasing amounts of biomaterials such as titanium and polyethylene. Previous work has demonstrated that concentrations of IL-1, TNF-α, and IL-6 have been shown to be higher in granulomas harvested from focal osteolytic lesions when compared with those from linear lytic lesions. Again, however, the particle load is not known. It is quite possible that the more focal lesions, which are expansile and appear radiographically more aggressive, are the result of higher particle concentration in that particular local environment. This theory is supported by the fact that the focal osteolytic defects also contain more macrophages and more ultrahigh molecular weight polyethylene debris. Thus, the particle burden may be another important factor that determines the radiographic appearance of the osteolysis. The pathologic process appears to be similar in both types of defects; however, a continuum may exist. With higher particle loads, more macrophages are seen and more bone-resorbing factors are produced. With higher particle loads the ability of the system to contain itself via fibroblast function, creating a collagen matrix to wall off the granuloma, may also be limited. Additional support for the importance of the macrophage in this process comes from in situ hybridization studies. These studies have demonstrated that IL-1 β protein is bound to both macrophages and fibroblasts; however, the messenger ribonucleic acid was detected in macrophages only.

In terms of the inflammatory potential of orthopaedic implant wear debris from commonly used materials, it appears that any biomaterial when exposed to macrophages in culture has a capacity to induce release of a variety of bone resorption factors; cobalt-chromium-aluminum alloy appears to be the most cytotoxic. Polymethylmethacrylate has been shown to inhibit DNA synthesis and appears to be more cytotoxic than polyethylene particles. Cellular toxicity is dose-dependent. The release of bone-resorbing factors in general is also dependent on partial concentration as well.

The size of the particles used in the cell culture may also influence the cellular response. In contrast to large particles, polymethylmethacrylate particles that were phagocytosable were stimulatory to macrophages, leading to the release of TNF-α. Fine particles also appeared to be more stimulatory in general than coarse particles.

The likelihood that osteolysis will develop in any given hip replacement is at this time difficult to predict. Factors that have been associated with an increased risk of developing osteolysis include young patient age, increased activity level, and a diagnosis of developmental dysplasia of the hip and osteonecrosis. It is unlikely that these specific diagnoses put patients at risk for the development of osteolysis. It is more likely that these diagnoses represent the patients who are relatively young and more active and therefore fall into another risk category. The risk of osteolysis definitely increases in proportion with polyethylene wear rates. The incidence of osteolysis has not been consistently associated with gender or weight.

Management of Osteolysis

The mainstay of management for periprosthetic osteolysis at this point in time is surgical intervention. Few data exist to indicate the optimum time to intervene. This decision depends on the fixation of the implant, patient symptoms, the degree of bone loss, and the location of the osteolytic lesion.

Revision of well-fixed cementless components with focal osteolytic lesions that occur with implant removal can result in significant damage to the remaining bone. A new treatment algorithm has been proposed for management of pelvic osteolysis and polyethylene wear in association with cementless porous-coated acetabular components. In type I, the metal shell is radiographically stable and the polyethylene liner is replaceable. For a liner to be replaceable it must meet several criteria, including commercial availability, intact metal shell and locking mechanism, satisfactory component position, and acceptable track record. In type II cases, the shell is stable both radiographically and at revision surgery; however, because of the inability to exchange the liner, the shell must be removed. Care must be taken in removing well-fixed porous-coated sockets in order to minimize damage to the remaining bone. Especially difficult is removal of the socket pressed against the medial wall. The surgeon should be prepared to suction the cup to avoid creating a major column defect or pelvic discontinuity. Following removal of the metal shell in a type II case, the defect is reconstructed based on available bone, and revision replacement is performed. In a type III case, the socket is unstable and has to be removed. Again, the reconstruction is based on the available bone.

Two- to 5-year results of revision operations of type I cases have been reported. These results support polyethylene liner exchange with debridement of lytic lesion. Two thirds of the lesions decreased in size over the follow-up period and another third completely resolved on radiographic evaluation. It is interesting to note that these results occurred regardless of whether the lesions were grafted or not. Femoral heads are downsized from 32 mm to 28 mm or 26 mm when possible.

More studies are necessary in other circumstances to delineate the best type of and time for intervention, especially when the implants are stable. It is important to remember that the majority of lytic lesions in stable components are asymptomatic, emphasizing the need for routine follow-up evaluation of patients who have undergone total hip replacement surgery. Finally, it may be possible in the future to retard the progression of these osteolytic lesions through pharmacologic intervention. A recent canine study has shown that alendronate prevents the development of osteolysis in a canine model. However, to date there are no data on the effect of bisphosphonates once osteolysis develops.

Annotated Bibliography

Besong AA, Tipper JL, Ingham E, Stone MH, Wroblewski BM, Fisher J: Quantitative comparison of wear debris from UHMW-PE that has and has not been sterilised by gamma irradiation. *J Bone Joint Surg* 1998;80B:340–344.

Age and irradiated polyethylene produce 6 times more volumetric wear and 34 times more wear particles per unit load when compared to polyethylene that is not sterilized.

Blaine TA, Pollice PF, Rosier RN, Reynolds PR, Puzas JE, O'Keefe RJ: Modulation of the production of cytokines in titanium-stimulated human peripheral blood monocytes by pharmacological agents: The role of cAMP-mediated signaling mechanisms. *J Bone Joint Surg* 1997;79A:1519–1528.

The authors use a variety of pharmacologic strategies to inhibit the release of cytokines and demonstrated that stimulation of human blood monocytes by titanium is regulated by normal signaling pathways.

Crowninshield RD, Jennings JD, Laurent ML, Maloney WJ: Cemented femoral component surface finish mechanics. *Clin Orthop* 1998;355:90–102.

The relationship between stem surface finish, band strength, and particle production is delineated.

Graeter JH, Nevins R: Early osteolysis with Hylamer acetabular liners. *J Arthroplasty* 1998;13:464–466.

The authors reviewed 78 patients with Hylamer liners at a mean 3.8 years after surgery; 11.5% of the radiographs demonstrated osteolysis greater than 1 cm^2. One patient had required a revision 4 years after surgery for severe acetabular and femoral lysis and 1 revision was pending.

Jasty M, Goetz DD, Bragdon CR, et al: Wear of polyethylene acetabular components in total hip arthroplasty: An analysis of one hundred and twenty-eight components retrieved at autopsy or revision operations. *J Bone Joint Surg* 1997;79A:349–358.

Multiregression analysis showed a significant relationship between head size and volumetric wear. Wear also correlated with failure.

Joshi RP, Eftekhar NS, McMahon DJ, Nercessian OA: Osteolysis after Charnley primary low-friction arthroplasty: A comparison of two matched paired groups. *J Bone Joint Surg* 1998;80B:585–590.

A high wear rate, component loosening and osteolysis were associated factors. Osteolysis was 3 times more common in men than women.

Kobayashi A, Freeman MA, Bonfield W, et al: Number of polyethylene particles and osteolysis in total joint replacements: A quantitative study using a tissue-digestion method. *J Bone Joint Surg* 1997;79B:844–848.

The authors concluded that the most critical factor in the pathogenesis of osteolysis is the concentration of polyethylene particles accumulated in the tissue.

Lee SH, Brennan FR, Jacobs JJ, Urban RM, Ragasa DR, Glant TT: Human monocyte/macrophage response to cobalt-chromium corrosion products and titanium particles in patients with total joint replacements. *J Orthop Res* 1997;15:40–49.

Peripheral blood monocytes from patients who had a total hip replacement produced significantly more IL-1 and PGE_2 compared to normal controls when challenged with titanium and chromium orthophosphate particles. This data suggests that the patients with the total hip replacements were sensitized to the metal particles.

Livingston BJ, Chmell MJ, Spector M, Poss R: Complications of total hip arthroplasty associated with the use of an acetabular component with a Hylamer liner. *J Bone Joint Surg* 1997;79A:1529–1538.

The authors observed radiographic signs of accelerated wear as early as 1 to 3 years after surgery. The mean wear polyethylene wear rate reported with Hylamer was 0.27 mm per year. It was also noted that the wear rate was significantly higher when mated with a femoral head made by another manufacturer compared with the wear rate when the socket was mated with a head made by the same company that made the liner.

Maloney WJ, Herzwurm P, Paprosky W, Rubash HE, Engh CA: Treatment of pelvic osteolysis associated with a stable acetabular component inserted without cement as part of a total hip replacement. *J Bone Joint Surg* 1997;79A:1628–1634.

Two- to 5-year follow-up study of polyethylene liner exchange with and without bone grafting of acetabular osteolysis with stable shells shows no failure with decrease in size of the lytic lesions in two thirds of the cases and resolution in an additional third.

Manlapaz M, Maloney WJ, Smith RL: In vitro activation of human fibroblasts by retrieved titanium alloy wear debris. *J Orthop Res* 1996;14:465–472.

This study demonstrated that fibroblasts exposed to titanium alloy wear particles become activated and release proinflammatory mediators that influence bone resorption supporting the hypothesis that the fibroblasts may play a role in particle-mediated osteolysis.

Morscher EW, Hefti A, Aebi U: Severe osteolysis after third body wear due to hydroxyapatite particles from acetabular cup coating. *J Bone Joint Surg* 1998;80B:267–272.

The authors report on 6 revisions of hydroxyapatite-coated polyethylene cups at 9 to 14 years after successful primary arthroplasty in which hydroxyapatite granules were embedded in the articulating surface of the polyethylene with abrasive wear of the cup.

Schmalzried TP, Szuszczewicz ES, Northfield MR, et al: Quantitative assessment of walking activity after total hip or knee replacement. *J Bone Joint Surg* 1998;80A:54–59.

An electronic digital predominator was used to record the number of steps taken by patients who had at least 1 total hip or knee replacement. The average was approximately 0.9 million cycles per year; however, the variation was great, differing by approximately 45-fold from the most to least active patient.

Shanbhag AS, Hasselman CT, Rubash HE: Inhibition of wear debris mediated osteolysis in a canine total hip arthroplasty model. *Clin Orthop* 1997;344:33–43.

In an animal model of osteolysis, oral bisphosphate therapy was shown to inhibit the development of wear debris mediated bone resorption.

Silverton CD, Jacobs JJ, Rosenberg AG, Kull L, Conley A, Galante JO: Complications of a cable grip system. *J Arthroplasty* 1996;11:400–404.

The authors point out the complications of multifilament cables with fraying, fragmentation, and metallic debris generation.

Wang A, Polineni VK, Stark C, Dumbleton JH: Effect of femoral head surface roughness on the wear of ultrahigh molecular weight polyethylene acetabular cups. *J Arthroplasty* 1998;13: 615–620.

The authors report that roughening of the femoral heads by an order of magnitude results in a twofold to threefold increase in wear. They also point out that the much wider clinical variation of wear cannot be fully explained by variations of surface roughness.

Yao J, Cs-Szabo G, Jacobs JJ, Kuettner KE, Glant TT: Suppression of osteoblast function by titanium particles. *J Bone Joint Surg* 1997;79A:107–112.

Phagocytosable titanium particles significantly decreased gene expression for collagen synthesis in osteoblast-like cells.

Yoon TR, Rowe SM, Jung ST, Seon KJ, Maloney WJ: Osteolysis in association with a total hip arthroplasty with ceramic bearing surfaces. *J Bone Joint Surg* 1998;80A:1459–1468.

The authors demonstrated significant acetabular and femoral osteolysis in the absence of bone cement and polyethylene. Examinations of the tissues revealed abundant ceramic particles.

Zicat B, Engh CA, Gokcen E: Patterns of osteolysis around total hip components inserted with and without cement. *J Bone Joint Surg* 1995;77A:432–439.

The patterns of osteolysis around cemented and cementless components are delineated by a retrospective review of radiographs.

Nakashima Y, Sun DH, Trindade MC, et al: Signaling pathways for tumor necrosis factor-alpha and interleukin-6 expression in human macrophages exposed to titanium-alloy particulate debris in vitro. *J Bone Joint Surg* 1999;81A:603–615.

The mechanisms of macrophase activation by titanium particles from the components of implants are discussed, and the signaling pathways involved in particle-mediated release of cytokines are identified.

Chapter 22
Results of Cemented Total Hip Replacement

Introduction

Total joint arthroplasty has been one of the major successes of human endeavor in the 20th century. In particular, the surgery of total hip replacement has held center stage in the specialized field of artificial joint reconstruction. A review of the literature on total hip arthroplasty (THA) provides an interesting perspective into the evolution of the various facets of this area of surgery. This process has consistently focused on improving the longevity of the arthroplasty, and has spanned infection, implant failure, component fixation, and bearing surfaces in isolation or in combination. Ever since the introduction of the concept of low friction arthroplasty by Sir John Charnley in the early 1960s, bone cement fixation continues to be regarded as the 'gold standard' for the evaluation of modern technology in the quest to improve the longevity of THA. This chapter will highlight the milestones of the development of cemented THA, evaluate the improvements in various facets of the procedure, and attempt to predict the future directions of research and development that seek to improve the long-term results. The results of the femoral component and acetabular component will be presented in two distinct sections in order to clarify and emphasize the relevant improvements in both components of cemented THA.

Cemented Femoral Components

Stages in Cementing Technique

As current understanding goes, there are three so-called generations in cement technique that warrant clarification. The conventional (first-generation) cementing technique involved manual digital packing of cement into an unplugged femur and acetabulum as popularized by Charnley. In addition, the femoral implants inculcated narrow medial margins and sharp edges (Muller femoral stem), varying surface roughness (Ra values) and were made of materials such as stainless steel (316L) or cast chromium-cobalt alloy, which, in combination with the stem geometry of the time, resulted in a significant risk of implant fracture. Needless to say, the results left much to be desired. Second-generation cementing techniques were then introduced and improved in the 1980s. They included plugging the femoral canal, pulsatile lavage, and cement delivery in a retrograde fashion with a cement gun. They used femoral components made of stronger forged superalloys with broad medial borders, rounded edges, and a collar. Although these improvements increased the longevity of these implants, research and development continued. The so-called 'third-generation,' or modern cementing technique has reduced the porosity of cement by centrifugation and vacuum mixing, and introduced cement pressurization devices, cement centralization devices, and femoral component surface modifications such as smooth, polished stems or precoating plus a rough surface. Although the benefits of the modern techniques still warrant critical evaluation, they may lead to further improvements and yet another generation in cement technique.

Definition of Failure and Evaluation of Results

The ambiguity in the literature with regard to the evaluation of the medium-term and long-term results of THA has been clarified in recent years. The definite evidence of cemented femoral component loosening includes (1) implant subsidence on serial radiographs, (2) change in implant position in the cement mantle, (3) progressive global radiolucency, (4) cement mantle fracture, and (5) implant fracture.

The accepted end points in survivorship studies should include revision surgery for all causes, clinical failure (painful arthroplasty), and radiographic (mechanical) failure. It is imperative that reports on the longevity of hip arthroplasty in general, and cemented hip implants in particular, should clearly mention these parameters of failure and the duration of follow-up. In this way, comparison across the various series and reports will provide surgeons with a more accurate assessment of the role of various factors in the survivorship of the various implants.

A summary of the results of first-generation cementing techniques is provided in Table 1. The long-term results focused attention on the high incidence of aseptic loosening

Table 1
Femoral stem results with first-generation cement techniques

Author (Year)	Hips (Final)	Follow-up (Years)	Revision Rate	Radiographic Loosening
McCoy (1988)	100 (40)	15.3	5%	7%
Joshi (1993)	218 (166)	16	14%	–
Neumann (1994)	241 (103)	17.6	8.3%	30%
Schulte (1993)	330 (98)	20	3%	7%
Wroblewski (1993)	1,324 (20)	20	6%	–
Kavanagh (1994)	333 (112)	20	16%	36%

of the femoral component (range 30% to 40% at 10 years) and high incidence of osteolysis (range 5% to 10% at 10 years). The process of osteolysis was erroneously attributed to bone cement (the origin of the term 'cement disease') and this led surgeons in the early 1980s to look to cementless fixation as a possible solution. However, nearly a decade of debate and the development of cementless fixation of femoral components has unearthed problems of thigh pain, concerns about the extent of porous coating of femoral stems, extensive disuse osteoporosis of the proximal femur, and an increased incidence of osteolysis on follow-up. These problems led to the development of the concepts of 'particle disease' and 'lysis without looseness' and the issue of wear; and to efforts to improve cement techniques that had already stood the test of time.

Table 2
Femoral stem results with second-generation cement techniques

Author (Year)	Hips (Final)	Follow-up (Years)	Revision Rate	Radiographic Loosening
Ranawat (1995)	236	9	2.1%	1.3%
Harris (1990)	105	11.2	1.9%	2.9%
Bourne (1998)	195	12	3%	2%
Barrack (1992)	50	12	0%	2%
Madey (1997)	356	15	1%	3%
Mulroy (1995)	162	15	2%	4.3%
Smith (1998)	161	18	5%	6%

Improvements in the results of cemented femoral components in THA with the introduction of second-generation cementing techniques are outlined in Table 2. A comparison of Tables 1 and 2 confirms a reduction in the incidence of femoral loosening by an order of magnitude (range 2% to 3% at 10 to 15 years) and in the incidence of femoral osteolysis, which in one report was as low as 0%. The results are comparable in the long-term evaluation of cemented femoral stems in patients aged 50 years or less. The new cementing techniques also improved survival of cemented revision hip arthroplasty in the medium-term. The Swedish Hip registry has confirmed the improved results in implant survival with the use of second-generation techniques.

The results of third-generation cementing techniques are even more encouraging, at least in the short- to medium-term. The few early reports are mixed as well as encouraging. The projected benefits must still be proven in long-term follow-up, but cautious optimism is not unfounded at this time. The low incidence of femoral osteolysis and superior radiographic results, when compared to cementless fixation, bodes well for cemented femoral implants in THA, especially in patients aged 60 years and older.

Failure Mechanisms

The modes of failure on cemented femoral components include pistoning of the stem or cement mantle, medial midstem pivot, calcar pivot, and bending cantilever mode. The radiographic categories of implant fixation in cementless implants have also been described. The mechanisms of failure of cemented femoral and acetabular components appear to be different. This process is mechanical in origin in the case of femoral failure, but biologic in nature in the failure of the acetabulum. Debonding at the cement-metal interface occurs initially, with an accompanying development of high peak stresses in the cement mantle. Thin cement mantles and cement mantle defects predispose the fixation to early failure. The resultant fracture of the cement mantle compromises the stability of the femoral implant. The biologic process then takes over as the particulate debris gains access to the endosteal bone. The ensuing chemomediator inflammatory response is the final common pathway that causes bone resorption, formation of a fibrous membrane, and further loosening.

Osteolysis

Bone resorption occurs around the implant as a result of the inflammatory response to the wear debris at the cement-bone interface. This process, previously referred to as 'cement disease,' prompted the research in the development of cementless implants. The persistence of osteolysis in the cementless components focused attention onto wear debris rather than cement as the cause of the osteolysis, and the term 'particulate disease' was coined. Autopsy studies as well as animal in vivo and in vitro studies have confirmed the role of chemomediators such as interleukin-1 (IL-1), tumor necrosis factor (TNF), and prostaglandin E_2 (PGE_2) as the substances responsible for bone resorption by the activated macrophages and giant cells. It may be possible that drugs directed at these mediators or at the cells that produce them might help prevent or reduce the osteolytic response.

A review of the literature provides an insight into the role of multiple factors that affect the long-term results of cemented THA. The complex interactions between the various factors and the relative role of each determine the medium-term and long-term results. The factors that play a role in the survivorship of cemented femoral implants in THA can be broadly categorized as patient factors, technique factors, design features, and material properties.

Patient factors that govern longevity of cemented femoral hip components include age of the patient, gender, body weight, activity levels, and quality of bone. The detrimental effects of male gender and body weight greater than 75 kg (165 lb) on survival of cemented femoral components have been confirmed. Patients with lower activity levels, such as older patients and patients with rheumatoid arthritis, have better longevity of cemented femoral components. Studies of Charnley THA showed better femoral stem survival in patients with dysplastic hips and rheumatoid arthritis compared to those with degenerative joint disease. The low incidence of femoral component revision or radiographic loosening in patients with rheumatoid arthritis has also been reported, although the function in this group of patients was inferior to that in patients with cemented femoral stems for other diagnoses. In patients with osteonecrosis, the Mayo Clinic experience of cemented THA has shown a significantly higher rate of mechanical failure compared to those with degenerative joint disease at a mean follow-up of 17.8 years, especially in patients younger than 50 years of age at the time of the index surgery.

A main issue of debate in the 1980s focused on the problem of young (35 to 60 years of age) patients in the context of survival of hip arthroplasty implants. This issue concerned the fixation of the femoral component with or without cement in the young patient. Although the results of first-generation cement techniques were unsatisfactory (failure rates in the range of 30% to 40%), subsequent improvements in stem design and cement techniques have improved the longevity of cemented femoral implants. A review of the long-term results of these improved techniques (second-generation) has revealed no detrimental effect of age in terms of durability of fixation (Table 3). The long-term results of cemented femoral components in patients younger than 50 years of age are essentially similar to those in the older age group (Tables 2 and 3).

The excellent long-term results of cemented femoral components in both young and older patients, as discussed earlier, have been made possible by improvements in various technical factors. The radiographic criteria for excellent cementing of femoral components have been well established. The attainment of sound cement-bone interlock is the most important factor in attaining good survivorship results in cemented femoral implants. This fact is supported by clinical correlation in the case of C2 and D cement grades. The results of A and B cement grades need to be evaluated with well-designed studies in order to substantiate the claim of improvement of the longevity of cemented femoral implants. The surgeon plays the pivotal role in achieving this interlock, and the solid primary stability of the implant determines its longevity. The various technical measures required include thorough preparation and cleaning of the bone interface using water pik lavage, a dry, cancellous bone bed using hypotensive anesthesia and dry packing, the use of a competent intramedullary plug, a gun to facilitate retrograde filling,

Table 3
Femoral stem results in younger patients (< 50 years)

Author (Year)	Hips (Final)	Follow-up (Years)	Revision Rate	Radiographic Loosening
Mulroy (1997)	47	15	2.1%	–
Joshi (1993)	218	16	14%	–
Sullivan (1994)	89	18	2.2%	6%
Callaghan (1998)	93	20 +	5%	8%

a proximal seal during cement pressurization, and the use of cement of appropriate viscosity and porosity. Although the optimal depth of cement penetration into the bony interstices is unknown, the importance of pressurization in achieving interdigitation of cement into the cancellous bone is well documented. The Swedish Hip Registry has confirmed significant improvement in implant survival with the use of each of these measures, which have a direct impact on cement pressurization and, consequently, on cement-bone macroscopic and microscopic interlock.

Centralizer

The importance of a minimum cement mantle of 1 to 2 mm has been confirmed by cement mantle finite-element analysis. This has translated into the well-known clinical association between cement mantle thickness less than 1 to 2 mm and cement fracture, osteolysis, and femoral component loosening. The concept of femoral component alignment (< 2° varus or valgus) has thus gained importance in avoiding the problem of an inadequate cement mantle. The issue of maintaining a minimum cement mantle thickness and the integrity of the cement mantle has focused surgical technique on the use of a cement centralizer. The methods available include the use of surgical expertise (free hand), proximal centralizer devices, midstem devices, distal centralizer devices, or a combination. The proximal centralizer devices have evolved from button-shaped spacers to modular ring-shaped centralizers mounted on the proximal stem immediately below the collar, which overcome the problem of femoral cavity-implant mismatch when the component is anteverted or the buttons embed into weak cancellous bone. Distal centralizers have tended to be multivaned, modular devices inserted onto the distal tip of the prosthesis. A randomized study evaluating a distal centralizer device showed that the group with centralizers had significantly improved cement mantles and neutral stem alignment. The group without centralizers tended to attain a varus stem alignment and inferior cement mantles.

In a report on the long-term performance of modular proximal and distal centralizing devices at a mean follow-up of 5.7 years, 93% of the femoral stems were implanted within 2° and 20% within 1° to 2° of neutral alignment. An adequate cement mantle was present in 92% of cases and, notably, fractures of the distal centralizer occurred in 6% of stems. These fractures were associated with misalignment of the stem and inadequacies of the cement mantle. In addition, 9% of the cases showed plastic deformation of the distal centralizer, and 7% of the cases confirmed impingement between the distal centralizer and the intramedullary plug. The evolution of centralizers continues with the development of different methods, materials, and midstem devices. The clinical sequelae of centralizer fractures are currently unknown, and the effect on medium-term results is not significant. However, the advantages of centralizer use in longer survivorship remain to be proved.

Porosity Reduction

The idea of porosity reduction in bone cement has been driven by in vitro studies on the fatigue strength of polymethylmethacrylate. These studies have demonstrated the significant benefit to the fatigue strength of bone cement with vacuum mixing and centrifugation in its preparation. Although both methods reduce pores or voids in the cement, centrifugation has been found to prevent the larger more problematic voids. Although various authors confirm the greater benefit of centrifugation compared with vacuum mixing in the short-term results, the significance of porosity reduction in vivo continues to be debatable. A report questioning the significance of porosity reduction in increasing the longevity of cemented femoral implants discussed the possibility that porosity reduction may be detrimental, because pore-free cement has a tendency to shrink during polymerization, which may compromise the implant-cement and cement-bone interfaces. The extrapolation of in vitro cement fatigue strength testing may not be suitable to the cyclical loading regimes that occur in vivo when the patient is not load bearing. These periods without load allow the bone cement to undergo the phenomenon of stress relaxation and, thus, affect its fatigue strength. The controversy of the role of pores in the prevention or development of cement cracks is another challenge to the concept of porosity reduction. In spite of extensive retrieval studies, various researchers have failed to prove conclusively that cement fractures are associated with cement pores. Another issue is the absence of evidence in the literature to show the significant difference in the revision rates with and without porosity reduction. The difficulty of performing a prospective, randomized study to evaluate the effect of porosity reduction on conventional bone cement and to compare it with high-fatigue strength cement may prevent the resolution of the controversy of the role of porosity reduction.

Another issue that has recently come to light on cement flow experiments is the accumulation of significant porosity about the distal stem with the use of the distal centralizers. The proposed hypothesis for the phenomenon is the development of voids in the wake of each fin as it traverses the cement mantle. It is proposed that the aerodynamics of the centralizer draw the pores in the proximal cement mantle into the distal regions and introduce blood and fat into the cement-stem interface. The trade-off between distal stem centralization and detrimental increased distal cement porosity warrants further evaluation.

Design Features

The design features of the cemented femoral stem have evolved with time and include issues such as modularity, offset, metallurgy, collar, and surface finish. The metallurgy of the cemented femoral stems has markedly improved from cast chromium-cobalt and cast stainless steel to present day superalloys such as forged chromium-cobalt or forged titanium alloy. It is thus possible to confirm that this development has essentially eliminated stem fracture. Developments in the design of neck diameters and stem offset ranging from 37 to 44 mm have also provided the balance between avoiding stem breakage, optimization of the biomechanics, and avoidance of impingement. The issue of optimal head diameter and modularity is more a problem of wear. Although the effects of wear have been proven to compromise the longevity of cemented femoral components, especially with the use of a larger femoral head, the focus of this chapter being fixation, this topic will not be discussed herein.

The debate of the role of a collar in cemented femoral components remains unresolved. Proponents of the fixed fulcrum concept cite the importance of a collar in cement mantle pressurization and reduction of implant micromotion and loosening. In opposition, proponents of the concept of implant subsidence, who favor collarless designs, cite difficulty to obtain and maintain calcar contact, proximal calcar stress shielding, and resorption and secondary debris generation between the collar, cement, and calcar. Both designs have provided acceptable long-term results and continue to be used.

Surface Finish/Precoat

The debate of the role of surface finish in survival of cemented femoral components also continues. The role of bone cement in femoral implant fixation is central to the conflicting perspectives. The two proposed mechanisms by which cement provides implant fixation to bone are adhesion of the implant to cement and the intrinsic stability of implant to cement geometry, which involves the concept of creep and stress relaxation of bone cement. Creep is defined as the time-dependent deformation of bone cement under a constant load. This property is attributed to the viscoelastic nature of bone cement and varies with time, environment, temperature, and changes in load. The phenomenon of creep in bone cement contributes to stress relaxation, which is defined as the change in stress with time under a constant strain (deformation). The end-result of stress relaxation is the reduction of tensile stresses, which prevents fatigue of the cement. Thus, fixation of cemented femoral components can be viewed as a result of cement-metal interface attachment or cement-metal interface motion. Needless to say, both modes have proven records in clinical settings, and femoral components with surface roughness (Ra) values ranging from 1.7 to 570 microinches (0.04 to 14.5 micrometers) have been implanted with acceptable outcomes. It is worth bearing in mind that contemporary cemented femoral components have surface roughness (Ra) values ranging from 1.7 to 170 microinches (0.04 to 4.25 micrometers).

A review of the literature has confirmed the success of the original polished Charnley prosthesis. The early 1970s saw the introduction of numerous stems in the United States with varying surface finishes. By the mid 1970s, the stems had a variety of surface roughness. This transformation of surface finish was not supported by the appropriate in vitro or in vivo studies. The importance of surface roughness was brought to the fore by the efforts of researchers who confirmed a higher rate of stem loosening with the matte surface. At about the same time, other authors reported 15-year results equal to the original Charnley prosthesis and expounded the benefit of bonding at the cement-implant interface. In addition, an increased incidence of stem loosening in rougher stems has been documented, and another study, although unable to show an increased revision rate in the rougher stems, did find significantly more femoral osteolysis in these patients.

The issue of surface roughness in improving the results of cemented femoral components has been further complicated by the debate of the role of precoating of these implants. The rationale for precoating implants is based on in vitro results of the weakness of the cement-metal interface compared with bulk cement itself. The precoating of the femoral component is designed to substantially reinforce this interface. Another fact that warrants mention is that stems with precoating require an Ra of 30 to 60 microinches (0.75 to 1.5 micrometers). The results in favor of the precoated implants are limited to a medium-term follow-up of 5 to 10 years and confirm a revision rate of less than 1%. In contrast, other reports in the literature reveal a different picture, with higher rates of failure of fixation, ranging from 5% to 7.6% within 10 years. The failures in these reports differed in that the cases in one series failed at the cement-bone interface, while those in other series failed at the cement-implant interface. In addition, most components that failed showed inadequate cement mantles.

Critical reviews of the various series, including rough stems and precoated stems, confirms that comparison between the series is complicated by the effects of different factors in varying combinations. In view of the multifactorial nature of the problem, the role of precoating in increasing the survival of cemented femoral implants can only be evaluated via a prospective randomized-blinded study with sufficient numbers and adequate follow-up to provide adequate statistical power.

In contrast to the controversy of the effect of surface finish and precoating in the context of cement-metal interface attachment, the issue of a smooth surface finish is pivotal to the concept of cement-metal interface motion as the basis of stability in cemented THA. A review of the evolution and results of the Exeter (Howmedica International, Staines, UK) cemented femoral component provides a diametrically opposite perspective of an elegant concept of cemented femoral implant stability. The concepts of a collarless double-taper geometry, polished surface finish, use of a centralizer, and the phenomenon of implant subsidence, cement creep, and stress relaxation is central to well-proven long-term results in the context of cemented femoral components. The importance of the surface finish was abundantly evident when the surface finish was changed from polished to matte in second-generation implants, with well-documented increased loosening rates. The weaknesses of these reports have been the change in the surface without a scientific basis and the absence of a prospective randomized comparative study. However, the documented long-term track record of the original design and the results of the third-generation of Exeter implants, which reverted back to the smooth polished surface finish, illustrate the point that alterations in the design of the stem may decrease rather than increase the survival of prostheses.

Conclusion

Factors that play a role in the longevity of femoral stems in THA continue to be evaluated and design improvements made to enhance the long-term survival of the implants. In order to ascertain the role of the different factors in the aseptic loosening of femoral stems in cemented and cementless THA, a critical appraisal of the short-term (5 to 8 years) and long-term (10 to 15 years) results is vital.

The short- and long-term results of femoral components in THA are influenced by a host of factors that include patient factors, design features, material factors, evaluation criteria, and duration of follow-up. Technical factors have a major bearing on the short-term and subsequent long-term results of the femoral component. These include an adequate cement mantle; avoidance of blood, marrow, and tissue fluids at the cement-implant and cement-bone interfaces; and the attainment of an ideal macroscopic and microscopic cement-bone interlock. Important patient factors include age, gender, patient weight, activity levels, and quality of the host bone. The design features that have a bearing on the longevity of femoral stems include head diameter and surface finish, torsional resistance of the stem (cross-sectional geometry of the proximal and distal stem), offset of the stem and neck length, stem surface finish, and others. Material factors, including quality of polyethylene, use of metals such as forged chromium-cobalt alloys, and cement parameters such as mantle and interlock, are coming into prominence in longer follow-up reports.

The problem of multiple factors and the relative contribution of each or a combination thereof in the loosening of femoral implants in THA is complex. Thus, it is extremely difficult to assess conclusively the role of a single factor. Only a well-controlled prospective randomized study could provide an insight into the role of a single parameter. In addition, attaining a large enough number of cases and a sufficiently long duration of follow-up (> 20 years) to provide the study with a suitable power at a defined level of significance is a major hurdle to the endeavor.

In spite of the difficulties in the accurate and reproducible evaluation of the different facets of cemented THA, the long-term results of cemented femoral stems may not be significantly improved by femoral stem surface finish and/or precoating and cement porosity reduction techniques. However, it is abundantly clear that the success of cemented femoral implants in long-term review is determined by the quality of the cement mantle, which depends on a combination of factors mainly involving implant design and cementing techniques. Hence, in order to attain the goal of a hip arthroplasty lasting the lifetime of the recipient, the direction of future research needs to focus on the issues of femoral stem centralization and improvements in the quality and reproducibility of cement techniques.

Cemented Acetabular Components

Since the pioneering efforts of John Charnley, bone cement techniques in socket fixation have undergone refinements, especially in the past decade. The critical evaluation of the various studies on cemented sockets has been clouded by ambiguity with regard to the definitions of failure. Terms such as possible, probable, and definite loosening have had varied connotations and meanings among different authors. Inconsistency in the end points for reporting clinical and radiographic failure is just as frequent. Clinical failure has been previously defined as revision of the acetabular component for any reason. The reported clinical failure rate of cement socket fixation ranges from less than 10% to 23% at 17 to 20 years follow-up (Table 4). Use of critical parameters

Table 4
Cemented acetabular component results at 17 to 20 years

Author (Year)	Prosthesis	Hips (Final)	Revision Rate	Radiographic Loosening
Wroblewski (1992)	Charnley	57	–	54%
Schulte (1993)	Charnley	98	10%	22%
Kavanagh (1994)	Charnley	69	16%	17%
Sullivan (1994)*	Charnley	89	13%	37%
Smith (1998)	CAD/Harris Design II	65	23%	26%
Callaghan (1998)	Charnley	93	19%	15%

*< 50 years of age

of radiographic failure, defined as presence of global radiolucency or migration of the acetabular component greater than 3 mm, has confirmed a radiologic failure rate of 25%. The main factor in the development of early aseptic loosening, ie, within 10 years, is failure to achieve sound micro and macro interlock at the time of surgery. Later failure involves both mechanical and biologic factors as a consequence of a histiocytic response to the wear debris.

The 10- to 15-year follow-up of THA has brought the issues of implant fixation and wear to the forefront. This chapter addresses both of these issues in the setting of the cemented all-polyethylene socket in THA.

Rationale of Socket Survival in THA

Currently available data seem to confirm that the cause of failure of the acetabular component in THA is not related to the type of fixation (cemented or cementless) but rather to the quality of the bond achieved. The host response to polyethylene wear particles is the driving force behind the mechanism that leads to aseptic loosening of the acetabular component and osteolysis around the noncemented cup in THA. The two mechanisms of aseptic loosening of the cemented acetabular component are mechanical and biologic. The biologic mechanism is believed to predominate and involves a macrophage response to polyethylene wear debris. This macrophage response leads to the resorption of trabecular bone at the bone-cement interface and the formation of a fibrous membrane. This fibrous membrane manifests as an apparent radiolucency on radiographs, confirming loosening of the acetabular components. The factors that determine the extent of bone resorption include the size, number, and type of the polyethylene particles, as well as the rate of production and the host response to these particles.

The authors propose a multifactorial causation for the failure of the acetabular component in THA. The important parameters that govern the durability of the socket include surgical technique, thickness of the polyethylene, amount of polyethylene wear (volumetric), and the host response to the wear debris. The contribution of these factors varies, although each may play a major role in the failure mechanism.

The issue of wear of the polyethylene in conventional THA has been brought to the forefront by data revealing an annual production of billions of polyethylene particles even under the circumstances of normal wear (Mode 1-undamaged head articulating against undamaged polyethylene). The production of wear particles caused by a third body wear mechanism will consequently be many times greater. It has been suggested that the histiocytic response to the polyethylene particles is unavoidable and leads to bone resorption and osteolysis at the interface. This manifests as a radiolucent line in the setting of the all-polyethylene cemented socket with type III or C fixation and osteolysis in well-fixed cemented (type I and II) and cementless sockets. It is important to draw attention to the manifestation of the bone resorption not only around the socket but also in the proximal femur. This phenomenon of reactive osteolysis around the femoral component, especially with the higher wear rates noted in noncemented sockets, has the potential to cause extensive bone loss, aseptic loosening of both components, and earlier failure in cementless THA.

At the cellular level, the proposed hypothesis for the development of osteolysis at the bone-implant interface involves the release of inflammatory mediators by the macrophages in response to wear particle debris. The chemical mediators that have been proposed to be responsible for the stimulation of the osteolytic reactions involve PGE_2, collagenases, and cytokines such as TNF and IL-1 and IL-6. These chemomediators stimulate the osteoclasts, osteoblasts, and macrophages that are finally responsible for bone resorption at the interface and the resultant bone loss and implant loosening.

The literature supports the fact that wear is greater in metal-backed acetabular components. The major contributing factors to increased wear in noncemented acetabular components are modularity, and therefore an additional bearing surface, lower polyethylene thickness, and femoral heads of larger diameters. The reported wear rates in noncemented acetabular components are 1 to 5 times greater than in cemented all-polyethylene components. However, a radiostereometric analysis (RSA) showed no significant differences in the wear rates in uncemented and cemented sockets using 22-mm diameter femoral heads followed for a minimum of 5 years. Based on the premise that the host response to the wear particles is the final common pathway in component loosening and osteolysis, it would be reasonable to assume that the problem will be more serious in noncemented sockets due to the factors mentioned previously.

Indications

The authors recommend the use of the cemented, all-polyethylene socket in THA as the implant/technique of choice for patients who are 60 years old or older, and whose life expectancy is estimated to be 15 to 20 years or less. Use of cemented, all-polyethylene socket is not advocated in the presence of extensive cyst formation or excessive bleeding, in dysplastic or rheumatoid patients, or for sockets with a reamed diameter of 48 mm or less.

Cement Technique

The implantation of a cemented, all-polyethylene socket demands a critical appraisal of the radiographs to assess the bony anatomy and architecture, the degree of acetabular dysplasia, and the presence of bone cysts. The orientation of the acetabular component is another factor that needs to be addressed during implantation. The interteardrop line is used as the reference, because it has the advantage of reproducibility and is also a true reference bony landmark at the time of surgery. The angle of desired inclination is determined by using a line at 45° to the interteardrop line, drawn from a point 1 cm lateral to the teardrop. This line, which meets the roof of the acetabulum in the anterosuperior region, is a good indicator of the amount of acetabular dysplasia present, and also provides the surgeon with a reference for socket inclination at the time of implantation.

The diameter of the implant can be more accurately templated from the lateral view of the hip, which facilitates the measurement of the crucial anteroposterior diameter of the bony acetabular socket. The use of serial standardized socket templates provides the surgeon with a fairly accurate idea of desired socket orientation and the size of the implant that is most likely to be used. The surgeon should bear in mind the possibility of varying magnifications on the lateral radiograph associated with the technical difficulties associated with attainment of a standardized view.

The major advantage of cemented THA is the attainment of immediate rigid fixation of both the acetabular and femoral components. This situation is most amenable to immediate full weightbearing status, which allows faster rehabilitation and ambulation without support. This optimal goal can be achieved with an excellent cement-bone bond. Meticulous attention to detail is necessary to achieve a rigid fixation of the implant to the bone. These details include the use of hypotensive epidural anesthesia, preparation of the acetabular bed, mixing and pressurization of the cement, and proper insertion of the acetabular component.

Factors in Initial Cement Fixation

The priorities at various stages in the implantation of an optimal cemented socket will be highlighted by the consideration of the stepwise procedure. At the outset, it is recommended that hypotensive epidural anesthesia is advisable in order to provide a well-controlled dry bed of cancellous bone. The proposed benefits include better penetration of cement into the prepared cancellous bed, thorough curettage of bone cysts, and prevention of an organized hematoma and subsequent fibrous membrane formation at the bone-cement interface, as such a membrane has the risk of allowing passage of wear debris.

The meticulous preparation of the acetabular bed is the most critical factor that is entirely surgeon-dependent. The investment of time in the development of a reproducible technique at this phase of the operation will go a long way in ensuring an excellent cement-bone interface in socket implantation. During the reaming of the acetabulum, care and attention should be paid to the provision of 80% to 100% coverage of the socket without violation of the medial wall. Serial reaming using incremental diameters of reamers should ensure a uniform cement mantle at least 2 to 5 mm thick following appropriate selection of the acetabular component. It is also the current recommendation to preserve the subchondral bone, and for this reason, reaming is performed until the cancellous 'blush' of the ischium and pubis is just visible.

The selection of the acetabular component should take into consideration the resultant polyethylene thickness. The critical thickness advocated is a minimum of 8 mm at all points of the articular surface. It stands to reason that when the outer diameter is 50 mm or less, a 22-mm femoral head would ensure adequate polyethylene thickness. In the case of an outer diameter of 50 mm to 60 mm, a femoral head of 28 or 26 mm would provide the optimal situation of adequate polyethylene, reduction in contact stresses and linear wear, and ensuring a good head-neck ratio for stability of the hip.

The issue of the macrolock is addressed by increasing the

surface area available by using a high-speed burr to create keyholes approximately 5 to 8 mm in diameter and 8 to 10 mm deep in the ischium and pubis. Multiple smaller keyholes placed in the remaining portion of the bony socket markedly facilitate the cement-bone interlock. Bone cysts, if present, are thoroughly curetted and debrided of all soft-tissue membranes, and the sclerotic walls of the cysts are burred down until cancellous bone is accessed. The final step includes a thorough lavage of the prepared bony socket, using water pick irrigation. The bed is then dried carefully with sponges and manual pressure.

The cement is mixed and allowed to stand until it has attained a doughy consistency. The wad of cement is implanted into a thoroughly dried acetabular bony socket and is pressurized into the bony interstices, using an air-filled rubber bladder, for 1 minute. This step is crucial in achieving both the macro- and microlock at the cement-bone interface. The all-polyethylene acetabular component is placed into the cement bed at 40° to 45° of lateral opening and 15° of anteversion. Minor adjustments are performed in order to attain the desired optimal position of the implanted socket, and constant pressure is maintained until the cement cures.

Results

A perspective of the long-term survival of cemented, all-polyethylene acetabular sockets can be attained by further evaluation of the cohort of 236 cemented sockets in 202 patients previously reported, implanted by the senior author between January 1978 and December 1983. We have reported clinical survivorship for all sockets to be 98% at 12 years. A recent evaluation of the clinical survivorship of this group has confirmed revision of the acetabular component in a further 3 cases, resulting in a clinical survivorship of 96.6% (confidence interval + 1%) at a mean of 15 years.

Discussion

The problems of fixation and wear of the components in total joint arthroplasty continue to plague the surgeon in the quest to increase the durability and survival of these artificial articulations. Although newer technologies are being researched, their success is tempered with unforeseen problems of their own. At the time of their introduction in the early 1980s, the proponents of noncemented devices were convinced that the elimination of cement would conclusively solve the problem of aseptic loosening. However, the test of time has confirmed the role of wear particles, the phenomenon of chemomediators and the accompanying inflammatory response resulting in bone resorption at the interface of the bone and the implant. This process manifests itself as radiolucent lines and progresses to global radiolucency and socket migration visible on radiographs in the case of cemented sockets fixation. In well-fixed cemented and cementless acetabular components, it is manifested by bone resorption and osteolysis. In addition, the detrimental factors in cementless acetabular components include a thinner polyethylene liner due to the metal acetabular shell, increased wear at the liner-cup junction, easy access of wear debris through the screw holes, and poorly designed machined polyethylene inserts. These factors compound the compromised situation especially in the early stages; when the bone-implant seal is at best tenuous and possibly vulnerable to a chemomediator attack. Unfortunately, the problem is not helped by the fact that these noncemented components are often implanted in younger, more active, and heavier patients, which further increases the volumetric wear. This fact is borne out in the alarming rate of osteolysis in the cementless acetabular components at intermediate follow-up.

The failure of the acetabular component continues to play a major role in the survivorship of THA, especially in the younger, more active, and sometimes heavier patient. Early failure of the acetabular component results from instability of the bone-implant interface. In the case of cemented sockets, this instability is caused by a poor initial microinterlock and macrointerlock at the bone-cement interface; in cementless sockets the failure of bone in-growth is paramount. Failure to achieve a sound bone-implant seal predisposes the host bone to the attack of the histiocytic response to the wear particles. It is relatively easier to attain a solid bone-implant seal in cementless sockets, and it is technically less demanding than the implantation of the optimal cemented acetabular component. In addition, the modularity of the noncemented acetabular component provides the benefit of easier exchange should revision become necessary.

Although debate continues to rage among the two proponents with regard to the fixation of the acetabular component in THA, the medium-term (10-year) results for both methods of fixation are comparable. This belief, although backed up by the literature, should be tempered by the growing concern of the alarming rates of radiographic osteolysis in the so-called well-fixed cementless acetabular components.

Direct and accurate comparison of the two methods of acetabular component implantation is flawed by variables in patient, surgeon, and implant. However, a reasonable prediction of the need for revision surgery due to failure of the acetabular component at 10 years would yield a rate in the region of 5%. Unfortunately, the extension of this prediction of the revision rates to 15 and 20 years is more likely to yield figures in the region of 15% to 25%, with osteolysis in the cementless socket constituting a definite link to failure of these components.

It is well known that prior experience continues to play a

major role in the direction that modern-day research takes. The possibility of developing new and wear-resistant polyethylene is exciting. Other alternate bearing surfaces, such as metal-on-metal or ceramic-on-ceramic articulations, may resolve the debate of socket fixation in favor of cementless acetabular components. It is not inconceivable that improved polyethylene and hard bearing surfaces have the potential to alter the wear characteristics and hence the problem of aseptic loosening of the acetabular component. The added advantage of modularity in noncemented acetabular sockets is a definite plus both in primary and revision THA. Until such time that newer, more reliable bearing surfaces are used commonly, the molded all-polyethylene socket is a good method of fixation for patients between 60 and 80 years of age.

Annotated Bibliography

Reporting Results in Total Hip Arthroplasty

Ranawat CS, Rothman RH: Editorial: All change is not progress. *J Arthroplasty* 1998;13:121–122.

This editorial emphasizes the importance of well-designed, prospective, randomized studies to evaluate the results of newly designed implants. It also stresses the need for adequate end points for survivorship analysis in terms of reoperation, clinical failure, and radiographic failure. In addition, the benefit of long-term results in the assessment of the durability of an implant warrants close scrutiny.

Factors in Longevity of Total Hip Replacement

Creighton MG, Callaghan JJ, Olejniczak JP, Johnston RC: Total hip arthroplasty with cement in patients who have rheumatoid arthritis: A minimum ten-year follow-up study. *J Bone Joint Surg* 1998;80A:1439–1446.

The 10-year results of 106 cemented total hip arthroplasties in patients with adult-onset rheumatoid arthritis confirmed an overall revision rate of 7% and revision for aseptic loosening in 2% of cases. The rate of acetabular radiographic loosening was 8% and femoral radiographic loosening was 2%. However, in this group of patients functional results were inferior when compared to cases with total hip arthroplasty for other diagnoses.

Ortiguera CJ, Pulliam IT, Cabanela ME: Total hip arthroplasty for osteonecrosis: Matched-pair analysis of 188 hips with long-term follow-up. *J Arthroplasty* 1999;14:21–28.

A matched pair study of cemented Charnley total hip arthroplasty comparing the results in osteonecrosis and degenerative joint disease at 10 years showed a comparable outcome in both groups in patients over 50 years of age, although the dislocation rate was higher in cases with osteonecrosis. Significantly higher rates of mechanical failure in patients with osteonecrosis and those younger than 50 years of age warrants caution when recommending cemented total hip arthroplasty for this group of patients.

Sochart DH, Porter ML: The long-term results of Charnley low-friction arthroplasty in young patients who have congenital dislocation, degenerative osteoarthrosis, or rheumatoid arthritis. *J Bone Joint Surg* 1997;79A:1599–1617.

The 25-year results of 226 Charnley cemented total hip arthroplasties in different patient populations with a mean age of 31.7 years showed that femoral component survival was 89% in dysplastic hips, 85% in rheumatoid arthritis, and 74% in degenerative joint disease. Acetabular component survival was highest in the patients with rheumatoid arthritis (79%) in comparison to the overall mean of 68% survival. However, patients with rheumatoid arthritis had the highest incidence of trochanteric nonunion (15%) and mortality (43%).

Cement Mantle Grades

Berger RA, Kull LR, Rosenberg AG, Galante JO: Hybrid total hip arthroplasty: 7- to 10-year results. *Clin Orthop* 1996;333:134–146.

Consecutive hybrid total hip arthroplasties (150) with a cemented precoated femoral stem and using modern cementing techniques was evaluated at a mean of 103 months. Aseptic loosening of the femoral occurred in 2 cases, both with inadequate cement mantles (C2 or D grades), 1 of which underwent revision. Two patients developed acetabular osteolysis without loosening. The probability of both components surviving 10 years was 96.9%, 98.6% for the acetabular component and 98.4% for the femoral component.

Dowd JE, Cha CW, Trakru S, Kim SY, Yang IH, Rubash HE: Failure of total hip arthroplasty with a precoated prosthesis: 4- to 11-year results. *Clin Orthop* 1998;355:123–136.

176 hybrid total hip arthoplasties using third-generation cement techniques with a mean follow-up of 6.3 years showed femoral component failure in 15% of cases, with an average time to revision of 3.9 years. None of the acetabular components failed. Poor cement mantles (C and D grades) and distal cement mantle deficiencies are significant predictors of femoral failure. The early failure developed at the cement-bone interface, while cement-metal debonding was a late development. Problems with strengthening the cement-prosthesis interface has been shown to lead to early failure of the cement-bone interface, especially in the face of poor cement mantles.

Mulroy WF, Estok DM, Harris WH: Total hip arthroplasty with use of so-called second-generation cementing techniques: A fifteen-year-average follow-up study. *J Bone Joint Surg* 1995;77A:1845–1852.

The grading system of the cement mantle in the femur has been improved with the introduction of grades C1 and C2. This report included 149 patients with 162 primary total hip arthroplasties implanted using second-generation cementing techniques and evaluated at a minimum of 14 years. Of the 90 surviving patients, the revision rate for femoral components was 2% and the rate of radiographic failure was reported as 7%. In contrast, acetabular components revealed a higher rate of loosening, with a revision rate of 10% and a radiographic loosening rate of 42%. A correlation between the prevalence of femoral component loosening and cement grade, especially C2, was statistically significant.

Cement Technique and Outcomes

Herberts P, Malchau H: How outcome studies have changed total hip arthroplasty practices in Sweden. *Clin Orthop* 1997;344: 44–60.

This article is a comprehensive review of the epidemiology of total hip replacement in Sweden, based on data available from the Hip Registry. Results were demonstrated to have improved with time, with a sequential reduction in the cumulative frequency of revision for aseptic loosening after 10 years from 8% for 1979 to 4.3% for 1985. The effects of patient-related factors, implant-related factors, and surgical/cementing techniques have been statistically analyzed, using risk ratios to provide a comprehensive review of the role of these factors in the outcomes of cemented total hip arthroplasty.

Centralizer

Berger RA, Seel MJ, Wood K, Evans R, D'Antonio J, Rubash HE: Effect of a centralizing device on cement mantle deficiencies and initial prosthetic alignment in total hip arthroplasty. *J Arthroplasty* 1997;12:434–443.

A randomized study of 60 consecutive cemented femoral components implanted with and without a distal centralizer device has confirmed the benefit of the centralizer in avoiding cement mantle deficiencies and attaining of neutral alignment of the femoral component.

Goldberg BA, al-Habbal G, Noble PC, Paravic M, Liebs TR, Tullos HS: Proximal and distal femoral centralizers in modern cemented hip arthroplasty. *Clin Orthop* 1998;349:163–173.

A retrospective review of 100 primary cemented centralized (proximal and distal devices) femoral components using third-generation cement techniques with a mean follow-up of 5.7 years confirmed no aseptic loosening and 91% satisfactory alignment and cement mantle thickness. Fracture of the distal centralizer occurred in 6% of stems with poor cement mantles and stem misalignment. The impact of centralizer fracture and deformation on aseptic loosening warrants observation.

Maltry JA, Noble PC, Kamaric E, Tullos HS: Factors influencing pressurization of the femoral canal during cemented total hip arthroplasty. *J Arthroplasty* 1995;10:492–497.

In vitro studies to determine the role of different factors in femoral cement pressurization during cemented hip arthroplasty are presented. The variations in volume of cement delivered, volume of the intramedullary canal, peak pressures generated, ability of the devices to maintain the pressure, as well as competency of intramedullary plugs, determine the depth of cement penetration into the cancellous bone of the femur.

Noble PC, Collier MB, Maltry JA, Kamaric E, Tullos HS: Pressurization and centralization enhance the quality and reproducibility of cement mantles. *Clin Orthop* 1998;355:77–89.

In vitro testing of 5 designs of intramedullary plugs in resisting migration during pressurization of the cement has shown the weakness of most available devices in larger canals greater than 12 to 14 mm with a failure rate of 6% to 7% at cement pressures in excess of 50 psi. The role of distal centralizers in the production of air bubbles around the tip of the femoral stem is demonstrated. The improvements warranted in the pressurization and centralization devices are highlighted.

Porosity of Cement

Ling RS, Lee AJ: Porosity reduction in acrylic cement is clinically irrelevant. *Clin Orthop* 1998;355:249–253.

This article evaluates the available literature on the effect of porosity reduction of bone cement on the results of primary total hip arthroplasty. The in vivo behavior of acrylic cement differs from in vitro laboratory data, and migration studies cast doubt on the effect of fatigue failure in aseptic loosening of hip implants. The benefit of porosity in cement stress relaxation is discussed and the role of porosity reduction in improving the longevity of cemented femoral components is questioned, as various other factors may play a role in the results of cemented total hip arthroplasty. The difficulties of a prospective, randomized, controlled study preclude easy resolution of the controversy.

Surface Roughness

Berger RA, Kull LR, Rosenberg AG, Galante JO: Hybrid total hip arthroplasty: 7- to 10-year results. *Clin Orthop* 1996;333: 134–146.

One hundred thirty-nine patients with 150 consecutive hybrid total hip arthroplasties using a precoated femoral component and contemporary cement technique were reported at a mean of 103 months follow-up. Aseptic loosening developed in 2 patients (1.3%), of whom 1 underwent revision surgery. Both patients had suboptimal cement mantles. The probability of implant survival at 10 years was predicted as 96.9% for both components, 98.6% for the acetabular component, and 98.4% for the femoral component in patients with hybrid total hip arthroplasty.

Callaghan JJ, Forest EE, Goetz DD, Johnston RC, Sporer SM: Total hip arthroplasty in the young adult. *Clin Orthop* 1997;344: 257–262.

This study compared the results of primary cemented total hip arthroplasties performed between 1979 and 1986 with a series of primary hybrid total hip arthroplasties performed between 1986 and 1991 in patients younger than 50 years of age. The high revision rate for aseptic loosening of the hybrid femoral components with a higher surface roughness (18%), compared to the cemented femoral components with a polished surface (5%), led the authors to modify the femoral component to a polished surface finish and a stem geometry similar to the Charnley flat back component.

Callaghan JJ, Tooma GS, Olejniczak JP, Goetz DD, Johnston RC: Primary hybrid total hip arthroplasty: An interim followup. *Clin Orthop* 1996;333:118–125.

This study reports the results of primary hybrid total hip replacement in degenerative joint disease in 131 consecutive hips (118 patients), using the uncemented Harris-Galante acetabular component and the cemented Iowa precoated femoral component. At a mean follow-up of 8 to 9 years, the revision rate of the femoral component for aseptic loosening was 6.1% and rate of radiographic loosening was 6.9%. In contrast, 0% of the acetabular components were clinically or radiographically loose.

The authors continue to recommend hybrid total hip arthroplasty using a femoral component with design modifications that include a smoother surface.

Clohisy JC, Harris WH: Primary hybrid total hip replacement, performed with insertion of the acetabular component without cement and a precoat femoral component with cement: An average ten-year follow-up study. *J Bone Joint Surg* 1999;81A: 247–255.

The results of 107 patients with 121 primary hybrid total hip arthroplasties using a precoat femoral component and comtemporary cement technique were reported at a mean follow-up of 120 months. One femoral component was revised for aseptic loosening, and there was radiographic evidence of osteolysis in the proximal femur in 7 cases and the distal femur in 5 cases. The cases with osteolysis were stable and asymptomatic. The results, based on 10 years data, have led the authors to recommend the cemented Precoat femoral stem.

Collis DK, Mohler CG: Loosening rates and bone lysis with rough finished and polished stems. *Clin Orthop* 1998;355:113–122.

This article presents the 27-year experience of cementing femoral components with varying surface roughness. Although the patient groups evaluated varied, a higher incidence of osteolysis on radiographs was seen with rough stems. The authors, however, were unable to show a higher rate of revision for aseptic loosening in femoral components with a rough surface.

Crowninshield RD, Jennings JD, Laurent ML, Maloney WJ: Cemented femoral component surface finish mechanics. *Clin Orthop* 1998;355:90–102.

The effects of surface finish on the results of cemented femoral components are evaluated based on in vitro push-out and abrasion testing. The effects of surface roughness on cement-metal interface attachment or cement-metal interface motion is discussed in relation to aseptic loosening. Also emphasized are the wide variations in the surface roughness of the different femoral implants used at the present time.

Harris WH: Hybrid total hip replacement: Rationale and intermediate clinical results. *Clin Orthop* 1996;333:155–164.

This article presents intermediate-term results (6.6 years follow-up) of 65 consecutive hybrid total hip replacements with a precoated femoral compenent, in patients with a mean age of 61 years. The revision rate of the femoral and acetabular conponents for aseptic loosening was 0%, emphasizing the intermediate term benefit of precoating.

Woolson ST, Haber DF: Primary total hip replacement with insertion of an acetabular component without cement and a femoral component with cement: Follow-up study at an average of six years. *J Bone Joint Surg* 1996;78A:698–705.

This report is a retrospective study of a consecutive group of hybrid, primary total hip arthroplasties (110 patients, 121 hips) using precoated femoral components, performed between 1985 and 1989 with a mean follow-up of 6 years. Overall, the revision rate was 5% for clinical or radiographic loosening of the femoral component, and 8% had endosteal lysis of the femur. In contrast, the revision rate for loosening of the acetabular component was 0%. The cement-bone interface was found to be the site of failure in patients with clinical or radiographic evidence of femoral loosening, especially in the presence of an inadequate cement mantle.

Acetabulum

Cement Technique

Ranawat CS, Deshmukh RG, Peters LE, Umlas ME: Prediction of the long-term durability of all-polyethylene cemented sockets. *Clin Orthop* 1995;317:89–105.

This retrospective study evaluates 236 cemented all-polyethylene acetabular components and uses a standardized scoring system to provide a correlation between the rate of aseptic loosening and the early radiographic appearance of the bone-cement interface. At a mean follow-up of 9 years, the rate of clinical failure was 0.8%, the rate of radiographic migration was 3%, and the rate of progressive global radiolucency was 3.4%. In addition, evaluation of postoperative radiographs, revealed a loosening rate of 2.2% for well-fixed sockets and a rate of 14.4% in poorly fixed sockets, confirming the predictability of survival of cemented all-polyethylene acetabular components based on the initial bone-cement interface that is achieved.

Ranawat CS, Peters LE, Umlas ME: Fixation of the acetabular component: The case for cement. *Clin Orthop* 1997;344: 207–215.

This article provides clarification of the definitions of acceptable end points in evaluating the long-term results of cemented total hip arthroplasty, especially cemented acetabular components. Volumetric wear of the all-polyethylene cemented socket is compared to metal-backed cemented and cementless sockets. The long-term failure of the acetabular component is due to mechanical and biological factors as a consequence of the histiocytic response to wear debris. The radiographic manifestation is global radiolucency when the socket is loose and osteolysis when it is well fixed either in cemented or noncemented sockets. The importance of meticulous surgical technique, organization of the surgical team and hypotensive anesthesia is emphasized as necessary for success of the cemented all-polyethylene socket, especially in patients older than 60 years of age with degenerative joint disease.

Acetabular Wear

Jasty M, Goetz DD, Bragdon CR, et al: Wear of polyethylene acetabular components in total hip arthroplasty: An analysis of one hundred and twenty-eight components retrieved at autopsy or revision operations. *J Bone Joint Surg* 1997;79A:349–358.

This study is an analysis of the wear in 128 cemented acetabular components retrieved either at autopsy or at revision surgery. The mean rate of volumetric wear, determined with a fluid-displacement method, ranged from a mean of 35 mm^3 per year in all-polyethylene sockets to 94 mm^3 per year in metal-backed components. Multivariate regression analysis showed a significant relationship between the size of the femoral head and the mean annual rate of volumetric wear, which represents a 7.5% to 10% increase in the rate of wear for every 1-mm increase in the size of the femoral head. The estimated median annual rate of wear was significantly higher in the metal-backed acetabular components.

Osteolysis in Cementless Total Hip Arthroplasty

Engh CA Jr, Culpepper WJ II, Engh CA: Long-term results of use of the anatomic medullary locking prosthesis in total hip arthroplasty. *J Bone Joint Surg* 1997;79A:177–184.

The authors report on the 10-year results in 167 patients (174 hips) with a mean age of 55 years of the anatomic medullary locking cementless hip system. The rate of survival at 12 years was 0.97 ± 0.02 (mean and standard error) for the femoral component and 0.92 ± 0.03 for the socket. There was a significantly higher rate of osteolysis and reoperation in younger patients in whom radiographic appearance of progressive wear was the common development.

Onsten I, Carlsson AS, Besjakov J: Wear in uncemented porous and cemented polyethylene sockets: A randomised, radiostereometric study. *J Bone Joint Surg* 1998;80B:345–350.

Using radiostereometric analysis the authors evaluated the wear in 95 hips at a mean of 5 years randomized for either a Harris-Galante or Charnley acetabular components and a cemented, 22-mm head monobloc Charnley stem. This is the only report showing no difference in the wear rate of cementless cups compared to cemented all-polyethylene cups at 5 years.

Classic Bibliography

Barrack RL, Mulroy RD Jr, Harris WH: Improved cementing techniques and femoral component loosening in young patients with hip arthroplasty: A 12-year radiographic review. *J Bone Joint Surg* 1992;74B:385–389.

Bartel DL, Bicknell VL, Wright TM: The effect of conformity, thickness, and material on stresses in ultra-high molecular weight components for total joint replacement. *J Bone Joint Surg* 1986; 68A:1041–1051.

Bono JV, Sanford L, Toussaint JT: Severe polyethylene wear in total hip arthroplasty: Observations from retrieved AML PLUS hip implants with an ACS polyethylene liner. *J Arthroplasty* 1994; 9:119–125.

Buechel FF, Drucker D, Jasty M, Jiranek W, Harris WH: Osteolysis around uncemented acetabular components of cobalt-chrome surface replacement hip arthroplasty. *Clin Orthop* 1994; 298:202–211.

Cooper RA, McAllister CM, Borden LS, Bauer TW: Polyethylene debris-induced osteolysis and loosening in uncemented total hip arthroplasty: A cause of late failure. *J Arthroplasty* 1992;7: 285–290.

Fowler JL, Gie GA, Lee AJ, Ling RS: Experience with the Exeter total hip replacement since 1970. *Orthop Clin North Am* 1988; 19:477–489.

Harris WH: Is it advantageous to strengthen the cement-metal interface and use a collar for cemented femoral components of total hip replacements? *Clin Orthop* 1992;285:67–72.

Hernandez JR, Keating EM, Faris PM, Meding JB, Ritter MA: Polyethylene wear in uncemented acetabular components. *J Bone Joint Surg* 1994;76B:263–266.

Jasty M, Maloney WJ, Bragdon CR, O'Connor DO, Haire T, Harris WH, : The initiation of failure in cemented femoral components of hip arthroplasties. *J Bone Joint Surg* 1991;73B: 551–558.

Ling RS: The use of a collar and precoating on cemented femoral stems is unnecessary and detrimental. *Clin Orthop* 1992;285: 73–83.

Malchau H, Herberts P, Ahnfelt L: Prognosis of total hip replacement in Sweden: Follow-up of 92,675 operations performed 1978-1990. *Acta Orthop Scand* 1993;64:497–506.

Oishi CS, Walker RH, Colwell CW Jr: The femoral component in total hip arthroplasty: Six to eight-year follow-up of one hundred consecutive patients after use of a third-generation cementing technique. *J Bone Joint Surg* 1994;76A:1130–1136.

Ranawat CS, Beaver WB, Sharrock NE, Maynard MJ, Urquhart B, Schneider R: Effect of hypotensive epidural anaesthesia on acetabular cement-bone fixation in total hip arthroplasty. *J Bone Joint Surg* 1991;73B:779–782.

Rockborn P, Olsson SS, : Loosening and bone resorption in Exeter hip arthroplasties: Review at a minimum of five years. *J Bone Joint Surg* 1993;75B:865–868.

Schmalzried TP, Kwong LM, Jasty M, et al: The mechanism of loosening of cemented acetabular components in total hip arthroplasty: Analysis of specimens retrieved at autopsy. *Clin Orthop* 1992;274:60–78.

Chapter 23

Cementless Primary Total Hip Arthroplasty

Uncemented hip implant designs were widely introduced in the 1980s, primarily in an attempt to improve the durability of total hip arthroplasty (THA) and to avoid the implant loosening and associated bone destruction seen with some cemented arthroplasties. Experience over the past decade with the at times bewildering array of different implant designs and materials used for cementless systems has demonstrated an equally wide range of success rates, failure modes, and problems. Although some failure mechanisms may be associated with a specific cementless design, other problems, such as particulate-generated osteolysis, have been revealed to be common to nearly all systems to some degree, whether cement fixed or cementless. In the face of excellent short-term pain relief with nearly all total hip designs, and variable intermediate to long-term durability, cost issues have recently been brought into sharp focus by a medical climate increasingly affected by economic concerns.

In a study of costs (rather than charges) for primary THA at a Boston medical center, actual costs between 1981 and 1990 rose 46.5%. Adjusted for inflation, this translates into a real increase of only 1.9% over that 10-year period. However, costs associated with the implant grew 212%, an inflation-adjusted real increase of 117% during the same time frame. The generally higher costs of uncemented systems has helped accentuate this trend and has resulted in some criticism based on the economics of the use of uncemented implants in certain patient subgroups, such as those on Medicare. However, in a recent study, when the lower costs of a cemented implant were added to the incremental costs of the cement, equipment for use of cement, supplies, and extra operating time needed for cemented arthroplasty, the actual expense for the hospital was slightly higher for a cemented hip replacement than for an uncemented THA. This suggests little initial economic advantage of one method over the other. It is important to bear in mind that the least expensive implant in the long run is the one that lasts the longest. In a report from the Norwegian Arthroplasty Registry, using Charnley results as a standard, the cost of the higher revision rates seen in many of the 200 largely untested implant designs used in Norway up to 1994 was calculated at $1.7 million U.S. dollars per year. The high economic and social costs associated with failure in revision surgery make a focus on long-term results even more important in the face of economic pressures.

Implant survivorship until radiographic loosening, symptomatic loosening, and revision have been used to judge durability of results for a specific device. It is also necessary to include osteolysis rates, because osteolysis, when present, is usually progressive and adversely affects long-term implant survivorship. Reported results have varied greatly for different uncemented implants and frequently show differences in durability between the socket and stem of the same implant system. Multiple design strategies have emerged out of an era marked by what has probably been too great a tolerance for a trial-and-error approach to implant validation. The often successful achievement of stable fixation of many of these implants to bone over the first decade postimplantation has been marred by increasing problems with polyethylene wear and particulate-generated osteolysis, in virtually all systems. These issues are emerging as the main concerns regarding long-term performance of these devices beyond the first decade.

Femoral Component Results

Reliable femoral fixation has been documented as attainable with a variety of cementless femoral designs in which aseptic loosening rates are under 0.5% per year over the first decade (Table 1). Some much less successful designs have also been introduced and subsequently abandoned, and a review of these results is also of interest. In other cases, second- and even third-generation versions of designs have been introduced to try to address perceived shortcomings with first-generation designs. Several features mark the variation between the femoral component designs that have been used

The author or the departments with which he is affiliated has received something of value from a commercial or other party related directly or indirectly to the subject of this chapter.

Table 1
Cementless femoral stem results

Stem*	(Design Features)	Study Location (Date)	No. of Hips	Years of Follow-up	Revision: Stem Loose	X-ray Results	Comment
AML	(Straight, Co-Cr$_1$ fully porous coated)	Alexandria, VA (1998)	507	5–14 (8.7)	1.2%	Of the unrevised-96% bone ingrown, 3.7% stable fibrous, 12.7% stem lysis, 25% stress shielding.	Originator's series; 1.4% reop for stem lysis with loose wear and lysis main concerns long-term.
		Seoul, Korea (1998)	52	11–12 (11.3)	2%	55% stem lysis	Main long-term socket wear and lysis.
APR-I	(Anatomic, titanium, proximal patch coating)	Los Angeles, CA (1997)	100	5–9.4 (6.7)	11%	41% lysis in unrevised hips. 70% progressive loss of fixation.	Oritingator's series 3% reop for lysis with stem loosening. Design abandoned.
APR-II	(Anatomic, titanium, circumferential proximal porous coating)	Los Angeles, CA (1996)	148	2–5 (3.4)	0%	0% loose	2nd generation. 1 revision for osteolysis.
Harris-Galante	(Straight, titanium mesh pads proximal)	Chicago, IL (1992)	121	3–6.2	3.3%	9% loose, 8% stable but with lysis distal	Originator's series. Design abandoned.
Identifit	(Intraoperative custom made smooth titanium implant with longitudinal grooves)	Columbus, OH (1995)	74	1–3.8 (2.6)	23%	Another 5% failed clinically and subsided = 28%. Mechanical failure mean subsidence for series = 0.6 mm (range 0–2.3 cm)	High failure rate despite 100% ave fill of proximal femur and >90% fill distally. Design abandoned.
Mallory-Head	(Straight, titanium, tapered, proximal plasma spray coating, roughened midstem)	Columbus, OH (1996)	177	0.6–8.5 (6.3)	3%	2% lucencies over 2 mm (incomplete)	Originator's series.

over the past 15 years. These include material used for fabrication of the implant, shape of the stem, distal extent of the porous coating or surface treatment, circumferential extent of implant coating (whether circumferential or discontinuous patch type coating), type of implant coating, and the use of modular versus nonmodular implants. All of these various design characteristics can potentially affect results and must be borne in mind when interpreting the results as stated in specific clinical reports on a particular device.

Implant Material

Successful results over the first decade have been reported using implants fabricated from both cobalt chromium and titanium. However, theoretical advantages that exist for implants with a lower modulus of elasticity with regard to potential stress shielding of bone would seem to favor use of titanium. Finite element studies showing as much as a twofold reduction in proximal femoral loading after bone ingrowth with an extensively porous-coated chromium-cobalt stem point to the potential for major bone remodeling. Recent studies regarding the stress shielding of bone around hip implants have shown reductions of 9% to 34% in bone density, as measured by dual energy x-ray absorptiometry (DEXA), in the proximal femur of patients with extensively coated chromium-cobalt stems. These remodeling changes, documented in sequential studies during the initial

Table 1 continued
Cementless femoral stem results

Stem*	(Design Features)	Study Location (Date)	No. of Hips	Years of Follow-up	Revision: Stem Loose	X-ray Results	Comment
Omniflex	(Straight, titanium, porous pads)	Indianapolis, IN (1994)	88	2–5.2 (3.5)	3.4%	7% loose and unrevised. 6.5% lysis	Total mechanical failure rate = 12%. Design abandoned.
Omnifit-HA	(Straight, titanium, proximal HA coated)	Multicenter (1998)	316	5.6–9.9 (8.1)	0.3%	0% loose, unrevised, 28% proximal lysis, no distal lysis.	Lysis in zones 1, 7, 8, 14 proximally the only cancer
PCA	(Anatomic, CoCr, proximal bead porous coated)	Multicenter Swedish (1997)	539	(6–8)	7.6% (loose and lysis)	22.1% subsided, 9.6% femoral lysis	Rapid progression of lysis between 3–7 years follow-up.
		Washington, DC (1995)	100	Minimum 7	2.0%	5% unstable, 13% femoral lysis	33% of femoral lesions progressed
S-ROM	(Straight, modular titanium, proximal porous, distal fluted)	Toronto, Canada (1993)	48	3–6	0%	0% loose, 1 incomplete proximal lucency	No modularity related problems noted.
Taperloc	(Straight, titanium, tapered proximal plasma spray)	Neenah, WI (1997)	145	8–12.5 (10)	0.7%	3% unstable, 3% stable fibrous, 6% femoral lysis	Main long-term issue: wear and lysis.
Trilock	(Straight, CoCr, wedge fit, tapered, 60% proximal sintered head coating)	Philadelphia, PA (1999)	71	Minimum 10 (11.5)	0%	5% loose, 3.2% lysis, all proximal	No lysis distal to lesser trochanter.

* AML, Trilock (DePuy, Warsaw, IN); APR-I, APR-II (Intermedics, Austin, TX); Harris-Galante (Zimmer, Warsaw, IN); Identifit (Thackery, Leads, England): Mallory-Head, Taperlock (Biomet, Warsaw, IN); Omniflex, Omnifit (Osteonics, Allendale, NJ); PCA (Howmedica, Rutherford, NJ); S-ROM (Joint Medical Products, Johnson & Johnson, Raynham, MA)

months following operation, stabilized by 1 year postsurgery and remain unchanged thereafter. Even higher reductions have been seen on DEXA in proximal femoral bone density for large-diameter cemented stems, with the least reductions observed seen in proximally porous-coated stems coupled with a horizontal collar designed to load the medial calcar region. These measured changes must be interpreted with some caution because ipsilateral disuse changes have been documented to occur in the entire limb. A recent study demonstrated proximal tibial and distal femoral bone loss of 15% to 16% following hip arthroplasty in the same limb, with changes around the hip of 34% suggesting an overriding disuse effect separate from those produced by the implant in many of the studies previously cited. Clinical success rates for relatively long, stiff chromium-cobalt, chrome extensively porous implants, such as the AML (DePuy, Warsaw, IN), rival or, in many cases, exceed those reported over the first decade with smaller more flexible titanium implants. Thus, it is not possible to show a clear advantage of lower modulus titanium implants over chromium-cobalt stems on the basis of available clinical series (Table 1).

Implant Shape

In general, implant designs have consisted of straight stems, with varying degrees of proximal to distal tapering on the anterior-posterior and medial-lateral projection, or have involved curved or anatomic implants, which attempt to match the intramedullary anatomy of the proximal femur. Despite significant past efforts at achieving accurate fit and fill of the proximal femur, the availability of anatomic implant designs has not proven to be a great advantage, and a number of very successful nonanatomic straight-stemmed implants that rely on varying degrees of machining and preparation of the proximal femur are available. Although satisfactory intermediate-term results have been reported with some anatomic implant designs, these have tended to be second-generation versions of the original implant on which they were based. Examples include the APR I versus APR II (Intermedics, Austin, TX) and original PCA stem versus more recent PCA E series (Howmedica, Rutherford, NJ), in which improved results have been reported. Several straight, highly tapered implants, which depend on proximal fixation and purposely avoid medullary fixation, have proven to be highly successful at up to 10 years postimplantation. These results have been seen for implants manufactured from chromium-cobalt and titanium, as demonstrated by the reported series for the Mallory head (Biomet, Warsaw, IN), Taperloc (Biomet, Warsaw, IN), and Trilock-lock (DePuy, Warsaw, IN) examples (Table 1).

Extent of Porous Coating

Surface treatments and porous coatings have been applied at all levels along the length of various implants from very proximal limited areas of porous coating to devices with extensive coating along the entire length of the implant. Extensive experience with the fully porous-coated chromium-cobalt AML implant has documented the highly reliable long-term fixation achievable with this approach, which relies on a scratch-fit interface with the diaphysis of the upper femur and intentionally facilitates distal fixation and load transfer past the proximal metaphyseal portion of the bone. It is important to note that with achievement of stable long-term fixation of the device, major clinical issues with the long-term performance of this implant relate to polyethylene wear and osteolysis. Some degree of stem lysis was seen in 12.7% of implants in one series at a mean of 8.7 years. Despite radiographic evidence of stress shielding in a quarter of these hips, no clinically evident problems have been reported from these changes at up to 14 years post-implantation. Equivalent results have been achieved with some proximally porous-coated implants of both titanium and chromium-cobalt, so long as the porous coating or surface treatment has been applied circumferentially (see Table 1).

Circumferential Versus Noncircumferential Porous Coating

This is an example of one design parameter that appears to be of critical importance with regard to long-term durability of fixation achieved and the extent of osteolysis observed in response to polyethylene wear. In the series recently reported and summarized in Table 1, 3 implant designs have experienced unacceptably high rates of stem loosening and periprosthetic osteolysis: the APR I, the Harris-Galante (Zimmer, Warsaw, IN), and the Omniflex (Osteonics, Allendale, NJ). Each of these implants is a noncircumferentially porous-coated device. The anatomic-shaped, titanium, proximally patch porous-coated APR I was marked by an 11% stem loosening rate, a 41% periprosthetic osteolysis rate, and a 3% reoperation rate for osteolysis about well-fixed femoral components after a mean of 6.7 years. Similarly, the straight-stem titanium Harris-Galante implant with wire mesh pads and smooth gaps between the porous pad portions proximally demonstrated a 9% rate of loosening, a 3.3% rate of revision for stem loosening, and an 8% incidence of significant lysis around stable stems at only 3 to 6.2 years follow-up. Similar observations with the Omniflex implant with titanium pads proximally help highlight the adverse effects of facilitated polyethylene particulate transport along nonporous, smooth portions of uncemented femoral components even when solid bone ingrowth to the porous-coated portions has occurred elsewhere on these devices.

Type of Coating

A review of recent reports of intermediate to long-term results reveals the successful use of a variety of surfaces for facilitation of bone attachment. The type of metal used for the stem influences the available options, with sintered beads frequently being employed in chromium-cobalt stems, such as the PCA or Trilock-lock, and plasma spray methods and wire mesh employed in titanium stems, such as the Mallory head, Taperloc, and Harris-Galante designs. Hydroxyapatite (HA) coating has been used with smooth or roughened stem substrates, and also as an overlay in combination with various porous surfaces. Available results suggest that all of these strategies can prove successful in providing for bone attachment and secure long-term fixation. Some experimental animal studies have shown increased strength of attachment when HA coatings are used, and radiographic studies have suggested improved attachment and loading to the proximal femur in HA stems. However, limited clinical data support preferential use of any one particular porous material or surface treatment. Exceptional results have been reported with an HA coating over the proximal portion of a smooth titanium stem at up to 10 years in a multicenter study of the Omnifit implant (Osteonics, Allendale, NJ), in which only one case of loosening was seen out of 316 hips. However, a separate study that compared a proximally porous anatomic design used with and without an HA coating showed no demonstrable benefit with regard to fixation or clinical results imparted by the HA. Available results do suggest that theoretical concerns about resorption of the HA coating, loss of fixation, and facilitation of wear of the joint by third-body particulate from the coating itself have proved groundless, at least over the first decade following implantation of such devices. Thus, available studies provide little in the way of clinical data to strongly support preferential use of one particular material or porous coating over any other, and they suggest that other design factors may be more important in explaining observed differences.

Modularity

Modular heads, available for virtually all designs mentioned, have become a routine aspect of femoral component manufacture. In addition, modular tips for some uncemented designs, such as the Omniflex, and modular body portions for implants, such as the S-ROM (Joint Medical Products, Johnson & Johnson, Raynham, MA) have been used. Several reports over the past 5 years have focused attention on the potential adverse effects of modular connections on femoral components, with the main issue being corrosion at the interface, particularly between dissimilar metals such as a cobalt-chromium head and titanium trunion of the stem. Corrosion, fretting, and the generation of particulate metallic debris may have direct effects on local tissues but may also serve as a third-body particulate within the articulation. This latter concern is greater with modular heads than with modular connections more distant from the actual articulation itself. Evidence suggests that corrosion occurs in many of these connections but is more common when mixed alloy head-neck couples are used. One recent retrieval study showed corrosion ranging as high as 35% for mixed metal implants, whereas only 9% to 10% of single alloy components showed similar changes at a mean of only 2 years postimplantation.

Uncemented Acetabular Component Results

Recently reported intermediate-term results at up to a decade following implantation of uncemented acetabular components have documented failure rates from aseptic cup loosening of less than 0.5% per year (Table 2). A current report of one of the most widely used uncemented acetabular components, the Harris Galante I, demonstrated no loosening radiographically at 5 to 10 years postimplantation. The only revisions performed in this study were required for femoral component loosening in 4.4% of the cases. This cup, which has a titanium shell, titanium wire mesh surface for ingrowth of bone, multiple adjunctive screws, and employs a modular polyethylene acetabular insert, was associated with a very low rate of marginal osteolysis (1%). Similarly impressive results were reported recently for a chromium-cobalt implant with a beaded surface and supplemental screw fixation through peripheral flanges. Revision for loosening occurred in 1.4% with radiographic loosening evident in 4% at a mean of 12 years postimplantation. In contrast to these very excellent outcomes, high rates of failure have been seen with some other design approaches. For example, a 6% to 25% revision rate for aseptic loosening has been reported for titanium-threaded cups at mean follow-up of 4.5 to 6 years, and the surgeons who authored this report have abandoned use of this type of implant. Durability of fixation of these devices is multifactorial and relates to a host of features, including not just the implant design, but also patient- and surgeon-related factors. Nonetheless, it is of interest to review the apparent effect of design differences, as reflected in some of the most successful and least successful long-term series recently reported.

Implant Material

Analogous to the pattern seen and results reported for femoral stems, successes and failures exist for both cobalt-chromium and titanium devices. Other factors relating to implant design seem to be of greater importance, because use of identical materials in 2 different devices (the ARC cup and the PCA cup), both manufactured during the same era by the same company, resulted in very different intermediate to long-term performance (Table 1). In the case of the PCA cup, significant problems with polyethylene wear, osteolysis, and implant loosening were observed on the acetabular side. In 2 series, revision for acetabular loosening at between 5 and 6.8 years mean follow-up was required in 11% and 13.2% of cases, even though initial results of these procedures were very good. The main concern of the authors of one of these reviews for these devices after 6 years is stated to be polyethylene wear and osteolysis. By a minimum 7-year follow-up, lysis, noted around 4% of cups and 13% of stems, correlated with increased polyethylene wear and young age at operation. In contrast, the ARC cup was associated with a low rate of cup loosening (1.4%), 4% incidence of radiographic loosening, and only 4% pelvic osteolysis rate at a mean 12 years postsurgery. Femoral head size and polyethylene thickness are probably critical factors helping to explain the difference in performance of some of these seemingly similar implants. In a review of 63 PCA hips with 26-mm heads compared to 97 hips with 32-mm heads, a major difference was found in the incidence of osteolysis. In the group receiving 26-mm heads no osteolytic lesions were observed at 3 to 6.9 years follow-up, whereas 25.7% of hips receiving 32-mm heads demonstrated osteolytic lesions on radiograph. All osteolytic lesions occurred in individuals not only with a 32-mm head but with a metal shell with an outside diameter of 52 mm or less. This is a striking demonstration of the contribution of thin polyethylene within the acetabular insert to the develop-

Table 2
Cementless acetabular component results

Cup*	Design Features	Study Location (Date)	No. of Hips	Years of Follow-up	Revision: Cup Loose	X-ray Results	Comment
ARC	Cobalt chrome, beaded, peripheral flanges + screws	Boston, MA (1988)	72	(12)	1.4%	4% loose 4% pelvic lysis	Materials identical to PCA, differs in design.
Harris-Galante I	Titanium wire mesh, multiple screws	Chapel Hill, NC (1996)	136	5–10 (7)	0%	0% loose 1% marginal osteolysis	Only versions were for femoral loosening (4.4%).
Mecring	Titanium, threaded	The Hague, Netherlands (1995)	411	3–7 (4.5)	6%	25% loose or migrated	Device abandoned.
T-TAP	Titanium, threaded	Madison, WI (1994)	68	5–9 (6)	25%	13% not yet revised but loose; thus 38% mechanical failure rate	Device abandoned.
PSL	Smooth hydroxy-apatite-coated versus porous, beaded versions of the same titanium cup	Multicenter (1998)	316	5.6–9.9 (8.1)	2.7% porous 11.9% HA coated	Of unrevised cups only 3 unstable (2 HA coated). Osteolysis in 5%	Same HA stem used for both cups with 0.3% loosening rate.
PCA	Cobalt-chrome, beaded with peripheral pegs	Newcastle on Tyne, UK (1994)	241	2–9 (5)	11% (loose ± lysis)	36% osteolysis around the cup. 11% loose beads	8 yr survivorship 57%, design abandoned.
		Swedish Multicenter (1997)	539	(6.8)	13.2% revised (all causes)	17.8% of cups loose or migrated >5 mm	61% survivorship at 7 yrs.
		Washington, DC (1995)	100	Min. 7	4% revised or reop recommended (lysis + loose)	Lysis around 4% of cups and 13% of stems	Main concern post 6 yrs = wear + lysis.
LSF	Cobalt-chrome, beaded with screws	New Orleans, LA (1997)	160	5–8	5% (loosening or lysis)	11% pelvic lysis	All retrievals: Backside poly to screw bead wear.
Trispike	Cobalt-chrome, porous with three spikes	Seoul, Korea	52	11–12 (11.3)	15%	38% lysis of cup and stem. 17% lysis stem only.	Wear was 2-12 mm, averaged 29 mm/yr and ranged up to 1.04 mm/yr max.

*ARC, PCA (Howmedica, Rutherford, NJ); Harris-Galante I (Zimmer, Warsaw, IN); Mecring (Mecron, Berlin, Germany); T-TAP (Biomet, Warsaw, IN); PSL (Osteonics, Allendale, NJ); LSF (Implant Technology, Secaucus, NJ); Trispike (DePuy, Warsaw, IN)

ment of a problem that had otherwise been linked to this cup design in general. Catastrophic failure of polyethylene liners is also possible in uncemented acetabular components when liner thickness is inadequate. In a report of 10 cases of modular polyethylene liner wear through to the metal backing or linear fracture, the authors found that all were in components with polyethylene thickness less than 5 mm.

Implant Shape

There is less variability in potential implant shapes on the acetabular side than on the femoral side. Given the hemispherical configuration of the acetabular cavity, the majority of acetabular components are hemispherical and available in incremental sizes. However, there has been recent work at developing more elliptical designs in order to attempt to engage the bone around the periphery of the acetabulum in a more secure fashion. Typically, some degree of under-reaming of the acetabular cavity is carried out to facilitate a tight connection. This form of adjunctive fixation may help reduce dependence on the screws, fins, or pegs that are employed in some other designs. Under-reaming of the acetabular cavity is not without risk. Laboratory experiments have shown that potential for fracture of the acetabular rim existing when under-reaming of greater than 2 mm is carried out for hemispherical cups. It is important to note that even in the laboratory, these cracks may not be visible on radiographs with the cup in place. Intraoperative fractures associated with implantation of porous acetabular components have been reported and can adversely affect outcome.

Adjunctive Fixation

Uncemented designs have typically employed screws through holes in the hemispherical cup, peripheral pegs, spikes, or fins as adjuncts to press-fitting of the acetabular component, in order to encourage stable cup positioning pending bone ingrowth. The most popular technique has been the use of multiple screws, usually through the cup, but in some designs at the periphery through the rim or flanges. While this method of fixation has proven effective and is associated with some of the most durable results reported, risks exist with the drilling and placement of screws. Posteriorly, the sciatic nerve is at risk, and anteromedially vascular injury is a concern. Serious hemorrhage and even death is possible if screws placed in the anterior-superior or anterior-inferior quadrant of the acetabular cavity penetrate to the intrapelvic vasculature. Concerns also exist regarding the potential for screws to serve as a source of particulate debris, and as a means of facilitating access of this debris to surrounding bone.

Type of Implant Coating

It is interesting to note the effect of different coatings on identical implant designs, allowing assessment of this factor as an independent variable. One such study of the PSL cup (Osteonics, Allendale, NJ) involved comparison of a smooth HA-coated cup to a porous-beaded version of the same design. At a mean follow-up of 8.1 years in a large multicenter trial, marked differences were seen in performance of these 2 implants despite their being inserted in combination with the same HA-coated stem in all cases. While the HA-coated stem performed well, with an aseptic loosening rate of 0.3%, the HA-coated acetabular component required revision for loosening in 11.9% of cases compared with only 2.7% for the porous version of the cup. The authors of this study speculate that the mechanical conditions provided by the HA-coated cup were insufficient to allow bony attachment. Subsequent studies combining the HA coating with screws and threads have shown improved performance of this coating under those different mechanical conditions. Recently reported results document the difficulty in proving any significant advantage of titanium wire mesh over chromium-cobalt beads. Excellent long-term results have been reported with both the titanium Harris Galante I and the chromium-cobalt ARC cup (Howmedica, Rutherford, NJ). Yet the ARC cup has a beaded surface, manufactured by the same company, similar to that of the PCA cup. The PCA cup has not performed nearly as well as the other two, with reports of 11% to 13% revision rates for loosening and osteolysis at mean follow-up periods of 5 to 7 years. In the Swedish Multicenter Study of the PCA hip, in 17.8% of 539 hips implanted, the cups were loose or had migrated more than 5 mm at follow-up. Survivorship at 7 years was calculated to be only 61%. Thus, widely variable results have been observed with very similar porous surfaces, and very similar results have been observed with very different surfaces.

Modularity

The issue of modularity is important with regard to acetabular components and may very well affect durability of these implants. In a study of the LSF hip (Implant Tchnology, Secaucus, NJ) at 5 to 8 year follow-up, 5% of cups required revision because of loosening or lysis, and 11% had pelvic osteolytic type lesions. Of particular note, with regard to the issue of modularity, was the presence in all retrieved cases of backside polyethylene wear and abrasion by the screw heads. These findings raise concerns about the modular interface on the backside of polyethylene inserts as potential sources of polyethylene particulate. The presence of modularity and the gaps that exist between the polyethylene insert and metal shell may allow for motion or pumping at this interface, which may facilitate passage of polyethylene particulate through any screw holes in the cups to the implant-bone interface behind the acetabular component. Retrieval studies have shown granulation tissue with giant cells and metal and polyethylene debris in screw holes of uncemented cups. Despite significant efforts by manufacturers to improve polyethylene insert locking mechanisms and to increase congruency and contact areas of these inserts, concerns still exist regarding potential contribution to the development of osteolytic lesions in these devices. These issues are of particular concern with regard to cementless implants because they are used in the youngest, most active patients undergoing hip arthroplasty. In 1 review, most patients developing osteolysis were on average 10 years younger than those who failed to show evidence of lysis, and most patients with radiographic evidence of osteolysis were asymptomatic. This finding reinforces the absolute necessity of regular radiographic follow-up of all such arthroplasty patients. Concerns have been raised about uncemented modular acetabular components versus cemented cups with regard to the rate of polyethylene wear seen and the potential for cup migration. An important recent study compared hips randomized to receive either an uncemented Harris-Galante cup or a cemented Charnley cup, in combination with a monoblock cemented Charnley stem in all hips. Wear, evaluated at 5 years postsurgery, was found to be the same in the HG cup and Charnley groups, when all other compounding variables, such as head size, stem type, patient age, and activity, were controlled.

Uncemented THA Results in Selected Patient Subgroups

Experience with hip arthroplasty over the past 30 years has suggested that certain patient subgroups seem to be at increased risk for perioperative and postoperative complications and have a higher likelihood of subsequent component loosening and revision. Factors that appear to affect implant survivorship and performance adversely have been young age, high activity level, and certain medical conditions that diminish the patient's ability to withstand the stress of surgery. Recent information has emerged regarding intermediate to long-term results of uncemented hip arthroplasty in a number of groups of potential interest.

Age Younger Than 50 Years

Several reports that have used the age of 50 years and younger as the cut-off for examining results of uncemented hip arthroplasty in younger patients have shown encouraging results. In contrast to the significantly higher rates of implant loosening seen in young patients with cemented arthroplasty, particularly on the acetabular side, it appears that at least intermediate-term results, up to a decade postimplantation, can be highly successful in terms of achieving stable implant fixation. In a report of 79 hips in which the HG-I cup (Zimmer, Warsaw, IN) had been used, at a mean of 8.8 years no instances of cup loosening were seen by radiographic assessment, and implant survivorship at 10 years was calculated at 98.8% despite a mean age at surgery of 37 years. Osteolysis around the cup was observed in 7.4% of cases, however, and in all the cases that required revision surgery on the acetabular side (1.3%), the cause was periprosthetic osteolysis. Similar durable results have been seen with femoral fixation using extensively porous-coated stems and proximally fixed HA-coated implants in young patients. In a review of 174 hips replaced in patients with a mean age of 37.6 years with extensively porous-coated femoral components, at a mean of 8.3 years the vast majority of revision surgeries required were for problems related to a suboptimal acetabular component design, whereas revision for stem loosening was necessary in only 1.1% of cases. Radiographic assessment suggested bony fixation in 96% of stems, stable fibrous fixation in 3.4%, and unstable implant conditions in only the 1.1% that required revision. Likewise, in a review of 152 HA-coated implants at 6.4-year mean follow-up, no instances of radiographic loosening or revision for stem loosening were seen, despite an average patient age at surgery of 39 years. Only one case of medullary osteolysis was seen around these circumferentially HA-coated implants, although 32% of cases did show marginal osteolysis in Gruen zones 1 and 7 proximally adjacent to the femoral component. These results document that when validated implant designs have been used, the main issues with regard to uncemented fixation on both the acetabular and femoral sides in young patients center on polyethylene wear and periprosthetic osteolysis. When suboptimal designs are used, particularly in those with less than ideal conditions at the articulation with regard to wear, failure rates increase considerably. In a review of 41 hips replaced using titanium heads at the articulation, 7.3% of cups were revised at a mean of 5.3 years in a group of patients averaging age 42 at the time of surgery. A suboptimal cup design and locking mechanism used along with use of a titanium head resulted in a 49% incidence of significant polyethylene wear, 29% acetabular osteolysis, and a 14.6% incidence of cup loosening. Thus, in young, active patients, use of a less than optimal or unproven implant design can involve serious risks.

Juvenile Inflammatory Arthritis

Not all young patients experience increased risks of implant failure, however, because the disease process contributing to the need for hip arthroplasty may also produce significant restrictions in patient activity level. In a review of 29 patients who underwent arthroplasty for juvenile inflammatory arthritis, despite a very young average age of 21 years at the time of surgery, extremely durable fixation results were reported, with no revisions for component loosening at 4.4 years. The main challenges in this patient subgroup were related to small dimensions and altered anatomy, particularly on the femoral side. Excellent pain relief and improvement in function were obtained in this patient population, and ongoing limitations in activity were related primarily to disease effect on other joints.

Sickle-Cell Disease

Another potentially challenging group of patients are those with sickle-cell disease. Although limited clinical experience has been reported in the literature, in a recent review of 16 hips undergoing 7 primary and 8 revision procedures, no instances of loosening either radiographically or at the time of subsequent revision surgery were observed. Three of 16 did require reoperation for osteolysis, however, again pointing out the fact that, particularly in young patients, issues of wear and osteolysis are of prime concern.

Osteonecrosis

Results of cemented arthroplasty have repeatedly been shown to be less durable in patients with osteonecrosis (ON) than in those with osteoarthritis. There is some evidence to suggest that the potential exists to improve on these results using uncemented implants, although outcomes remain extremely design sensitive. In a review, 53 patients with ON were compared with 155 patients with osteoarthritis. All patients were younger than 50, and all received an HA-coated femoral stem. At a mean of 6.8 years (minimum 5 years) follow-up, the stem loosening rate radiographically was zero for both groups, and no revisions were required for stem loosening. Problems centered on the acetabular side, where suboptimal component design resulted in a mechanical failure rate of 10% for the ON group and 7.5% for the osteoarthritis group. Osteolysis was seen in another 7% of cases. In another study that compared 29 osteoarthritic patients with 29 patients with ON, at a mean of 7 years follow-up no difference was seen in fixation using uncemented implants in the 2 groups, with revision for loosening required in only one patient in the series who happened to have ON.

By contrast, in a recent review of 98 cases at 7.3 years postsurgery, use of a noncircumferentially porous-coated femoral component was associated with a very high failure rate when coupled with a less than ideal acetabular component design, which experienced accelerated polyethylene wear. Revision for loosening was necessary in 21% of cases. Thus, as with other demanding patient subgroups, hip arthroplasty in patients with ON places significant demands on the implant design. Use of components with an established track record for durable long-term performance is recommended.

Obesity

Conventional wisdom has held that failure rates for hip arthroplasty should be higher in patients who are obese because of the increased loads anticipated through the implant during the course of every day activity. In fact, accumulated data indicate that these individuals, perhaps related to a lower than average activity level overall and a diminished number of loading cycles to the implant, experience no higher incidence of implant loosening risk than unselected patient series. In a review of 60 obese patients with a body mass index greater than 30, comparison was made to 142 nonobese patients. At 4 years average follow-up, no difference was observed in overall results with regard to radiographic loosening or incidence of osteolysis. Although there may be some prolongation of surgery times and some slight increase in blood loss, obesity by itself does not constitute a contraindication to hip arthroplasty. Many of these patients, because of prevailing bias against performing surgery in the face of obesity, are markedly disabled prior to arthroplasty and are extremely grateful for the dramatic improvement in pain relief experienced as a result of the surgery. Preoperative medical consultation is important in this patient subgroup, particularly for those with a body mass index over 40. With morbid obesity, weight reduction efforts are of major importance, but more from a general medical standpoint than related to any arthroplasty performed.

Prior Therapeutic Pelvic Radiation

One patient subgroup at very high risk for implant loosening are those patients who have experienced previous therapeutic radiation. In a review of 9 patients who had undergone prior pelvic radiation, despite use of the Harris Galante I acetabular component, 22% required reoperation for implant loosening at only 3.1 years average follow-up, and double that number, 44%, were radiographically loose. This extremely high fixation failure rate for an implant, which otherwise has a loosening rate approaching zero over the first decade, highlights the marked adverse effect that prior therapeutic radiation can have on the ability of the bone to respond biologically at the implant interface. Although this high failure rate is distressing, there is as yet no published information to suggest better results with any other reconstruction strategy. Still these results have led some to consider use of cemented implants in combination with antiprotrusio devices at the time of primary hip arthroplasty in these patients.

Summary

Success or failure after THA is the culmination of a complex interplay of multiple factors, including underlying disease process, patient-specific factors, implant and design factors, and surgeon-controlled, technique-dependent factors. While the best designed device can be caused to fail by what may seen on the surface to be small changes in surgical methodology or technique, design factors can also doom even the most expertly performed reconstruction. Recently reported intermediate to long-term results of uncemented hip arthroplasty reported here have documented the potential for durable, long-term fixation to bone with these implants, while other studies of similar or shorter duration have resulted in the discontinuance of specific implant designs, modification of some others, and continuing efforts at validation of still others. The main recurrent concern overshadowing the most successful of these series relates to polyethylene wear and particulate-induced osteolysis of bone around implants with longer term follow-up. The future durability of these and similar implants will depend on the rates and severity of these wear-related changes. Design efforts should and will continue to focus on ways to minimize particulate load to the joint while preserving the very successful fixation results achieved with many of these uncemented implant designs.

Annotated Bibliography

Barrack RL, Folgueras A, Munn B, Tvetden D, Sharkey P: Pelvis lysis and polyethylene wear at 5-8 years in an uncemented total hip. *Clin Orthop* 1997;335:211–217.

This study documents results of 160 primary uncemented porous-coated total hip arthroplasties involving a chromium-cobalt acetabular component of hemispherical design with a sintered bead porous coating implanted with screws and articulating with a 32-mm chromium cobalt head. While no acetabular revisions had been performed at 2 to 4 year follow-up and there were no instances of pelvic lysis noted, by 5 to 8 years follow-up expansile pelvic lytic lesions had occurred in 11% of cups with 5% requiring revision. Abrasion of the screw head against the back side of the polyethylene liner was seen in all retrieved cases. This study documents a relatively high rate of development of osteolytic lesions during the intermediate follow-up time frame between 5 and 8 years, raising concerns about the long-term performance of this and similar systems.

Berger RA, Jacobs JJ, Quigley LR, Rosenberg AG, Galante JO: Primary cementless acetabular reconstruction in patients younger than 50 years old: 7- to 11-year results. *Clin Orthop* 1997; 344:216–226.

The authors report on 79 consecutive Harris-Galante I acetabular components inserted in patients younger than age 50 years. The average age at surgery was 37 (range 20 to 49 years). Average follow-up was 106 months. There were no cases of aseptic loosening. Two cups were revised during femoral revision and 2 excessive worn polyethylene liners were exchanged, with one acetabular osteolytic area debrided and grafted. All these procedures involved retention of the metal shell. At final follow-up all 72 acetabular cups were radiographically stable with acetabular osteolysis noted in 7.4%. Polyethylene wear was inversely related to patient age. Ten-year survival of the acetabular reconstruction by the Kaplan-Meier method was 98.8%.

Bryan JM, Sumner DR, Hurwitz DE, Tompkins GS, Andriacchi TP, Galante JO: Altered load history affects periprosthetic bone loss following cementless total hip arthroplasty. *J Orthop Res* 1996; 14:762–768.

The authors used dual energy x-ray absorptiometry (DEXA) to measure periprosthetic distal femoral and proximal tibial bone mass in the affected and opposite limbs of 8 patients who had undergone unilateral total hip arthroplasty 10 years earlier using a cementless porous-coated titanium stem. Gait analysis was also used to assess asymmetry and lower limb loading. The study data demonstrate that local stress shielding affecting the prosthesis is also influenced by the global effect of decreased loading of the limb and that both contribute to the overall bone loss seen. Thus, previous studies have probably overestimated the apparent magnitude of periprosthetic bone loss due to the implant by as much as 50%.

Capello WN, D'Antonio JA, Feinberg JR, Manley MT: Hydroxyapatite-coated total hip femoral components in patients less than fifty years old: Clinical and radiographic results after five to eight years of follow-up. *J Bone Joint Surg* 1997;79A: 1023–1029.

One hundred thirty-three patients (152 hips) who underwent total hip arthroplasty using an HA-coated femoral stem with an average age of 39 years at surgery (range, 16 to 49 years) were reviewed at minimum 5 years postsurgery (mean, 6.4 years; range, 5 to 8.3 years). All stems demonstrated osteointegration radiographically. The study results show that hydroxyapatite-coated femoral components can achieve excellent and stable fixation in young patients with the only worrisome radiographic changes relating to marginal osteolysis due to particulate debris from the articulation.

Dorr LD, Lewonowski K, Lucero M, Harris M, Wan Z: Failure mechanisms of anatomic porous replacement: I. Cementless total hip replacement. *Clin Orthop* 1997;334:157–167.

The authors report on the results of 100 consecutive primary total hip arthroplasties performed by a single surgeon at an average 6.7 years follow-up. Use of the implant was limited to those in whom a satisfactory intraoperative fit could be obtained. At final follow-up revision had been required in 16% with a mechanical failure rate of 11%. Seventy percent of hips had progressive loss of fixation. Loss of fixation correlated with younger patient age, higher patient activity level, metaphyseal fill of less than 90% and increased polyethylene wear and associated osteolysis. The acetabular component remained well fixed in 97% of hips. The authors concluded that the failure rate was unacceptably high and the use of this implant has been abandoned.

Dowdy PA, Rorabeck CH, Bourne RB: Uncemented total hip arthroplasty in patients 50 years of age or younger. *J Arthroplasty* 1997;12:853–862.

This study documents the results of uncemented THA in patients 50 years or younger. Forty-one hips in 36 patients were reviewed at 5.3 years mean follow-up. Average age at implantation was 42 years. At follow-up, 49% of cases demonstrated evidence of polyethylene wear with significant acetabular lysis in 12 of these 20 hips. Five cups were definitely loose and one possibly loose. Three patients underwent revision for acetabular loosening and/or osteolysis. The authors concluded that although the femoral stem design was excellent, the suboptimal cup design and locking mechanism, combined with use of a titanium femoral head, resulted in high rates of wear and osteolysis.

Furnes A, Lie SA, Havelin LI, Engesaeter LB, Vollset SE: The economic impact of failures in total hip replacement surgery: 28,997 cases from the Norwegian Arthroplasty Register, 1987-1993. *Acta Orthop Scand* 1996;67:115–121.

Up to January 1994 approximately 200 different implant combinations were used during THA in Norway. Five thousand five hundred hip arthroplasties were performed each year, at a total annual cost of approximately $70 million. The authors focused on the economic consequences of the use of inferior primary hip arthroplasty designs. They used the Charnley prosthesis inserted with high viscosity, antibiotic-containing cement as their standard and compared other implant subgroups to this. Compared to the reference Charnley arthroplasty group, the group of all other primary hip arthroplasties resulted in incremental costs of approximately $1.7 million per year due to the higher revision rates experienced.

Havelin LI, Espehaug B, Vollset SE, Engesaeter LB: Early aseptic loosening of uncemented femoral components in primary total hip replacement: A review based on the Norwegian Arthroplasty Register. *J Bone Joint Surg* 1995;77B:11–17.

This report from the Norwegian Arthroplasty Registry covers 24,408 primary total hip replacements inserted between 1987 and 1993 in that country. Thirteen percent (2,907) were performed with uncemented femoral components. The authors compare the results of eight different designs, each of which was used in more than 100 patients.

Havelin LI, Vollset SE, Engesaeter LB: Revision for aseptic loosening of uncemented cups in 4,352 primary total hip prostheses: A report from the Norwegian Arthroplasty Register. *Acta Orthop Scand* 1995;66:494–500.

This Norwegian Arthroplasty Registry study covers the years 1987 to 1994, during which 5,021 primary hip replacements were performed with uncemented acetabular components. Survivorship until revision for aseptic loosening was performed for the 11 most common implant types. Overall cumulative revision for acetabular components was 3.2% after 5 years and 7.1% after 6 years, but with large differences noted between designs.

Jacobs JJ, Kull LR, Frey GA, et al: Early failure of acetabular components inserted without cement after previous pelvic irradiation. *J Bone Joint Surg* 1995;77A:1829–1835.

This study explored the effect of previous irradiation of the pelvis on acetabular component survival when the cup had been inserted without cement during the course of a primary total hip arthroplasty. Of 11 patients (12 hips), 3 died before 1 year, leaving 9 hips studied at an average of 37 months postsurgery. At the time of follow-up, 3 of the 9 cups had migrated, of which 2 required revision. One additional component demonstrated progressive radiolucency without clinical symptoms. Thus 4 of 9 cups (44%) had experienced failure of fixation to bone. This study documents the high mechanical failure rate associated with use of porous-ingrowth components on the acetabular side in cases of patients who had undergone previous irradiation.

Kim Y-H, Kim J-S, Cho S-H: Primary total hip arthroplasty with the AML total hip prosthesis. *Clin Orthop* 1999;360:147–158.

This report involves 50 patients (52 hips) who received the uncemented AML femoral stem with a four-fifths porous coating and a 3-spike uncemented cup. Average age at surgery was 47.6 years, with diagnoses of osteonecrosis in 18, osteoarthritis in 16, fracture of the femoral neck in 14, ancient sepsis in 3, and posttraumatic arthritis in 1. Wear ranged from 2 to 12 mm on the socket side with an average of 3.3 mm and an annual wear rate of 0.29 mm. The maximum wear rate observed was 1.04 mm/year. This study documents satisfactory results of the AML femoral component but excessive wear and resulting osteolysis related to the acetabular component. The authors conclude that these results mandate close ongoing radiographic assessment of these and similar patients for the development of osteolytic lesions and/or component migration related to wear of the acetabular component.

Kronick JL, Barba ML, Paprosky WG: Extensively coated femoral components in young patients. *Clin Orthop* 1997;344:263–274.

This report covers 174 hips in 154 patients who were age 50 years or younger at the time of primary hip arthroplasty at 8.3-years follow-up. Mean age at surgery was 37.6 years (14 to 50 years). Nine percent had severe stress shielding, and 7.5% experienced acetabular failure. Of 174 fully coated stems, 99.4% had stable fixation, with 96% showing bone ingrown patterns, and 3.4% a stable fibrous fixation pattern. In 1 hip (0.6%), fixation was not stable. Two stems (1.1%) had been revised. The overall rate of osteolysis was 4%.

Latimer HA, Lachiewicz PF: Porous-coated acetabular components with screw fixation: Five to ten-year results. *J Bone Joint Surg* 1996;78A:975–981.

This report covers 136 consecutive hip arthroplasties using the Harris-Galante-I acetabular component reported at a mean of 7 years postsurgery (range, 5 to 10 years). Line-to-line reaming was used prior to inserting the acetabular component in this single surgeon series. Fixation was supplemented with 3 to 6 screws (mean, 4 screws). There were no radiographically loose cups at final follow-up and no revisions for loosening. No cup had radiolucent lines in all 3 acetabular zones. Four percent had radiolucencies in 2 zones and 25% had radiolucencies in 1 zone. Asymptomatic osteolysis at the rim of the acetabular component was seen in only 2 hips (1%) at a mean follow-up of 7 years, with polyethylene wear averaging 0.1 mm/year overall. The only revision procedures required in this series of 136 cases were due to femoral loosening, noted in 6 cases.

McLaughlin JR, Lee KR: Total hip arthroplasty with an uncemented femoral component: Excellent results at ten-year follow-up. *J Bone Joint Surg* 1997;79B:900–907.

This report of 138 patients (145 hips) documents experience with the Taperloc uncemented femoral component at an average of 10 years (range 8 to 12.5 years) postsurgery. Eighty-seven percent were good or excellent at final follow-up, 7% fair, and 6% poor. Radiographically, 94% demonstrated bone ingrowth, 3% were believed to have stable fibrous, and 3% unstable implant fixation. Femoral osteolysis was noted in 6%, but major lysis was present in only 1 case. One femoral stem was revised for aseptic loosening, 1 for sepsis, and 3 other well-fixed stems were removed during the course of an acetabular revision. These results from a single surgeon series demonstrate that excellent results are achievable with this design at 10 years postimplantation.

Smith SE, Estok DM II, Harris WH: Average 12-year outcome of a chrome-cobalt, beaded, bony ingrowth acetabular component. *J Arthroplasty* 1998;13:50–60.

This report of 72 hips (67 patients) reconstructed with a chromium-cobalt component with sintered ingrowth beads and peripheral flanges for screw fixation involves the ARC cup produced by Howmedica (Warsaw, IN). This cup is of interest in that with regard to the materials used it is identical to the PCA cup produced by that same company. The 2 designs differ only with regard to cup design. The results of this series were compared to reported results for the PCA in order to define the effect of the cup design differences. Average follow-up for the ARC cup was 12 years, with 3 cups (4%) requiring revision at an average of 8.5 years postsurgery. Aseptic loosening was the cause of revision in one case, component malposition and recurrent dislocation were the reasons for the other two. Incidence of acetabular loosening was 4%, pelvic lysis occurred in 4%. This is in contrast to the reported rates of acetabular revision with the PCA component which have ranged as high as 11% at 2 to 10 years, with aseptic loosening rates as high as 30% at substantially shorter time frames.

Classic Bibliography

Callaghan JJ, Heekin RD, Savory CG, Dysart SH, Hopkinson WJ: Evaluation of the learning curve associated with uncemented primary porous-coated anatomic total hip arthroplasty. *Clin Orthop* 1992;282:132–144.

Coventry MB: Lessons learned in 30 years of total hip arthroplasty. *Clin Orthop* 1992;274:22–29.

Engh CA, Glassman AH, Suthers KE: The case for porous-coated hip implants: The femoral side. *Clin Orthop* 1990;261:63–81.

Goldring SR, Clark CR, Wright TM: Editorial: The problem in total joint arthroplasty: Aseptic loosening. *J Bone Joint Surg* 1993;75A:799–801.

Hernandez JR, Keating EM, Faris PM, Meding JB, Ritter MA: Polyethylene wear in uncemented acetabular components. *J Bone Joint Surg* 1994;76B:263–266.

Huiskes R: Failed innovation in total hip replacement: Diagnosis and proposals for a cure. *Acta Orthop Scand* 1993;64:699–716.

Rorabeck CH, Bourne RB, Laupacis A, et al: A double-blind study of 250 cases comparing cemented with cementless total hip arthroplasty: Cost-effectiveness and its impact on health-related quality of life. *Clin Orthop* 1994;298:156–164.

Wiklund I, Romanus B: A comparison of quality of life before and after arthroplasty in patients who had arthrosis of the hip joint. *J Bone Joint Surg* 1991;73A:765–769.

Chapter 24
Hybrid Total Hip Replacement

Introduction

In hybrid total hip replacement, the femoral component is inserted with cement and the acetabular component is inserted without cement. This concept was introduced in the early 1980s, when clinical results demonstrated the reliable durability of cemented femoral components and the unacceptable early aseptic loosening rates (as high as 50% in some series) seen in cemented all-polyethylene sockets. Finite element analysis revealed that placing a metal backing behind the socket polyethylene reduced the stresses seen at the prosthesis-cement-bone interface. Cementless and cemented metal-backed components were introduced to solve the early acetabular aseptic loosening problem. Although cemented metal-backed components have proven to be a clinical failure, certain cementless acetabular sockets have had reported early mechanical failure rates of 0% to 2%. Mechanical failure is defined as the number of hips requiring revision plus the number of components considered radiographically loose.

The decade of the 1990s has focused on refinement of the cemented femoral designs and the technique of how they are placed. Improved polyethylenes, alternative bearing surfaces, more conforming acetabular socket designs, and innovative medical therapies are being introduced to solve the most troublesome problem facing long-term success in hybrid total hip arthroplasty (THA): particulate debris-induced osteolysis.

The Cemented Femoral Component

Design Characteristics and Mechanisms of Failure

Long-term success of femoral components depends on a complex interplay of prosthesis geometry, surface coating, cement, and surgical technique. Initiation of failure in cemented femoral components is a mechanical event, with debonding of the prosthesis from the cement. Debonding from the cement-metal interface causes peak stresses within the cement mantle to increase significantly. Torque produced during walking and stair climbing produce these peak stresses proximally and at the tip, and these stresses are high enough to initiate cracks within the mantle. Once the mantle has been compromised mechanically, biologic processes become more important. As a result of debonding and cement fracture, stability of the stem is compromised, and wear particles have access to endosteal bone, leading to focal osteolysis. Previous to these events, the femoral side is considered to have a high resistance to particles flowing through the periprosthetic joint space, as compared to the acetabulum. Stem instability leads to micromotion within the mantle, generating a large volume of additional debris.

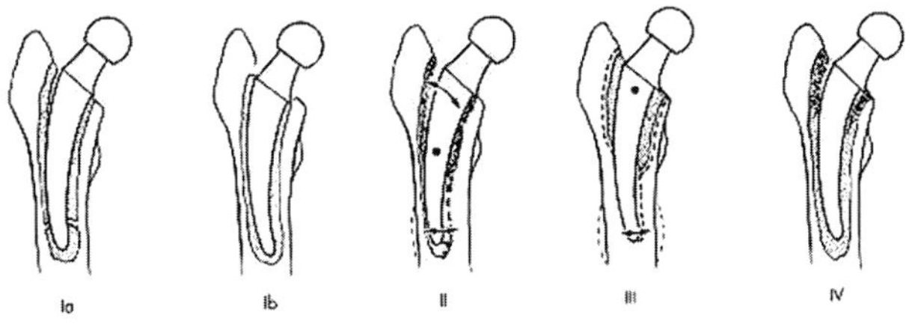

Figure 1

Modes of failure for a cemented femoral component. I: Subsidence of the stem within the cement mantle. II: Subsidence of the stem and cement within the bone. III and IV: Diaphyseal and calcar pivot. V: Cantelever.

Component geometry affects the way stresses are delivered to the cement mantle (Fig. 1). Previous designs with sharp corners were found to initiate cement cracks adjacent to these points. Finite element studies have shown that tapered stems with an additional taper at the tip result in the most efficient pattern of mantle stress distribution. The presence of a collar delivers stress to the calcar, possibly avoiding calcar absorption and reducing stresses seen in the proximal cement mantle. However, significant debate exists about whether or not the presence of a collar has clinical significance. Short-term reports comparing collarless and collared designs have shown no difference with respect to clinical or radiographic scores. One study of 98 hips showed that calcar collar contact was obtained in 74% of cases immediately following implantation. At 2 years, 76% of cases had lost calcar contact.

Roughened (bead-blasted, matte-finish), methacrylate precoat, and highly polished surfaces are all in use currently in hybrid hip arthroplasty. Early designs had a polished surface, whereas more recent stems have rougher surface finishes. Smooth implants have lower fixation strengths, however, with interface motion between the stem and the cement, less debris is generated to contribute to focal osteolysis.

Roughened surface stems enhance the strength of the cement-metal interface. Although these stems may have a lower probability of interface motion, much more debris is generated if motion does occur. A review of long-term studies describing the clinical success of polished and roughened stems suggests that surface composition is but one variable in the multifactorial etiology of aseptic loosening. When compared with other designs, components with proximal precoating with methacrylate have shown inferior results. One recent study reported a 1% stem fracture rate at 10 years. Other studies have reported early mechanical failure rates as high as 26% at 5 to 8 years.

Radiologic Evaluation

Evaluation of radiographic stability is reported using the zonal analysis described by Gruen (Fig. 2). The femur is divided into 7 zones on the anteroposterior radiograph and has been modified to include 7 zones on the lateral radiograph. As defined by Harris, a continuous radiolucent line at the cement bone interface in all zones is considered probably loose. If the line occupies 50% to 99% of the interface it is considered possibly loose. However, autopsy studies have cast doubt on the significance of these radiolucencies on the femoral side. Adaptive bone remodeling forms a second inner cortex adjacent to the cement mantle, indistinguishable on radiograph. Between the inner and outer cortex, a second medullary canal forms, which is responsible for the radiolucency on radiograph. In contrast to the lucency seen on the acetabular side, which contains fibrous tissue, the lucency caused by adaptive bone remodeling is nonprogressive and has not been found to have a role in aseptic loosening. Definite loosening is present if one of the following is seen: implant subsidence greater than 2 mm based on serial postoperative radiographs, new cement-metal radiolucency, cement mantle fracture, or implant fracture. Radiostereographic methods have been shown to detect femoral migration as small as 0.02 mm. Early subsidence greater than 1.2 mm has been shown to be an early predictor of loosening. When compared with serial postoperative radiographs, radionucleotide imaging and hip arthrogram show no additional benefit.

Quality of the cement mantle has been classified radiographically by Barrack and Harris. In class A, there is complete filling of the proximal femur, with no distinguishable border between the cement and the bone. Class B shows near complete filling, with a noticeable demarcation between cement and bone. In class C1, there is an incomplete cement mantle in the proximal femur, with greater than 50% of the cement-bone interface demonstrating radiolucencies. Class C2 mantles have areas in which the cement thickness is less than 1 mm, or the prosthesis is up against the bone. Class D mantles have gross deficiencies or multiple large voids. Anteroposterior and lateral postoperative radiographs should be used to grade the mantle. Class C and D mantles have been shown to have greater rates of aseptic loosening, but there is high interobserver variability in cement mantle grading.

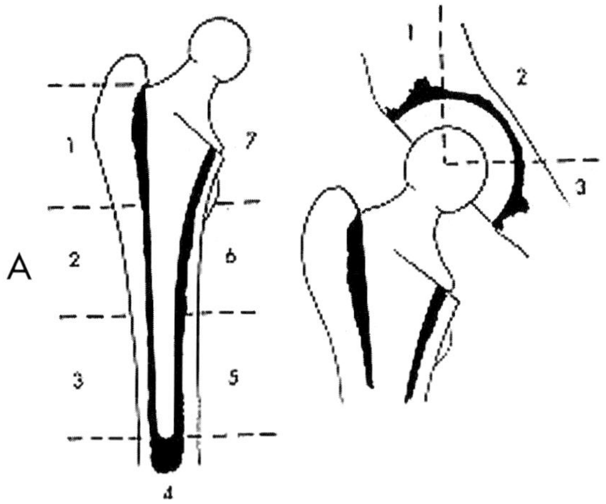

Figure 2

A, Gruen zones I–VII for radiographic analysis of a cemented femoral component. **B**, DeLee and Charnley radiographic zones for evaluating an acetabular component.

Cement Technique

Fixation of femoral components with polymethylmethacrylate has undergone significant advancement since its introduction. First-generation cement technique, introduced by Charnley, involved finger packing doughy cement into an unplugged femoral canal. Many components of that period were manufactured from stainless steel and contained a narrow medial side and sharp borders. Long-term results demonstrating 30% to 40% aseptic loosening rates have been reported in multiple studies at 8 to 10 years.

Second-generation technique included plugging the femoral canal, cleaning the canal with a pulsatile lavage, followed by retrograde injection of bone cement with a cement gun. Excellent 20-year follow-up results have recently been published for this technique. A 5% aseptic loosening rate has been reported in 161 hips in which a bead-blasted monoblock stem was used. Aseptic loosening rates of 6% and 7% have been reported in other series of 330 and 333 hips respectively. Polished and smooth stems were implanted in these studies.

Third-generation technique involves all aspects of the second-generation approach plus porosity reduction (vacuum mixing and centrifugation), pressurization of the cement mantle, and surface modifications of the femoral components (grit blasting, polymethylmethacrylate precoating) to enhance the prosthesis-cement interface. In vitro studies of centrifugation have shown pore sizes to be reduced from 400 microns to 200 microns. Ultimate tensile strength was increased 24%, while ultimate compressive strength increased 136%. Vacuum mixing has shown similar results. Porosity reduction takes on importance due to analysis of failed femoral components that have demonstrated cement fracture propagation through pores. In a report of 100 consecutive arthroplasties using third-generation technique, with 6- to 8-year follow-up, a mechanical failure rate of 1% was reported. However, no long-term clinical results are available for third-generation technique that show an advantage over second-generation technique. Based on the results seen in the second-generation technique studies, extremely large numbers of patients followed 20 years will be required to indicate any significantly greater clinical efficacy.

Fourth-generation technique includes all aspects of third-generation technique plus the addition of proximal and distal femoral cement centralizers. Finite element analysis has demonstrated that cement stresses are highest at the most proximal and distal portions of the cement mantle. Varus or valgus placement of the femoral component greater than 5° significantly increases stresses within the cement mantle by reducing cement mantle thickness in Gruen zones 5 and 6. Numerous clinical studies have implicated excessive valgus or varus positioning within the cement column as a predictor of failure. One report demonstrated that 50% of mechanical failures in a cohort of patients had a prosthesis placed in 5° of varus or greater. One recent study of 100 consecutive patients using fourth-generation technique showed that 93% of stems were within 2° of neutral alignment, with no cases of mechanical failure at 5.7 years.

Surgical Technique

Careful preoperative planning is necessary for proper selection of components and restoration of limb length (Fig. 3). The femoral template should allow a minimum of 2 mm of cement mantle aligned in a neutral position. Based on the projected center of hip rotation, which corrects for limb length if needed, the length of the femoral osteotomy from the lesser trochanter is measured to allow correct selection of femoral offset and prosthesis neck length. Width of the stem centralizer and cement plug can also be determined at this time. The distance from the lesser trochanter to the center of hip rotation should be recorded and used as a guide for establishment of intraoperative leg-length equality. While taking these measurements, it is important to note the relative internal/external rotation of the femur as evidenced by the profile of the lesser trochanter. Distortions in the lesser trochanter/center of hip rotation measurement and femoral offset may be present.

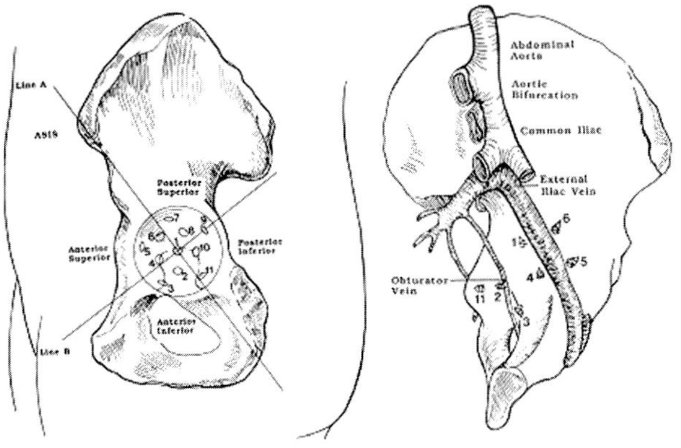

Figure 3

Lateral and medial view of the pelvis showing the safe zones for acetabular screw placement.

During performance of a posterior approach to the hip, the short external rotators, posterior hip capsule, and quadratus femoris are tagged for future repair. Once the hip is dislocated, the neck osteotomy is measured based on the preoperative template. After the acetabular component is placed, femoral exposure is obtained with a flexion-adduction-internal rotation maneuver. A full and unimpeded view of the proximal femur is obtained with a femoral neck retractor placed under the anterior femoral neck, as well as retractors placed on the medial and lateral borders of the femur. Soft tissue present at the junction of the femoral neck and greater trochanter should be removed. Entrance into the femoral canal is performed with a box-cutting tool to lateralize the opening into the greater trochanter. Next, a canal finder is placed in a neutral position into the femoral diaphysis, with care taken not to perforate the cortex. The femur is reamed and broached appropriately to the correct size, always cognizant of keeping the instruments lateral to ensure neutral and not varus placement of the final component. Proper anteversion is considered aligned with the patient's posterior femoral neck. Once the final broach is placed, the appropriate neck and trunion offset trials are placed and measurement of the lesser trochanter-center femoral head is taken and compared with the preoperative template. Over-lengthening can be assessed intraoperatively with the rectus femoris tightness test, which is flexion of the knee and extension of the hip, after the trial reduction. Any osteophytes on the anterior femoral neck should be removed to prevent instability.

Once satisfactory stability is noted, the trial femoral components are removed and the appropriate sized canal plug placed 1 cm distal to the tip of the prosthesis. To avoid a femoral fracture, the plug should not be placed with excessive force. When cementing of the prosthesis is imminent, the anesthesiologist should be made aware to anticipate the possible hypotension caused by the methacrylate monomer. The canal is then cleansed with a pulsatile lavage and packed with a dry sponge. During this time the cement is mixed, noting the ambient temperature and humidity of the room to gauge the time needed for curing. At approximately 4 minutes from the initiation of mixing, the cement is injected retrograde with the cement gun, allowing the pressure within the canal to push the nozzle of the gun out, rather than introduce air to the canal by pulling on the handle. The cement column should be proximally pressurized to create sufficient mantle in Gruen zones 1, 6, and 7. In vitro research has shown that a cement pressure of 20 psi produced a cement intrusion depth of 2.2 mm for Simplex-P and 1.4 mm for Palacos cements, respectively. There are concerns with proximal pressurization with respect to excessive introduction of cement monomer into the circulation, causing fat embolism and bone necrosis. The prosthesis should be inserted in neutral position to the appropriate depth and pressure applied until the cement is cured to avoid expulsion of the component as the cement expands during polymerization. After placement of the femoral head and final reduction, careful repair of the posterior structures is performed. The tagging sutures of the structures described earlier are drawn up through drill holes in the posterior aspect of the greater trochanter. In a prospective review of hundreds of patients receiving a posterior approach, repair of the piriformis, conjoint tendon, and quadratus femoris reduced the dislocation rate to 1%.

The Cementless Acetabular Component

Design Characteristics

Once early failures of cemented polyethylene sockets became common, research into the development of metal-backed components was initiated. Early biomechanical studies demonstrated that stresses seen at bone-cement-prosthesis interface were markedly reduced in metal-backed sockets as well as more evenly distributed. It was suspected that the increased interface stresses seen in cemented all-polyethylene components caused cement fatigue leading to early mechanical loosening. Cementless metal-backed, cemented metal-backed, and press-fit smooth metal-backed acetabular components were developed as a consequence of this theory. Recent evidence has refuted the mechanical theory of the initiation of acetabular loosening. Autopsy studies in patients with a cemented all-polyethylene acetabular component indicated that the interface between the cement and bone was being invaded by soft tissue, starting at the periphery. In pull-out studies, the greater the egress of this soft-tissue front from the periphery towards the dome, the less force required to remove the component. Analysis of this soft-tissue front has described a fibrous stroma with various inflammatory cells and cytokines, including activated macrophages, lymphocytes, and interleukins. This tissue corresponds to the linear radiolucent lines seen in all-polyethylene acetabular components. Based on this information, the initiation of loosening in acetabular components is considered a biologic event.

Early and late clinical results of metal-backed cemented components have been universally disappointing. Multiple authors have reported mechanical failure rates of 40% to 50% at 10 years. One study with a minimum 15-year follow-up reported an 86% rate of failure. Press-fit smooth metal-backed components, anchored to the acetabulum with a central peg, were a universal failure in all studies conducted. Based on this data, these designs are no longer recommended for use in THA.

Design features of metal-backed sockets have evolved over the last 10 to 15 years. Current implants are composed of either titanium alloy or cobalt-chromium with a variety of coatings added to obtain biologic fixation. In vitro studies have shown titanium to be more biologically compatible, as evidenced by an increased ability of cells to spread and adhere to the surface. However, no studies have demonstrated titanium to be a better choice of metal over cobalt-chromium in the design of metal-backed acetabular components. Many initial designs had a hemispherical outer radius, but a hexagonal inner geometry in which the polyethylene articulated. This caused edge loading of the polyethylene at the periphery with significant subsequent early failure. Examples of this include the ACS cup design of DePuy and the Universal cup by Biomet. Other first-generation cups had an inner hemispherical radius, which has served as the model of cup designs today. Current designs are ultraconforming, which maximize metal and plastic contact with a simple and stable locking mechanism. The goal is to minimize the motion between the metal-plastic junction to effectively transfer stress and reduce wear. Potential areas of concern regarding "backside wear" particle generation are sharp edges along the locking mechanism, screw heads (fretting against the screw hole, wearing against the polyethylene), and empty screw holes. This phenomenon takes on importance due to the high shear stresses seen at the polymetal interface. A comparison of various designs with regard to backside wear concluded that designs that limited the number of screw holes and polished the inner surface of the metal shell generated the least amount of wear. Other studies have demonstrated that 71% of the load across the liner-shell interface is borne by the locking mechanisms. Both in vitro and finite element analysis studies have documented between 8.5 and 12.8 µm of polyethylene extrusion through fenestrations in the metal backing.

Fixation coatings available include sintered beads, titanium plasma spray, titanium wire mesh, and hydroxyapatite (HA). The optimal pore size to enhance bone ingrowth is 150 to 250 µm. Autopsy studies in components that were considered well-fixed showed that approximately 25% to 45% of the superior surface was ingrown with bone. Most of the ingrowth was located in the posterosuperior portion or around screw holes. Dual geometry (larger radius of curvature around the periphery compared to the dome), spikes, peripheral fins, and threads have been introduced to enhance initial fixation. One study compared the extraction and lever-out forces required to remove commercially available acetabular cup geometries. Included in the study were 1 and 2 mm oversized hemispherical cups and various dual geometry designs. Dual geometry cups required significantly more force to extract, but 2 mm oversized hemispherical components had greatest resistance to torque. No differences have been shown between spikes or peripheral fins in implant stability or clinical results.

Surgical Technique

Meticulous preoperative planning is essential for successful results in hip arthroplasty. Acetabular templating should restore the anatomic center of hip rotation, allow adequate coverage of the component within the socket, and assist in equalizing leg lengths. Oversizing the metal-backed shell requires excessive bone stock removal, leaves a greater portion of the shell uncovered, and will lengthen the extremity by lowering the center of hip rotation. No more than 30% of the prosthesis should be uncovered by acetabular bone. If greater than 30% uncoverage is anticipated or encountered during the procedure, placement of a femoral head autograft should be considered. Bulk allografting has not had favorable clinical results. Femoral head autografts have been shown at 5 years to have excellent clinical results, but data extending the review to 10 and 15 years have shown a steady drop-off in clinical success. Recent long-term data on grafts supporting cemented acetabular components have demonstrated younger age and greater than 50% of cup coverage as indicators of failure. Short-term data on grafts supporting 30% to 50% of metal-backed components have been favorable, but no long-term data are currently available. It must be noted, however, that bone graft providing coverage of a metal shell does not grow into the prosthesis to provide biologic fixation. During placement of an autograft, it should be placed into a bleeding surface to enhance healing. The graft is fixed into position with cancellous screws or bolts. It should be noted that larger diameter screws may cause the graft to split. Once the graft is in position, it should be reamed progressively until the graft is congruent with the host acetabulum.

Whichever surgical approach is used, excellent circumferential exposure of the acetabulum is necessary. All remnants of the acetabular labrum should be removed by sharp dissection, and the contents of the pulvinar within the condyloid fossa extracted to identify the medial wall of the acetabulum. Adequate retraction of the femur will allow unimpeded reamer positioning during preparation of the socket. The first reamer should be medialized until it abuts, but does not penetrate, the medial wall of the acetabulum. This allows for restoration of the anatomic center of hip rotation. Subsequent reamers should be placed in the position in which the prosthesis is to be placed, which is in 20° of anteversion and 45° of abduction. Cups placed at 60° have been found to generate more linear polyethylene wear than cups placed at ~45°. Reaming should remove all remnants of articular cartilage and penetrate into the subchondral bone until an excellent bleeding bed is noted. The metal shell selected should measure no more than 2 mm larger than the last sized reamer employed during preparation of the socket. In a study of the incidence of fracture and the force required to seat components, which were 2 mm and 4 mm oversized, the forces required to seat the cups were 2,000 N and 4,000 N, respectively. The group oversized by 4 mm had a fracture rate of 93% noted in cadaver specimens. Force should be applied until the shell can be visually confirmed against the bone, or an audible pitch change is noted during insertion. Gaps left behind 2 mm oversized metal sockets have been shown at 2 years to disappear either by superior socket migration or bone replacement. Acetabular trials may be used to assess whether adequate rim fit will be obtained during placement. If the rim fit is in question or the patient is osteopenic, acetabular screws should be inserted to supplement fixation. Anatomic studies have shown that screws placed in the anterior superior and anterior inferior quadrants of the cup may compromise the external iliac vein and obturator artery, respectively. Posterior screw placement (in screws > 25 mm) may injure the sciatic nerve or the superior gluteal artery. Care should be taken to seat the screws completely, so that the screw heads do not wear against the backside of the polyethylene. Once the metal shell has been inserted, circumferential exposure of the acetabulum should be obtained and all soft-tissue remnants removed from the rim so that the full seating of the polyethylene is not disturbed. Acetabular osteophytes that cause impingement during range of motion should be removed.

Radiologic Evaluation of Uncemented Sockets

DeLee and Charnley devised the radiographic classification system for acetabular components. Martell and associates revised the classification by subdividing DeLee zones II and I. The socket should be evaluated for linear radiolucencies and cavitary osteolytic lesions. Linear radiolucencies of 2 mm or greater are considered significant. Based on serial radiographs, the socket is considered stable if a nonprogressive radiolucency is seen in 2 or fewer zones, with no evidence of superior socket migration, eccentric polyethylene wear, or change in the angle of inclination of the cup. Definite acetabular component migration has been considered to be horizontal or vertical migration greater than 2 to 3 mm or a change in the opening angle of the cup greater than 5°. Meaningful measurements can only be made from radiographs that are comparable with respect to magnification and positioning. Due to positioning difficulties, all subsequent radiographs should be compared to the first postoperative film, not the radiograph obtained in the recovery room. Differences in magnification can be determined by x-ray markers or by comparing the size of the femoral head. Positioning on an anteroposterior pelvic film can be compared by the profiles of the obturator foramen. Recommended intervals for radiographic follow-up should be the first postoperative visit, 6 months, and then annually.

Polyethylene Wear and Osteolysis

Osteolysis induced by wear particles continues to be the most serious problem affecting long-term success of hybrid THA. "Effective joint space" is the term used to define the area around the prosthetic interfaces, which is exposed to circulating joint fluid containing wear particles. The sources of these particles include submicron polyethylene head on cup wear debris, cement particles, backside wear debris between the polyethylene and the metal liner, and metal debris from trunion-head articulations and acetabular screw head-metal shell motion.

Wear within the polyethylene socket has been shown to be relatively high within the first 4 to 5 years after implantation, with rates reported as high as 0.4 mm/yr in cemented, noncemented, and hybrid hip arthroplasty alike. This "wearing in" phenomenon is related to the small mismatch in curvature between the head and socket. The distance that the head slides, rather than rotates, has been shown to relate directly to the amount of wear. Once the head has worn into the socket so that the two are concentric, wear rates drop significantly. One recent study compared the wear rates of different manufacture's polyethylene, using heads from other companies. Wear rates were different for a particular polyethylene, depending on which company's femoral head was used. The authors believed that the small differences in manufacture's tolerances were responsible. Volumetric wear is greatest in 32-mm heads, while linear wear is most prevalent in sockets where 22-mm heads are used. Ceramic heads have been found to have an extremely low coefficient of friction on polyethylene and low wear rates in several studies. However, they are expensive ($700) and have been associated with fracture. Ceramic-on-ceramic articulations have been investigated as an alternative-bearing surface with excellent short-term clinical results. However, one recent long-term report of this combination in 102 hips demonstrated a 22% incidence of femoral osteolysis. Histologic analysis of the soft-tissue membrane around the revised stems revealed ceramic material ingested by activated macrophages.

Sterilization technique has been shown to greatly affect the way in which polyethylene inserts wear. Gamma radiation has an effect of crosslinking the polyethylene molecules together if it is carried out in an inert atmosphere. Research has shown that the degree of cross-linking within a polyethylene insert correlates with decreased wear particle generation. However, concerns are being raised regarding the material's decreased fracture toughness, which will predispose the insert to brittle fractures. The material has shown excellent wear characteristics on wear simulators and short-term clinical trials, however, no long-term data are available. Current sterilization techniques include radiation under ethylene oxide, argon, and nitrogen. Great efforts are taken to avoid the presence of oxygen during the sterilization process to avoid oxidation. Oxidation has also been found to have occurred in polyethylenes that have had too long a shelf life.

Multiple long-term results of cemented all-polyethylene acetabular components have reported a linear wear rate of 0.05 to 0.1 mm/year. The majority of literature demonstrates that wear in cementless metal-backed polyethylene sockets is greater than in cemented sockets. Wear rates in metal-backed liners have been shown to be 0.1 to 0.7 mm/year. Socket wear in hybrid hip arthroplasty must be analyzed on a design-specific basis. Various cup designs differ with respect to polyethylene conformity, thicknesses, and locking mechanisms. Designs created with superior clinical success have reported wear rates of 0.15 to 0.25 mm/year. It is currently recommended to have a thickness of at least 6 mm of polyethylene in a metal-backed socket liner.

Strategies for reducing the volume of polyethylene wear particles have also focused on improving polyethylene.

Hylamer M is an example of improved polyethylene. In vitro studies showed it to be an excellent bearing material, with reduced wear compared to conventional polyethylene. However, clinical results have demonstrated significant problems with Hylamer with regard to excessive wear, with subsequent osteolysis and early revision. One recent study on 78 patients with Hylamer liners reported a 11.5% incidence of cavitary osteolytic lesions greater than 1 cm. Two patients required revision for lysis, and a fracture through a lesion in the greater trochanter occurred in another.

Osteolysis remains the most significant problem affecting long-term success of THA. Not surprisingly, metal-backed cup designs, which had the least amount of polyethylene wear, had lesser amounts of osteolysis. Incidence of lysis is dependent on each specific design. In summary, the amount of polyethylene wear in uncemented sockets is at least double that seen in cemented ones. The patterns of lysis are different, and only long-term studies will show whether these issues will become clinically important.

Results of Hybrid THA

Intermediate results (5 to 8 years) of hybrid hip arthroplasty are very encouraging, particularly with respect to performance of the acetabular component. Multiple studies have reported mechanical failure rates of 0 to 2% at 5 to 8 years. This is significant improvement over the results seen in cemented cups, especially in the younger patient. Data have recently been published on 45 hips in patients younger than 50 years of age. They reported no cups to be radiographically or clinically loose. More careful analysis of cemented socket survivorship data shows that patients with inflammatory arthritis display loosening rates of 50% to 100% at 15 year follow-up. While no long-term data are available for cementless sockets in patients with rheumatoid arthritis, early to intermediate results show loosening rates of 2% to 5%.

One study has been published describing greater than 10 year results on hybrid arthroplasty. They reported on 52 consecutive hips followed for an average of 12.3 years. None of the stems were loose. Only 1 cup was considered radiographically loose, but it was functioning well. Pelvis lysis was seen in one cup, whereas a 21% incidence of femoral osteolysis was seen.

Annotated Bibliography

Cemented THA With Contemporary Cementing Techniques

Madey SM, Callaghan JJ, Olejniczak JP, Goetz DD, Johnston RC: Charnley total hip arthroplasty with use of improved techniques of cementing: The results after a minimum of 15 years of follow-up. *J Bone Joint Surg* 1997;79A:53–64.

This study evaluated a group of 357 consecutive THAs. Among the 142 hips in 130 patients alive at minimum 15-year follow-up, the rates of femoral and acetabular revision for aseptic loosening were 2% and 10%, respectively. The combined rates of aseptic loosening and/or revision for loosening were 5% on the femoral side and 22% on the acetabular side.

Mulroy WF, Estok DM, Harris WH: Total hip arthroplasty with use of so-called second-generation cementing techniques: A fifteen-year-average follow-up study. *J Bone Joint Surg* 1995;77A: 1845–1852.

One hundred two hips in patients alive for a minimum of 14 years following standard cemented primary THAs using a grit-blasted femoral component with second-generation cementing technique were evaluated. Two femoral components (2%) underwent revision for aseptic loosening. Another 7% of femoral components were loose radiographically, but were not revised. Of the 81 all-polyethylene acetabular components, 10% were revised. An additional 42% were loose radiographically.

Barrack RL, Mulroy RD Jr, Harris WH: Improved cementing techniques and femoral component loosening in young patients with hip arthroplasty: A 12–year radiographic review. *J Bone Joint Surg* 1992;74B:385–389.

Fifty primary cemented total hip replacements were evaluated at a mean 12-year follow-up (range, 10 to 14.8 years). No femoral component was revised for aseptic loosening, and only 1 was loose radiographically. In contrast, 11 patients (22%) underwent revision for loosening of the cemented acetabular component, and another 11 acetabular components were loose radiographically.

Cementless Acetabular Replacement Results

Smith SE, Estok DM II, Harris WH: Average 12-year outcome of a chrome-cobalt, beaded, bony ingrowth acetabular component. *J Arthroplasty* 1998;13:50–60.

Seventy-two hips were evaluated following insertion of a cobalt-chromium porous-coated acetabular component at an average 12-year follow-up (range, 10 to 13.3 years). Overall, 3 acetabular components were revised. The total incidence of aseptic loosening of the acetabular component was 4% (3 components). The loosening rate was significantly less than the 42% loosening rate noted by the same surgeon with cemented acetabular components at similar follow-up.

Kim YS, Callaghan JJ, Ahn PB, Brown TD: Fracture of the acetabulum during insertion of an oversized hemispherical component. *J Bone Joint Surg* 1995;77A:111–117.

Fifteen fresh and 15 embalmed cadaveric acetabuli, 52, 54, 56, or 58 mm in diameter, were prepared for insertion of hemispherical porous-coated acetabular components oversized by 2 mm or 4 mm. The average force required to seat components oversized by 2 mm and 4 mm was 2,000 N and 3,000 N, respectively. Acetabular fractures developed in 93.3% of the 4 mm oversized group, and in 26.7% of the 2 mm oversized group. Of the 18 fractures noted, only 15 could be detected radiographically.

Schmalzried TP, Wessinger SJ, Hill GE, Harris WH: The Harris-Galante porous acetabular component press-fit without screw fixation: Five-year radiographic analysis of primary cases. *J Arthroplasty* 1994;9:235–242.

One hundred twenty-two primary THAs with insertion of an oversized porous-coated acetabular component without screws were followed for an average of 56 months (48 to 66 months). There were no acetabular fractures, no component was revised, and no component was radiographically loose.

Surgical and Cement Technique

Berry DJ, Harmsen WS, Ilstrup DM: The natural history of debonding of the femoral component from the cement and its effect on long-term survival of Charnley total hip replacements. *J Bone Joint Surg* 1998;80A:715–721.

Two hundred and ninety-seven consecutive Charnley THAs followed for a minimum of 20 years, or until death or revision, were evaluated. Early debonding between the cement and superolateral aspect of the stem and cement with a radiolucency of less than 2 mm was not associated with hip pain or mechanical loosening. A radiolucent line greater than 2 mm at this location was associated with poorer results.

Ebramzadeh E, Sarmiento A, McKellop HA, Llinas A, Gogan W: The cement mantle in total hip arthroplasty: Analysis of long-term radiographic results. *J Bone Joint Surg* 1994;76A:77–87.

Eight hundred thirty-six cemented femoral components were reviewed at a mean follow-up of 9 years to evaluate the relationship between cement mantle thickness, medullary canal fill and stem alignment, and long-term radiographic outcome. Neutral and valgus stems had better results than stems placed in more than 5° varus. Stems with 2-mm to 5-mm cement mantles in Gruen zones 6 and 7 and greater than 50% canal fill had the best outcomes.

Patient Factors

Chmell MJ, Scott RD, Thomas WH, Sledge CB: Total hip arthroplasty with cement for juvenile rheumatoid arthritis: Results at a minimum of 10 years in patients less than 30 years old. *J Bone Joint Surg* 1997;79A:44–52.

Thirty-nine patients (66 hips) with a diagnosis of juvenile rheumatoid arthritis underwent cemented THA and were evaluated after an average 15.1-year follow-up. The femoral revision rate was 18% and the acetabular revision rate was 35%. The 15-year survivals of the femoral and acetabular components were 85% and 70%, respectively, with revision as an end point.

Jacobs JJ, Kull LR, Frey GA, et al: Early failure of acetabular components inserted without cement after previous pelvic irradiation. *J Bone Joint Surg* 1995;77A:1829–1835.

Eight patients (9 hips) who had undergone insertion of a porous hemispherical acetabular component without cement following prior pelvic irradiation were alive at an average 37-month follow-up. Of the acetabular components in this series, 44% were loose or had undergone revision surgery for loosening.

Hybrid Hip Replacement Results

Berger RA, Kull LR, Rosenberg AG, Galante JO: Hybrid total hip arthroplasty: 7- to 10- year results. *Clin Orthop* 1996;333: 134–146.

One hundred fifty consecutive primary hybrid THAs with femoral components inserted with contemporary cementing technique and hemispherical porous acetabular components inserted without cement were followed for 7 to 10 years. Aseptic loosening was noted in 2 femoral components (1.3%). Aseptic loosening occurred in 2 acetabular components(1.3%), and 2 additional components had acetabular osteolysis without loosening.

Callaghan JJ, Tooma GS, Olejniczak JP, Goetz DD, Johnston RC: Primary hybrid total hip arthroplasty: An interim followup. *Clin Orthop* 1996;333:118–125.

One hundred thirty-one consecutive primary hybrid THAs with with femoral components inserted with contemporary cementing technique and hemispherical porous acetabular components inserted without cement were followed for 8 to 9 years. Eight femoral components (6.1%) were revised for aseptic loosening. No acetabular components were revised for aseptic loosening, and none had migrated.

Goldberg VM, Ninomiya J, Kelly G, Kraay M: Hybrid total hip arthroplasty: A 7- to 11-year followup. *Clin Orthop* 1996;333: 147–154.

One hundred and twenty-five consecutive primary hybrid THAs with femoral components inserted with contemporary cementing technique and hemispherical porous acetabular components inserted without cement were followed for an average of 8.6 years (range, 7 to 11 years). One femoral component was revised for aseptic loosening, and a second was radiographically loose. No acetabular components were loose or were revised for aseptic loosening.

Lewallen DG, Cabanela ME: Hybrid primary total hip arthroplasty: A 5- to 9-year followup study. *Clin Orthop* 1996;333: 126–133.

One hundred fifty-two consecutive primary hybrid THAs with femoral components inserted with contemporary cementing technique and hemispherical porous acetabular components inserted without cement were followed for 5 to 9 years. Three hips (2.2%) underwent revision for aseptic loosening of the femoral component, 1 for acetabular loosening(0.7%), and 1 for dislocation (0.7%).

Smith SE, Harris WH: Total hip arthroplasty performed insertion of the femoral component with cement and the acetabular component without cement: Ten to thirteen-year results. *J Bone Joint Surg* 1997;79A:1827–1833.

Fifty-two consecutive primary hybrid THAs with femoral components inserted with contemporary cementing technique and hemispherical porous acetabular components inserted without cement were followed for 10 to 13 years. Two hips were revised for late recurrent dislocation without loosening. No femoral or acetabular components were loose radiographically, and none were revised for loosening. Pelvic osteolysis was noted in 2% of cases; femoral osteolysis was noted in 15% of cases.

Sporer SM, Callaghan JJ, Olejniczak JP, Goetz DD, Johnston RC: Hybrid total hip arthroplasty in patients under the age of 50: A 5- to 10-year follow-up. *J Arthroplasty* 1998 13: 485–491.

In a consecutive series of 45 total hip replacements using the Harris-Galante I acetabular cup and the Iowa grit-blasted methylmethacrylate precoated stem in 37 patients under the age of 50, 5- to 10-year results are described. No acetabular components and 8 femoral components (18%) were revised for aseptic loosening. The total mechanical failure rate was reported as 24% on the acetabular side and 0% on the acetabular side. Excessive failure of the femoral side was attributed to early debonding of the femoral component from the cement and the roughened surface finish applied.

Woolson ST, Haber DF: Primary total hip replacement with insertion of an acetabular component without cement and a femoral component with cement: Follow-up study at an average of six years. *J Bone Joint Surg* 1996;78A:698–705.

One hundred twenty-five consecutive primary hybrid THAs with femoral components inserted with contemporary cementing technique and hemispherical porous acetabular components inserted without cement were evaluated at an average 6-year follow-up. Four hips underwent revision for aseptic loosening of the femoral component. No acetabular components underwent revision for loosening, and none were loose radiographically.

Chapter 25
Revision Total Hip Replacement

The orthopaedic surgeon who chooses to perform revision total hip replacement (THR) faces several technical challenges. The patients are often elderly and debilitated, with compromised soft tissues and inadequate metabolic reserves. A multitude of problems, such as component loosening, instability, leg length inequality, fracture, or infection, may need to be resolved. Existing bone stock may be only slightly less than that encountered in the primary situation or woefully inadequate.

Meticulous preliminary planning is critical to ensure a successful procedure. In addition to technical expertise, a vast array of specialized instruments, implants, and bone graft reserves are required.

A variety of cemented and cementless implants are currently available. Neither type is appropriate in all situations, but instead should be selected depending on the patient's age, activity level, remaining bone stock, and reason for revision. It is estimated that more than 120,000 THRs are performed each year in the United States, and 18% of these are revision cases.

Mechanisms of Failure

Material Failure

The materials used to construct THR implants must be able to sustain loads of 2 to 3 times body weight with routine activities of daily living, with peak loads approaching 6 to 8 times body weight. The materials must be biologically inert and have acceptable wear rates to minimize the generation of wear debris. High-density polyethylene has been in use since Charnley introduced low friction arthroplasty in 1959, and remains the most commonly used articulating surface. Because of improved manufacturing techniques of the materials, polyethylene wear has been markedly diminished by minimizing the deleterious effects of oxidative degradation, aging, and polyethylene fusion defects. Despite these advances, osteolysis induced by polyethylene debris remains a major cause of implant loosening and revision.

Earlier total hip designs used stems made of stainless steel or cast cobalt chrome that were susceptible to fatigue fracture after years of service. The possibility of stem fracture has been diminished, but not completely eliminated, by stronger alloys of stainless steel, forged cobalt chrome, and titanium. Implants used in revision THR must be even more durable because of the presence of more extensive porous coating, the number of modular attachments, and less support from existing bone stock.

Loss of Fixation

Bone cement (polymethylmethacrylate) has been in use for the last 40 years to anchor both femoral and acetabular components. Cement works best where there is good interdigitation into the surrounding cancellous bone bed that allows for optimal transfer of weightbearing stresses between the bone and implant. When cement is subjected to high stresses over time, it may undergo fatigue failure, resulting in fracture, fragmentation, and ultimately osteolysis and/or implant loosening. Long-term success with cemented THR is possible for primary replacement, with failure rates ranging from 5% to 50% for the acetabular component and 2% to 32% for the femoral component at 11 to 22 years follow-up. The prospect for long-term fixation with cement for revision surgery is much less encouraging. When an implant and cement are removed during a revision, a great deal of the cancellous bone may be lost. In a laboratory model using cadaver bone to simulate cemented revisions, the interface shear strength between bone and cement dropped to 20% of that found in a primary THR and finally to 6.8% of the primary situation with a second revision. The interior of the acetabulum and femoral canal are usually quite sclerotic at the time of revision. Increased oozing from the bone occurs after removal of the thickened interface membrane. Because of this it may be extremely difficult to achieve excellent cement interdigitation, jeopardizing long-term success, unless removal of a

The author or the department with which he is affiliated has received something of value from a commercial or other party related directly or indirectly to the subject of this chapter.

neocortex uncovers residual cancellous bone.

Cementless THR was introduced to eliminate the potential failure of bone cement and hopefully achieve longer-lasting fixation. Even with primary THR, cementless replacement is doomed to failure if intraoperative stability is not obtained, and if subsequent bone ongrowth is inadequate. These problems are greatly compounded in the revision situation because of segmental and cavitary defects of the acetabulum or femur coupled with osteoporosis that make it not only more difficult to achieve initial stability but also increase the risk of intraoperative fracture.

Mechanical Failure

Despite the use of sound materials to construct the implants and the ability to achieve fixation with either cement or bone ingrowth, failure may occur because of poor implant design. The polyethylene must be of adequate thickness, preferably 6 mm or more, to avoid excessive wear and osteolysis. A 32-mm head will increase the volume of polyethylene debris generated, even with adequate polyethylene thickness, when compared to heads with a smaller diameter. Modular components increase the treatment options available, but also increase the risk of catastrophic dissociation and the generation of particulate metal debris. Metal ingrowth pads or hydroxyapatite surfaces may delaminate from the implant and constitute yet another source of particulate debris.

Wear Debris

It may be possible to achieve long-term fixation with either cement or by bony ingrowth and yet experience failure secondary to the generation of wear debris. This problem is the major obstacle to long-term success. The debris particles may consist of polyethylene, bone cement, metal, or ceramic. The use of a modular implant may increase the risk of debris generation. Once liberated, the particles incite an inflammatory reaction and cell-mediated response that can cause osteolysis and implant loosening. Revision surgery is often performed with modular implants and cerclage cables or trochanteric grips that facilitate surgery, but pose an additional risk of debris generation.

Infection

The risk of infection over the life of an implant in primary THR is approximately 1%. In revision surgery, this risk is at least twice as high. The possibility of infection should always be considered, especially when an implant loosens prematurely. The detection of occult infection with appropriate laboratory studies and hip aspiration, if indicated, should be attempted prior to revision surgery. Treatment of the infected THR is discussed in detail in Chapter 17.

Instability of the Components

Recurrent dislocation is a major cause of early revision. The risk of dislocation is much higher following revision THR because of compromised soft tissues and poor muscle strength. If a trochanteric osteotomy results in nonunion, the incidence of postoperative dislocation increases dramatically. An acetabular component that is placed too vertical, with excessive anteversion, or with any degree of retroversion, may result in instability. Care must be taken to remove peripheral acetabular osteophytes, especially along the anterior edge; otherwise, impingement can cause dislocation. Impingement of the greater trochanter against the back of the acetabulum or a prominent posterior edge of the acetabular component can lead to anterior instability. If uncemented components are used, inadequate bone stock of either the acetabulum or femur may lead to postoperative migration of the implants and recurrent instability. Unrecognized fractures of the acetabulum and femur can have the same result. If femoral offset is not recreated or if excessive shortening results, soft-tissue tension may not be adequate to maintain stability. If an adduction contracture goes unrecognized and is not corrected by adductor tenotomy, it will be very difficult for the patient to abduct sufficiently in the postoperative period, leading to increased instability, especially with hip flexion. Reoperation for dislocation is most successful when the cause for underlying instability is identified and corrected.

Periprosthetic Fracture

In a series from the Mayo Clinic, periprosthetic fracture was second only to aseptic loosening in causing revision. Fractures may be divided into those occurring intraoperatively and postoperatively. Femoral fractures are more common than those of the acetabulum. In primary cemented hip replacement, the estimated incidence is < 1% for cemented but in the range of 3% to 20% for uncemented femoral components. In the revision situation, the incidence increases to 6% or less with cemented but is as high as 40% with cementless implants. The incidence of acetabular fracture associated with cementless implants in primary cases seems to be greater than with cemented cases and is usually caused by excessive force used to seat the socket, especially with under-reaming of the acetabulum. Intraoperative fracture of the acetabulum has been reported less frequently than femoral fracture in revision cases, due in part to the "line to line" acetabular reaming performed in most series.

The incidence of postoperative femoral fracture is estimated to be at 0.1% to 2.5% over the life of the implant. Advanced age, osteoporosis, and osteolysis are factors that contribute to fracture susceptibility. Minimally displaced fractures of the acetabulum can be treated conservatively with protected weightbearing until fracture healing occurs. Displaced fractures will require implant revision and/or open reduction and internal fixation of the fracture. A useful classification scheme describes not only the anatomic location of the fracture, but also the status of stem fixation and existing bone stock and therefore considers the surgical tack to follow for different fractures. Femoral fractures may be divided into fractures involving the lesser or greater trochanter, fractures around the femoral stem with or without instability of the implant as a result of the fracture, and those occurring well distal to the femoral stem that may be treated with open reduction and internal fixation in a routine fashion.

Preoperative Assessment

Clinical Findings

Pain is the main presenting symptom in patients with component loosening. Nearly all patients with prosthetic joints will experience some aching or stiffness upon initiating ambulation after prolonged sitting. Patients with loose implants, however, will have persistent pain that makes any prolonged ambulation difficult. The pain may be located in the groin or thigh and radiate to the knee. Pain is especially worrisome if it has been present since implantation and may indicate either a smoldering infection or an implant that never had initial stability. The patient may have an antalgic component to their gait with associated thigh atrophy from disuse. An abductor lurch may or may not be present, depending on the biomechanical nature of the hip and the integrity of the abductor musculature. Patients may also report progressive shortening or rotation of the extremity, decreasing ambulation endurance, and a greater dependence on ambulatory aids. Range of motion may become compromised, making it increasingly difficult to perform activities such as stair climbing or donning shoes. With catastrophic implant failure, these symptoms may appear suddenly and could be associated with crepitus if dissociation of the implants has occurred. Pain may also be caused by conditions such as bursitis, tendinitis, lumbar spine disease, abscess, and hernia. Patients with progressive shortening of the extremity may notice a progressive external rotation contracture as well.

Radiographic Studies

Standard views include anteroposterior views of the pelvis, the involved hip, and some type of true lateral view of the upper femur. The radiographs must be of sufficient quality to permit assessment of the bone stock and to determine the presence of any subtle radiographic changes, such as periosteal reaction and radiolucencies between cement and bone, cement and implant, and implant and bone. It is possible to note and quantify the extent of polyethylene wear based on the position of the femoral head in relation to the edge of the acetabular component. Current radiographs should be compared with previous radiographs whenever possible because this may document migration of either the acetabular or femoral component, which is pathognomonic for loosening. Radiolucencies that are progressive and surround the mantle of cemented implants are strongly predictive of loosening. Meaningful radiolucencies often have a reactive sclerotic line adjacent to the radiolucent area and can therefore be distinguished from the radiolucency resulting from normal rarification of adjacent cancellous bone. Other signs strongly suggestive of loosening of a cemented implant include cement fracture, radiolucency between the implant and cement mantle, and fracture of the femoral stem and/or acetabular polyethylene.

The radiographic criteria of both stable and unstable cementless femoral implants has been described. Stable femoral components should have bone apposition to the porous ingrowth surfaces with no intervening radiolucency. Proximal rarification ("stress-shielding") of cortical bone is not unusual. Endosteal "spot welds" are areas of bony condensation bridging the endosteal surface to the ingrowth area and are most common at the distal extent of the ingrowth pad. At times it may resemble a small flying buttress. Radiolucencies are commonly seen around the smooth distal portions of the stem and are of little consequence. Loose femoral and acetabular components may or may not exhibit implant migration, but commonly have radiolucencies adjacent to the bone ingrowth surfaces. With a loose, subsiding femoral component, it is not unusual to see a thick, bony pedestal bridging the endosteal surface at the tip of the implant. The bone surrounding loose migrating implants may show dramatic bony remodeling if present for many years.

Radiographs should also be carefully scrutinized for any evidence of implant fracture, shedding of the ingrowth surface, or osteolysis. Osteolysis may progress dramatically over the years with no overt clinical signs or symptoms. It is advisable that well-functioning implants be radiographed at least every 2 years, despite the lack of clinical symptoms, to assess the presence of progressive osteolysis.

Other Diagnostic Studies

Other radiographic views that may be helpful are Judet oblique views of the pelvis to assess the bone stock in the anterior and posterior columns. A cross-table lateral view is useful to assess remaining bone stock in the posterior column as well as the orientation of the cup in relation to the pelvis. Computed tomography (CT) scans of the pelvis and femur may help to visualize the remaining bone stock, despite the scatter interference from the metal implants. The CT scan may be combined with intravenous contrast to note the proximity of major vessels to loose implants. Magnetic resonance imaging has a limited role, but may be helpful in assessing periarticular soft tissues, especially in determining the cause of pain that is not implant-related. Bone scans in concert with indium-labeled white blood cell scans have been helpful in discerning between aseptic loosening and infection. The sine qua non in making the diagnosis of an infected THR is the aspiration arthrogram. The cell count of the aspiration fluid should be noted; if the white blood cell count is greater than 25,000/mm^3 and is predominately polymorphonucleocytes, then the implant is most likely infected. A Gram stain is helpful in that it may demonstrate the bacteria if present in sufficient quantity. The patient's peripheral white blood cell count is often normal in the presence of a deep-seated infection, but the erythrocyte sedimentation rate and C-reactive protein are usually elevated. If suspicions remain regarding infection during the time of revision, an intraoperative frozen section may be performed. More than 10 white blood cells per high-powered field is considered to be strongly suggestive of acute inflammation. If the frozen section, in combination with intraoperative findings, is suggestive of infection, then it may be prudent to obtain multiple intraoperative cultures of the soft tissues along with abundant tissue for histologic examination and to postpone implantation until the patient's status is elucidated. It is wise to obtain multiple samples when culturing for infection. The difficulty arises when an organism is cultured that is commonly a contaminant. If such an organism is cultured and only 1 specimen was obtained, then it may not be clear whether or not the hip is truly infected.

Surgical Treatment

General Considerations

A critical step in the execution of any procedure is the preoperative planning, and this is especially true in revision THR. If the operation was performed at another facility, the operative note should be obtained, to note the type of implants used and the conditions encountered at the time of surgery. Areas of missing bone, such as cortical windows, may not be readily apparent from the radiographs. By knowing the type of implants in place, it may be possible to obtain specialized extraction tools. If the femoral stem is not to be revised, new modular femoral heads for the stem should be available because it may be necessary to adjust the length or offset or the head may be damaged. It is helpful to know whether stems have a modular head or monoblock design. It is important to know whether or not the acetabular component is modular, and if so, an understanding of the locking mechanism is necessary. New acetabular polyethylene liners should also be available, even if a change of the acetabular component is not anticipated. Excessive polyethylene wear or damage to the socket during the revision may make it necessary to revise the polyethylene liner.

Templating of the radiographs is a key component of preoperative planning. Templates of the implants to be used should be available. The proposed size of the implant to be used is determined. It is helpful to have some determination of femoral neck length that can be measured on the radiograph and corroborated intraoperatively. Measuring the distance from the top of the lesser trochanter to the center of rotation is a handy reference technique. In the event that the lesser trochanter is missing, some other bony landmark can be chosen, such as the relation of the center of rotation to the tip of the greater trochanter. If a transfemoral approach or extended trochanteric osteotomy is contemplated, it is helpful to measure the distance from the tip of the greater trochanter to the distal extent of the osteotomy, based on the exposure necessary to remove the stem and/or cement. It is possible to predict the effect implants of different size will have on the overall leg length. The difference between the current location of the center of the femoral head and its proposed relocation, in relation to a fixed point on the femur, will help to determine the contribution of the femoral component to leg length. In a similar fashion, if the center of rotation is currently high in relation to the acetabulum and is then brought back down to a more anatomic position closer to the teardrop, then the effect on leg length must also be determined. It should be noted whether sufficient femoral offset will be recreated with the new implants, or whether specialized implants (lower neck/shaft angle or enhanced offset stems and cups) are necessary.

Equipment

When performing revision THR, it is necessary to have on hand not only the equipment available to do the job but items that may be necessary should things take an unexpected turn. Specialized tools are necessary to remove implants and cement. These include pneumatic drills and burrs, flexible osteotomes, cement chisels and splitters, stem extractors for either monoblock implants or for modular stems following removal of the femoral head, and cobalt-chrome cerclage cable and clamps used to reattach the greater trochanter. Bone graft, both morcellized and large structural pieces, must be on hand to augment bony deficiencies. If the implants are to be cemented, powdered antibiotic such as tobramycin can be incorporated into the cement to lessen the chance of infection. Ultrasonic tools are quite helpful for use in thermal removal of bone cement. The segmental cement extraction system ("seg-ces") can be used to remove an intact cement mantle in 1- to 2-cm pieces by placing new cement into the old cement mantle to anchor the extraction rod and thus remove the old cement with the new. If a large blood loss is anticipated, a centrifugal cell washer can be used to aspirate and recycle the patient's red blood cells. An image intensifier and radiolucent table are quite helpful if there is an extensive amount of cement to be removed far distal in the femoral canal. This enhances the correct placement of power instruments and helps to minimize the chance of cortical perforation. Long curved chisels, powered either by hand or pneumatically, can be used to break up the interface behind the acetabular component and facilitate cup extraction.

Implant Selection

After careful evaluation of the radiographs, it must be determined whether one or both of the components is to be revised. Implant loosening can usually be determined prior to surgery and well-fixed implants need not be revised. Rarely, it may be necessary to remove a well-fixed femoral component, especially a monoblock design, to have sufficient exposure for acetabular revision. A new implant can be cemented into the old cement mantle if it is intact.

The Femoral Side

A classification system of bone loss patterns encountered in revision THR is quite helpful in preoperative planning. It should be noted that the classification may change once the bone condition is assessed at surgery. A number of classifications schemes are available. The American Academy of Orthopaedic Surgeons® (AAOS) Committee on the Hip proposed a classification in 1993 (Outline 1). It covers both revision and primary situations. In addition to a description of defect types, there are also subclasses for defect location and the overall quality of remaining bone. Although thorough, the numerous subclasses make its application somewhat unwieldy.

A discussion of the various reconstruction options is easier with a simplified classification such as the one proposed by Mallory in 1988 (Outline 2, Figure 1). This classification seeks to guide implant selection based upon remaining bone stock. A type I defect has an intact cortex, and cancellous bone remains in the upper metaphysis. A type II defect likewise has an intact cortex but has lost most of the cancellous bone. In type III defects, cortical bone loss is now apparent.

Outline 1

The American Academy of Orthopaedic Surgeons® classification of femoral deficiencies in total hip arthroplasty

I. Segmental deficiencies
- Proximal
  - Partial
    - Anterior
    - Medial
    - Posterior
  - Complete
- Intercalary
- Greater trochanteric

II. Cavitary deficiencies
- Cancellous
- Cortical
- Ectasia

III. Combined segmental and cavitary deficiencies

IV. Malalignment
- Rotational
- Angular

V. Femoral stenosis

VI. Femoral discontinuity

(Reproduced with permission from D'Antonio J, McCarthy JC, Bargar WL, et al: Classification of femoral abnormalities in total hip arthroplasty. *Clin Orthop* 1993;296:133–139.)

Outline 2

The Mallory classification of femoral bone deficiency in revision total hip replacement

I. Cortical tube intact, cancellous bone is present.

II. Cortical tube intact, cancellous bone is absent.

IIIA. Cortical deficiency extending to the lesser trochanter.

IIIB. Cortical deficiency extending to between lesser trochanter and isthmus.

IIIC. Cortical deficiency extending to the level of the isthmus.

(Reproduced with permission from Mallory TH: Preparation of the proximal femur in cementless total hip revision. *Clin Orthop* 1988;235:47–60.)

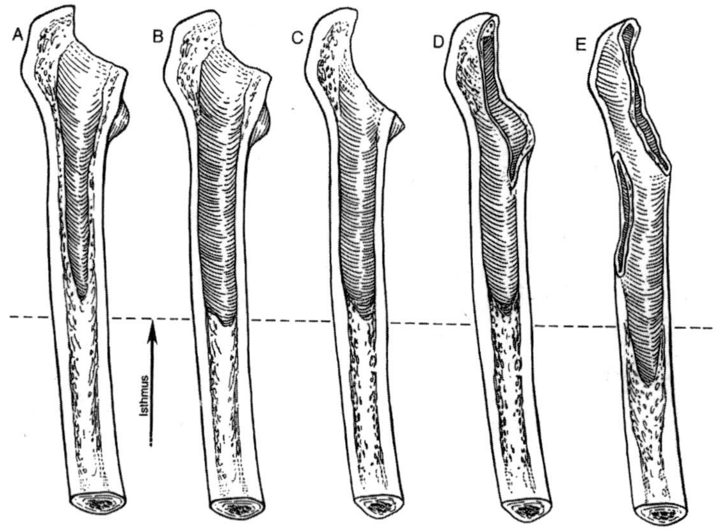

Figure 1

Mallory's classification of femoral bone loss in revision. **A**, Type I. **B**, Type II. **C**, Type IIIA. **D**, Type IIIB. **E**, Type IIIC. (Reproduced with permission from Buly RL, Nestor BJ: Revision total hip replacement, in Craig EV (ed): *Clinical Orthopaedics*. Philadelphia, PA, Lippincott Williams & Wilkins, 1999.)

In the type IIIA defect, there is bone loss down to the level of the lesser trochanter. In the type IIIB defect, cortical bone loss extends below the lesser trochanter and in the IIIC defect, cortical bone loss extends down to the level of the isthmus. With a knowledge of the type and amount of bone present with which to work, it then must be determined whether to use a cemented or cementless implant. In the type I defect, because a fair amount of bone remains, it should be possible to achieve a good result with either type of stem. With increasing degrees of cortical bone loss, specialized implants such as calcar replacement stems may be necessary along with strut or proximal femoral allografts to make up bone deficiencies. With the type IIIB defect, fortunately enough bone still remains above the isthmus, so that it is possible to achieve stable fixation by pressing a cementless implant into the converging bone in this location. The type IIIC defect presents a problem. It may be impossible to anchor a fully coated stem distally because of the divergent femoral canal below the isthmus. Specialized implants may be necessary along with a proximal femoral allograft.

The Acetabular Side

As in the femur, it is helpful to have a classification scheme for bone defects. The AAOS proposed a classification system in 1989 with segmental and/or cavitary defects along with special categories for pelvic dissociation and arthrodesis (Outline 3). The Paprosky classification is specific for failed THR and assesses the severity of bone stock loss and the ability of the acetabulum to contribute to implant stability (Outline 4, Figure 2). In this system, the need for various types of bone graft (morcellized or structural) can be predicted. As with the femoral classification, the true status may not be apparent from radiographs and modification may be required at surgery. A type 1 defect is one in which there is minimal osteolysis with very little migration of the acetabular component. In the type 2 defect, there is superior migration of the cup, but less than 2 cm. The type 2A defect has superomedial migration with the upper rim of the ilium remaining intact. In the type 2B defect, migration is superolateral with segmental loss of the upper rim. The type 2C defect has teardrop lysis, indicating loss of the medial wall. In the type 3 defects, structural allograft or metal augmentation are necessary to replenish the missing bone

Outline 3

The American Academy of Orthopaedic Surgeons® classification of acetabular deficiencies in total hip arthroplasty

I. Segmental Deficiencies
- Peripheral
  - Superior
  - Anterior
  - Posterior
- Central (Medial wall absent)

II. Cavitary Deficiencies
- Peripheral
  - Superior
  - Anterior
  - Posterior
- Central (Medial wall intact)

III. Combined Deficiencies

IV. Pelvic Discontinuity

V. Arthrodesis

(Reproduced with permission from D'Antonio JA, Capello WN, Borden LS, et al: Classification and management of acetabular abnormalities in total hip arthroplasty. *Clin Orthop* 1989;243:126–137.)

Outline 4

The Paprosky classification of acetabular bone deficiency in revision total hip replacement

1. Minimal lysis or component migration.

2A. Superior-medial migration < 2 cm.

2B. Superolateral migration < 2 cm.

2C. Teardrop lysis, loss of medial wall.

3A. Migration > 2 cm, ischial lysis present.

3B. Same as 3A plus disruption of Köhler's line, indicative of profound medial loss. Pelvic dissociation may be present.

(Reproduced with permission from Paprosky WG, Perona PG, Lawrence JM: Acetabular defect classification and surgical reconstruction in revision arthroplasty: A 6-year follow-up evaluation. *J Arthroplasty* 1994;9:33–44.)

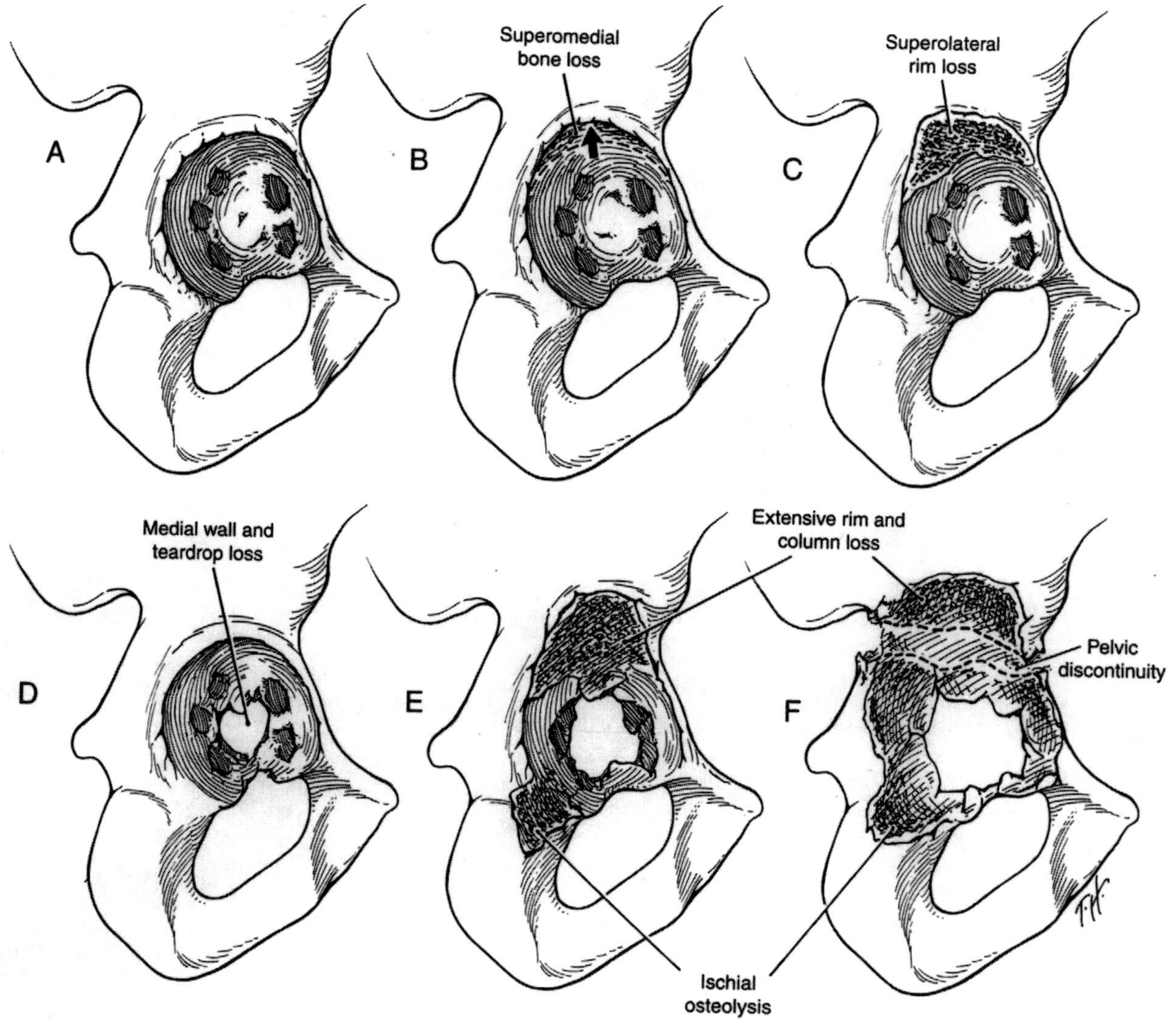

Figure 2

Paprosky classification of acetabular bone loss in revision total hip replacement. **A**, Type 1. **B**, Type 2A. **C**, Type 2B. **D**, Type 2C. **E**, Type 3A. **F**, Type 3B. (Reproduced with permission from Buly RL, Nestor BJ: Revision total hip replacement, in Craig EV (ed): *Clinical Orthopaedics*. Philadelphia, PA, Lippincott Williams & Wilkins, 1999.).

stock. The type 3A defect has more than 2 cm of superior migration along with osteolysis of the ischium, indicative of posterior column loss. In the type 3B defect, Köhler's line is disrupted, adding significant medial loss to the picture, and therefore a profound global detriment. As in the type I femur, the type 1 acetabular defect can be handled with either a cemented or cementless hemispherical cup because of the minimal bone loss. In the type 2 defects, uncemented hemispherical cups may be used if the remaining rim is sufficient to provide intraoperative stability of the implant. The type 2B defect is oblong-shaped and may require a similarly shaped implant, or it can be managed with structural bone graft to replace the socket in anatomic position. Alternatively, a regular implant may be placed at a high hip center, obviating the need for specialized implants or structural graft. Screws and/or plates may be necessary for internal fixation of larger structural bone grafts for segmental defects. If there is insufficient host rim to stabilize the uncemented implant or if there is insufficient bone to provide bone ingrowth, then a cemented cup should be used, preferably with some type of metal reinforcement ring. The type 3 defects require structural allograft. If there is pelvic discontinuity, antiprotrusio cages can be used as a large plate to span the defect, with screws above and below the socket to provide continuity from the ilium to the ischium. Pelvic reconstruction plates can also be used in the effort to restore pelvic stability. Bone grafting, usually a combination of structural and morcellized and, at times, entire acetabular allografts, are required to augment the large bone defects encountered.

Surgical Approaches

The hip joint can be exposed by a number of different techniques and the key is for the surgeon to choose the approach that is the most comfortable to use. The old incision should be used whenever possible to avoid wound healing problems. The anterior and posterior flaps are then meticulously elevated off the vastus lateralis, greater trochanter, and abductor musculature. In order to avoid the complications inherent with trochanteric osteotomy, it is possible to then proceed with either an anterolateral or posterior approach into the hip joint. With the anterolateral approach (Hardinge, transgluteal) the abductors are elevated off the anterior aspect of the greater trochanter and the abductor muscle fibers are split longitudinally, with care taken to avoid injury to the superior gluteal nerve. The femoral head is then dislocated anteriorly with external rotation of the leg. A meticulous repair of the abductors is necessary to prevent limp and weakness. Conversely, with a posterior approach, the femoral head is dislocated posteriorly with flexion and internal rotation. In the posterior approach, the capsule and external rotators usually cannot be separated and are peeled down in a long, continuous layer off the back of the greater trochanter.

If the exposure is still inadequate with either approach, a release of the capsule on the contralateral side can be performed either from within or outside the joint to increase mobility. By careful elevation of the capsule from the periphery of the acetabular component and by elevating the capsule off the femoral neck, it is usually possible to gain sufficient exposure to perform revision of the implants. Attempts should be made to leave the psoas tendon intact on its insertion onto the lesser trochanter.

If exposure is still inadequate despite these measures or if the abductor muscle sling must be retensioned as in problems with recurrent dislocation, it is then necessary to osteotomize the greater trochanter. This can be done with the classic trochanteric osteotomy, in which the greater trochanter is detached from the femur with the abductor musculature insertions left intact. The greater trochanter is mobilized in a cephalad direction to gain additional exposure of the hip joint and lateral side of the ilium. Alternatively, a trochanteric slide can be performed in which the greater trochanter is osteotomized but the vastus lateralis origin, along with the abductor musculature, is left intact on the greater trochanter. In this manner, the greater trochanter is now a bipedicle fragment and the anchoring effect of the vastus lateralis helps to prevent cephalad migration, should the trochanter fixation fail. With either type of trochanteric detachment, the femoral head can be dislocated in either the anterior or posterior direction.

At times it may be necessary to gain additional exposure to the femoral canal to remove extra long stems that are cemented or stems with extensive porous coating. In these situations it may be futile to attempt removal with exposure alone at the most proximal end of the femur. Another good indication for this type of approach is with type IIIB and IIIC femoral defects in which the proximal bone loss is so extensive that it is much easier to proceed with implant and cement removal through a controlled opening of the lateral femoral cortex. If limited access is needed, it may be more prudent to proceed with fenestrations in the cortical bone to gain access to broken stem tips or fragments of remaining cement. However, if a much more extensive exposure is needed, the options are then a transfemoral approach or an extended trochanteric osteotomy. In the extended trochanteric osteotomy, the entire greater trochanter is elevated but the distal osteotomy is made much further down the shaft instead of just below the vastus ridge. With the transfemoral approach, the greater trochanter is split in the coronal plane and the posterior half of the greater trochanter remains attached to the rest of the femur. With either technique, the lateral third of the femur is then opened in an anterior direction and the vastus lateralis is kept attached to the lateral bone fragment to maintain vascularity. The exposure is exceptional with either approach. The lateral cortical bone is then repaired after implantation with cerclage cables and augmented with bone graft if necessary.

Surgical Technique: Acetabulum

Complete exposure of the acetabulum should be performed before attempting implant removal. Grossly loose cemented implants may be easily removed from the cement mantle, following which the cement mantle can be broken into pieces and removed. It may be much more difficult to remove uncemented implants, even if they do not have stable bone ingrowth. The modular polyethylene liner should be removed if present and screws removed from inside the metal shell. Curved cement chisels are then passed around the backside of the socket with great care taken to avoid injuring the neurovascular structures on the medial side, especially if there is a significant medial wall defect. The cup should be completely freed up before attempting removal so that the extraction of segmental pieces of acetabular bone stock can be avoided. A threaded insertion tool can help to facilitate removal. Otherwise, an offset punch may be used to impact on the upper edge and flip the cup downward for extraction. If it is still impossible to remove the cup, a high-speed drill with a diamond wheel can be used to section the cup into pieces to facilitate removal. At this point the bony defects are assessed and a decision is made whether to use cemented or cementless implants. All of the acetabular membrane should be removed. There will often be cavitary defects containing cement and/or membrane if iliac, pubic, or ischial anchoring holes had been used at the original surgery. Care must be taken in removing large cement fragments that have extruded through the medial wall or fine mesh "Mexican hats" because they may be close to or adherent to the iliac or obturator vessels. If they do not represent an impediment to implant insertion, it may be more prudent to leave them in place and proceed with the reconstruction. If it is necessary to remove components or cement located medial to the quadrilateral plate, the pelvic vessels are at significant risk. An approach has been described in which a retroperitoneal approach is performed first and the major vessels are isolated with loops. The hip is then entered and the implants removed.

For the type 1 defect, use of an uncemented hemispherical socket that obtains purchase on the rim is possible. Alternatively, a new socket may be cemented into place. Morcellized bone graft should be packed into cavitary defects. Acetabular reamers are used to freshen the bony surface and remove irregularities, leaving a bed of healthy, bleeding bone. If an uncemented cup is used, it may be desirable to select a cup that is 2 mm larger than the last reamer to obtain press fit stability. Screw augmentation may be necessary into the ilium or ischium if adequate press fit stability is not achieved.

For the type 2 deformities, larger bone deficiencies must be addressed. Large cavitary defects, including a deficient medial wall, can usually be handled with morcellized bone graft. Deficiencies of the acetabular wall or columns will usually require structural allograft. Femoral head, distal femur, or proximal tibia allografts may be used, depending on the configuration of the defect. A high-speed burr can be used to shape the bone into a shape that straddles the deformity and can then be secured with internal fixation. Alternatively, elliptical-shaped defects can be managed with oblong-shaped cups or uncemented cups with modular metal augments, which will fill the bony defect and bring the center of rotation to a more anatomic position near the teardrop. The last option is to use smaller, uncemented components, placed at a high hip center and then make up for the leg length inequality by using femoral components with an increased neck length. It has been estimated that successful bone ingrowth into porous components can be achieved if the sockets have at least 40% to 50% of their ingrowth surface area adjacent to host bone.

In the type 3 defects, structural allografts are almost always required and the degree of bone loss associated with osteolysis can be so severe that true pelvic dissociation exists. With pelvic dissociation, there may be no remaining bone bridging the ilium above to the ischium below the acetabulum. In these cases, the only grafting option may be an acetabular transplant, which is sculpted to fit snugly against host bone and can then be secured with either pelvic reconstruction plates or by using a large reinforcement ring such as the Burch-Schneider ring, which can act as a large plate. The acetabular component is then cemented into the allograft, preferably into some type of metal reinforcement ring.

Constrained acetabular implants may be used if the soft tissues are so deficient that postoperative stability is in jeopardy. These implants have an altered liner that "captures" the femoral head, markedly increasing the force necessary for dislocation. With sufficient force, however, the implants will dissociate or the bone fixation may fail. The constrained nature of the implant may affect long term success because of the increased risk of loosening or polyethylene wear.

Femoral Reconstruction

After dislocation, enough of the capsule and soft tissue should be removed from the upper femur so that the leg can be rotated into the proper position and the upper femur delivered up out of the wound to allow implant removal and subsequent insertion. It is very common to have bony overgrowth of the greater trochanter, and all bone must be removed from above the shoulder of the implant to avoid fracturing off the greater trochanter during stem extraction. Loose femoral stems will usually come out of the cement mantle very easily, loop extractors for monoblock stems and specialized extractors that bolt onto a Morse taper facilitate stem removal. At times, the entire cement mantle may come out adherent to the stem, but in most cases a portion remains behind as a result of varying degrees of loosening and cement disintegration. If the cement mantle is extremely well fixed with no apparent defects, it may be possible to cement a new stem into the existing cement mantle, downsizing it just enough to allow a new cement layer around the stem. If the cement mantle must be removed, the technique of using a new cement with a threaded extractor (segmental cement extraction system, or "seg-ces", Zimmer, Warsaw, IN) works very well. The remaining cement mantle can also be chiseled out with specialized instruments, with the assistance of ultrasonic tools, pneumatic chisels, and high-speed drills.

With the removal of cementless implants, the stem may be extracted easily if stable bone ingrowth has never been achieved. Stems with bone ingrowth can be extremely difficult to remove. Flexible osteotomes or high-speed drills with wire tips can be used to disrupt the bone/implant interface to aid in extraction. With extensively-coated stems, or stems that are not loose and are precoated with polymethylmethacrylate (PMMA), it may be necessary to use one of the more extensile approaches to the femoral canal.

In the type I deformity, sufficient bone (including cancellous bone) remains behind to allow either cementing a new component or going with a cementless implant. A typical type I deformity is encountered following the removal of a painful, press fit hemiarthroplasty. Although cancellous bone remains in the upper metaphysis, it is usually behind a sclerotic rim of bone (neocortex) that must be freshened with reamers or rasps to allow access to the cancellous bone. A regular length implant may be cemented, with a longer length required only if cortical defects such as screw holes must be bypassed. For cementless implants, the bone is carefully reamed and broached and the uncemented implant inserted. All cementless implants must have intraoperative stability, not only to axial load but to rotation and bending stresses as well. Any cementless implant that does not achieve significant stability is doomed to failure. In any revision situation, it is desirous to have a contingency plan with another type of implant available. If stability cannot be achieved with a cementless implant, it may be necessary to cement the stem. If an uncemented implant is selected with only proximal porous coating, there may be just enough bony compromise to prevent absolute stability and therefore it is helpful to have stems with more extensive porous coating as a backup.

With the type II deformity, although the cortical tube remains intact, nearly all of the cancellous bone from the femoral canal has been lost. Because of the inability to achieve cement interdigitation, cemented implants may be less desirous. If the stem is to be cemented, it may be necessary to switch to a longer stem to have a large surface area with which to attain fixation. Going with a longer cemented stem does not restore bone stock and may make any subsequent re-revision even more difficult.

Uncemented implants can be used, provided the bone is sturdy enough to ensure the intraoperative stability necessary for long-term success. Primary uncemented stems are designed for use in the normal femur without extensive bone loss. In the revision situation, the bone is more compromised and the porous ingrowth surfaces may need to be more extensive. There should be some mechanism to achieve a tight fit both distally and proximally. In the situation of a revision with a loose stem that had been present for years, the upper femur may have remodeled into retroversion. Uncemented stems, such as the S-ROM, (DePuy/Johnson & Johnson, Warsaw, IN) which allow independent placement of the porous ingrowth sleeve and femoral stem are extremely useful to adapt to the abnormal anatomy. Type II defects are also very amenable to impaction grafting. With this technique, the femoral canal is filled with firmly packed morcellized allograft. A metal stem is then cemented into the impacted bone graft and this bone incorporates with time to restore depleted bone stocks.

With the type III defect, more extensive bone grafting and modified implants may be necessary. With the IIIA defect, cortical bone loss extends down to the level of the lesser trochanter and the use of napkin ring allografts for this type of deformity has been described. There has not been a high success rate associated with these grafts. An alternative is to use specialized calcar replacement stems that will sit securely on the remaining medial calcar. These stems may be inserted either with or without cement. Uncemented varieties usually require a longer, coated, metaphyseal segment in order to achieve stability and bony ingrowth. A number of these stems now have available bolts or grips that securely anchor the greater trochanter to the femur and implant. With both type II and IIIA defects, it may be necessary to use an extensively porous-coated stem, if that is the only means by which to achieve implant stability and ingrowth.

With the type IIIB defects, the degree of cortical destruction has now extended below the lesser trochanter, but fortunately, bone below the old prosthesis bed, just above the isthmus, is spared. It may be impossible to use conventional cemented stems because of difficulty in anchoring the stems in the proximal femur. Stems with porous coating limited to the proximal segment are also unsuitable. Long, uncemented stems with extensive porous coating are extremely useful in this type of reconstruction. The distal femoral canal can either be machined with flexible reamers or with straight, tapered reamers to accept either a long, curved, porous-coated implant or a straight, tapered implant with flutes and a roughened titanium surface. Cortical strut allograft can be used to bridge cortical defects and to help restore bone stock. If cement is to be used, it may be necessary to use an entire proximal femoral allograft, cement the stem into the allograft, and to either secure it into the distal femur with an uncemented fluted or press-fit implant or by cementing a long stem into the host bone. Impaction grafting is difficult in this situation because there is an incompetent cortical tube to contain the morcellized bone graft. A transfemoral approach or extended trochanteric osteotomy with grafting not only facilitates implant removal, but also helps to restore proximal femoral bone stock.

With the type IIIC defect, use of an extensively-coated porous stem is much more difficult because the only remaining bone sufficient to anchor the implant is now below the isthmus where the femoral canal is divergent. This makes it very difficult to achieve stable implant bone apposition except at the very top of the cortical tube. A massive proximal femoral allograft is still an option in this situation. A "hybrid" alternative is to cement a long porous-coated stem distally to achieve initial implant stability following a transfemoral or extended osteotomy approach. The remaining proximal femoral bone is crushed around the porous-coated implant, augmenting it with strut allograft and morcellized bone as necessary, to achieve additional fixation to the implant and to help restore proximal femoral bone stock. The results of this technique have not been reported in the literature, but it is one of the options available in these cases of profound bone loss. Tobramycin can be added to the cement at 1.2 g per 40 mg of PMMA powder to lessen the chance of postoperative infection.

Rehabilitation

Patients should be mobile as quickly as possible after surgery, preferably during the first postoperative day. Patients with cemented components can bear weight as tolerated with the exception of impaction grafting, in which partial weightbearing may be delayed until some consolidation of the bone graft takes place, usually after 6 to 12 weeks. With an uncemented femoral component, unless it is a type I deformity with extremely stable fixation, it may be more prudent to proceed with toe-touch weightbearing to prevent subsidence and stem rotation until bony ingrowth occurs, about 6 weeks postimplantation. With an uncemented socket, the patients can bear weight as tolerated, provided that there is excellent bony support for the socket. With less than optimal fixation, or with use of a structural allograft, it may be necessary to restrict weightbearing for 6 to 12 weeks until additional bony consolidation occurs. With a straightforward posterior approach, no special protection of the abductor mechanism is required. If, however, a trochanteric osteotomy or slide was performed, or if an anterolateral approach was used and repair of the abductor mechanism was less than optional, the patient should maintain restricted weightbearing for at least 6 weeks and active abduction exercises should be prohibited during this period. Patients will usually use a walker or crutches until they regain sufficient muscle strength to ambulate with a cane, anywhere from 3 to 12 weeks after surgery. An abduction brace is used if there are concerns regarding hip stability and is used for 6 to 12 weeks after surgery until there has been enough healing of the pericapsular tissues to prevent dislocation.

Complications

Preoperative planning is imperative to avoid complications. Reading the operative note from the previous surgery is extremely helpful. It is beneficial to run through a checklist of necessary equipment and the steps of execution prior to surgery to avoid intraoperative surprises. All of the equipment that may be necessary, along with the required implant and types of bone graft, should be determined beforehand.

Whatever surgical technique is necessary should be used to expose the implants and revise them expeditiously. Without sufficient release of the soft tissues, it may not be possible to restore the required leg length and offset to enhance stability and improve biomechanics. It is important to assess the degree of hip abduction possible after reimplantation; if insufficient, a percutaneous adductor tenotomy is helpful.

If a trochanteric osteotomy or a trochanteric slide is performed, it is necessary to release the pericapsular scar tissue so that the trochanter can be positioned properly, especially if leg lengthening is necessary. In the event of an old trochanteric nonunion with proximal migration, this is especially important to allow reattachment and to permit adequate hip adduction postoperatively.

The risk of intraoperative periprosthetic fracture is higher in the revision case as compared to primary THR. Osteopo rosis is often present. The acetabulum or femur may be fractured during removal of implant and cement or may fracture upon insertion of implants, especially uncemented implants, which require a tight fit. In cases of severe osteoporosis, a femur may fracture with dislocation maneuvers. Long cement chisels and high-speed burrs may perforate the femur. Perforations that are unrecognized may lead to cement extrusion or postoperative periprosthetic fracture because of the presence of stress risers. Fluoroscopy with the use of power tools helps prevent perforation, especially when attempting to remove cement from the depths of the femoral canal. If possible, cortical defects should be bypassed with a femoral component that is longer by at least 2 canal diameters. Femoral perforations should also be covered with cortical onlay graft to heal the defect.

Vascular injuries are much more common in revision surgery because of the degree of dissection necessary for reconstruction, and the proximity of large pelvic vessels to the acetabular component in cases of protrusio. A CT scan with intravenous contrast and/or arteriogram should be performed in the event of a large protrusio deformity or if it is necessary to remove a large cement mass medial to the quadrilateral plate. In a series of 27 cases, safe removal of medial displaced implants and cement was achieved by using a double incision approach. A retroperitoneal approach was made to isolate the iliac vessels. Next, a hip incision was made and the components removed. In this fashion, if brisk bleeding is encountered, control of the vessels could be quickly achieved. When inserting acetabular screws with uncemented acetabular components, it is vital to avoid the anterior cup quadrants to protect the iliac vessels and the obturator neurovascular bundle. Injury to the major nerves about the hip is a devastating complication and can be caused by excessive tension on the soft tissues, inappropriate placement of retractors, laceration, pressure from hematoma, or heat from extruded cement. Injury to the superior gluteal nerve can be prevented by avoiding dissection greater than 5 cm above the tip of the greater trochanter with a Hardinge approach. Lengthening of more than 4 cm has been associated with an increased risk of stretch injury to the sciatic nerve. Somatosensory evoked potential monitoring has been used in the past in an effort to monitor nerve function and minimize the chance of iatrogenic nerve injury. More recently, electromyographic monitoring has been reported to be beneficial in acetabular fracture surgery and is quite useful in hip replacement revision surgery, especially if it is necessary to remove hardware and reconstruct the posterior wall.

Leg length inequality can hamper patient function if severe enough and may cause considerable patient dissatisfaction. With profound shortening, it may not be possible to achieve leg length equality. As part of the preoperative planning it is helpful to be aware of any true leg length inequality as well as any apparent leg length inequality secondary to scoliosis or pelvic tilt. Most implant systems, and especially revision implant systems, make it possible to fine-tune the leg length with a variety of modular implants. Reliable bony landmarks may be absent in revision surgery. A helpful technique is to measure changes in leg length from a fixed point on the pelvis, marked by a Steinmann pin, to a mark made on the fascia of the vastus lateralis or other femoral landmark. By noting the difference before and after implantation, it is possible to approximate the effect on overall leg length.

As can be imagined, the risk of dislocation is much higher after revision surgery, compared to primary THR, because of diminished muscle strength, inadequate soft tissue, and more extensive surgical dissection. Dislocation rates are higher in revision surgery than in primary surgery and are even higher with nonunion of the greater trochanter. A trochanteric osteotomy may not be required in most revision cases but is helpful to enhance stability if the soft tissues are lax. Intraoperative range of motion testing is certainly not foolproof or completely predictive of postoperative stability, but is helpful to obtain a sense of overall implant stability. The physician should check for anterior instability with hip extension and external rotation. It should be possible to flex the hip beyond 90° without dislocation and to achieve at least 30° of internal rotation at 90° of flexion before dislocation occurs. Instability increases dramatically with an acetabular component that has been placed too vertically or into any degree of retroversion. A cup with excessive anteversion may lead to anterior instability. It is necessary to not only fine-tune leg length, but offset as well to maintain the proper soft-tissue tension. Increasing lateralization of the femoral component will help to tighten the soft tissues and increase stability without adding excessive leg length. This can be achieved with cups that add several millimeters of lateralization or with femoral components that have a few millimeters of lateralization built into the component or with stems that have a lower neck shaft angle (in the range of 125° to 130°) to achieve the same effect. Constrained cups are available that have either a hooded polyethylene insert to cover more of the femoral head with an external metal locking ring or a bipolar head component that is contained within a larger polyethylene bearing and external metal locking ring to contain the femoral head once engaged. These devices may be helpful in cases of recurrent dislocation, which have been refractory to more conventional approaches such as bracing or trochanteric advancement. A population of recurrent dislocators achieved a success rate of 96% with a constrained acetabular insert. While effective at reducing the incidence of dislocation, these implants increase the complexity of the articulation and run the risk of failure from dissociation or accelerated polyethylene wear and therefore should be considered as an approach of last resort.

Heterotopic ossification can mar an otherwise excellent reconstruction by significantly reducing range of motion and functional improvement if severe enough. Patients at risk (those with previous heterotopic ossification, ankylosing spondylitis, or diffuse idiopathic skeletal hypertrophy) should be identified and extra efforts taken to prevent ossification. Prophylaxis can be achieved with either nonsteroidal anti-inflammatory drugs such as indomethacin or with radiation therapy to the periarticular soft tissues. Doses as low as 700 cGy have been documented to be effective at preventing heterotopic ossification and have also been reported to be effective if given in a preoperative dose.

Results

In assessing the results of THR revision, several issues must be considered. Some measure of outcome success must be employed to assess the results of reconstruction. Certainly the most valuable studies are those with long follow-up times. Studies with a high percentage of patients lost to follow-up may be suspect because it is not possible to determine how many of those lost to follow-up eventually went on to failure. In any series, the definition of "failure" must be determined. Certainly any re-revision must be viewed as a failure, but failures must also include reconstructions that have become loose and will go on to require revision, should the patient live long enough and remain sufficiently active. The degree of bone loss in the femur and acetabulum should be stated; otherwise, meaningful comparisons between studies may not be possible.

Cemented Total Hip Revision

There is considerable evidence that THR in the primary situation performed with cement can yield extremely good results in the long term, especially on the femoral side. With revision THR, the situation is much different. Following removal of the components in revision surgery, the bone of the acetabulum and femur are often very sclerotic, making cement interdigitation difficult, and overall bone quality is often greatly compromised. There may be considerable bony deficiencies, making the overall volume of bone available for fixation even more diminished.

The earliest series of revision hip replacements were done with standard-sized components inserted with "first-generation" cement techniques. In one series, the results of 110 revisions performed both in New York and Boston were reported. At an average of 3.4 years, 1.8% of the acetabular components and 5.4% of the femoral components required revision. An alarming frequency of radiolucent lines were noted. In a subsequent follow-up study of the same patients at 8.1 years, the overall failure rate had risen to 29%.

In another study of 66 patients with an average follow-up of 2.1 years, revision rates of 3% for acetabular component and 9% for the femoral component were noted. However, radiographic failures were seen in an additional 71% and 29%, respectively. In another series of 166 patients with an average follow-up of 4.5 years, the acetabular revision rate was 2.5%, the femoral revision rate 6%, and radiographic failure rate 53% and 44%, respectively. In a study with reference to the femoral component alone, of 112 patients at 6.5 years of follow-up, stem revision was required in 3.6% with only an additional 7.7% showing radiographic evidence of loosening.

The age of the patient at the time of revision surgery can play a role, because younger patients are much more active and therefore more likely to fail. In a series of patients from Sweden, all of whom were younger than age 55 years, 67 patients were studied at an average of 4 years' follow-up. Twenty-one percent of patients required a revision with an additional 36% demonstrating radiographic loosening. A follow-up study of the same patients was extended to an average of 10 years. A total of 83% had either undergone revision or demonstrated radiographic loosening. The authors recommend alternative solutions in younger, active patients. Results can be somewhat better in older patients. In a series of 60 patients at 5 to 14 years' follow-up and an average age of 71, the overall loosening rate was 18.5% for cups and 29% for stems with a survivorship of 85% at 14 years, with 4 of 60 patients undergoing revision for loosening. In an effort to attain better fixation with significant proximal loss, others have suggested using a longer cemented stem. In a study of 110 hips at 5 years minimum of follow-up (average, 6.7 years) there was a 12% failure rate along with a 16% incidence of perforation and a 5% fracture rate. The difficulty in removing cement from the depths of the femur in the next revision should be kept in mind.

Improved cementing techniques have been shown to be beneficial in improving survival of the femoral component in primary cemented THR. The same seems to hold true in the revision situation. In a series of 47 hips, reviewed at a minimum 10-year follow-up, the femoral revision rate was 9.5% with an overall radiographic failure rate of 26%. This was seen as well in another series of 38 hips reported at a minimum 10-year follow-up, the femoral revision rate was 10.5% with an additional 10.5% shown to be radiographically loose. Another study, of 110 patients at 4.6-year follow-up, showed a femoral revision rate of 3.6% with an overall radiographic loosening rate of 5%. A study from England reported on the use of the Charnley cemented stem in 351 femoral revisions over a 16-year period, average 6-year follow-up. Femoral revision rate was 5.7% with an additional 7.1% radiographically loose. The results were better when improved cement techniques were used.

Other studies have not demonstrated a benefit with "modern" techniques. In a series of 139 patients reported at 3.6 years, the revision rate was 8.6% with an overall radiographic failure rate of 16%.

The prognosis is even more guarded with a second or third cemented revision. One series reported 45 cases that underwent a second revision and 7 cases that had a third revision done, at an average follow-up of 3 to 3.5 years. Despite the relatively short follow-up, mechanical failure was present in 24% and 29%, respectively.

In the face of severe bone loss, the desire to use cement may have to be coupled with techniques to restore or augment existing bone stock. Techniques using morcellized allograft bone (impaction grafting) have been described for both acetabular and femoral reconstruction. A series of 88 hips were revised for cavitary or segmented defects of the acetabulum and reviewed at 5.7 years' follow-up. Metal reconstruction mesh was fashioned to contain the morcellized bone at either the periphery of the segmented defect or at the depth of a cavitary defect, after which an acetabular component is cemented in place. At follow-up, there were 4 revisions and 6 cases of radiographic failure for an overall failure rate of 11.4%. This study has been extended to an average follow-up of 11.8 years for 62% of the cases (minimum 10-year follow-up) with 37 cavitary defects and 23 combined cavitary/segmented defects. There were 5 revisions and 4 radiographic failures with an overall survival rate of 90%.

An alternative method for cemented acetabular revision is to use metal reinforcement rings. An acetabular reinforcement ring was used in 27 cases reported at an average follow-up of 7.2 years (5 to 10 years). Migration of the implant was seen in 44% of cases, and in 50% of cases with segmental bone defects. The best results were obtained when there was intimate host bone contact by the ring.

For the deficient femur, impaction grafting is gaining popularity as a means to enhance bone stock. Morcellized bone is tightly impacted into the femur above a distal restrictor and then a stem is cemented into the mantle of morcellized bone. One series reported 60 cases with 2 to 5 years' follow-up. There was some degree of subsidence of the stem within the cement mantle in 48% of cases, yet only 7% showed subsidence of the cement/graft composite within the cortical tube. Two failed because of sepsis, 3 from fracture of the femur, and 3 required cup exchange. Although preliminary results are promising in that they may provide a reliable way to augment bone stock, the high incidence of subsidence is disturbing and longer follow-up is required to ensure continued stability of the stem. Another study of 79 cases treated with this technique revealed an 11% incidence of massive subsidence (greater than 10 mm) with an additional 11% showing subsidence to a lesser degree.

In cases of massive bone loss, there may be little choice other than the use of substantial structural bone graft in addition to morcellized bone graft. Cavitary acetabular defects, such as the Paprosky type 1, can usually be managed with morcellized graft, even if substantial in size. Cases with large segmental defects or acetabular dissociation may require structural graft. Uncemented acetabular components may be considered if at least 50% of the component can be placed on viable host bone; otherwise, a cemented acetabular component is preferred. One study reported on the results of 67 minor column defects at 7.1 years with an 86% success rate. For the major column defects, 107 cases were reported at an average of 7.1 years follow-up. The success rate fell to 55% in this series but results were better when a metal reinforcement ring or cage had been used. With this type of construct, 7 out of 8 were successful, with the one failure caused by infection. The long-term prognosis for structural allografts for the acetabulum remains guarded. In a series of 15 allografts and 55 autografts at an average of 16.5 years, there was an incidence of socket loosening of 66% and 60%, respectively. Although the grafts could heal to host bone reliably, after many years graft revascularization and subsequent resorption would lead to collapse. There may be no other alternative to structural graft in these severe cases and the bone that does incorporate may make subsequent revision easier.

An alternative to structural graft is to use a larger version of the acetabular reinforcement ring, the Burch-Schneider antiprotrusio cage with flanges that lie against the ilium and ischium. The cage is secured with screws, bone graft is placed behind the shell and a polyethylene socket is cemented. One series reported on the use of the cage in 42 cases at an average follow-up of 5 years (range, 2 to 11 years). There was an overall failure rate of 24%, divided evenly between infection and aseptic loosening. In another study of 28 cases, the average follow-up was 33 months. Eighty percent reported minimal or no pain and remained community ambulators. Fourteen percent of the cages had migrated, but none required revision.

With massive bone loss of the proximal femur, structural allograft can be used in concert with a long stem that is cemented only to the allograft. A step-cut is used at the junction of allograft and host bone to provide additional rotational stability along with bone grafting of the junction and application of any remaining proximal bone to the allograft. In a large series of 200 cases that had been followed for at least 2 years, the success rate was 85% and the revision rate was 12.5%.

Cementless Acetabular Reconstruction

Because of the very high incidence of radiographic loosening following cemented acetabular revision, there has been a growing trend toward cementless fixation. Two studies reinforce the notion that cementless fixation may indeed be superior. One study reported the results of 129 hips followed for an average of 44 months. Eighty percent of the cases required morcellized autograft or allograft packed into defects. The revision rate was 5%, caused by either infection or instability. There were no cases of aseptic loosening. This study was updated in 1996 with an average follow-up of 8.3 years. None of the cases were revised for loosening or demonstrated migration. Another study with longer follow-up at 7 years (range, 5 to 12 years) reported the results in 57 hips. None were revised or awaiting revision and there was no evidence of radiographic loosening, despite use of bone graft in 79%. These results strongly suggest that cementless acetabular components offer the best revision solution in the intermediate term. In a similar study of 140 hips with an average follow-up of 41 months, bone grafting was also required in 91% of cases. There were only 2 cases of aseptic loosening, both in the face of severe bone loss and pelvic discontinuity.

As in the case of cemented revision, structural allograft may be necessary with large segmental defects or pelvic discontinuity. Sixty-seven distal femoral allografts used in cases of Paprosky type 3A or type 3B defects were studied at an average of 6.1 years. Failure occurred in 3 of the 48 3A defects and in 7 out of 11 of the 3B defects. Twenty of the 3B defects were treated instead with acetabular transplant. After 32 months, there were only 2 failures, both for infection. The authors recommend a distal femur for the type 3A defect but prefer an acetabular transplant for the 3B defects. Uncemented shells may be used if approximately 40% to 50% of the component can be placed against host bone. Otherwise, the cup should be cemented.

An alternative technique in the face of superior segmental defects is to use uncemented components placed at a high hip center. The advantage in this situation is that structural allograft is not required and the majority of the implant can be placed against host bone. The downside is that the anatomic hip center is not restored, the greater trochanter may need to be advanced distally, and a calcar replacement type stem should be used to equilibrate leg length. In a study evaluating the high hip center, 49 revisions were done at a hip center averaging approximately 3 cm higher than normal. In the majority of cases, small acetabular implants were required. There were no cases of revision for loosening; 3 cups had a complete radiolucent line. Despite the high hip center, it was possible to lengthen the leg in the majority of cases.

The other alternative to the high hip center is to use jumbo uncemented components. The cups are stabilized on the remaining acetabular rim and cavitary defects are filled with morcellized bone. One review of 19 cases employing cups in the range of 70 to 80 mm was reported at an average of 10 years' follow-up. One case was revised for sepsis; none were revised for loosening.

A novel approach is to use specialized implants such as oblong cups or bilobed modular components to maximize the host implant contact area and restore the hip center to an anatomic position and equilibrate leg lengths.

Cementless Femoral Reconstruction

The difficulties in achieving good cement interdigitation into bone with cemented revision has been discussed. Second- and third-generation cement techniques may improve results but, as with acetabular components, there is a growing trend toward uncemented implants. There are 2 schools of thought. The first is to use extensively-coated implants and achieve distal fixation in all cases of femoral revision. The second is to use proximally coated implants in order to recreate a normal stress distribution in the femur and hopefully to prevent the problems with long-term stress shielding.

Several studies have demonstrated good results with an extensively-coated stem. One series of 174 hips were followed for an average of 7.4 years with a minimum 5-year follow-up. The revision rate was 5.7% with an additional radiographic loosening of 1.1% for an overall failure rate of 6.9%. Survivorship was 91% at 9 years. Failures were attributed to an undersized femoral component. Another study reported the results of 175 hips followed at an average of 5 years. Ninety-six percent of the components remained in place, 4 were revised for painful loosening, 2 as part of a resection arthroplasty and 1 for infection. Eighty-three percent were considered to be bony ingrown, 16% as being stable fibrous and 1.7% as having unstable fibrous ingrowth. Severe stress shielding was seen in 8% of cases.

In a large series of 297 revisions at an average follow-up of 8.2 years, a long, curved, fully-coated implant was used along with an extended proximal femoral osteotomy in a large number of cases. The mechanical failure rate was reported at

2.4%. In revisions with 90% or greater canal fill, subsidence was less than 2%. For those with canal fill averaging 75%, subsidence was greater than 2 mm with an average of 7 mm. It was recommended that at least 4 cm or preferably 6 cm of "scratch fit" intimate contact be obtained in the endosteum of the distal femur.

Concerns about stress shielding, especially with larger diameter stems, along with the difficulty of removing an extensively coated stem, keep the interest level in proximally-coated implants high. However, cementless femoral revision with proximally-coated implant has been less predictable. One problem is that a number of earlier uncemented revision stems were simply longer versions of a primary type stem that made intimate contact between the proximal porous coating and host bone difficult to achieve. One study of 375 hips using 6 different stem designs, at an average follow-up of 4.7 years, had only a 58% survival rate at 8 years; this rate dropped to only 20% if radiographic loosening was considered. An additional study reported an 8.7% revision rate and 20% radiographic loosening rate in 69 hips using a bowed stem (Osteonics, Allendale, NJ) at 2.8 years. In addition, there was a 46% fracture rate.

Discouraging results were reported in a study of 49 hips at an average follow-up of 65 months (range, 48 to 87 months) with the BIAS (Zimmer, Warsaw, IN) stem, a long, bowed titanium stem that lacks circumferential porous coating. Four percent were revised, but an additional 45% demonstrated progressive subsidence. Survival was 96% at 6 years with revision as the end point, but only 37% with subsidence as the end point.

Better results have been obtained with a proximally-coated titanium calcar replacement type stem using cortical strut onlay allograft when necessary. Six revisions were required for a 3% failure rate with 98% union rate of the strut grafts. However, another study using the same implant reported their results in 52 hips at 4- to 6-year follow-up. Ten percent of the stems were revised for aseptic loosening and another 14% showed radiographic evidence of loosening. However, 11 of the 12 failures occurred in cases with moderate to severe proximal bone loss, and therefore may represent improper selection in these types of cases. A 40% incidence of femoral fracture was reported.

An alternative type of implant is a modular stem with a variety of implant sizes available proximally for each distal diameter. In this fashion, the bone can be machined with a better proximal as well as distal fit, while the modular sleeve can be oriented independently of the stem to maximize contact and stability. In a series of 52 hips, using the S-ROM (DePuy/Johnson & Johnson, Warsaw, IN) stem, reported at 3 years, there was a 10% mechanical loosening rate. However, most of these had profound bone loss and 22% required structural femoral allograft as well. In another series of 104 hips with the same implant at 2- to 8-year follow-up, there was a 5.8% incidence of revision and radiographic loosening, with 82% having good or excellent hip scores.

A smaller study of 34 patients with the same implant was reported at an average of 51 months' follow-up. Eighty-eight percent had either slight or no pain, 1 stem was revised for infection and all but 1 of the remainder demonstrated radiographic evidence of stable bony ingrowth.

Summary

Preoperative planning is the key to success in THR. The surgeon must have command of all the various approaches necessary to not only expose the hip but to allow insertion of the proper implants. It is necessary to assess the degree of bone deficit and be prepared to correct the defects with either morcellized or structural bone graft. The implants must be stable on completion of surgery and can be inserted with or without cement, depending on the situation. Bone augmentation of defects is especially important in the younger patient so that there may be more and not less bone to work with on the next revision.

Annotated Bibliography

Aribindi R, Barba M, Solomon MI, Arp P, Paprosky W: Bypass fixation. *Orthop Clin North Am* 1998;29:319-329.

The results of 297 revisions with an average follow-up of 8.2 years are reported with a long curved, extensively-coated stem. The mechanical failure rate was 2.4%. The benefits of an extended trochanteric osteotomy are elucidated.

Cabanela ME: Reconstruction rings and bone graft in total hip revision surgery. *Orthop Clin North Am* 1998;29:255-262.

This study outlines the role of various metal reinforcements rings and cages in cases of severe bony deficiency of the acetabulum.

Cameron H: Experience with proximal ingrowth implantation in hip revision surgery. *Acta Orthop Belg* 1997;63(suppl 1):66-68.

One hundred four proximally-coated modular stems were inserted with an average follow-up of 2 to 8 years. The combined revision and radiographic loosening rate was 5.8%.

Cameron HU: Modified cups. *Orthop Clin North Am* 1998;29: 277-295.

The technique of using oblong, uncemented acetabular components as an alternative to structural bone graft for segmental defects of the acetabulum is demonstrated.

Chandler HP, Ayres DK, Tan RC, Anderson LC, Varma AK: Revision total hip replacement using the S-ROM femoral component. *Clin Orthop* 1995;319:130-140.

This study reports on the use of a modular proximally-coated stem in 52 hips, at an average follow-up of 3 years. Extensive bone defects required the use of structural allografts in 22 cases (42%). Mechanical loosening was present in 9.6%.

Elting JJ, Mikhail WE, Zicat BA, Hubbell JC, Lane LE, House B: Preliminary report of impaction grafting for exchange femoral arthroplasty. *Clin Orthop* 1995;319:159-167.

The use of impaction grafting for femoral revision in 60 patients is reported at an average of 2 to 5 years. Forty-eight stems subsided an average of 2.8 mm inside the cement mantle with a 7% incidence of subsidence within the cortical tube. A 13% revision rate was noted for sepsis, femoral fracture, and cup exchange.

Gross AE, Duncan CP, Garbuz D, Mohamed EM: Revision arthroplasty of the acetabulum in association with loss of bone stock. *J Bone Joint Surg* 1998;80A:440-451.

The authors report their results with cavitary defects and segmented defects of the acetabulum. Cavitary defects had a 90% success rate at 6.8 years. The minor column defects had a success rate of 86% at 7.1 years, while the major column defect cases had a success rate of 55% at 7.1 years.

Gross AE, Hutchison CR: Proximal femoral allografts for reconstruction of bone stock in revision arthroplasty of the hip. *Orthop Clin North Am* 1998;29:313-317.

Results of 200 proximal femoral structural allografts were reported at a minimum of 2 years' follow-up. The incidence of revision was 12.5% with a "successful" outcome seen in 85%.

Jasty M: Jumbo cups and morsalized graft. *Orthop Clin North Am* 1998;29:249-254.

Nineteen cases with a "jumbo" cup (70 to 80 mm) were reported at an average of 10 years' follow-up. One cup was removed for sepsis; none were revised for loosening. The author believes that this technique is a good alternative to structural bone grafting.

Katz RP, Callaghan JJ, Sullivan PM, Johnston RC: Results of cemented femoral revision total hip arthroplasty using improved cementing techniques. *Clin Orthop* 1995;319:178-183.

"Second-generation" techniques were used in 47 hips with a minimum of 10 years' follow-up. The revision rate was 9.5%, with an overall failure rate of 26.1%.

Lachiewicz PF, Poon ED: Revision of a total hip arthroplasty with a Harris-Galante porous- coated acetabular component inserted without cement: A follow-up note on the results at five to twelve years. *J Bone Joint Surg* 1998;80A:980-984.

The authors extended a previous study of patients who underwent a cementless revision of the acetabulum with the Harris-Galante socket. Average follow-up was 7 years (range, 5 to 12 years). No patients had undergone revision or were awaiting revision, and there was no radiographic evidence of loosening despite the use of bone grafting for defects in 79% of cases.

McLaughlin JR, Harris WH: Revision of the femoral component of a total hip arthroplasty with the calcar-replacement femoral component: Results after a mean of 10.8 years postoperatively. *J Bone Joint Surg* 1996;78A:331-339.

The use of a cemented calcar replacement stem is reported, mostly for proximal medial bone loss. Thirty-eight hips were followed at an average of 10.8 years (5.8 to 16.6). Twenty-one percent were revised with an additional 11% demonstrating radiographic loosening. Having only 1 size available generated suboptimal cement mantles and a higher incidence of cement loosening.

Moreland JR, Bernstein ML: Femoral revision hip arthroplasty with uncemented, porous-coated stems. *Clin Orthop* 1995;319: 141-150.

An extensively-porous coated stem was used in 175 cases, an average 5-year follow-up. Most stems achieved either a bone ingrowth or stable fibrous ingrowth, 96% of the stems remain in place. There were 7 revisions, and severe stress shielding was seen in 8%.

Mulliken BD, Rorabeck CH, Bourne RB: Uncemented revision total hip arthroplasty: A 4- to-6-year review. *Clin Orthop* 1996; 325:156-162.

The results of 52 cementless revisions were reported at 4- to 6-year follow-up. Femoral revision was performed with a long titanium stem with proximal porous coating. Six percent of sockets showed radiologic loosening but none required revision. However, 10% of stems required revision with an additional 14% showing radiologic loosening. Eleven of the 12 failures were in femora with grade 3 or 4 bone loss. The intraoperative fracture rate of the femur was 40%. Alternative stem types were recommended in cases of severe proximal bone deficiency of the femur.

Mulroy WF, Harris WH: Revision total hip arthroplasty with use of so-called second-generation cementing techniques for aseptic loosening of the femoral component: A fifteen-year-average follow-up study. *J Bone Joint Surg* 1996;78A:325-330.

The results of 43 cemented femoral revisions were reported at an average follow-up of 15.1 years. Twenty percent were revised. An additional 6% were radiographically loose for an overall failure rate of 26%. "Second-generation" techniques on the femur improved results compared to other long-term studies.

Paprosky WG, Bradford MS, Jablonsky WS: Acetabular reconstruction with massive acetabular allografts, in Pritchard DJ (ed): *Instructional Course Lectures 45*. Rosemont, IL, American Academy of Orthopaedic Surgeons, 1996, pp 149-159.

The authors reported on the use of distal femoral allograft in 67 cases and acetabular transplant in 20 cases. Acetabular transplants were recommended in the most severe (type 3B) deformities whereas distal femoral allografts were sufficient for type 3A deformity.

Peters CL, Rivero DP, Kull LR, Jacobs JJ, Rosenberg AG, Galante JO: Revision total hip arthroplasty without cement: Subsidence of proximally porous-coated femoral components. *J Bone Joint Surg* 1995;77A:1217-1226.

The authors reported on cementless femoral revision in 49 hips, followed an average of 65 months (range, 48 to 87 months) with a long curved titanium stem with proximal ingrowth pads. While only 4% had been revised at follow-up, a total of 45% had progressive subsidence. Survival at 6 years was 96% with revision as the end point but only 37% when considering revision plus subsidence. The authors do not recommend the use of a noncircumferentially coated titanium stem that does not achieve adequate apposition of host bone to porous coating.

Petrera P, Trakru S, Mehta S, Steed D, Towers JD, Rubash HE: Revision total hip arthroplasty with a retroperitoneal approach to the iliac vessels. *J Arthroplasty* 1996;11:704-708.

A technique is described for revision surgery in which the iliac vessels are at risk for injury. A retroperitoneal approach is performed with dissection of the iliac vessels and placement of silicone loops. The wound is closed temporarily and the revision total hip is performed. If bleeding is encountered, tensioning the loops allows for control of hemorrhage and rapid exposure of the vessels. No significant complications were reported in 23 cases.

Raut VV, Siney PD, Wroblewski BM: Revision for aseptic stem loosening using the cemented Charnley prosthesis: A review of 351 hips. *J Bone Joint Surg* 1995;77B:23-27.

This study reported on the use of various models of the Charnley stem for cemented femoral revision in 351 hips at an average follow-up of 6 years. Twenty stems (5.7%) had been revised, and another 25 (7.1%) showed some radiographic evidence of loosening. Survivorship was 97% at 8 years, 92% at 11 years. As techniques changed over the course of the study, the authors believed that the important features in attaining a long lasting result were the use of a cement plug, achieving a uniform cement mantle, and excavating into the lesser trochanter to achieve additional fixation in cancellous bone.

Shinar AA, Harris WH: Bulk structural autogenous grafts and allografts for reconstruction of the acetabulum in total hip arthroplasty: Sixteen-year-average follow-up. *J Bone Joint Surg* 1997; 79A:159-168.

Ten of 15 structural allografts used for revision surgery failed at an average of 16.5 years. The greater the coverage of components by allograft bone, the higher the failure rate. In most cases, some bone did incorporate, making re-revision easier.

Silverton CD, Rosenberg AG, Sheinkop MB, Kull LR, Galante JO: Revision of the acetabular component without cement after total hip arthroplasty: A follow-up note regarding results at seven to eleven years. *J Bone Joint Surg* 1996;78A:1366-1370.

This study extends the follow-up of Padgett's study from 1993 to 8.3 years (range, 7 to 11 years) in 115 hips. While an additional 6 hips required revision in the intervening years, none were revised for acetabular loosening. No cups demonstrated radiographic migration, although 5% did have a complete radiolucent line. Suvivorship was 87% at 9 years.

Slooff TJ, Schreurs BW, Buma P, Gardeniers JW: Impaction morcellized allografting and cement, in Cannon WD Jr (ed): *Instructional Course Lectectures 48*. Rosemont, IL, American Academy of Orthopaedic Surgeons, 1998, pp 265-274.

Impaction grafting technique of the acetabulum was reported in 88 hips at 5.7 year follow-up, the combined revision and radiographic loosening rate was 11.4%.

Weber KL, Callaghan JJ, Goetz DD, Johnston RC: Revision of a failed cemented total hip prosthesis with insertion of an acetabular component without cement and a femoral component with cement: A five to eight-year follow-up study. *J Bone Joint Surg* 1996;78A:982-994.

Sixty-one hybrid revisions (uncemented socket, cemented stem) were compared with all cemented revisions done by the same surgeon at a follow-up of 5 to 8 years. Forty-nine hips were available for follow-up evaluation. Both populations had about the same overall femoral failure rate of 8% and 9% respectively; however, survival of the acetabular component was markedly better in the hybrid group with an overall failure rate of 2%, compared to 30% in the group done entirely with cement. The authors conclude that although cemented femoral revision with "second-generation" techniques produce reasonable results, cemented acetabular revision should be abandoned.

Younger TI, Bradford MS, Magnus RE, Paprosky WG: Extended proximal femoral osteotomy: A new technique for femoral revision arthroplasty. *J Arthroplasty* 1995;10:329-338.

An extended femoral osteotomy is described that facilitates implant and cement removal and implant positioning. A high healing rate was noted and a modification of the postoperative regimen was not required.

Classic Bibliography

Callaghan JJ, Salvati EA, Pellicci PM, Wilson PD Jr, Ranawat CS: Results of revision for mechanical failure after cemented total hip replacement, 1979 to 1982: A two to five-year follow-up. *J Bone Joint Surg* 1985;67A:1074-1085.

Head WC, Wagner RA, Emerson RH, Jr, Malinin TI: Revision total hip arthroplasty in the deficient femur with a proximal load-bearing prosthesis. *Clin Orthop* 1994;298:119-126.

Kavanagh BF, Ilstrup DM, Fitzgerald RH, Jr: Revision total hip arthroplasty. *J Bone Joint Surg* 1985;67A:517-526.

Lawrence JM, Engh CA, Macalino GE: Revision total hip arthroplasty: Long-term results without cement. *Orthop Clin North Am* 1993;24:635-644.

Padgett DE, Kull L, Rosenberg A, Sumner DR, Galante JO: Revision of the acetabular component without cement after total hip arthroplasty: Three to six-year follow-up. *J Bone Joint Surg* 1993;75A:663-673.

Pak JH, Paprosky WG, Jablonsky WS, Lawrence JM: Femoral strut allografts in cementless revision total hip arthroplasty. *Clin Orthop* 1993;295:172-178.

Pellicci PM, Wilson PD Jr, Sledge CB, et al: Long-term results of revision total hip replacement. A follow-up report. *J Bone Joint Surg* 1985;67A:513-516.

Schutzer SF, Harris WH: High placement of porous-coated acetabular components in complex total hip arthroplasty. *J Arthroplasty* 1994;9:359-367.

Tanzer M, Drucker D, Jasty M, McDonald M, Harris WH: Revision of the acetabular component with an uncemented Harris-Galante porous-coated prosthesis. *J Bone Joint Surg* 1992;74A:987-994.

Section 3
The Knee

Chapter 26
Knee Joint: Anatomy and Biomechanics

Chapter 27
Evaluating the Arthritic Knee

Chapter 28
Nonarthroplasty Alternatives in Knee Arthritis

Chapter 29
Biomechanics of Total Knee Design

Chapter 30
Fixation in Total Knee Replacement: Bone Ingrowth

Chapter 31
Surgical Principles of Total Knee Replacement: Incisions, Extensor Mechanism, Ligament Balancing

Chapter 32
The Knee: Rehabilitation

Chapter 33
Evaluation of Results of Total Knee Arthroplasty

Chapter 34
Long-Term Results of Total Knee Replacement

Chapter 35
Complications Associated With Total Knee Arthroplasty

Chapter 36
Revision Total Knee Replacement

Chapter 26
Knee Joint: Anatomy and Biomechanics

Introduction

The stability and mobility of the knee are dependent on complex interactions between the shape of the articulating surfaces, passive soft tissue surrounding the joints, and active muscle contraction. A change in one of these fundamental components (articular surface, ligaments, or muscle function) can produce profound changes in the function of the other structures of the knee joint. Advances in reconstructive procedures, as well as increasing demands for improved function following treatment, have required a better understanding of the interaction between the fundamental anatomy of the knee and biomechanical function. There is a particular need for an improved understanding of the dynamic function of the knee joint. This chapter will focus on the interrelationships between knee anatomy and the functional biomechanics of the knee joint. The fundamental anatomy and passive biomechanics of the knee joint have been well described, but new information is being generated on the dynamic interaction between active muscle contraction and the passive characteristics of the joint.

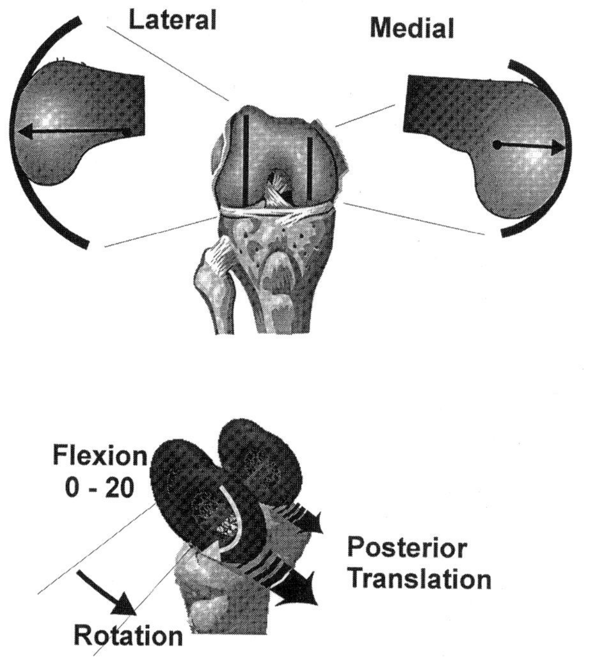

Figure 1

The distal curvature of the lateral femoral condyle is larger than that of the medial femoral condyle. As a result, during the early ranges of knee flexion, the femur rotates externally and translates posteriorly a greater distance on the lateral tibial articular surface than on the medial tibial articular surface. This coupling of rotation with flexion as the femur approaches full extension has been described as "screw-home" movement.

Passive Motion and Tibiofemoral Joint Anatomy

Passive motion is generated from external forces acting on the segments adjacent to the knee joint in the absence of active muscle contraction. The forces that act under these conditions are much lower than the type of forces generated during dynamic functions, such as walking. The majority of the information on the passive mechanics of the knee comes from studies using cadaver material, anatomic dissection, and mathematical models. This information is useful, but it cannot always be extrapolated to the interpretation of dynamic function, because the dynamic forces generated by the muscles are sometimes nearly an order of magnitude greater than the passive ligamentous restraint forces.

The passive motion of the knee joint is governed by the geometry of the articular surfaces and by restraint of the passive soft tissue surrounding the joint. For example, consider the motion of the tibiofemoral joint. The distal radius of the lateral and medial femoral condyles is substantially different (Fig. 1). The radius of a circle placed through the distal portion of the medial femoral condyle is approximately one half that of the lateral femoral condyle. The asymmetric geometry of the femoral condyles can be related to some important intrinsic biomechanical characteristics of the knee joint. Passive flexion between 0° and 20° of flexion involves primarily rolling motion (as opposed to sliding motion). Thus for the same angular change (flexion) the condyle with the larger radius will move further than the condyle with the

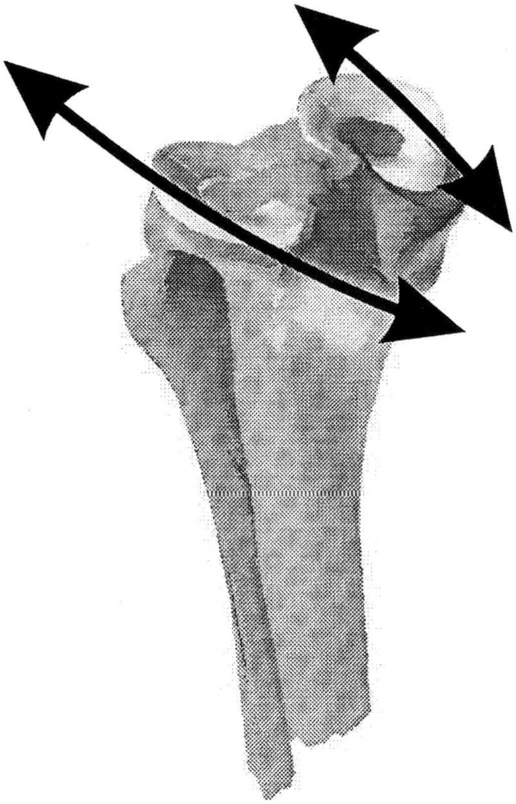

Figure 2

Its attachment permits the lateral meniscus greater mobility than the medial meniscus. This increased mobility of the lateral meniscus allows greater movement of the lateral femoral condyle in early flexion as described in Figure 1.

smaller radius. Consequently, as the knee flexes from a fully extended position, the lateral femoral condyle will roll posteriorly further than the medial femoral condyle. This coupling of motion between flexion and rotation of the knee has been observed during passive motion and described as the "screw-home" movement. It should be noted that this movement takes place because passively the femoral condyle rolls over the surface of the tibia between 0° and 20° of flexion. When a wheel rolls without sliding, there is a 1:1 correspondence between the point of contact on the femur and its adjacent point on the tibia. Therefore, the lateral femoral condyle with the larger radius will travel further during rolling. Beyond 20° of flexion, and during activities where the movement of the femur with respect to the tibia is influenced by external forces such as active muscle contraction, the femur can slip relative to the tibia. Passively, beyond 20° of flexion, the relative femoral tibial movement is dominated by slip at the interface between the femur and the tibia.

Meniscal Function

The lack of conformity between the articular surfaces is mediated by the presence of the menisci. Both menisci are thicker at the periphery and become thin towards the center of the joint. On cross section they have a wedge-like appearance. Load bearing is an important function of the menisci. Strong evidence exists that the menisci support a large fraction of the load on the knee joint. In addition, they distribute this load between the lateral and medial surfaces of the knee. The menisci also provide anterior-posterior stability to the knee. The medial meniscus has been described as the secondary restraint to anterior tibial displacement in the absence of the anterior cruciate ligament. The medial meniscus is more securely attached to the surface of the tibia and has less mobility than the lateral meniscus. Both menisci are fixed to the tibia at their anterior and posterior horns while the rest of the structure is freely mobile.

The relatively greater mobility of the lateral meniscus is consistent with the difference in the motion of the lateral and medial femoral condyles. The mobility of the lateral meniscus allows for the increased movement of the lateral femoral condyle (in early flexion) relative to the medial femoral condyle (Fig. 2). This interaction between the geometry of the femoral condyles and meniscal function is one of many examples of the close functional interaction between the anatomic structures of the knee.

Cruciate Ligaments

The cruciate ligaments play a central role in modulating the dynamic interactions between many of the anatomic structures that determine knee function; therefore, the cruciate ligaments play a fundamental role in the overall function of the knee joint. It is useful to examine the functional role of the cruciate ligaments relative to the other constituents of the knee joint. The absence of one or both of these ligaments will substantially change the mechanics of walking and the performance of other activities of daily living, such as stair climbing.

The anterior and posterior cruciate ligaments are located in the center of the knee joint and provide primary restraint to anterior-posterior movement of the knee. The anterior cruciate ligament (ACL) attaches to the posterior portion of the medial surface of the lateral femoral condyle in the form of a segment of a circle. It is oriented slightly oblique to the vertical, with the anterior side straight and the posterior side convex. The tibial attachment of the ACL is in front of and lateral to the interior tibial spine. While the primary role of the ACL is to provide anterior restraining forces, it also resists varus-valgus rotation of the tibia, especially in the absence of the collateral ligaments. In addition, this ligament resists internal rotation of the tibia.

The posterior cruciate ligament (PCL) originates at the lateral aspect of the medial femoral condyle and inserts on the most prominent aspect of the intercondylar area of the tibia. Its femoral attachment is shaped like a segment of a circle horizontally directed with the upward boundary of attachment horizontal and the lower boundary convex and parallel to the lower articular margin of the condyle. The main function of the PCL is to resist posterior translation of the tibia relative to the femur. The PCL provides approximately 95% of the total restraining force against posterior translation of the tibia when the knee is at 90° of flexion. Recent studies of ligament morphology have demonstrated that the PCL increases in cross-sectional area from its tibial attachment to its femoral attachment. Conversely, the ACL decreases in area from its tibial attachment to its femoral attachment. The PCL cross-sectional area is approximately 50% greater than that of the ACL at the femoral attachment and 20% greater at the tibial attachment. The PCL is also divided into 2 functional components: the anterior lateral, which is taut in knee flexion, and the posterior medial which is taut in knee extention. The anterior lateral component is stiffer and stronger than the posterior medial component.

Functional Role of the Cruciate Ligaments

The cruciate ligaments appear crossed when viewed in the sagittal plane, and their function has often been related to the mechanics of a 4-bar linkage. However, the cruciate ligaments are crossed in 3-dimensional space, and their behavior is more like that of elastic cables that provide an envelope of stability and motion. For example, at any angle of knee flexion, a range of possible anterior-posterior translations are possible. It has been shown that in a neutral position the passive knee joint will move within a certain range without noticeable resistance to applied loads. This region can be considered as a region of extremely low stiffness or high mobility of the knee joint. This envelope of stiffness or flexibility varies with the angle of knee flexion. At full extension, the envelope of motion is quite small and the knee remains quite stable. At full extension, the ACL is completely tensed. Then, as the knee flexes, portions of the ligaments relax. The PCL begins to tighten as the knee flexes beyond 40° of flexion. Thus, as the knee flexes from full extension, the envelope (anterior-posterior motion) increases. At approximately 20° of flexion, there is a minimum of restraint to anterior-posterior motion of the knee. The changing envelope of stability at the knee is important from a functional viewpoint. At full extension, the knee is passively stable, allowing for standing posture with a minimal amount of muscular demand. During dynamic activities, such as walking, (where the knee typically flexes to approximately 20° during midstance) the ligaments are relatively relaxed and the dynamic stability is provided by large muscle forces generated by muscle contraction.

The interaction between the orientation of the cruciate ligaments and the cam-like shape of the femoral condyles are the primary determinates of how the knee changes its passive stability with flexion. The interaction between the cam-shaped geometry of the femoral condyles and the orientation of the cruciate ligaments is illustrated in Figure 3. In full extension, the sagittal plane orientation of the ACL is approximately 30° with respect to the joint line while the PCL is more horizontal. As the knee flexes to 90°, the ACL becomes horizontal and the PCL becomes perpendicular to the joint line. Thus, when the knee is flexed, the PCL provides distraction stability to the knee. This function is likely important for activities that involve deep flexion, such as squatting, where knee flexion can exceed 130°.

The cruciate ligaments influence stability and motion in planes other than the sagittal plane. In particular, the attachment of the PCL on the lateral portion of the medial femoral condyle relative to its tibial attachment orients the ligament obliquely in the frontal plane (Fig. 4). This oblique orientation of the PCL is compatible with the asymmetry in the geometry of the distal femoral condyles. As previously described (Fig. 1) the femur rolls posteriorly during flexion from full extension. Since the distal curvature of the lateral femoral condyle is larger, the lateral femoral condyle will move posteriorly a greater distance than the medial femoral condyle. As a result, the femur will rotate externally with flexion relative to the tibia. This axis of rotation is compatible with the oblique orientation of the PCL and permits mainte-

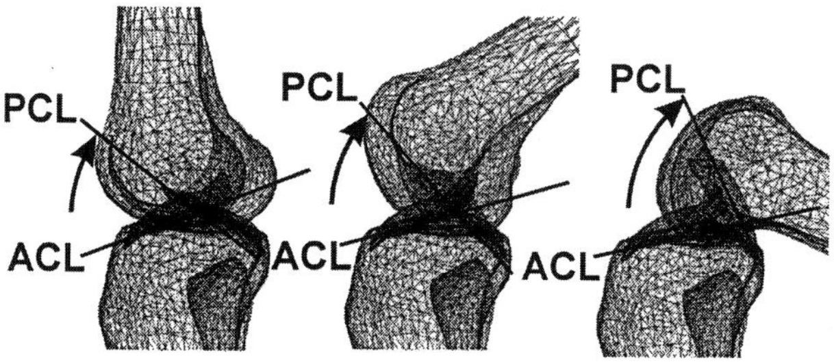

Figure 3

The anterior and posterior cruciate ligaments (ACL, PCL) change orientation as a function of knee flexion. The PCL orientation is approximately perpendicular to the tibial surface in deep flexion.

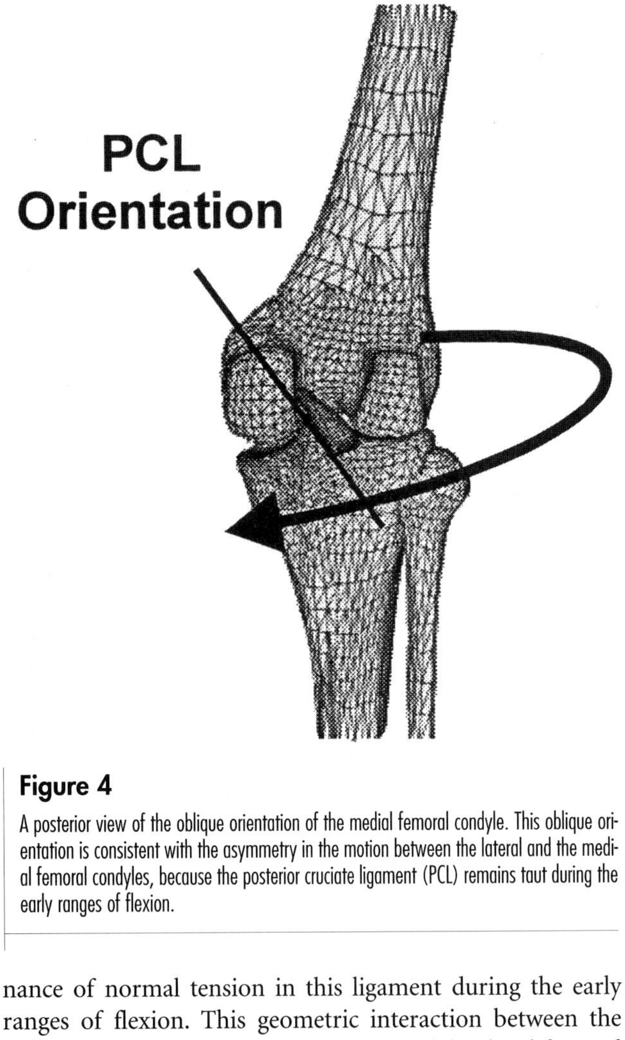

Figure 4

A posterior view of the oblique orientation of the medial femoral condyle. This oblique orientation is consistent with the asymmetry in the motion between the lateral and the medial femoral condyles, because the posterior cruciate ligament (PCL) remains taut during the early ranges of flexion.

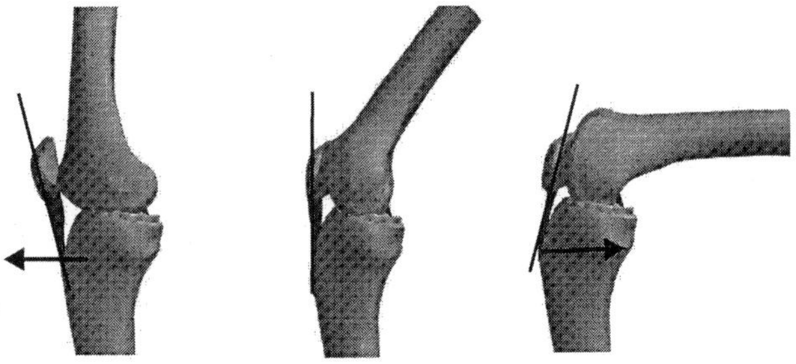

Figure 5

This illustration of the changing directional pull of the patellar ligament as the flexion of the knee changes shows how the ligament pulls the tibia anterior in early flexion and posterior in late flexion.

nance of normal tension in this ligament during the early ranges of flexion. This geometric interaction between the anatomy of the PCL and the geometry of the distal femoral condyles is likely an important consideration in the design of knee replacements in which retention of the PCL is considered. Clearly, the interaction with the femoral condyles and the orientation of the cruciate ligament play a fundamental role in the function of the knee joint.

Dynamic Interactions of the Cruciate Ligaments

It has also been shown that the cruciate ligaments interact with the active patterns of muscle contraction during such functional activities as walking and stair climbing. It has been observed that there is an interaction between the direction of pull of the extensor mechanism on the tibia and the functional role of the ACL and PCL. When the knee is near full extension, the patellar ligament places an anterior pull on the tibia (Fig. 5). This anterior pull is normally resisted by the ACL. In the absence of the ACL, the tibia would move forward until the forces would be balanced by secondary restraints to anterior displacement, such as the medial meniscus. Patients with ACL-deficient knees tend to lose strength in the quadriceps muscle due to disuse. It has also been shown that patients with long term ACL-deficient knees tend to adapt a gait that avoids or reduces the level of quadriceps contraction. If this is the case, their gait reduces the anterior force generated by quadriceps muscle contraction when the knee is near full extension, thus minimizing the strain on secondary restraints, such as the medial meniscus. This type of gait adaptation involves reprogramming the patterns of locomotion in a manner that alters the patterns of contraction between the quadriceps and hamstrings during this early stance phase of the gait cycle. This observation again illustrates the importance of an understanding of the dynamic function of the knee in the context of relating the roles of the passive and active structures of the joints.

Another example of the dynamic adaptation seen in patients with functional loss of one or more of the cruciate ligaments is associated with total knee replacement design. Retention of the PCL has been shown to biomechanically provide appropriate femoral rollback during stair climbing. The functional differences between the PCL-retaining and sacrificing designs have been related to the differences in the normal posterior movement of the femur on the tibia (rollback), with flexion (Fig. 6). Normally, when the knee flexes, the lever arm (distance between tibiofemoral contact and patellar ligament) of the quadriceps increases. If rollback does not occur, the quadriceps muscles will have a reduced lever arm. Abnormal rollback is one explanation for the reduced quadriceps movement associated with loss of the PCL, because reduced rollback would shorten the lever arm of the quadriceps muscle. Rollback must occur prior to the time during the stair climbing cycle when maximum demand is placed on the quadriceps. Maximum quadriceps demand is

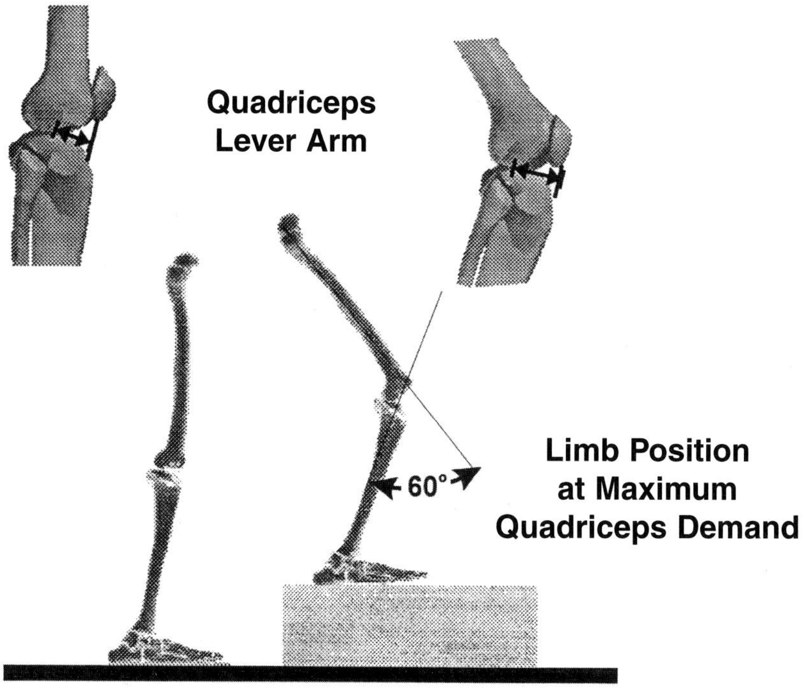

Figure 6

An illustration of the position of the knee joint (approximately 60° flexion) where the quadriceps exert maximum contractile force while ascending the stair. The rollback of the femur on the tibia provides an increased lever arm for the quadriceps muscle at 60° of knee flexion.

During normal function, the patella contacts the trochlear surface of the femur initially at approximately 10° of flexion along the narrow band across the medial and lateral facets of the inferior margin of the patella. With increasing flexion, the contact area moves proximally on the patella. The contact area increases with knee flexion. At approximately 90° of flexion, the tendinous band of the quadriceps shares in load transmission from the extensor mechanism to the femoral trochlea. After 120° of flexion, the articular surface of the patella is in contact with the femoral condyles.

The changing contact between the patella and the femoral trochlea mechanically alter the force transmission characteristics of the patellofemoral joint. The first transmission characteristics of the patellofemoral joint change as a function of knee flexion, because the location of contact between the patella and the femoral trochlea change with flexion. Therefore, the patellofemoral trochlea interaction does not behave mechanically as a pure pulley mechanism in which the entire quadriceps force is transferred from the

between 50° and 60° of flexion during stair climbing (Fig. 6). Most PCL-substituting designs use cam postmechanisms that engage later in flexion and thus do not provide the normal rollback associated with a functioning PCL.

Patellofemoral Mechanics

The previous section described a dynamic interaction between the orientation of the patellar tendon and the cruciate ligaments. As illustrated in Figure 5 the extension mechanism acting through the patella will produce an anterior pull when the knee is near full extension and a posterior pull when the knee is flexed. Again, the interdependence of the various anatomic structures that make up the knee joint is evident when these dynamic interactions are examined from a dynamic viewpoint. Clearly, there are secondary pathologic changes in the patellofemoral joint that result from cruciate ligament injuries. In addition to the classical understanding of the function of the patellofemoral joint, there are important dynamic interactions that must be considered when attempting to understand both normal and pathologic function of the knee joint.

quadriceps muscle to the tibia. The patellofemoral joint is capable of transferring the greatest quadriceps force to the patellar tendon when the knee is near full extension. As the knee moves from 15° to 90° of flexion, the amount of quadriceps force transferred to the patellar tendon decreases by approximately 40%. The reduction in extensor forces transferred across the patellofemoral joint is mitigated by tibiofemoral rollback that takes place between 0° and 20° of flexion. As a result of the rollback between the femur and the tibia, the knee's ability to generate an extensor moment increases up to approximately 40° of flexion.

An examination of the contact force between the femur and patella (retropatellar force) during various activities of daily living (Fig. 7) demonstrates that the retropatellar forces can be described as a function of knee flexion. When the knee is near full extension, the magnitude of retropatellar force is relatively low. As flexion increases between 0° and 40°, the retropatellar force increases, reaching a maximum between 60° and 90° of flexion.

The stability of the patella is governed by the congruency of the shape of the retropatellar surface with the femoral trochlea. The area of contact between the patella and the femoral trochlea changes with flexion in a manner that pro-

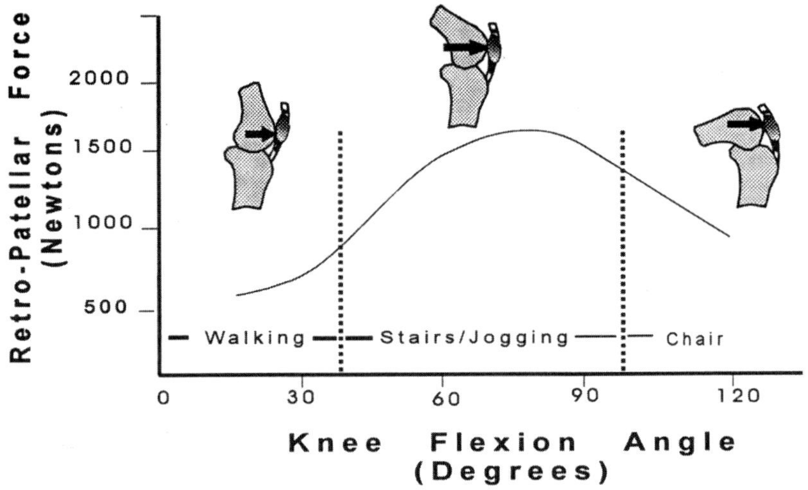

Figure 7

The force on the retropatella varies with flexion angle and activity. Typically, the largest forces occur between 40° and 100° of flexion. This curve was derived from Huberti and Hayes. (Reproduced with permission from Huberti HH, Hayes WC: Patellofemoral contact pressure: The influence of q-angle and tendofemoral contact. *J Bone Joint Surg* 1984; 66A:715–724).

duces varying amounts of patellar stability. The more prominent portion of the lateral femoral trochlea provides increased lateral stability to resist the natural tendency for the lateral pull of the extensor mechanism. The orientation of the femoral trochlea follows the laterally directed pull of the extensor mechanism with an oblique orientation relative to the mechanical axis (Fig. 8). The femoral trochlea also has a broader opening proximally and funnels the patella distally to a very narrow conforming contact. Thus, as the patella moves from a contact position near full extension where loads are relatively low to a contact position at angles that exceed 40° of flexion, both the conformity of the patella with the femoral trochlea and the contact area increase. This interrelationship between movement of the patellofemoral contact and the anatomy of the patellofemoral joint has important biomechanical and clinical implications. Clearly, in the flexed position, where the retropatellar surface experiences its greatest forces, a high degree of conformity as well as contact area is mechanically efficient for maintaining stability and minimizing contact stresses on the retropatellar surface. It can also be seen that conditions leading to patella baja or patella alta can alter the naturally optimal relationships between stability and contact area in a manner that can lead to either dislocation or abnormally high contact stresses on the retropatellar surface and to subsequent degenerative changes to the patellofemoral joint.

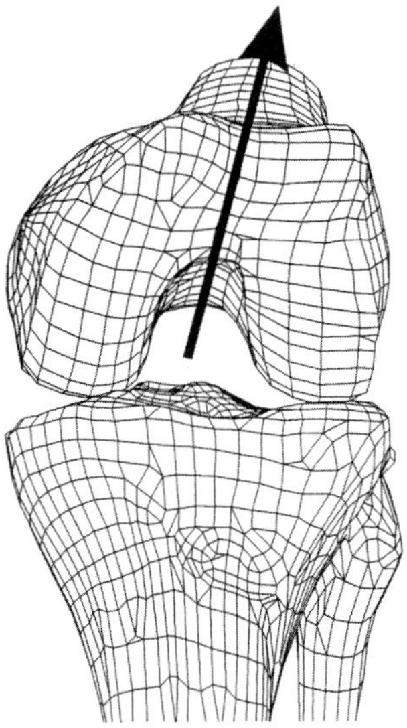

Figure 8

Orientation of femoral trochlea relative to the long axis of femur.

It has been shown that the shape and curvature of the femoral trochlea can influence function during stair climbing. In a study, patients with two types of total knee replacement that differed primarily in the shape of the femoral trochlea demonstrated significant differences in stair climbing function. The group that had an anatomically shaped femoral trochlea had near-normal function during stair climbing. The second group, in which the normal curvature of the femoral trochlea was nonanatomic, did not achieve normal stair climbing. The functional differences between the groups appeared to correspond to a larger curvature of the femoral condyle in the nonanatomic group. It appeared that patients were sensing excessive strain in the soft tissue holding the patella in place when the patella was tracking over the more prominent nonanatomic trochea (Fig. 9).

Collateral Ligaments of the Knee

The medial and lateral passive stability of the knee depends primarily on the collateral ligaments. As previously discussed, the cruciate ligaments provide secondary stability to transverse movement of the knee. This type of stability is extremely important, because the dynamic loads during walking tend to place a substantial varus thrust on the knee. The muscles that cross the knee also act to stabilize the knee to these types of loads. The medial collateral ligament (MCL) and the lateral collateral ligament (LCL) function differently, and it is useful to examine their anatomic characteristics relative to their functional roles. The MCL has both vertical and oblique fibers. The anterior fibers, which are contained in the superficial portion of the ligament and originate primarily at the medial epicondyle of the femur, consist of heavy, vertical-

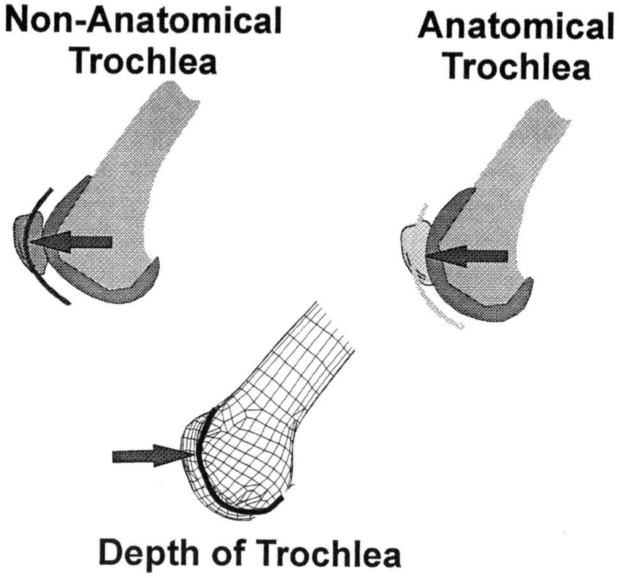

Figure 9

An illustration of a comparison between nonanatomic trochlea and anatomic total knee replacement trochleas, compared with a normal trochlea. Patients with a nonanatomic trochlea have some abnormal characteristics during stair climbing (Reproduced with permission from Andriacchi TP, Yoder D, Conley A, Rosenberg A, Sum J, Galante JO: Patellofemoral design influences function following total knee arthroplasty. *J Arthroplasty* 1997;12:243–249.)

ly oriented fibers that run distally to an insertion on the medial surface of the tibia. The tibial insertion is immediately posterior to the insertion of the pes anserinus. The posterior oblique fibers originate from the femoral epicondyle and are attached to the tibia immediately inferior to the posterior tibial articular surface with an attachment to the medial meniscus. During flexion of the knee, the superficial vertical fibers of the MCL remain taut while the oblique fibers are relaxed. In extension, the anterior fibers are relaxed while the posterior fibers are tensed. The deep fibers of the MCL extend from the femur to the midpoint of the peripheral margin of the medial meniscus and the tibia. Clearly, the primary function of the MCL is to restrain valgus rotation of the knee joint. It should be noted that the femoral insertion of the MCL is posterior and superior to the geometric rotational axis of the medial condyle. As a result of its femoral attachment, the longitudinal fibers become tense in extension and are relaxed with flexion.

The LCL resists the normal adduction moment that occurs during the walking cycle. The origin of the LCL runs from the outer surface of the lateral condyle to the head of the fibula. Its femoral attachment is superior and posterior to the geometric center of curvature of the lateral condyle. As a result, its longitudinal fibers become tense in extension and are slackened during flexion.

Dynamically, the knee also achieves stability through the contraction of the muscles that cross the joint. The active and passive knee stabilizers interact dynamically during walking. The knee can achieve dynamic stability in the absence of passive stability using muscle contraction during activities such as gait. Muscle contraction can increase the stiffness of the knee joint to varus or valgus loading while unloading the passive soft-tissue structures. The mechanism for dynamically stabilizing the knee to varus or valgus loading can be seen by considering the forces and moments that act at the knee and by calculating the required internal muscle, passive soft-tissue, and articular natural forces necessary to balance these external forces. Typically, during walking there is a tendency for the lateral side of the knee to open, resulting in a pivoting throughout the medial femoral condyle. In the absence of any muscle contraction, this varus thrust would be resisted primarily by tension in the lateral collateral ligaments in conjunction with tension in any of the passive lateral structures of the joint. However, if quadriceps force due to muscle contraction is present, there is an additional stabilizing motion associated with the momentum of the quadriceps relative to the medial femoral condyle contact location on the tibia. This synergistic action between muscle contraction and dynamic stability of the knee is commonly seen during activities such as walking, where the substantial loads generated tend to destabilize the knee.

Summary

The in vivo mechanics of the knee joint depend on a complex set of interactions between the geometry of the articular surfaces, passive soft-tissue restraints, and active muscle contraction. Future improvements in knee joint reconstructive procedures will require a better understanding of these complex interactions.

Annotated Bibliography

Andriacchi TP, Yoder D, Conley A, Rosenberg A, Sum J, Galante JO: Patellofemoral design influences function following total knee arthroplasty. *J Arthroplasty* 1997;12:243–249.

This study reported a relationship between a nonanatomic trochlea and abnormal function during stair climbing.

Banks SA, Markovich GD, Hodge WA: In vivo kinematics of cruciate-retaining and -substituting knee arthroplasties. *J Arthroplasty* 1997;12:297–304.

A fluoroscopic measurement technique has been used to provide detailed 3-dimensional kinematic assessment of knee arthroplasty function during a step-up activity. The results indicate that both prosthetic component selection and surgical technique have a significant effect on prosthetic knee kinematics during functional activities.

Covey DC, Sapega AA, Sherman GM: Testing for isometry during reconstruction of the posterior cruciate ligament: Anatomic and biomechanical considerations. *Am J Sports Med* 1996;24: 740–746.

This study reported that the change in the distance of linear separation between each pair of osseous fiber attachment sites of the posterior cruciate ligaments was measured and plotted as a function of the knee flexion angle from 0° to 120°. Data were collected under 4 sequential test conditions that had in common quadriceps relaxation, absence of tibial rotation forces, and horizontal femoral stabilization.

Delp SL, Kocmond JH, Stem SH: Tradeoffs between motion and stability in posterior substituting knee arthroplasty design. *J Biomech* 1995;28:1155–1166.

This study examined how changes in component geometry of posterior substituting knees affect tibiofemoral kinematics and prosthesis stability.

Dye SF: The knee as a biologic transmission with an envelope of function: A theory. *Clin Orthop* 1996;325:10–18.

This study demonstrated that the knee can be characterized as a complex set of asymmetrical moving parts acting together as a living biologic transmission. The purpose of this system is to accept, transfer, and dissipate loads generated at the ends of the long mechanical lever arms of the femur and tibia. In this analogy, the various ligaments represent sensate adaptive linkages, the articular cartilages represent bearings, and the menisci, mobile sensate bearings within the transmission.

Farahmand F, Senavongse W, Amis AA: Quantitative study of the quadriceps muscles and trochlear groove geometry related to instability of the patellofemoral joint. *J Orthop Res* 1998;16: 136–143.

This was a quantitative study of the major anatomic structures associated with instability of the patellofemoral joint: the quadriceps muscles and the femoral trochlear groove. Photographic "skyline" views of the trochlear groove produced data showing that, contrary to popular belief, the trochlear groove did not deepen in the area contacted by the patella with progressive knee flexion.

Fox RJ, Hamer CD, Sakane M, Carlin GJ, Woo SL: Determination of the in situ forces in the human posterior cruciate ligament using robotic technology: A cadaveric study. *Am J Sports Med* 1998;26:395–401.

The authors examined the in situ forces in the posterior cruciate ligament as well as the force distribution between its anterolateral and posteromedial bundles. Using a robotic manipulator in conjunction with a universal force-moment sensor system, posterior tibial loads from 22 to 110 N were applied to the joint at 0° to 90° of knee flexion. The magnitude of the in situ force in the posterior cruciate ligament and its bundles was significantly affected by knee flexion angle and posterior tibial loading.

Harner CD, Xerogeanes JW, Livesay GA, et al: The human posterior cruciate ligament complex: An interdisciplinary study: Ligament morphology and biomechanical evaluation. *Am J Sports Med* 1995;23:736–745.

This study of the structural and functional properties of the human posterior cruciate ligament complex measured the cross-sectional shape and area of the anterior cruciate, posterior cruciate, and meniscofemoral ligaments in 8 cadaveric knees. The posterior cruciate ligament increased in cross-sectional area from tibia to femur. The meniscofemoral ligaments did not change shape in their course from the lateral meniscus to their femoral insertions.

Hilding MB, Lanshammar H, Ryd L: Knee joint loading and tibial component loosening: RSA and gait analysis in 45 osteoarthritic patients before and after TKA. *J Bone Joint Surg* 1996;78B: 66–73.

In this prospective study of gait and tibial component migration in 45 patients with osteoarthritis treated by total knee arthroplasty, the authors reported a relationship between gait with increased flexion moments and tibial component loosening.

Ishii Y, Terajima K, Terashima S, Koga Y: Three-dimensional kinematics of the human knee with intracortical pin fixation. *Clin Orthop* 1997;343:144–150.

Knee motion was measured with an instrumented spatial linkage fixed with intracortical Kirschner wires. This technique allows an accurate description of the relative angular and linear movements between the tibia and femur without the effect of skin movement relative to the bone and without the effect of changing muscle volume. Motion of the tibia relative to the femur was described in terms of 3 clinically meaningful rotations and 3 translations between full extension and 60° flexion.

Mommersteeg TJ, Blankevoort L, Huiskes R, Kooloos JG, Kauer JM: Characterization of the mechanical behavior of human knee ligaments: A numerical-experimental approach. *J Biomech* 1996;29:151–160.

This report showed that during knee-joint motions, the fiber bundles of the knee ligaments are nonuniformly loaded in a recruitment pattern, which depends on successive relative orientations of the insertion sites. These fiber bundles vary with respect to length, orientation, and mechanical properties. As a result, the stiffness characteristics of the ligaments as a whole vary during knee-joint motion. The purpose of the study characterized this variable mechanical behavior and verified the hypothesis that it is essential to consider the ligaments of the knee as multi-bundle structures in order to characterize fully their mechanical behavior.

Ritchie JR, Bergfeld JA, Kambic H, Manning T: Isolated sectioning of the medial and posteromedial capsular ligaments in the posterior cruciate ligament-deficient knee: Influence on posterior tibial translation. *Am J Sports Med* 1998;26:389–394.

This study demonstrated that the superficial medial collateral ligament is the structure responsible for a decrease in posterior tibial translation in the posterior cruciate ligament-deficient knee.

Sakane M, Fox RJ, Woo SL, Livesay GA, Li G, Fu FH: In situ forces in the anterior cruciate ligament and its bundles in response to anterior tibial loads. *J Orthop Res* 1997;15: 285–293.

This study reported the in situ forces in 9 human anterior cruciate ligaments as well as the force distribution between the anteromedial and posterolateral bundles of the ligament in response to applied anterior tibial loads ranging from 22 to 110 N at knee flexion angles of 0° to 90°. The nonuniformity of the anterior cruciate ligament under unconstrained anterior tibial loads was demonstrated.

Stiehl JB, Abbott BD: Morphology of the transepicondylar axis and its application in primary and revision total knee arthroplasty. *J Arthroplasty* 1995;10:785–789.

This study revealed that the center of the knee was determined as the depth of the anterior intercondylar groove. The transepicondylar axis (TEA) is an important landmark that, from this study, is virtually perpendicular to the mechanical axis of the lower extremity and parallels the knee flexion axis. Femoral component rotation and joint line positioning in total knee arthroplasty can be determined using the TEA.

Stiehl J, Komistek RD, Dennis DA, Paxson RD, Hoff WA: Fluoroscopic analysis of kinematics after posterior-cruciate-retaining knee arthroplasty. *J Bone Joint Surg* 1995;77B: 884–889.

Fluoroscopic methods were used to study the kinematics of the knee in 47 patients with total knee arthroplasty and 4 control subjects with normal knees while performing a single-leg deep-knee bend.

Taylor SJ, Walker PS, Perry JS, Cannon SR, Woledge R: The forces in the distal femur and the knee during walking and other activities measured by telemetry. *J Arthroplasty* 1998;13: 428–437.

The forces and moments in the shaft of a distal femoral replacement were measured by telemetry for a subject during different activities, and calculations were then made of the forces at the knee. The axial force showed a small peak at heel-strike followed by 2 main peaks during stance.

Classic Bibliography

Ahmed AM, Burke DL, Hyder A: Force analysis of the patellar mechanisms. *J Orthop* 1987;5:69–85.

Ahmed AM, Burke DL, Yu A: In vitro measurement of static pressure distribution in synovial joints: Part II. Retropatellar surface. *J Biomech Eng* 1983;105:226–236.

Ahmed AM, Chan KH, Shi S, Lanzo V: Correlation of patellar tracking motion with the articular surface topography. *Trans Orthop Res Soc* 1989;14:202.

Amis AA, Dawkins GP: Functional anatomy of the anterior cruciate ligament: Fibre bundle actions related to ligament replacements and injuries. *J Bone Joint Surg* 1991;73B:260–267.

Andriacchi TP, Galante JO: Retention of the posterior cruciate in total knee arthroplasty. *J Arthroplasty* 1988;(suppl 3):S13–S19.

Andriacchi TP, Galante JO, Fermier RW: The influence of total knee-replacement design on walking and stair-climbing. *J Bone Joint Surg* 1982;64A:1328–1335.

Berchuck M, Andriacchi TP, Bach BR, Reider B: Gait adaptations by patients who have a deficient anterior cruciate ligament. *J Bone Joint Surg* 1990;72A:871–877.

Draganich LF, Andriacchi TP, Andersson GB: Interaction between intrinsic knee mechanics and the knee extensor mechanism. *J Orthop* 1987;5:539–547.

Gollehon DL, Torzilli PA, Warren RF: The role of posterolateral and cruciate ligaments in human knee stability: A biomechanical study. *Trans Orthop Res Soc* 1985;10:270.

Heegaard J, Leyvraz PF, Van Kampen A, Rakotomanana L, Rubin PJ, Blankevoort L: Influence of soft structures on patellar three-dimensional tracking. *Clin Orthop* 1994;299:235–243.

Huberti HH, Hayes WC: Patellofemoral contact pressures: The influence of q-angle and tendofemoral contact. *J Bone Joint Surg* 1984;66A:715–724.

Insall JN, Kelly MA: Anatomy, in Insall JN, Windsor RE, Scott WN, Kelly MA, Aglietti P (eds): *Surgery of the Knee*, ed 2. New York, NY, Churchill Livingstone, 1993, pp 1–20.

Kapandji I (ed): *The Physiology of the Joints: Annotated Diagrams of the Mechanics of the Human Joints*, ed 2. Edinburgh, Scotland, Churchill Livingstone, 1970, vol 2.

Lafortune MA, Cavanagh PR, Sommer HJ III, Kalenak A: Three-dimensional kinematics of the human knee during walking. *J Biomech* 1992;25:347–357.

Markolf KL, Mensch JS, Amstutz HC: Stiffness and laxity of the knee: The contributions of the supporting structures. A quantitative in vitro study. *J Bone Joint Surg* 1976;58A:583–594.

Noyes FR, Schipplein OD, Andriacchi TP, Saddemi SR, Weise M: The anterior cruciate ligament-deficient knee with varus alignment: An analysis of gait adaptations and dynamic joint loadings. *Am J Sports* 1992;20:707–716.

Chapter 27
Evaluating the Arthritic Knee

Introduction

The evaluation of the arthritic knee encompasses a broad spectrum of criteria. Depending on the age of the patient and the severity of the symptoms, different therapeutic treatments may be considered. Because of the variety of possible treatments, it is important to have an accurate assessment of patient-provided as well as clinically obtained information in order to allow the physician and patient to discuss the most appropriate therapeutic treatment to meet the patient's expectations.

History

The patient's history provides most of the subjective data used in the evaluation. The examiner should attempt to quantify the patient's level of symptomatology from patient-provided information and from objective observations. This information should be collected in 4 different dimensions: the severity of pain, the impact of symptoms on daily life, the impact of pain on the patient's lifestyle, and the prior history of treatment.

Patients vary in the ways they describe their symptoms. Their most common complaint is knee pain. Categories such as mild, moderate, and severe should be considered to quantify the severity of the patient's symptoms during different activities. Assessing the level of pain during walking, standing, and climbing stairs determines the impact of the arthritic condition in activities typical of daily living. Asking if the patient experiences pain during periods of inactivity or sleep will determine if they have rest pain. In addition to documenting the severity of the pain, it is important to quantify the impact of symptoms on the patient's daily activities. This can be done by detailing their ability to walk distances before stopping, determining how many stairs they can climb, evaluating the level of assistance they need on getting up from a chair, and determining their need for ambulatory aids.

Assessing the impact of the knee pain on the patient's lifestyle is also important. Some patients may not be incapacitated in activities of daily living, but their symptomatology prevents them from pursuing a satisfying quality of life. Recreational activities, such as sports and traveling, may be significantly affected. If the patient is working, the impact of the arthritic knee on employability must be considered. Finally, documentation of the efficacy of prior treatments, including the length of use of nonsteroidal anti-inflammatory agents, the number of steroid injections, and the results of previous surgical procedures, is essential in determining the appropriate therapeutic regimen for the patient.

Physical Examination

The physical examination of the arthritic knee is composed of observation, palpation, and manual assessment. The examination of an arthritic knee has 2 purposes. The first is to corroborate the patient's symptoms taken during the medical history. The second is to recognize deformities that may impact the selection of treatment. Because most arthritic processes involve 1 or more deformities, it is important to identify these deformities and assess the impact of the treatment on the deformity. As the number and severity of the deformities increases, the options for treatment decrease. Total knee replacement and osteotomy are the only treatment methods available that will address deformities caused by arthritis. Because patients may have other ongoing processes or deformities in the lower extremity that are affected by an existing arthritic condition, it is important to evaluate the entire extremity. These extremity deformities or disease processes may also have an impact on therapy selection.

Observation

Observation of the patient is critical for identification of problems. The patient's gait should be assessed prior to total knee arthroplasty (TKA) because certain gaits are associated with specific medical histories. The finding of an antalgic gait may corroborate a history of arthritis. Ligamentous instabilities may be present in a patient who walks with a thrust.

The presence or absence of prior scars is important in planning a surgical procedure. Existing incision scars can create wound-healing problems that may increase the likelihood of infection. Assessment of the severity of these soft-tissue problems should be planned preoperatively. The 2 most common methods for covering soft-tissue defects are muscle flaps, in the case of large defects, or, in less severe cases, skin expansion devices. Deformities in the extremity from prior trauma and congenital or developmental diseases may affect the use of instrumentation during osteotomy or TKA. Signs of poor vascularity of the feet should be noted, as well as deformities of the hindfoot and forefoot, because these can affect landmarks used for the TKA techniques and instrumentation.

Observation of alignment on physical examination can be difficult. The patient's body habitus can obscure the true alignment of the extremity. Even though the alignment should be observed, more exact measurements can usually be obtained from standing radiographs.

Palpation

Palpation of the arthritic knee allows the physician to determine areas of pain and crepitus. The induction of pain during palpation of the medial and lateral joint lines is typical of the arthritic knee. The feeling of crepitus, particularly during movement of the patellofemoral joint, is not atypical. An assessment of the extremity pulses is valuable in determining the extent of vascular disease in the extremity. Lack of distal pulses may jeopardize the ability of the skin to heal after a surgical procedure. Preoperative evaluation of vascular health is of the utmost importance.

The active knee range of motion should be recorded. It is not unusual for arthritic knees to have decreased flexion and flexion contractures. Any deficiencies in the extensor mechanism should be noted. Patients with extensor lags may expect a prolonged rehabilitation period after a surgical procedure. These patients can then be properly informed and their postoperative expectations modified. It is not uncommon for these patients to have limited postoperative gains in range of motion. If a patient has a significant flexion contracture, it may be necessary to resect more distal femur or perform a posterior capsular release to obtain full extension in the operating room.

Range of Motion

The physical examination of the knee should begin by measuring the range of motion of the knee. This must be done both actively and passively to evaluate the function of the extensor mechanism. It is uncommon for the arthritic knee to have an extension lag. If present, it could be a sign of neurologic disorder or previous trauma, and a diagnostic workup should be considered. Flexion contractures are common to arthritic knees. Flexion contractures of more than 10° may be an indication against osteotomy. During TKA, flexion contractures of less than 10° usually do not require additional attention during the TKA. However, contractures of more than 10° may require additional bony resection from the distal femur and/or a posterior capsular release. There are different techniques for releasing the posterior capsule. The surgeon must be careful to avoid injury to the vascular structures situated posterior to the lateral compartment. Resecting the distal end of the femur is safer than performing a posterior capsular release; however, the surgeon is constrained by the insertion of the collateral ligaments. Excessive bony resection above the collateral ligament insertions may result in ligamentous instability, requiring a constrained prosthesis. At times, resecting up to the collaterals may compromise some of the posterior fixation on the condyles and may require the addition of a stem on the femoral condyle.

Ligament Examination

The ligament examination of the arthritic knee is similar to that of a nonarthritic knee. The information derived from the examination is not only diagnostic, but also affects intraoperative decisions on ligamentous balancing. Ligamentous instability may be a contraindication to treating the patient with an osteotomy.

The concept of ligamentous balancing during TKA was introduced in the late 1960s. Experience with hinged devices and high transfer force loads to the bone-cement interface of the prostheses led to the concept that ligament tensioning was needed to lengthen the life of the implant and decrease forces at the bone-cement interface. In the presence of competent ligaments, hinged prostheses are not needed. The concept of releasing the contracted collateral ligament to correct alignment while still maintaining a competent ligament was introduced in the early 1970s. These 2 concepts remain the cornerstones of modern TKA.

Medial Collateral Ligament Over 90% of arthritic knees are in varus alignment. As the arthritic process progresses, the medial collateral ligament (MCL) tends to contract and the lateral collateral ligament (LCL) tends to lengthen. Preoperative evaluation of the tightness of the MCL will determine the degree of medial collateral release needed to achieve appropriate ligamentous balancing. Absence of medial collateral stability may indicate the need for a semiconstrained prosthesis. The degree of medial collateral competence can be tested by applying a valgus stress to a knee positioned at 30° of flexion. In this manner, the examiner can estimate the amount of release necessary to bring the knee back to normal alignment. The knee can also be tested in full extension. If the varus alignment corrects with valgus stress, significant medial collateral and posterior cruciate compromise has occurred. However, this is quite rare.

Lateral Collateral Ligament Valgus arthritic deformities are less frequent than varus deformities. In the valgus knee, the

LCL and its associated structures contract and the MCL lengthens. By applying a varus stress to a knee positioned at 30° of flexion, the examiner can gauge the need for release of the lateral structures to achieve ligamentous balancing and correct alignment. If the knee opens up to varus stress in full extension, the lateral structures may have been significantly compromised and use of a constrained prosthesis may be warranted.

Cruciate Ligaments Although there is significant controversy in the literature about the preservation of the posterior cruciate ligament (PCL) during TKA, most contemporary designs resect the anterior cruciate ligament. A history of a PCL injury may induce a cruciate-retaining surgeon to have a cruciate-substituting design as a backup. Unfortunately, it is difficult to estimate the function of these ligaments preoperatively because most arthritic knees have a significant amount of bony stability. This stability is caused by the loss of cartilage-producing congruent bony surfaces inherently stable in the anteroposterior plane and by the development of osteophytes.

The competency of the PCL can be ascertained by performing a posterior drawer test. The knee is bent to 90° and a posterior force is directed on the tibia. The examiner's thumbs can be placed on the edge of the tibia. Usually the tibial plateau is about 1 cm prouder than the femoral condyles with the knee flexed at 90°. The amount of posterior instability can be gauged by the degree of motion of the tibia with respect to the femur. The tightness of the PCL should be determined at the time of the arthroplasty. A PCL that is too tight can lead to limited flexion and increased wear of the polyethylene. If the ligament is too loose, it can cause inappropriate rollback and early wear of the polyethylene.

Imaging

Imaging techniques can be used in the care of the arthritic knee for diagnostic purposes, for preoperative planning, and for postoperative evaluations. Conventional radiographs are the most commonly used imaging method. Other modalities such as fluoroscopy, computed tomography (CT), nuclear medicine, and magnetic resonance imaging (MRI) can be helpful in the evaluation and treatment of specific conditions.

Conventional Radiography Standing anteroposterior views are used to delineate overall alignment and loss of joint space in the femoral tibial articulation. Long bone films can be useful in further detailing alignment, particularly in the presence of skeletal deformities, prior trauma, or other joint replacements. Occasionally, 45° posteroanterior radiographs can be used to increase the sensitivity of standard anteroposterior views in determining joint-space narrowing. Lateral radiographs can depict the loss of joint space in the patellofemoral joint and reveal the presence or absence of posterior osteophytes formation. Patellofemoral views (Merchant, sunrise) demonstrate the loss of joint space in the patellofemoral joint and patellar alignment on the trochlea. Tunnel views of the knee can be helpful in evaluating loose bodies, osteochondritis dissecans, condylar fractures, and osteonecrosis of the knee.

These radiographs can also be used postoperatively in the evaluation of a surgical procedure or diagnostically during the evaluation of failed implants. Conventional radiography can reveal radiolucent lines, implant malposition, component breakage, advanced polyethylene wear, patellar and periprosthetic fractures, and osteolysis.

Fluoroscopy The use of conventional radiography for documenting radiolucent lines around implants has its shortcomings. Because of the complex geometry of the implants and the need for parallel views of these geometries, many investigators use fluoroscopy as a means of documenting radiolucent lines. Fluoroscopy is the best imaging technique for assessing the bone-cement interface on an implant because it allows for the perfect positioning of the radiographic beam parallel to the implant's edge. It has also been used postoperatively by investigators to assess the amount of rollback of the femoral component on the tibial component in different total knee designs.

Fluoroscopy is also used in combination with computerized analysis of joint spaces to assess the progression of arthritic changes. This method can be used to assess the quantitative effect on cartilage of disease-modifying osteoarthritic drugs.

Computed Tomography CT has a limited role in the care of the arthritic knee. It has not been helpful in delineating early cartilaginous abnormalities. After knee replacement, CT has a limited role diagnostically because of the interference caused by the metallic implants.

Nuclear Medicine Nuclear medicine studies may be useful in the postoperative evaluation of the arthritic knee. Technetium bone scans, gallium scanning, and indium white blood cell scanning have been used to aid in the diagnosis between aseptic loosening and infection of knee implants. Their sensitivity and specificity vary significantly in the medical literature. Their cost-effectiveness has come into question, because they can only be used to infer, not to definitely diagnose an infection. The definitive diagnosis of an infected implant is by means of a positive culture.

Magnetic Resonance Imaging Despite its advantages in multiplanar imaging and soft-tissue contrast over other radiographic modalities, the use of MRI in the care and treatment of the arthritic knee is questionable. Even though it may be more sensitive than plain radiographs in determining cartilaginous abnormalities, it can still underestimate the extent of cartilaginous damage. Arthroscopy is considered to be the most sensitive technique in evaluating cartilage. Unfortunately, because interpretation of the views obtained under arthroscopy are subjective and can vary from surgeon to surgeon, it is difficult to measure cartilaginous damage qualitatively and quantitatively.

Scoring Techniques

Historic Perspective

The development of the modern TKA can be dated back to the 1960s. The polycentric knee, designed by Frank H. Gunston, introduced the use of 2 cemented polyethylene tibial components articulating with 2 cemented femoral components. Over time, prostheses with varying degrees of tibiofemoral conformity were introduced, and different philosophies regarding the sacrifice of the ACL and PCL emerged. As a result, a variety of methods for evaluating TKA performance were developed by investigators. Investigators have standardized reporting methods by selecting the ones they found most useful. The Hospital for Special Surgery Knee Score and the Knee Society Score have emerged as the most widely used standards for reporting TKA results.

Over the last several years there has been interest in developing another method to measure the results of medical therapeutics. Some of this methodology, commonly known as outcome studies, was developed to evaluate the results of a particular treatment from the patient's perspective. Outcome studies in total joint arthroplasty are composed of 2 basic measurements; a health status questionnaire (the Medical Outcomes Study Short Form 36 [SF-36]) and a pain and function questionnaire. The health status questionnaire attempts to measure the patient's quality of life. The Western Ontario and McMaster Osteoarthritis Index or WOMAC score has been used by the Patient Outcome Research Team at the University of Indiana in their evaluation of TKA.

Total Knee Replacement Scores

The 2 most commonly used scores for reporting of the results of knee arthroplasty in the medical literature are the Hospital for Special Surgery Knee Score (HSS Knee Score) and the Knee Society Score (KS Score). The Knee Society Score can be thought of as a derivation of the HSS Knee Score, because it incorporates most aspects of the HSS Knee Score and was created at a later date. The HSS Knee Score and the KSS Score are evaluations performed by an observer (usually a health care professional) through an interview and physical examination. Both of these tests assess and reward points for pain, function (walking and stair climbing), range of motion, muscle strength, ligamentous stability, alignment, flexion contractures, extension lag, and the use of ambulatory aids. The Knee Society Score adds a categorical score to differentiate patients according to their functional impairment with relation to medical infirmity or other affected joints in the body. The American Medical Association in their *Guides to the Evaluation of Permanent Impairment* uses a modification of the Knee Society Score to assess TKAs.

The Western Ontario and McMaster Universities Osteoarthritis Index (WOMAC Score)

Originally designed to test the effectiveness of nonsteroidal anti-inflammatory agents in the treatment of osteoarthritis, the WOMAC Score was chosen by the Patient Outcome Research Team at the University of Indiana to study total knee arthroplasty. It is based on a questionnaire that is completed by the patient without the help or intervention of the health care provider. The questions relate to difficulties the patient has in performing activities of daily living. It has proven to be an effective and reproducible vehicle in medical research.

The HSS Knee Score, Knee Society Score, and WOMAC Score are the most authoritative measures of the outcomes of TKA evaluations. The HSS Knee Score and the Knee Society Score are interview based and are dependent on a physical examination. The 2 main weaknesses of these scores are that they are subject to examiner bias and that the physical examination parameters can carry a significant amount of interobserver discrepancies. However, they provide more detailed information about the physical dynamics of the prosthesis than the WOMAC Score. As a result, the HSS Knee Score and the Knee Society Score are more powerful tools when used to compare specific dynamics of the prosthesis.

Although the HSS Knee Score and the Knee Society Score differ in organization and technique from the WOMAC Score, the 3 scales have been proven to correlate well with each other in their measurement of total knee replacement outcomes.

Uses of Total Knee Replacement Scores

Until recently, total knee replacement scores were used primarily by investigators to report the results of TKAs. Investigators evaluated the patient's preoperative function prior to TKA, and then compared these measures to postoperative scores at different postoperative times. In this manner, patient variables (comorbidities), as well as different types of prostheses, could be evaluated.

Over the last decade there has been increased pressure to decrease the cost of medical treatments. As a result, it has become increasingly important to evaluate the outcomes of different medical treatments. Outcome studies evaluate the change in the patient's quality of life as well as the therapeutic result. In 1989, the Agency for Health Policy and Research decided to fund several Patient Outcome Research teams to study different medical therapeutics. This type of research has 2 objectives: to document the value of a specific therapy relative to its cost and to determine its impact on the patient's quality of life. If this type of research is successful, the results may be used by government and, eventually, third-party payers to ration or direct medical care into more effective therapeutic means. Many providers are concerned that these data may eventually be used to judge the ability to deliver health care.

This has led many total joint physicians who previously had limited interest in keeping an objective measurement of the results of their TKAs to reevaluate their record-keeping. Because of concerns about the role of third-party payers in deciding health care providers, practitioners are starting to gather more outcome data.

There are different commercial products that collect a multitude of information, including some of the scales discussed in this chapter, financial data on the cost of the prosthesis, length of stay, and other parameters. Most of these products are computer database software that allow record keeping of significant variables. A variety of reports can be produced, allowing physicians to study their own data and become more competitive. Some programs allow practitioners to join a national data bank and compare their data to others in the country.

Most of these programs have been designed by physicians in conjunction with orthopaedic companies that have a concomitant interest in assuring that physicians who use their products stay competitive. Some companies will collect and analyze data at no charge for physicians who use their products. Others sell the software and allow physicians to use the data and reports as they wish. Unfortunately, this adds cost to business operations, because it usually requires a separate, dedicated computer system. If outcome data are required of all practitioners, business software packages will be developed that incorporate outcome data subroutines into their normal operations.

Annotated Bibliography

Doege TC, Houston TP (eds): *Guides to the Evaluation of Permanent Impairment*, ed 4. Chicago, IL, American Medical Association, 1995.

This American Medical Association publication provides objective information on how to evaluate permanent impairment for specific injuries. It is an essential tool for any physician involved in patient impairment evaluations.

Gold DA, Scott SC, Scott WN: Soft tissue expansion prior to arthroplasty in the multiply-operated knee: A new method of preventing catastrophic skin problems. *J Arthroplasty* 1996;11: 512–521.

The authors provide a surgical technique for treating patients who need a total knee arthroplasty and who have a high potential for skin complications. Excellent results were obtained without major problems.

Sun Y, Sturmer T, Gunther KP, Brenner H: Reliability and validity of clinical outcome measurements of osteoarthritis of the hip and knee: A review of the literature. *Clin Rheumatol* 1997;16: 185–198.

The authors summarize reliability and validity studies between different outcome measures and discuss the shortcomings of the studies performed to date. They conclude that the reliability and validity of clinical scores of hip and knee arthritis are limited and continued research in the area is needed.

Blackburn WE Jr, Chivers S, Bernreuter W: Cartilage imaging in osteoarthritis. *Semin Arthritis Rheum* 1996;25:273–281.

The authors discuss the current imaging techniques used in the diagnosis and evaluation of osteoarthritis. The review incorporates the advantages and disadvantages of each technique.

Stiehl JB, Komistek RD, Dennis DA, Paxson RD, Hoff WA: Fluoroscopic analysis of kinematics after posterior-cruciate retaining knee arthroplasty. *J Bone Joint Surg* 1995;77B: 884–889.

The authors fluoroscopically studied the rollback of posterior cruciate ligament-retaining implants in 47 patients. The implant did not reproduce normal posterior cruciate ligament kinematics in the study population.

Callahan CM, Drake BG, Heck DA, Dittus RS: Patient outcomes following unicompartmental or bicompartmental knee arthroplasty: A meta-analysis. *J Arthroplasty* 1995;10:141–150.

This study summarizes the literature describing patient outcomes following unicompartmental and bicompartmental knee arthroplasty; however, the authors believed that this was potentially due to patient selection criteria.

Chapter 28 Nonarthroplasty Alternatives in Knee Arthritis

Medical Therapy

Nonsteroidal anti-inflammatory drugs (NSAIDs) are the most common class of drugs used to alleviate the symptoms of osteoarthritis. While there are many drugs currently on the market, the differences in clinical efficacies between them are related more to reducing gastrointestinal (GI) side effects than to their ability to reduce inflammation. New strategies employed with these therapies have included the additional use of prostaglandin agonists as a separate drug or in combination with an NSAID. While this combination has been shown to modestly reduce the number of GI side effects, it is difficult to determine if it is worth their high cost. The adverse effects of these drugs have been studied extensively. The risk of bleeding, perforation, hospitalization, or death was found to be 3 times higher among NSAID users. From a study of 8,800 patients it was determined that 1% to 2% of NSAID users annually will develop a serious GI complication. Epidemiologic data estimate that NSAID-induced GI injury causes 7,600 deaths and 76,000 hospitalizations annually in the United States.

NSAID medications achieve their effect by inhibiting the conversion of arachidonic acid to prostaglandins that serve as key components in the inflammatory process. Two distinct forms of cyclooxygenase (COX), the prostaglandin synthase, have been identified, designated COX-1 and COX-2. COX-1 is the ubiquitous form of the enzyme found widely expressed in the body, including the GI tract, kidneys, and platelets. COX-2 is found in very low levels in normal tissues, but in very high levels in inflamed ones. Recent drug therapies aimed at selective COX-2 inhibition have been described. One recent study compared the GI effects of a COX-2 inhibitor with those of Naprosyn, using endoscopy as the outcome instrument. No patients receiving the COX-2 inhibitor developed gastric ulcers, while 19% of the patients receiving Naprosyn developed ulcers. They also reported no effect on platelet aggregation or thromboxane-2 levels compared with aspirin. A recent double-blind, placebo-controlled, multicenter study of 9,323 patients compared the clinical efficacy of Meloxicam (COX-2 inhibitor) and diclofenac. They found that differences in clinical efficacy, measured by visual analog scale, modestly favored diclofenac. However, the patients reported significantly fewer GI side effects on Meloxicam, including GI ulcers, dyspepsia, diarrhea, and abdominal pain. While the GI side effects were significantly reduced, renal safety profiles and liver function test abnormalities were equivalent to diclofenac.

Recent news reports have popularized oral glucosamine as a potent agent in the treatment of osteoarthritis. Manufacturers claim the drug works by maintaining the health of the hyaline cartilage. While there are anecdotal reports of clinical efficacy, to date there are no reliable well-controlled, double-blind trials to support using these drugs. There are also no descriptions of dosage guidelines or clinical safety trials.

Injections

Steroid injections of the knee have been a mainstay of nonoperative treatment of gonarthrosis. Glucocorticoids are well-known anti-inflammatory agents, although their mechanism of action is only partially understood. Steroids greatly decrease neutrophil migration into the inflamed joints. They prevent phagocytosis, lysosomal enzyme release, and the synthesis of several inflammatory mediators. Synthesis of prostaglandins and interleukin-1 has been shown to be reduced by as much as 50%. Intra-articular corticosteroids change the characteristics of synovial fluid, increasing its hyaluronic acid concentration and, thus, its viscosity, enabling it to increase the lubricating characteristics of synovial fluid. In patients with rheumatoid arthritis, gadolinium-enhanced magnetic resonance imaging has demonstrated an up to 68% reduction in synovial membrane and joint effusion volume 1 week after intra-articular injection of methylprednisolone.

There are a number of steroid preparations available for intra-articular use. Duration of effect is inversely proportional to solubility, with triamcinolone hexacetonide the least soluble and the longest acting. A survey of 2,000 members of the American College of Rheumatology showed favored preparations to be methylprednisolone (34.6%), triamcinolone hexacetide (31.2%), and triamcinolone acetonide (21.7%).

There are a number of side effects associated with corticosteroid injection. Systemic effects include suppression of the hypothalamic-pituitary-adrenal axis, decrease in plasma cortisol, and suppressed stress response to hypoglycemia. Steroid arthropathy, which results from the chronic use of intra-articular therapy, has been described. Steroids have been shown to have adverse effects on hyaline cartilage, including fibrillation, fissure formation, thinning of the cartilage layers, and denudation of bone. Microscopic analysis of chondrocytes has shown a progressive loss of endoplasmic reticulum, mitochondria, and Golgi apparatus with increasing number of injections. This resulted in a linear decrease in proteoglycan content and protein synthesis. Other complications reported with steroid injections of the knee include osteonecrosis of distant joints, infection, patella tendon rupture, and hypersensitivity reactions.

Viscosupplementation therapy with hyaluronic acid (HA) derivatives has gained popularity in recent years as a nonoperative treatment in patients with gonarthrosis. Treatment consists of removal of all joint fluid from the affected knee and injection of the hyaluronate derivative once a week for 3 to 5 weeks (depending on the preparation). The preparations commonly used are hylan G-F 20 (Synvisc) and sodium hyaluronate (Hyalgan). While its mechanism of action has not been elucidated, one recent report comparing baseline cartilage biopsies in patients who had undergone HA therapy demonstrated interesting morphologic differences. Statistically significant changes were seen in reconstitution of the superficial amorphous layer of the cartilage, improvement in chondrocyte density, and reduction in synovial inflammation.

Several peer-reviewed studies have shown little difference between hyaluronic therapy, steroid injections, and NSAID therapy. Others have shown significant improvements with HA, especially in scores related to pain and function. However, one recent double-blinded, placebo-controlled multicenter study of 240 patients found that active patients older than 60 years with moderate to severe arthritis were the group most likely to benefit from treatment with intra-articular hyaluronan injections. Selecting the correct patients is important, considering the $500 cost per patient. The most common complication of this therapy is injection-site inflammation and pain. No systemic effects or knee infections were reported in any of the studies. In an analysis of 495 injected knees, a 2.7% rate of adverse effects were seen per injection, 7% per joint after completion of therapy. The incidence of injection site irritation was influenced by the injection technique. Adverse effects per injection were reported as 5.2% with a medial approach in a partially bent knee, 2.4% with a direct straight injection, and 1.5% with a direct lateral approach.

Synovectomy

Open synovectomy was the traditional procedure of choice for patients with intractable synovitis and preservation of articular cartilage. This procedure is now reserved for patients with rheumatoid arthritis. A radical knee debridement and partial meniscal excision is usually performed. Recovery tends to be slow, with particularly prolonged knee joint stiffness and swelling. Several studies have demonstrated that, although patients improve in the short term, results deteriorate as time passes and the disease process progresses. In a long-term study of rheumatoid patients, results depended on the severity of the disease at the time of the open synovectomy. Eighty-three synovectomies were evaluated in 65 patients, with an average follow-up of 7 years. In patients with radiographic stage II disease, 18 had good results, 14 fair, and 8 poor, with 22 of the 40 knees requiring reoperation. In stage III disease, there was only 1 good result in 16 knees, and 11 of the 16 knees required total knee arthroplasty.

Arthroscopic knee synovectomy is the recommended method of removal of diseased rheumatoid synovium with cartilage preservation. Benefit from the procedure is multifold, including pain relief and improved range of motion from the synovial tissue removal and excision of mechanical problems, such as a torn or degenerated meniscus. Additionally, the extensive lavage that occurs with arthroscopic surgery may also remove debris and crystalline and immune complexes.

Surgical indications for synovectomy are severe pain, refractory to medical management for at least 4 to 6 months; preserved range of motion; and no signs of joint space involvement or significant deformity as seen on a radiograph. These indications hold true for synovectomy of all joints, not only the knee. Arthroscopic synovectomy is usually performed as an outpatient procedure. If the procedure is prolonged and multicompartmental, a suction drain may be used and the patient admitted overnight. Protective weight-bearing is recommended with crutches or a cane until pain and swelling subside. As knee joint swelling subsides, range of motion and strengthening exercises are advanced under the supervision of a physical therapist.

Results of this procedure have been encouraging in the short term. In one series of 22 synovectomies in 17 patients with rheumatoid arthritis followed for at least 4 years, there were 2 failures requiring knee replacement, and 2 patients required further arthroscopic synovectomy. There were 2 significant hemarthroses, which resolved without further surgical treatment. In a report on a series of open and arthroscopic procedures, 41 arthroscopic procedures had 83% good results at 3 years, but deteriorated to 46% at 8 years follow-up. Of 26 patients who underwent open synovectomy, 81% had good results at 3 years and 40% had good results at 8 years. This report supported the use of arthroscopic synovectomy in patients with early radiographic disease and documented the ease of recovery and reduced morbidity with the arthroscopic method. There is less postoperative pain, return to work is more rapid, and both knees can be operated on at the same time.

Chemical synovectomy has been used for nearly 50 years as a surgical alternative in patients with rheumatoid arthritis, in whom synovectomy has been indicated. This treatment modality has not been shown to be effective in the treatment of osteoarthritis. A comparison of the results of chemical synovectomy in patients with rheumatoid and osteoarthritis reported 74% good results at 1 year in patients with rheumatoid arthritis and 43% good results in patients with osteoarthritis. Multiple studies have reported similar results. A comparison of radiopharmaceutical therapy with triamcinolone injection found no difference between the two groups at 6 year follow-up. There are a number of safety concerns with this therapy. The greatest concern has been postinjection extra-articular radiation leakage to nontarget organs, including adjacent lymph nodes, liver, lung, and spleen.

In addition to reduction in the bulk of synovial tissue after synovectomy, it has been postulated that another theoretical advantage is the reduction in lysosomal enzymes and collagenases. One study, however, found only a minor reduction in lysosomal enzymes after synovectomy and no change in the amount of complement in the joint.

Valgus Bracing

Valgus bracing for medial compartment osteoarthritis was first introduced in 1989. These braces provide pain relief by reducing the load in the affected compartment and by providing improved knee joint stability and proprioception. These braces work by application of 3-point bending about the knee joint to produce a net medial force to increase the load taken up by the lateral compartment. Application of the medially directed force through the use of bladders, condylar pads, or straps (opposed by the proximal and distally directed lateral forces) is the feature that distinguishes one brace design from another.

Several clinical and biomechanical studies have provided evidence to support the concept of valgus bracing as a useful treatment in medial compartment osteoarthritis of the knee joint. One study demonstrated a 10% to 20% decrease in knee adduction moment in knees wearing the GII unloader brace through automated gait analysis. Pain and function scoring instruments measured before and after wearing the brace indicated that pain decreased by 48% and activities of daily living increased by 79%. Gait analyses reported the mean tibiofemoral angle to be decreased from 185.1° to 183.7°. Isokinetic muscle strength increased from 36.8 Nm to 42.8 Nm. Lateral movement of the center of gravity decreased with GII application in all patients studied. Clinical studies have shown encouraging results. A prospective analysis of 18 patients at 1 year follow-up reported a 39% reduction in pain experienced with activities of daily living. Before brace wear patients reported a walking tolerance of 51 minutes prior to the onset of pain. This time increased to 107 minutes at 1 year.

Valgus bracing of the knee for medial compartment gonarthrosis is not indicated for all patients with symptoms. The severity of the arthritis and limb deformity must be considered prior to its use. A patient with advanced arthritis or a varus alignment of 20° or greater probably will not receive much benefit. Analysis of the data suggests that the ideal candidate for this treatment would be a young, active patient who has failed medical therapy and arthroscopic lavage, but is too young to consider arthroplasty.

Arthroscopic Lavage and Debridement

Many studies have published supportive data for the use of arthroscopic lavage, debridement, and chondroplasty as effective treatments for knee arthritis. These procedures allow removal of inflammatory mediators (interleukins, metalloproteinases), degenerative cartilage, and meniscal fragments. There continues to be a debate whether these techniques provide placebo effect or actual therapeutic benefit. One recent pilot study randomized 10 patients, half to an arthroscopy group and half to a group in which only the portals were made, but no procedure was performed. All 5 patients who received the sham operation reported significant clinical relief at 6 months and would recommend the procedure to their friends and family. One report has documented minimum 10-year results after arthroscopic debridement. Eighty-three knees underwent the procedure for pain, which limited their function. Fifty-four patients (65%) did not require further surgery at latest follow-up and were satisfied with the results of the arthroscopic debridement. Patient satisfaction in this group averaged 8.6 on a 0 to 10 scale. Twenty-nine knees required total knee replacement (TKR) at an average of 6.7 years from the original debridement. Projected savings of $777,276 were reported for the 54 patients who did not receive an arthroplasty, by comparing the Medicare reimbursement of TKR ($19,730 excluding implant) verses arthroscopic debridement ($5,336).

Studies comparing arthroscopic debridement and needle lavage show slightly better results in the needle group (44% versus 58%). There does not appear to be a role for chondroplasty in the treatment of osteoarthritis. Data comparing arthroscopy with and without chondroplasty demonstrate significantly inferior results for chondroplasty. In one study, 50% of patients who underwent abrasion chondroplasty required total knee arthroplasty within 3 years.

Osteotomy

In the late 1970s, Mark Coventry established high tibial osteotomy and supracondylar femoral osteotomy as a treatment for gonarthrosis. The basic biomechanical concept is to realign the mechanical axis of the extremity in order to unload the arthritic anatomic compartment. Although total knee arthroplasty has enjoyed significant clinical success, there are clinical situations in which osteotomy is indicated. The last several years have produced long-term 15- to 20-year data on the survivorship of this procedure.

The mechanical axis and tibiofemoral angle is determined from full-length extremity radiographs. The mechanical axis is a line drawn from the center of hip rotation to the center of the ankle mortise. In normal patients, the line should pass through the knee slightly medial to the tibial spines. In the normal knee, 60% of weightbearing is achieved through the medial femoral condyle. The tibiofemoral angle is obtained by the intersection of the lines drawn along the anatomic axis of the femur and tibia. Normal is considered 5° to 7°. Medial compartment involvement with a varus deformity is treated with a valgus-producing tibial osteotomy; lateral compartment involvement with a valgus deformity is treated with a varus-producing femoral osteotomy.

High Tibial Osteotomy

Indications for high tibial osteotomy (HTO) include: (1) age < 60 years, (2) arthritis confined to one anatomic compartment, (3) 10° to 15° of varus deformity on weightbearing radiographs, (4) preoperative arc of motion of 90°, (5) flexion contracture < 15°, and (6) sufficient strength and motivation to use assistive devices and perform a rehabilitation program. Contraindications to HTO include: (1) narrowing of the lateral compartment cartilage, (2) lateral tibial subluxation greater than 1 cm, (3) medial compartment bone loss of more than 2 to 3 mm, (4) ligamentous instability, and (5) inflammatory arthritis. Although not strict contraindications, patients on workers' compensation or who have had a prior partial or complete menisectomy may not have as good results. The procedure seems particularly suited for younger, heavy individuals involved in heavy labor or athletics. The potential asymmetric appearance of the limb after correction needs to be communicated to the patient preoperatively, because unsatisfactory patient results could be obtained for purely cosmetic reasons.

Preoperative assessment should include a thorough history and physical examination. Range of motion, presence of contractures of the joint, and ligamentous stability should be documented. Careful examination of the hip, foot, and ankle should be performed. Examination of the patient's gait is very important. In a varus knee, the ground reaction force is directed medially, causing a varus thrust during weightbearing. The thrust may not be correctable by HTO. Some authors have used gait analysis for preoperative planning. One report stated that patients who walked with a decreased knee adduction moment preoperatively were likely candidates for clinical success. Recent literature has criticized traditional static radiographic preoperative planning, because the mechanical axis shifts medially during one-legged stance. Despite the high cost and limited availability of gait analysis, it remains a useful research tool. Some authors advocate the use of heel wedges, valgus braces, or casts to predict clinical success.

Meticulous preoperative planning is critical for proper surgical technique and good results. Methods described for obtaining correction in high tibial osteotomy include lateral closing wedge, medial opening wedge, and dome type. Closing lateral wedge osteotomy is the most popular method of obtaining correction. From the standing 3-ft extremity radiograph, the lines outlined in Figure 1 should be drawn. Line 1 is drawn through the medial third of the lateral plateau. This allows for the inclusion of 3° to 5° of overcorrection, which has been reported to be necessary for success. Lines 2 and 3 calculate the angle of correction.The height of the wedge needed on the lateral cortex to resect has traditionally been 1 mm for each angle of correction. Undercorrection has been associated with plateaus greater than 58 mm using this method. For larger plateaus, the formula, W = diameter of the plateau × 0.02 × angle of correction, has been employed effectively. The transverse osteotomy should be made 2 cm from the joint line. While performing the bone cuts, it is crucial not to penetrate the medial cortex. It should be used to hinge the osteotomy closed. Fixation of the osteotomy can be performed using 2 or 3 staples or a buttress plate. While no difference in nonunion rates has been noted between the two fixation methods, a higher infection rate has been reported for buttress plates (9.3% compared to 0.8%). Earlier range of motion and weightbearing is allowed with buttress plate fixation. Unrestricted correction requires untethering the fibula, which can be accomplished by osteotomizing the fibula, by fibular head excision with soft-tissue repair, or by release of the proximal tibia/fibula articulation. Fibular osteotomy increases the likelihood of a peroneal nerve palsy (Fig. 2). High-risk areas to the peroneal nerve are present 30 mm distal to the fibular head (superficial portion) and 60 to 150 mm from the fibular head (branch to the extensor hallucis longus).

Clinical Results

Established literature has documented excellent clinical results for HTO at 10 years. Predictors of clinical success have been valgus overcorrection of 5° to 7° and the degree of lateral compartment arthrosis at the time of surgery. Results have been shown to deteriorate with time. Recent 15- to 20-year data, published on 60 high tibial osteotomies, demonstrate a significant drop-off in clinical scores after 15 years. The study showed satisfactory results of 73% at 10 to 14 years, which decreased to 40% at 20 years. Recurrence of varus deformity was shown to average 3.3°. In agreement with previous literature, no correlation was seen between clinical results and return of varus deformity. Progression of medial and lateral arthrosis was reported as 69% and 67%, respectively.

Complications of HTO include nonunion (0% to 5%), patella baja and infrapatella scarring (80%), infection (1% to 9%), lateral ligament laxity, shortening of the limb, and predisposition to fracture because of the size of the proximal fragment. Peroneal nerve palsy (5%), popliteal artery laceration, and deep vein thrombosis have also been reported. It is currently recommended that prophylaxis against deep vein thrombosis be employed.

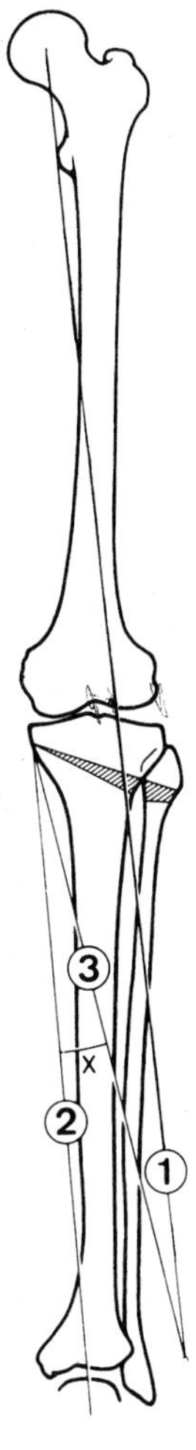

Figure 1

A full-length weightbearing radiograph is obtained. Line 1 is the predicted mechanical axis from the center of the femoral head passing through a portion of the lateral tibial plateau, which is measured to be between 30% and 40% of the lateral plateau width and extrapolated to the level of the projected position of the center of the ankle. Line 2 runs from the medial corticoperiosteal hinge or pivot point where the arms of the osteotomy will meet down to the center of the ankle. The angle X subtended by lines 2 and 3 is the desired amount of correction. (Reproduced with permission from Miniaci A, Ballmer, FT, Ballmer PM, et al: Proximal tibial osteotomy: A new fixation device. *Clin Orthop* 1989;246: 250-259.)

Supracondylar Femoral Osteotomy

A number of conditions can cause lateral compartment arthritis of the knee. The majority of patients with valgus knee deformity have primary lateral osteoarthritis, but rheumatoid arthritis, neurologic conditions (polio), collagen vascular diseases, or trauma can cause this problem as well. The incidence of primary lateral gonarthrosis is 5 times higher in women. The average age of symptomatic presentation is 55 to 60 years of age.

Indications for varus-producing supracondylar femoral osteotomy (SFO) include isolated lateral compartment arthrosis, valgus deformity less than 15° or valgus joint line tilt > 10°, 90° arc of range of motion, and < 10° flexion contracture, either posttraumatic or associated with osteoarthritis. Although significant osteoporosis is not a contraindication for SFO, care must be taken while attempting to achieve rigid fixation. Similar to HTO, SFO is best suited for stout, younger patients involved in heavy labor.

Careful preoperative planning is essential for SFO success (Fig. 3). Valgus alignment of the lower extremity is represented by a tibiofemoral angle > 12°, and a mechanical axis located through the midportion of the lateral plateau resulting in 80% of the force being distributed through the lateral compartment. The generally accepted recommendation is to correct the tibiofemoral angle to 4° to 6°. Based on finite element data, this should transfer 80% of the force distribution to the medial compartment. For rigid fixation, a 90° fixed angle blade plate should be used. Using proper summation pin technique, a guide pin should be placed 2.5 cm proximal and parallel to the joint line. Based on the full-length extremity weightbearing radiograph, the desired amount of correction is calculated as the angle formed between the blade plate and the lateral or medial femoral cortex, once the blade portion has been inserted in the distal femur. The plate may be applied medially or laterally. A midline incision may be used with a subvastus exposure of the distal femur with anterior reflection of the vastus medialis. After removal of the wedge of bone from the medial closing wedge osteotomy, the proximal femur may be inserted into the distal piece for greater stability. Plate application will assist in the reduction.

Clinical results from SFO have been reported as 90% suc-

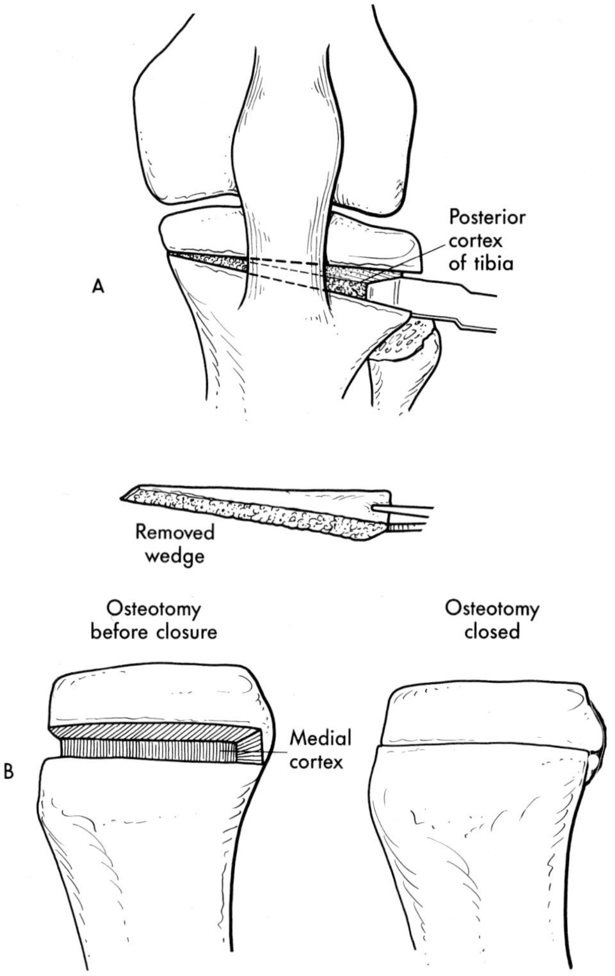

Figure 2

A, The bone wedge is cut to, but not through, the posterior cortex of tibia before its removal. **B**, The lower saw cut is deepened through the posterior cortex and the osteotomy wedge is closed as illustrated on the right. This permits the posterior lip of the bone above to override the cortex distal to osteotomy for stability. (Reproduced with permission from Slocum DB, Larson RL, James SL, Greinier R: *Clin Orthop* 1974;104:239.)

cessful at 5 years, based on Hospital for Special Surgery and Knee Society rating scores. One recent study reported a 90% satisfaction rate with the procedure, however, a 57% complication rate was reported: 48% required manipulation, 10% were infected, 19% had delayed or nonunion, and 5% had fixation failure. Best results were seen in patients who had less severe lateral gonarthrosis, adequate correction of the valgus deformity, and rigid fixation. Staple use appeared to be involved in the majority of manipulations and delayed unions. In a series of 49 consecutive SFOs, predicted survival before conversion to TKR was 87% at 7 years. There was no correlation between age, sex, tibiofemoral angle, and amount of correction. Removal of the implant improved the clinical result.

Total Knee Arthroplasty After Osteotomy

HTO is a useful procedure that can delay subsequent total knee arthroplasty by several years. Revision rates after HTO has been reported as 6% to 37%, with survival analysis depending on the length of follow-up. Reported success rates are comparable to those of revision procedures, with good to excellent results of 80% to 85% at intermediate follow-up. Problems encountered with TKA after HTO are patella infera (80%), offset of the tibial plateau from the shaft, location of skin incision, and patella tracking. More recent data support these findings. One recent study compared two groups of 60 patients (group A had a previous HTO, group B had a primary arthroplasty) with respect to Knee Society scores and operative complications. The primary arthroplasty group scored significantly higher with 88% rated excellent or good, compared with 63% for the post-HTO group. Significantly higher rates of tibial tuberosity elevation (11% versus 1.6%), lateral release (24% versus 1.6%), and proximal tibial valgus deformity (40% versus 14%) were seen in group A. No differences were described with respect to infection rates, allograft use, or postoperative manipulation under anesthesia. Among risk factors associated with poorer outcome of TKA after HTO are worker's compensation patients, absence of pain relief after HTO, multiple prior knee operations, and occupation as a laborer. Technical considerations to consider while performing this procedure have been described. They include proper skin incision to avoid skin slough, care in inverting the patella to

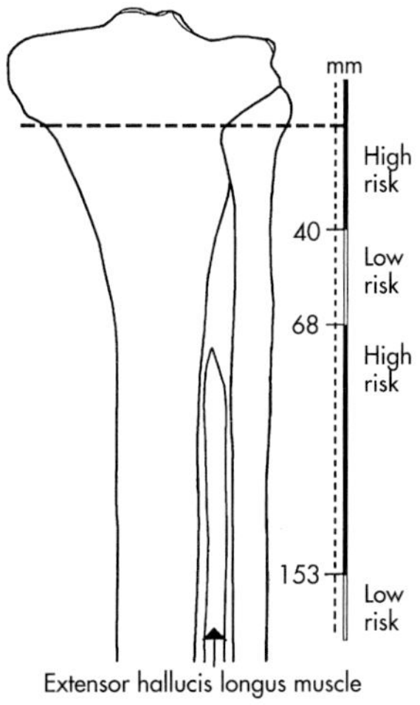

Figure 3

Coventry technique of the lower femoral osteotomy. The angle to be corrected is measured on preoperative roentgenogram, and the nail of the blade is driven into femoral metaphysis so that the plate will accomplish the desired correction when attached to the osteotomized femoral shaft. The wedge with the apical angle equal to the amount of correction is removed with osteotomy. (Reproduced with permission from Coventry MB: *J Bone Joint Surg* 1973;55A:23.)

avoid tubercle avulsion during exposure due to the patella baja, and care to avoid malalignment of the tibial component from the prior osteotomy.

Relatively little literature has been published regarding total knee arthroplasty after SFO. Although excellent clinical results, as high as 90%, have been reported, the numbers present in these studies are small. The major technical difficulty associated with the procedure is medial offset and relative varus orientation of the distal femur. This requires the use of extramedullary instrumentation for the distal femoral cut to restore anatomic valgus. Care should be taken if the femoral component to be used has stems.

Treatment of Isolated Cartilage Lesions

Defects in articular cartilage rarely heal spontaneously. Some patients do not develop clinical symptoms, but most eventually develop degenerative changes associated with the cartilage damage. The incidence of these lesions is believed to be very high, however, data from various studies vary widely. One recent study reported the incidence of articular cartilage injuries from 31,515 arthroscopies. They demonstrated 53,569 lesions in 19,827 patients. Grade III lesions of the patella were most common, while grade IV lesions were predominantly located on the medial femoral condyle. Seventy-four percent of patients had a single cartilage lesion, while 36% demonstrated no associated ligamentous or meniscal pathology. Other epidemiologic reports estimate that 35 million Americans of all ages have degenerative arthritis that has become progressive from either acute or chronic chondral injuries.

Partial-thickness lesions penetrate the articular cartilage but do not reach the subchondral bone. Full-thickness lesions reach down to the subchondral bone but do not penetrate it. Osteochondral lesions reach down through the subchondral bone layer. Partial- and full-thickness lesions have a minimal capacity for repair due to the lack of blood supply within hyaline cartilage. Nutrition is obtained from the pumping of nutrients within the synovial fluid, through the cartilage layers via hydrostatic pressure gradients produced during joint loading. Osteochondral defects heal with fibrocartilage tissue. The source of this repair tissue is pluripotential stem cells located within the bone marrow. Marrow stimulation techniques are designed to recruit these stem cells to participate in the repair process of partial and full-thickness cartilage defects.

Considerable research during the last several years has been aimed at using autogenous cartilage transplantation in the treatment of isolated cartilage lesions. The fibrocartilage present in the body's natural repair process has biomechanical properties different from those of hyaline cartilage, which predispose it to degeneration. Transplantation of cultured cells and autogenous grafts (mosaicplasty) are the current procedures most often employed to introduce hyaline cartilage to lesions. Osteochondral transplantation, periosteal/perichondral transplantation, artificial cartilage matrixes, growth factors (transforming growth factor B), and meniscal allografts are exciting new options, which are undergoing study for general use.

Marrow Stimulation Techniques

Subchondral Drilling

This technique calls for several 2.5-mm drill holes to be made within the cartilage defect after loose unsupported cartilage has been debrided. The holes allow blood supply to lay down a clot containing stem cells from which the fibrocartilage can form. Preoperatively, patients should receive a complete radiographic examination of the knee, including a posteroanterior view of the knee in 45° of flexion to check anterior and posterior joint space. If varus/valgus alignment or subchondral sclerosis is present, cartilage drilling will be ineffective. In one study of 78 patients, full- and partial-thickness defects were drilled. Sixty-one showed clinical improvement, 2 needed another arthroscopy for unrelated reasons, which demonstrated congruent fibrocartilage. To date, however, there are no long-term controlled studies for this procedure.

Microfracture

This procedure, popularized by Steadman, uses a manual awl technique to penetrate the subchondral bone. Preoperative assessment is similar to subchondral drilling. Indication for microfracture includes a full-thickness lesion in a weightbearing area between the tibia and femur, or associated with the patella and trochlea groove. Another indication is degenerative changes in a knee that has proper axial alignment. Loose or marginally attached cartilage fragments are debrided. Removal of the calcified cartilage layer is extremely important based on the basic science of this procedure. Excessive damage to the subchondral bone should be avoided. The technique calls for 3 to 4 holes to be made per square cm with specially designed angled arthroscopic awls. The awl technique avoids the thermal necrosis associated with mechanical drilling. The various angles available make hard-to-reach areas, such as the posterior femoral condyle, more accessible than with standard drilling techniques. Proper depth of penetration is seen when fat droplets are visualized emanating from the lesion. Patients are placed in continuous passive motion (CPM) immediately and are touch down weight bearing with crutches.

Two to 12 years clinical follow-up of 235 patients has recently been reported. At 3 to 5 years, 75% of patients were improved, 20% unchanged, 5% worse. Criterion of activities of daily living and strenuous work showed 67% of patients improved. At 7 years, pain was the parameter with the greatest improvement. Negative predictors of success included chronic lesions, age > 30 years, preoperative joint space narrowing, and no CPM following surgery. Patients with combined injuries fared better than patients with isolated chondral lesions. Histologically, the microfracture regenerated tissue was reported to be a hybrid of hyaline and fibrocartilage.

Chondrocyte Transplantation

Mosaicplasty

This procedure harvests osteochondral plugs from nonarticulating areas of the distal femur and places them into the cartilage defect. Potential problems of laboratory error and the significant cost of chondrocyte transplantation can be avoided. Defects < 2 cm have been treated with a variety of sized plugs ranging from 2.7 to 8.5 mm in size. Indications are similar to the marrow stimulation techniques, except lesions on the patella have been treated. The plugs obtained should measure 2.5 mm in length. Donor plugs are obtained from the lateral portion of the distal femur adjacent to the patellofemoral joint, as well as the intercondylar notch. Recent work has investigated the contact pressures at osteochondral donor sites in the knee. Significant pressures were registered at all sites from 0 to 110° of knee flexion, bringing into question whether or not these areas are truly nonweightbearing. The plugs most proximal on the lateral femur registered the lowest contact pressures.

Recent clinical data were reported on 57 patients undergoing mosaicplasty with minimum 3-year follow-up. Based on Hospital for Special Surgery knee scores, 91% of patients had a good or excellent result. Arthroscopic biopsies taken from the repair areas showed hyaline cartilage with areas of fibrous repair tissue interspersed between the plugs. Fibrocartilage was seen in the areas from which plugs had been taken.

Autogenous Chondrocyte Transplantation

In a report published in 1994 on 23 patients who underwent autogenous cultured chondrocyte transplantation, results at minimum 2-year follow-up showed that 14 of 16 patients who had a femoral condylar defect and 2 of 7 patients who had a patella defect had a good or excellent result. Biopsy results reported that 11 of 16 condylar lesions and 1 of the patella defects showed hyaline cartilage. Indications for the procedure in this study were patients with isolated femoral condylar, patella, and trochlea defects without other signs of degenerative arthritis. Full-thickness lesions treated ranged in size from 10 to 12 mm. The technique calls for obtaining a 12 mm by 5 mm full-thickness articular cartilage specimen from the superior aspect of the medial femoral condyle. This will supply ~250,000 cells, which are enzymatically digested and cultured for 3 weeks to obtain ~12 million cells. The cultured chondrocytes are replanted and covered with a periosteal flap recovered from the medial aspect of the proximal tibia. The flap is sutured into place with 6.0 vicryl after the lesion is debrided of granulation tissue. Special care is taken not to generate bleeding from the subchondral bone bed. The suture lines are coated with fibrin glue to ensure water tightness, and the cells are injected. CPM is started 12 to 24 hours after the procedure and is continued for 6 to 8 hours a day for 6 weeks. Weightbearing for the lesions on the femoral condyle is toe-touch for 6 weeks, advanced to full body weight by 12 weeks with use of one crutch. On the average it is 4 months before patients have discarded their assistive devices and are walking comfortably. At approximately 6 to 9 months, nonimpact activities, such as cycling and swimming,

Table 1
Results following chondrocyte transplantation

Lesion Location	No. of Patients	% Improved	% Not Improved
Femoral condyle	62	89%	31%
Femoral condyle +ACL repair	27	74%	26%
OCD	32	84%	16%
Patella	12	69%	31%
Trochlea	12	58%	42%
Multiple	53	75%	25%
Overall	219	78%	22%

ACL, anterior cruciate ligament; OCD, osteochondritis dissecans are encouraged. High-impact activities are allowed after graft hardness is similar to surrounding tissue, which takes 9 to 12 months. Larger lesions and osteochondritis dessicans can take up to 24 months to heal. Lesions on the trochlea are slower in the rehabilitation process and healing. Weightbearing status is allowed at full weightbearing with a knee immobilizer. Kneeling and squatting are not permitted until 12 to 18 months.

Long-term (2- to 10-year) follow-up of the first 219 patients treated in Sweden with chondrocyte transplantation was recently reported. The results are summarized in Table 1.

Histologic examination in 14 of 20 patients biopsied showed the presence of hyaline cartilage. Tissue type present correlated with clinical response in 85% of patients. Immunohistochemical analysis revealed that the repair tissue stained positive for aggrecans and type II collagen. A specially designed indentation probe performed measurements of the repair tissue stiffness. Baseline readings taken from normal hyaline cartilage measured an average of 3 N. Hyaline-like repair tissue averaged 2.80 N and the fibrous-like repair tissue measured 1.23 N.

In a multicenter, international observational series on 249 patients at 12-month follow-up and 50 patients at 24-month follow-up, improvement was seen in 78% of all study patients. The most promising results were seen in femoral lesions at 24 months, with 86% showing improvement. The mean defect size treated was 4.4 m^2.

Annotated Bibliography

Medical Therapy

Hawkey C, Kahan A, Steinbruck K, et al: Gastrointestinal tolerability of meloxicam compared to diclofenac in osteoarthritis patients: International MELISSA Study Group. Meloxicam Large-scale International Study Safety Assessment. *Br J Rheumatol* 1998;37:937–945.

The MELISSA study was a 28-day, large-scale, double-blind, randomized, international, prospective trial of 9,323 symptomatic osteoarthritic patients. Patients were randomized to receive either Meloxicam (COX-2 inhibitor) or diclofenac. Fewer GI adverse events were seen in Meloxicam (13%) compared to diclofenac (19%). Significantly less dyspepsia, nausea, abdominal pain and diarrhea were reported. No endoscopy verified ulcer was seen in the COX-2 inhibitor, while 4 were seen in the diclofenac group. There were 5 hospitalization days attributed to Meloxicam complications, compared to 121 with diclofenac. Differences in efficacy, as assessed by visual analog scales, consistently favored diclofenac. Significantly more patients discontinued Meloxicam because of lack of efficacy. Although the COX-2 inhibitor did display significantly fewer GI side effects, liver and renal safety profiles were similar.

Simon LS, Lanza FL, Lipsky PE, et al: Preliminary study of the safety and efficacy of SC-58635, a novel cyclooxygenase 2 inhibitor: Efficacy and safety in two placebo-controlled trials in osteoarthritis and rheumatoid arthritis and studies of gastrointestinal and platelet effects. *Arthritis Rheum* 1998;41: 1591–1602.

Four phase II trials are described to document the clinical efficacy of a COX-2 inhibitor. A 2-week osteoarthritis efficacy trial, a 4-week rheumatoid arthritis efficacy trial, a 1-week endoscopy study of GI mucosal effects, and a 1-week study on platelet function were performed. The 2 arthritis trials identified dosages, which were consistent in relieving symptoms compared to placebo. In the upper GI study, 19% of patients receiving Naprosyn developed gastric ulcers, while none in the COX-2 group or placebo did. No meaningful effects on platelets or Thromboxane-2 levels were seen with the COX-2 inhibitor. In all 4 trials, SC-58635 was well tolerated, with a safety profile similar to that of placebo.

Injections

Lussier A, Cividino AA, McFarlane CA, Olszynski WP, Potashner WJ, De Medicis R: Viscosupplementation with hylan for the treatment of osteoarthritis: Findings from clinical practice in Canada. *J Rheumatol* 1996;23:1579–1585.

A retrospective study of 1,537 injections in 336 patients involving 458 knees was performed. The overall response and the change of activity level were judged better or much better for 77% of the treated knees after the first course of treatment, and 87% after a second course. Local adverse effects were observed in 28 patients, with an overall rate of 2.7% adverse events per injection, 7% per joint, and 8.3% per patient. The incidence of adverse events is significantly influenced by injection technique: 5.2% adverse events per injection with a medial approach to a partially bent knee, 2.4% straight medial, and 1.5% straight lateral. Most events were a localized synovitis which abated with time.

Rozental T, Sculco TP: Intra-articular corticosteroids: An updated overview. *Am J Orthop*, in press.

Excellent overview of the indications and complications of intra-articular steroid injections.

Wobig M, Dickhut A, Maier R, Vetter G: Viscosupplementation with hylan G-F 20: A 26-week controlled trial of efficacy and safety in the osteoarthritic knee. *Clin Ther* 1998;20:410–423.

The efficacy and safety of Hylan G-F 20 was evaluated in a multicenter, double-blind trial in patients with chronic osteoarthritis of the knee. The study group (57 knees) received 3 intra-articular injections of Hylan 1-week apart. The control group (60 knees) received 2 ml of buffered saline. Using a visual analog scale, patients were assessed using the following clinical variables: pain during weightbearing, pain at rest during night, reduction of pain during the most painful movement of the knee, and treatment success. The differences between Hylan G-F 20 and saline treatment were statistically significant for all outcome measures. In the Hylan group, 56% of patients were free or nearly free of weightbearing pain 10-24 weeks after the last injection; compared with 13% in the control group. No adverse affects were reported.

Valgus Bracing

Lindenfeld TN, Hewett TE, Andriacchi TP: Joint loading with valgus bracing in patients with varus gonarthrosis. *Clin Orthop* 1997;344:290–297.

Eleven patients with isolated osteoarthritis of the medial compartment were fitted with a valgus brace and tested before and after brace wear with pain- and function-scoring instruments and by automated gait analysis. Biomechanical data was compared with 11 healthy control subjects. Scores from analog pain scales decreased 48% with brace wear, and function with activities of daily living increased 79%. Mean adduction moment decreased by 10%, within values recorded in healthy subjects.

Osteotomy

Bergenudd H, Sahlstrom A, Sanzen L: Total knee arthroplasty after failed proximal tibial valgus osteotomy. *J Arthroplasty* 1997;12:635–638.

The results of total knee arthroplasty were evaluated in 113 patients with gonarthrosis (14 patients with and 99 without prior operation with proximal tibial valgus osteotomy). There was no difference in the final result after follow-up periods of 4 to 9 years with respect to average Hospital For Special Surgery score, degree of knee flexion, and later knee revisions between the two groups. No difference was found in operative time, but a significantly greater blood loss and other postoperative complications were noted among the previously osteotomized group of patients; indicating a more complicated procedure for these patients compared with the nonosteotomized group of patients.

Cameron HU, Park YS: Total knee replacement after supracondylar femoral osteotomy. *Am J Knee Surg* 1997;10:70–72.

Cameron HU, Botsford DJ, Park YS: Prognostic factors in the outcome of supracondylar femoral osteotomy for lateral compartment osteoarthritis of the knee. *Can J Surg* 1997;40:114–118.

Forty-nine consecutive patients with unicompartmental osteoarthritis of the knee involving the lateral compartment had a supracondylar femoral osteotomy with blade plate fixation. A Knee Society score greater than 80 was obtained in 81% of patients, but in the function portion of the measurement only 30% had a similar score. Life-table analysis demonstrated the predicted survival before conversion to total knee replacement to be 87% at 7 years. There was no correlation with patient age, sex, femorotibial angulation, and amount of correction or time after the intervention. Removal of the fixation device improved the clinical result.

Mathews J, Cobb AG, Richardson S, Bentley G: Distal femoral osteotomy for lateral compartment osteoarthritis of the knee. *Orthopedics* 1998;21:437–440.

Twenty-one patients with lateral compartment osteoarthritis and valgus deformity of the knee underwent distal femoral osteotomy (medial closing wedge) between 1983 and 1993, with follow-up ranging from 1 to 8 years. Ten knees had plaster cast immobilization, 5 had fixation with 2 staples supplemented with a plaster cast, and 6 knees had rigid internal fixation with an AO blade plate. Fifty-seven percent had a satisfactory result using the Knee Society Clinical Rating. Fifty-seven percent also had a significant complication, including severe knee stiffness requiring manipulation under anesthesia (48%), nonunion/delayed union (19%), infection (10%), and fixation failure (5%). Five knees (19%) required TKR within 5 years of surgery. Satisfactory results were obtained only in those patients who had less severe degrees of osteoarthritis confined to the lateral compartment (grades I to III), adequate correction of valgus deformity (the anatomic axis within 2° from zero), and rigid internal fixation to permit postoperative early immobilization.

Phillips MJ, Krackow KA: High tibial osteotomy and distal femoral osteotomy for valgus or varus deformity around the knee, in Cannon WD Jr (ed): *Instructional Course Lectures 47*. Rosemont, IL, American Academy of Orthopaedic Surgeons, 1998, pp 429–436.

Excellent summation of the material with a detailed bibliography.

Rinonapoli E, Mancini GB, Corvaglia A, Musiello S: Tibial osteotomy for varus gonarthrosis: A 10- to 21-year follow-up study. *Clin Orthop* 1998;353:185–193.

Long-term results of 102 high tibial osteotomies for varus gonarthrosis are presented with average 15-year follow-up (range, 10 to 21 years). The results, assessed according to the scoring system of the Hospital For Special Surgery were excellent or good in 55% and fair or poor in 45%. Twenty-six patients in the current study were previously reported in 1986. In this group of 26 patients, excellent or good results decreased from 73% to 46%. No statistically different results were found according to the amount of correction. Loss of correction greater than 5° was observed in 11 knees. Clinical and survivorship data tend to deteriorate after 10 to 15 years consistent with prior studies. Excellent bibliography.

Takai S, Yoshino N, Hirasawa Y: Revision total knee arthroplasty after failed high tibial osteotomy. *Bull Hosp Jt Dis* 1997;56:245–250.

Twelve knees, which underwent revision total knee arthroplasty after failed high tibial osteotomy, were reviewed. The time from osteotomy to arthroplasty ranged from 9 months to 9 years. The average follow-up period after arthroplasty was 7 years. The patients were divided into 2 groups. Group 1 patients had the arthroplasty to relieve pain from recurrent varus deformity. Group 2 were patients who progressed to bi- and tricompartmental arthritis. No difference was found clinically between the groups. However, patella height was found to be significantly lower in group 1 compared to group 2.

Chapter 29
Biomechanics of Total Knee Design

Total knee replacement designs must provide for several key mechanical goals: appropriate function (kinematics, ranges of motion, and constraint); safe and effective transfer of large joint reaction loads to the surrounding bony structures; secure, permanent fixation of the implant components; and long-term wear resistance. The implant designer strives to meet these goals by choosing the shapes of the implant components and the materials from which they are fabricated. Important shape considerations include the geometries of the joint surfaces and the location and shapes of fixation structures such as pegs, stems, and porous coatings. Important material factors include mechanical and wear properties of the metallic alloys and ultrahigh molecular weight polyethylene (UHMWPE).

Unfortunately, design goals are not independent. For example, the shapes of the joint surfaces that create the best function for a knee replacement may adversely affect polyethylene wear. Thus, rational compromises must be sought. In this chapter, mechanical goals will be discussed in terms of these compromises using examples from a number of different types of knee implants (unicondylar, cruciate retaining, posterior stabilized, mobile bearing, and constrained). The orthopaedic surgeon must consider the limitations that these compromises can create on implant performance when selecting a specific design.

Function (Kinematics, Ranges of Motion, and Constraint)

The natural knee achieves a large range of motion in flexion and extension and appropriate constraint to varus and valgus angulation and internal and external rotation through a combination of bony and cartilage geometries, ligaments and joint capsule, and muscle action (see Chapter 26). Total knee replacements are designed to provide similar function primarily through the geometry of the femoral and tibial articulating surfaces in concert with remaining soft-tissue structures. Virtually all contemporary knees, for example, approximate the anteroposterior geometry of each femoral condyle using multiple radii, with larger radii to contact the tibial plateau near extension and smaller posterior radii to contact with the plateau as the knee flexes. Together with a constant radius for the tibial surface, this approach provides large contact areas in extension (for better wear resistance), and the opportunity for rollback of the femur on the tibia during flexion, providing a large range of motion (as in the natural joint).

Designs intended to rely more on ligaments for constraint require less-constrained articulating geometries. Examples include unicondylar knees, which must function in the presence of one or both cruciate ligaments, and posterior cruciate-sparing knee designs, which maintain the posterior cruciate ligament (PCL) as a natural means of generating posterior translation during flexion (thus allowing for a large range of motion). Articulating surface designs that restrict motion too greatly could compete with ligament function. The goal, therefore, is to match the constraint of the design with the function of the ligament. Whether this is possible from the basis of implant design or surgical technique has been controversial. Recent in vivo fluoroscopic studies of PCL-sparing designs have shown that kinematics are quite unpredictable, with knees often showing anterior, rather than posterior, femoral translation during flexion. These findings, together with concerns of wear (discussed below), have led some proponents to question the efficacy of these designs.

More constrained anteroposterior geometries can be used in designs that substitute for the PCL. Substituting for the PCL can provide both range of motion and joint stability and allows for more conforming surfaces without compromising kinematics. The geometric constraint of more curved articular surfaces (ie, with smaller radii of curvature) allows for controlled posterior femoral translation by designing the equilibrium position (the low point) of the tibial articulating surface to be posterior. Additional constraint is provided by a post and cam mechanism (hence the description "posterior stabilized" for such designs), although the necessary space for the mechanism requires more resection of femoral bone from the intercondylar notch. In contrast with PCL-sparing designs, posterior-stabilized designs have demonstrated well-controlled femoral translation during flexion in studies of in vivo kinematics using fluoroscopy. A concern that the moment applied to the tibial component by the femoral cam contacting the tibial post could exacerbate loosening has not materialized, and several posterior-stabilized designs have demonstrated excellent clinical results at more than a decade of follow-up.

In the medial-lateral direction, the design of the contacting geometry depends on the desired amount of rotational constraint (among other considerations). Two design approaches have emerged. Some designs consist of a single radius for each condyle of the femoral component and a single, slightly larger radius for each tibial plateau. Rotational laxity is limited in these designs, but the curved, conforming surfaces in the medial-lateral direction provide large contact areas, even when the joint load must be resisted totally by 1 condyle to resist varus-valgus moments (Fig. 1). Other designs use larger radii between the femoral and tibial components, resulting in flatter articulating geometries. These designs are not as rotationally constrained, but have less ability to resist varus-valgus moments without encountering high contact stresses at the edge of the plateau.

Mobile bearing knee designs have been advocated to create more naturally functioning (and, as discussed below, more wear-resistant) knee replacements than more conventional, fixed-bearing designs. The goal of a mobile bearing knee replacement is to separate the movement needed for function from the movement between the articulating surfaces. This is achieved by having 2 articulations: between the femoral and tibial components, and between the tibial component and a base plate fixed to the tibia. The mobile nature of the tibial component, either as a meniscal-type bearing or as a rotating platform, is intended to allow the soft tissues (muscles and ligaments) around the joint to control and constrain joint motion, thus imparting more natural kinematics. In meniscal types of mobile bearing designs, the optimal configuration is a single matching radius for the articulating surfaces of the femoral and tibial components. Such a configuration, however, requires too great a posterior displacement of the mobile bearing during flexion. The compromise is to have a femoral component with multiple radii (much like fixed bearing designs).

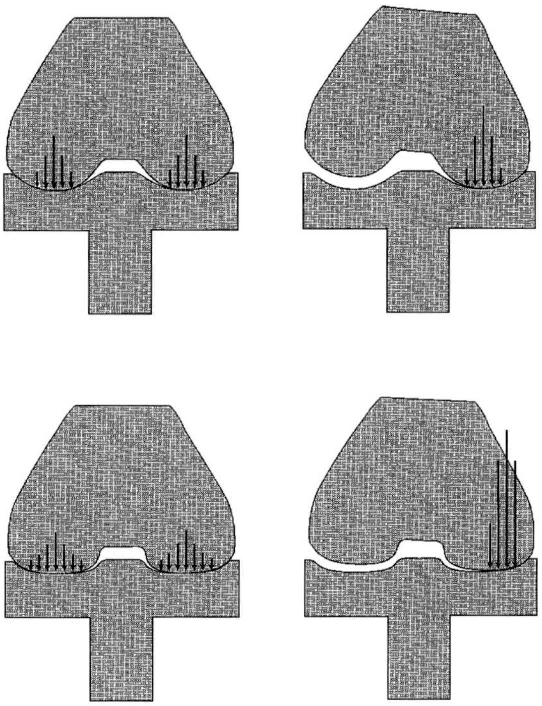

Figure 1

When load is shared evenly between both condyles, a condylar design with a single radius of curvature for the femoral and tibial components in the medial-lateral direction has a smaller contact area (top, left) than a flatter design with a larger central radius and small radii at the edge of the flat (bottom, left). But when the load is redistributed to 1 condyle, the single radius of curvature design maintains a large contact area (top, right), while the flatter design suffers edge loading on a much smaller contact area (bottom, right), causing large contact stresses. (Reproduced with permission from Burstein AH, Wright TM: *Fundamentals of Orthopaedic Biomechanics.* Baltimore, MD, Williams & Wilkins, 1994, p 205.)

Abnormal kinematics in mobile bearing designs have been demonstrated in fluoroscopic studies of knee patients. During a deep knee bend, as the knee flexed, the femur moved anteriorly relative to the tibia in half of the patients, while no motion was noted at the mobile bearing in the other half of the patients. These in vivo studies underscore the fact that soft tissues and the remaining (altered) knee anatomy cannot be relied upon to provide natural function, similar to the conclusion from the same types of studies in PCL-sparing implants that also employ unconstrained geometries in hopes that the remaining ligaments and soft tissues will provide normal function.

Load Transfer

Most primary total knee designs are surface replacements. The components of these implants do not rely on long intramedullary stems for fixation. Instead, the components cover the surfaces of the femur, tibia, and patella, thus transferring joint loads directly to the underlying cancellous bone. In this respect, the components mimic the way subchondral bone bears load in the natural joint. The distributed loads in the cancellous bone are gradually transferred to the cortical shell. An implant's ability to transfer load effectively is governed by how the joint reaction load is distributed over the articulating surfaces, how the implant deforms as a result of the load distribution, and how the load distribution and the implant deformation affect the load distribution to the bone-implant interface and the underlying bone.

Load distribution on the joint surface depends on the stiffness of the implant, (which in turn is controlled by its geometry and the elastic modulus of the material from which it is made), and the shape of the contacting surfaces. Consider, for example, a modern condylar total knee replacement (design A) with an 8-mm thick tibial component made from conventional UHMWPE with an elastic modulus of 1 GPa (Fig. 2). For comparative purposes, the relative peak contact stress with the load shared equally between the condyles has a value of 1.

In a second design (B), the same surface shapes and the same thickness are used, but the elastic modulus for UHMWPE is doubled to 2 GPa, as might be the case with an "enhanced" material, such as heavily cross-linked polyethylene. The increased modulus stiffens the implant, reducing the contact area and increasing the contact stress by 40%. In a third design (C) with conventional UHMWPE and the same thickness, the shapes of the contacting surfaces are made less conforming by increasing the medial-lateral radius of the tibial component by 2 mm. The decreased conformity increases the peak contact stress by 14%. Finally, consider a design (D) with the same curvatures and elastic modulus as A, but with a tibial component only 5 mm thick. In this case, the peak contact stress increases by 29%.

Conditions in which loads are not shared between the tibial plateaus must also be considered. For example, a varus or valgus moment applied across the joint in sufficient magnitude will cause the load to be totally concentrated on only 1 plateau. The load distribution induced by such a redistribution will again depend on the shapes of the contacting surfaces (Fig. 1). The change in the shape of the implant caused by the applied loads significantly affects load transfer to the cancellous bone. Most implant designs employ flat surfaces intended to conform against flat surfaces cut into the bone (the flat surfaces cut on the proximal tibia and the flat and chamfer cuts made on the distal femur). For loads to be transferred over as large an area as possible, the implant should deform as little as possible. When load is applied to 1 condyle of a conventional bicondylar plateau (Fig. 3, *A*), contact forces develop at the prosthesis-cancellous bone interface. The area over which the load is distributed at this interface, however, is larger than the contact area on the joint surface. A bending moment is created in the implant by this difference in distribution, causing the opposite plateau to bend upward. If the deformation is not resisted (such as with an interlocking surface on the bottom of the plateau for cement penetration or with screws to secure the component to the bone), separation will occur and no load will be transferred. If a means exists to resist deformation, tensile forces will develop across this interface.

For a unicondylar plateau (Fig. 3, *B*), the area over which the load is distributed at the interface is more nearly equal to that over which the contact force is distributed on the joint surface. The bending moment is much smaller than in the bicondylar case, and the tibial plateau transfers load to the bone-implant interface in an almost direct manner.

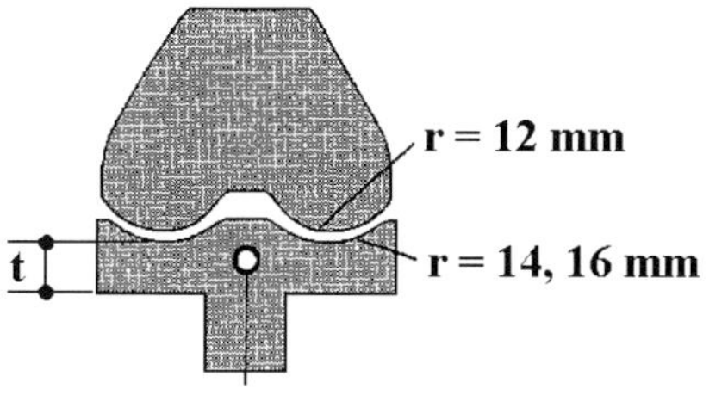

	(mm)	Modulus (GPa)	(mm)	Relative contact stress
A	8	1	12,14	1.00
B	8	2	12,14	1.40
C	8	1	12,16	1.14
D	5	1	12,14	1.29

Figure 2

Three factors affect contact stresses in total knee components: the elastic modulus of the ultrahigh molecular weight polyethylene (UHMWPE) (compare A and B), the conformity between the articulating surfaces (compare A and C), and the thickness of the UHMWPE (compare A and D). (Reproduced with permission from Burstein AH, Wright TM: *Fundamentals of Orthopaedic Biomechanics.* Baltimore, MD, Williams & Wilkins, 1994, p 204.)

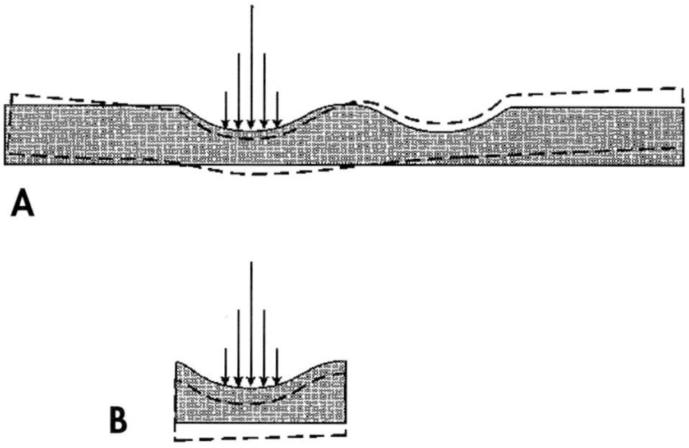

Figure 3

When the load is distributed over 1 condyle of a bicondylar tibial component, significant bending deformations occur (**A**), greater than in the unicondylar component which has a much smaller medial-lateral dimension (**B**). (Reproduced with permission from Burstein AH, Wright TM: *Fundamentals of Orthopaedic Biomechanics.* Baltimore, MD, Williams & Wilkins, 1994, p 206.)

Unfortunately, the sudden change in load distribution at the edges of the unicondylar plateau creates high shear stresses in the bone, which can cause bone fracture and subsidence and loosening of the implant.

In the natural knee joint, joint loads are distributed to the underlying cancellous bone over a very large area by the stiff subchondral bone. This bone is typically removed, however, in knee replacement surgeries, leaving the much more compliant and weaker cancellous bone. The bone becomes the weak link in the system, experiencing cyclic tensile and compressive stresses that approach the strength levels of the material. In an effort to more evenly distribute load to the cancellous bone and thus ensure that the stresses in any single region of the bone are minimal, most contemporary knee implants include a metallic base plate in the tibial component. The metal backing reduces the maximum compressive bone stresses, although the reduction is marginal when the loads are shared between the plateaus. A substantial reduction does occur, however, during severe situations, as when load is applied to just 1 plateau.

Although metal backing decreases the maximum compressive stress in the bone, it also increases the maximum tensile stress. Again, the increase is greatest for severe cases in which loads are applied unevenly to the plateaus. The opposite plateau of the metal-backed component tends to lift off from the cancellous bone, similar to the situation in the polyethylene implant (Fig. 3). It is important, therefore, in metal-backed designs as well to provide resistance to lift off (eg, with undercuts for cement penetration or with screws across the interface).

Although a metal backing is advantageous for load transfer, it presents additional design problems, including the need for secure, rigid attachment between the polyethylene insert and the metallic tray to prevent dissociation and to minimize wear between the insert and tray. Both the metallic tray and the UHMWPE insert must be of sufficient thickness to ensure strength and, in the case of the UHMWPE, to minimize wear. These are difficult design goals to meet, especially when considering that the amount of bone resected from the proximal tibia should also be minimized, and the joint line should be maintained in as near an anatomic position as possible. These problems, together with the added cost of a metallic tray, have caused some surgeons to advocate the use of all-UHMWPE tibial components for primary total knee arthroplasties, especially in elderly, low-demand patients.

The same biomechanical considerations apply to load transfer in femoral and patellar components. Load transfer in these 2 types of implant components has not been explored extensively, probably because fewer clinical problems are related to load transfer in these bones.

Fixation

Polymethylmethacrylate (PMMA) bone cement remains the "gold standard" for fixing total knee components to the surrounding bone, because loosening is a rare complication in most large, long-term clinical series, occurring less frequently than with total hip femoral components at comparable follow-up periods. Surgeons remain reluctant to use cemented prostheses in young active patients, however, and press-fit and porous-coated total knee replacements have been introduced with the aim of achieving stable biologic fixation without cement.

Design goals for cementless fixation are less clear than for cement fixation. The relationship between the way loads are transferred in the initial period after implantation and the subsequent extent and distribution of tissue ingrowth is often unpredictable, as is the subsequent remodeling that occurs in the surrounding bone. Stable initial fixation must be achieved for adequate tissue ingrowth to occur. Devices to provide this initial fixation include screws and pegs. Regardless of technique, however, a fibrous layer may form at the interface between the porous layer and the bone, further compromising fixation.

Whether fabricated from UHMWPE or metal, the pegs employed in contemporary cementless designs can be thought of as supplemental fixation. When pegs are located near the center of the tibia between the plateaus, they are coupled to much more porous and thus less stiff cancellous bone than is present under the plateaus. Because there is no stiff bone structure to accept loads transferred from the peg, little load sharing occurs between the peg and the bone. However, pegs do provide resistance to shear and torsional loads between the implant and the bone. Pegs incorporated under the plateaus can aid in fixation. However, bone often preferentially grows into such pegs when they are incorporated into porous-coated prostheses. Because the ingrowth occurs at the expense of adequate ingrowth into the rest of the bone-implant interface, fixation can be jeopardized.

Wear

Wear of the articulating surfaces of UHMWPE components in total knee replacements is inevitable. The large contact stresses experienced by the material even in highly conforming designs are sufficient to cause wear damage. Surface damage in turn generates polyethylene debris that accumulates in the soft tissues. Although osteolytic changes leading to loosening seem more rare in total knee replacements than in total hip replacements, minimization of the stresses responsible for the generation of this debris through the choice of geometry and UHMWPE material properties remains an important design goal in total knee arthroplasty.

Wear-damage modes observed in total knee replacements differ from those seen in total hip replacements. In total hip replacements, abrasive and adhesive wear mechanisms dominate, causing burnishing and scratching. In total knee replacements, pitting and delamination are often observed, and these damage modes result in large amounts of debris, although the particle sizes tend to be larger than those that result from burnishing and scratching. Pitting and delamination are caused by fatigue. The contact area moves over the tibial surface during functional loading of the knee, creating large cyclic stresses in the material that cause cracks to initiate and grow on and below the component surface.

Stress analyses (using, for example, the finite element method) of the contact problem in total knees have provided insight into factors that affect wear. The magnitudes and locations of the maximum principal stresses and the maximum shear stress that are probably associated with fatigue wear are affected by the conformity of the surfaces, by UHMWPE component thickness, and by the elastic modulus of the UHMWPE. These are the same design factors that affected load transfer (Fig. 2). More recently, dynamic analyses of the contact problem have demonstrated that substantial residual stresses are also generated by the moving contact area. The large contact stresses at or near the articulating surface are, therefore, further increased by the presence of the residual stresses that remain in the material, making the material even more prone to fatigue failure.

Conformity

Conformity affects both contact stresses and constraint. For example, posterior stabilized, total condylar type implants provide appropriate function by having 2 radii of curvature for the tibial component (1 in the anteroposterior direction and 1 in the medial-lateral direction) and 3 radii for the femoral component (2 in the anteroposterior direction, 1 intended to contact the tibia near extension and a smaller one for flexion, and a third in the medial-lateral direction). The conformity could be increased in either direction by making the tibial and femoral radii match more closely. Stress analysis shows that changing the conformity in the anteroposterior direction has little effect, allowing the geometry in this direction to be dictated more by appropriate flexion-extension motion than by wear considerations.

Conformity changes in the medial-lateral direction significantly affect both contact stress and constraint. The contact area could be maximized (and the stress minimized) if the femoral and tibial radii were made the same. This is the same situation as for PCL-sparing designs with highly conforming femoral and tibial components that were both flat in the medial-lateral direction. These surfaces presented no rotational constraint, but created unacceptable edge loading under varus and valgus moments (Fig. 1). Flat medial-lateral femoral and tibial surfaces cause the load to be concentrated over a very small area at the outer edge of 1 plateau, leading to locally high stresses both in the UHMWPE and the underlying cancellous bone. Meeting the design objective of ensuring appropriate kinematics for the PCL while ignoring the kinematic design objective of adequately resisting varus and valgus moments adversely affects both wear and fixation. Many contemporary PCL-sparing designs no longer have flat contact surfaces; instead, they have more curved, condylar surfaces. However, because it is not known how such surfaces interact with the PCL, PCL function in these joints is questionable.

Making the radii the same for the posterior stabilized, total condylar implant, which has curved surfaces, would significantly increase the rotational constraint provided by the implant. The surrounding soft-tissue structures would be unable to share torsional loads about the knee joint. With the torsional load resisted entirely by the prosthesis, increased stresses would be placed on the fixation interfaces, increasing the likelihood of loosening.

Appropriate condylar design, therefore, requires a compromise between 2 objectives: minimizing contact stresses to maximize wear resistance and minimizing fixation surface stresses to optimize fixation. Conforming surfaces provide rotational constraint that is inversely proportional to the radius. Smaller radii provide more constraint, while larger radii (ie, flatter surfaces) provide less resistance to rotation. The appropriate choice has been examined analytically by determining trade-offs between predicted static contact stress and constraint force. More comprehensive examinations of these trade-offs require more sophisticated dynamic analyses that include ligamentous constraints and more detailed material models for UHMWPE.

As discussed above, an alternative approach to avoid the compromise between contact and constraint that exists for fixed bearing designs is to use a mobile bearing. Mobile bearing designs have the potential advantage of minimizing constraint between moving parts within the tibial component, thus allowing for a high degree of conformity at both the articulating and mobile surfaces. From a wear standpoint, however, the advantages of increased conformity (and therefore potentially lower stresses) at the contact surface must be weighed against the creation of an additional articulation between UHMWPE and metal at the mobile bearing interface. Though mobile bearing interfaces are also highly conforming, they can undergo abrasive and adhesive wear such as occurs in total hip replacements, making osteolysis a concern. A more prevalent disadvantage, however, is a significant incidence of dislocations and bearing fractures, with clinical reports in the literature averaging more than 3%.

Thickness

The thickness of the UHMWPE portion of the tibial component is another important factor affecting stresses associated with wear in knee replacements. As thickness increases, polyethylene stresses decrease and become less sensitive to thickness (Fig. 4). For thick components, stresses show little sensitivity to UHMWPE thickness. For thinner components, however, a small change in thickness (for example, from 4 mm to 8 mm) creates a large decrease in stress. It is commonly recommended that a minimum UHMWPE thickness of 8 mm to 10 mm be maintained for tibial components, although the result will depend on the design of the articulating surfaces.

UHMWPE Properties

The elastic modulus of UHMWPE is an important factor in wear because it is the material property that most influences contact stress. The modulus of a metallic alloy, such as cobalt alloy, is 200 times that of UHMWPE, so that the femoral component is a rigid indenter compared to the UHMWPE tibial component. Therefore, the polyethylene modulus controls the stresses created by contact between the 2 components. Unfortunately, efforts to strengthen polyethylene to make it more resistant to failure usually have been accompanied by significant increases in elastic modulus. Past attempts at strengthening UHMWPE, such as adding carbon fibers, caused the modulus to double, causing contact stresses to increase and resulting in generally poorer wear behavior. Careful analysis and experimentation are required, therefore, to determine if increase in contact stress due to increased modulus overshadows any strength advantage of a stronger, higher modulus UHMWPE.

UHMWPE properties are also altered by radiation sterilization and exposure to oxidative environments. Molecular chain length is decreased and cross-links between chains are increased, causing density and elastic modulus to increase. The increased modulus results in even higher stresses and decreased wear resistance. Degradation has been implicated in severe wear of total knee components, although no clear correlation between degradation, increased wear, and clinical performance has been established.

A number of material factors influence degradation, including method of manufacturing and resin type. Recent evidence from analyses of retrieved UHMWPE tibial components has shown that implants directly molded from polyethylene powder were resistant to oxidative degradation after more than a decade of clinical use, while degradation in implants that had been machined from extruded bars showed degradation in as little as 4 years. The cause of this finding is currently unknown, as is the contribution of such resistance to improved wear behavior.

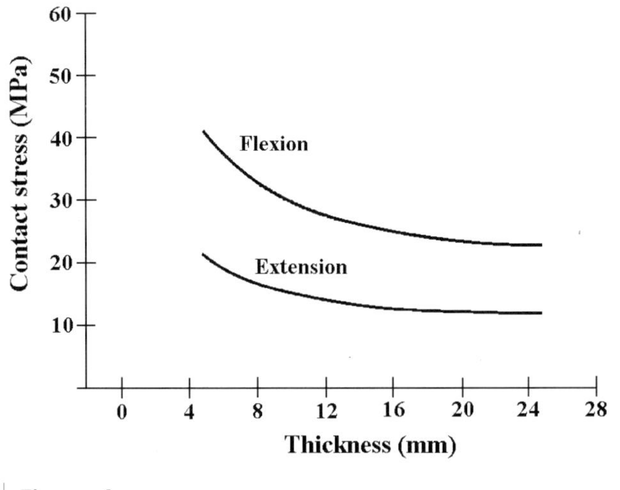

Figure 4

Contact stress plotted as a function of ultrahigh molecular weight polyethylene thickness for a condylar type knee replacement. (Reproduced with permission from Burstein AH, Wright TM: *Fundamentals of Orthopaedic Biomechanics.* Baltimore, MD, Williams & Wilkins, 1994, p 215.)

Additional Design Considerations for Revision Knee Replacement

Fixation

Revision surgery often raises additional concerns for fixation because of loss of bone stock, ligamentous instability, or a periarticular fracture. Bone defects may be filled with bone graft, bone cement, or metal. The biologic solution, using graft, is ideal, provided that the defect shape allows for containment of the graft and that the graft will not be required to bear load until sufficient healing has occurred. PMMA cement has the advantage of filling the defect intimately and creating an immediate mechanical bond to the surrounding bone, but it has minimal strength and obviously cannot remodel. Metallic implants can be an effective alternative. With careful preparation of the remaining bone to match the implant geometry, the metal provides an immediate stiff and strong load path. Most contemporary knee replacement systems incorporate wedges and inserts that can be attached to the tibial and femoral components at surgery to fulfill this role.

Long metallic intramedullary stems are a common part of modular knee implant systems. Long stems have been used as supplementary fixation, particularly in revision arthroplasty. The goal is to allow the fixation between the stem and the surrounding cortex to share bending and torsional loads. Ideally, the fixation between stem and bone should not be rigid axially, so that axial joint loads can still be transferred from the joint surfaces to the remaining cancellous bone under the tibial plateau. One approach is the use of a smooth fluted rod sized so that it is press-fit into the medullary canal. The contact between the flutes and the bone provide torsional resistance, and the press-fit allows bending moments to be shared between the stem and the bone. The smooth surface of the stem, however, does not allow axial loads to be shared. Few guidelines exist as to the precise nature of such fixation and how it is affected by the relative diameters and stiffnesses of the bone and stem and the length of the stem.

Constraint

The design goals for total knee replacement in the presence of inadequate or absent collateral ligament constraints must extend to provision of supplemental joint stability under the internal and external rotations and the varus and valgus angulations encountered during daily activities. Many of the early hinged designs of total knee replacements routinely sacrificed the collateral ligaments. Ligament function was replaced with a linked component. The significant incidence of loosening in these implants is often explained by the rigidity of the metal-to-metal hinge, which transferred the torsional load directly to the interfaces between the bone, cement, and prosthesis. Hinged designs have advanced considerably from these earlier times, incorporating metal-on-polyethylene bushings, "sloppy" hinge designs, and rotating mobile platforms all intended to provide appropriate rotational and varus-valgus constraint.

Constrained condylar knee replacements are used in the more common situation in which the collateral ligaments are still present but are incapable of providing adequate constraint. Constraint in this type of design is provided by a polyethylene central spine on the tibial insert that fits into a mating intercondylar box on the femoral component. Varus-valgus and rotational constraints occur by contact between the medial and lateral surfaces of the polyethylene spine and the corresponding surfaces of the metallic intercondylar box.

Despite the clinical success of constrained condylar implants, analysis of retrieved components often shows permanent medial-lateral deformation of the spine, consistent with large varus and valgus bending moments being resisted by this structure, and significant wear damage to the spine surfaces, even when the spine is reinforced by a metallic reinforcing post. Such findings emphasize that this type of constraint can provide only a portion of the rotational and varus-valgus stability to the knee. The surgeon must strive to balance the remaining soft tissues so that these structures continue to contribute to joint stability.

Patellofemoral Design

Patellar complications remain a significant problem in total knee replacement, although the extent to which complications such as instability and pain are influenced by the patellofemoral design is not well understood. The same design goals exist for this joint as for the tibiofemoral joint, namely function, load transfer, fixation, and wear resistance, as do the same compromises, for example, between constraint and wear. Components must provide an adequately constrained articulation over a large range of motion, while allowing for the complex relative displacement, tilt, and rotational movements between the remaining bony structures to which the components are fixed. In general, 2 designs for the patellar component have emerged in contemporary knee systems: simple geometries such as spherical, dome-shaped patellae, and more anatomic geometries that aim to recreate the facets of the natural patella. Advantages of the former are a relatively unconstrained patellofemoral joint when articulating against the anterior flange of the femoral component, ease of insertion with no concerns for rotational alignment, and relatively broad contact areas against the flange, at least near extension. Advantages of the latter are a more constrained patellofemoral joint with even larger contact areas, although surgical alignment becomes more important.

Femoral component designs for the flange also vary, from a symmetrical vertical groove to more anatomic grooves often with a few degrees of valgus inclination and a raised lateral border. The need for a more anatomic patellar component and asymmetrical designs remains controversial. Little experimental evidence exists, however, to demonstrate increased constraint provided in such designs compared to dome-shaped, symmetrical designs, and clinical performance does not generally demonstrate a difference. One problem in such comparisons is that factors other than shape impact performance. For example, the depth and inclination of the femoral groove significantly impacts both the constraint provided by the joint and the mechanics, as the moment arm and the working length of the quadriceps muscle are significantly altered.

Fixation of patellar components is typically with acrylic

bone cement. Supplemental fixation is required to resist torsional and shear loads across the implant-patellar interface and is usually provided by pegs on the anterior surface of the component and undercuts on the surface for cement penetration. Metal backing of patellar implants to allow for porous coatings for biologic fixation proved clinically unacceptable, with a high incidence of dissociation between the UHMWPE and metal components and excessive polyethylene wear.

Observations made on retrieved patellar components often reveal considerable wear and deformation. This is understandable, given the large joint contact loads and the small contact areas. Analytic studies, for example, demonstrate that stresses can exceed the yield strength of UHMWPE by as much as a factor of 4. While such damage may contribute to failure in extreme cases, the deformation of the contact surface also results in a more conforming situation. Contact stresses decrease and the patellar component contacts the femoral flange over more of the range of motion.

In posterior-stabilized and constrained condylar type implants, an additional design problem exists. These implants require an intercondylar box on the femoral component to accept the posterior-stabilized or constrained post of the tibial component. The intersection of the anterior box geometry and the base of the patellar flange can lead to an open volume into which soft tissue can grow after implantation of the device. The resulting entrapment of soft tissue during flexion and extension results in a "clunk" syndrome, as the trapped tissue pops out of this volume. In extreme cases, surgical intervention is necessary to relieve the problem. More recent designs have avoided this problem and improved the kinematics and contact pattern of the patellofemoral joint by extending the flange as far posterior as possible without interfering with the box geometry.

Annotated Bibliography

Design

Vander Sloten J, Labey L, Van Audekercke R, Van der Perre G: Materials selection and design for orthopaedic implants with improved long-term performance. *Biomaterials* 1998;19: 1455–1459.

Design and materials selection questions are considered in 2 case studies, 1 being that of a tibial component of a total knee prosthesis. Bioactive surfaces to enhance fixation are discussed as are the needs for better presurgical planning systems and advanced surgical tools.

Kinematics

Dennis DA, Komistek RD, Stiehl JB, Walker SA, Dennis KN: Range of motion after total knee arthroplasty: The effect of implant design and weight-bearing conditions. *J Arthroplasty* 1998;13:748–752.

Active and passive knee range of motion was determined in patients with normal knees and with PCL-sparing and posterior-stabilized implants. Patients with normal knees exhibited significantly greater knee flexion. Patients with posterior-stabilized implants demonstrated greater flexion than patients with PCL-sparing implants when measured in weightbearing, despite having less range of motion and lower clinical ratings preoperatively.

Stiehl JB, Dennis DA, Komistek RD, Keblish PA: In vivo kinematic analysis of a mobile bearing total knee prosthesis. *Clin Orthop* 1997;345:60–66.

Ten normal subjects and 10 patients with a PCL-sparing mobile bearing total knee performed deep knee bends under fluoroscopy to determine tibiofemoral contact positions. At flexion angles < 60°, femoral roll back was noted in both groups. Beyond 60°, normal knees continued to roll back, but mobile bearing knees moved anteriorly. Five mobile bearing knees had some movement of the bearings; the other 5 remained fixed.

Fixation

Stern SH, Wills RD, Gilbert JL: The effect of tibial stem design on component micromotion in knee arthroplasty. *Clin Orthop* 1997;345:44–52.

Rigid body mechanics were used to determine 3-dimensional motions of tibial components with no stem, a short 40-mm stem, and a long 75-mm stem under central, posterior, and medial loading. Longer stems were associated with increased micromotion, especially under eccentric loading. Cemented implants had more stable fixation, compared with noncemented implants.

Wear

Bartel DL, Rawlinson JJ, Burstein AH, Ranawat CS, Flynn WF Jr: Stresses in polyethylene components of contemporary total knee replacements. *Clin Orthop* 1995;317:76–82.

Contact stresses and strains were calculated for 8 contemporary knee designs. Finite element analysis was used for the minimum available polyethylene thickness with the knee in flexion. The greatest differences among designs was for the von Mises strain, which peaked beneath the surface. The differences in stresses were less notable because of the nonlinear UHMWPE material behavior. Advantages of more conforming surfaces and thicker polyethylene components were confirmed.

Bell CJ, Walker PS, Abeysundera MR, Simmons JM, King PM, Blunn GW: Effect of oxidation on delamination of ultrahigh-molecular-weight polyethylene tibial components. *J Arthroplasty* 1998;13:280–290.

Examination of retrieved UHMWPE knee implants showed that oxidation caused by postirradiation damage led to a subsurface band. Delamination cracks propagated through the band. In wear tests, delamination occurred in artificially aged UHMWPE only where bands had formed. Tensile and fatigue tests of oxidized UHMWPE showed a significant reduction in tensile strength and fatigue resistance compared to control material.

Estupiñán JA, Bartel DL, Wright TM: Residual stresses in ultra-high molecular weight polyethylene loaded cyclically by a rigid moving indenter in nonconforming geometries. *J Orthop Res* 1998;16:80–88.

Stresses in polyethylene knee components subjected to cyclic moving loads were examined using nonlinear finite element analysis. Differential plastic deformation under the UHMWPE surface led to tensile horizontal residual stresses at the surface and compressive stresses beneath the surface. Magnitudes of the residual stresses indicate their importance in wear mechanisms.

Furman BD, Ritter MA, Perone JB, Furman GL, Li S: Effect of resin type and manufacturing method on UHMWPE oxidation and quality at long aging and implant times. *Trans Orthop Res Soc* 1997;22:92.

Examination of retrieved and never implanted (but aged on the shelf) UHMWPE tibial components revealed that resin type and processing method had a significant effect on the amount of oxidation experienced by the implants. Implants made by direct molding of 1900 resin were much more resistant to oxidative degradation than previous measurements on implants made from other resins and processing methods.

Palmer SH, Morrison PJ, Ross AC: Early catastrophic tibial component wear after unicompartmental knee arthroplasty. *Clin Orthop* 1998;350:143–148.

Seven cases of a cohort of 32 unicondylar knee replacements that failed because of early catastrophic UHMWPE wear are reported. Possible reasons for failure include inadequate thickness, fusion defects as a result of the sterilization process, increased rotational freedom, and reduced conformity.

Sathasivam S, Walker PS: Computer model to predict subsurface damage in tibial inserts of total knees. *J Orthop Res* 1998;16:564–571

Finite element models were performed using multiple orientations of the femoral component predicted from gait analysis and a damage function analogous to strain energy density to predict where delamination wear would occur. Damage susceptibility was strongly influenced by implant design. The method is proposed as an improvement over static analyses and experiments in predicting wear damage.

Wright TM, Goodman SB (eds): *Implant Wear: The Future of Total Joint Replacement.* Rosemont, IL, American Academy of Orthopaedic Surgeons, 1996.

This monograph provides answers to several clinical, biologic, and bioengineering questions surrounding wear of total joint implants. The answers were drafted by invited attendees at an NIH/AAOS sponsored workshop and are supported by a comprehensive bibliography.

Mobile Bearing Implants

Matsuda S, White SE, Williams VG II, McCarthy DS, Whiteside LA: Contact stress analysis in meniscal bearing total knee arthroplasty. *J Arthroplasty* 1998;13:699–706.

Tibiofemoral contact stress was measured with fixed bearing and mobile bearing components in 5 cadaver knees at 0°, 30°, 60°, and 90° of flexion and at 15° of internal or external rotation. A mobile bearing surface offered an advantage with rotational malalignment. However, severe malalignment caused marked increases in stresses beneath the mobile bearing, which could cause deformity and subluxation.

Szivek JA, Anderson PL, Benjamin JB: Average and peak contact stress distribution evaluation of total knee arthroplasties. *J Arthroplasty* 1996;11:952–963.

Contact stress patterns and contact areas were experimentally measured in a number of contemporary knee implants. Contact areas varied depending on design. All designs had maximum stresses in excess of the yield strength of UHMWPE. The LCS mobile-bearing design had substantially lower patellofemoral contact stresses and larger contact areas, though peak contact stresses were in excess of 30 MPa in some areas at low flexion angles.

Patella

Andriacchi TP, Yoder D, Conley A, Rosenberg A, Sum J, Galante JO: Patellofemoral design influences function following total knee arthroplasty. *J Arthroplasty* 1997;12:243–249.

The influence of patellofemoral design was evaluated by testing 2 patient groups while walking, climbing stairs, and rising from a chair with knee implant designs that differed in femoral trochlear curvature. One design had a smaller patellar flange radius, causing the patella to articulate more anteriorly and distally than the second design, which had a larger radius. A significant functional difference occurred during stair climbing. The first group had a higher quadriceps moment during late stance phase and increased knee flexion, suggesting a relationship between a nonanatomic trochlea and abnormal function.

Chew JT, Stewart NJ, Hanssen AD, Luo ZP, Rand JA, An KN: Differences in patellar tracking and knee kinematics among three different total knee designs. *Clin Orthop* 1997;345:87–98.

Patellar rotation, tilting, lateral shift, and displacement in relation to the femoral groove center were measured in an in vitro study of cadaver knees with several knee designs implanted. No difference was found between the intact knee and the various implants regarding rotation, displacement, and lateral shift. All designs showed significant lateral tilting compared with the intact knee, suggesting the need for additional modification of implant geometry.

Elbert K, Bartel D, Wright T: The effect of conformity on stresses in dome-shaped polyethylene patellar components. *Clin Orthop* 1995;317:71–75.

Polyethylene stresses were examined in 2 patellar components, 1 with geometry of a newly manufactured dome-shaped component and 1 with geometry of a deformed and worn retrieved component. Stresses were more severe in the new component and were more severe than determined previously for tibiofemoral contact. For both models, stresses exceeded UHMWPE yield stress in most of the contact area, consistent with large amounts of deformation observed on many retrieved patellar components.

Classic Bibliography

Bartel DL, Burstein AH, Santavicca EA, Insall JN: Performance of the tibial component in total knee replacement: Conventional and revision designs. *J Bone Joint Surg* 1982;64A:1026–1033.

Bartel DL, Wright TM: Design of total knee replacements, in Petty W (ed): *Total Joint Replacement.* Philadelphia, PA, WB Saunders, 1991, pp 467–481.

Burstein AH, Wright TM: Biomechanics, in Insall JN, Windsor RE, Scott WN, Kelly MA, Aglietti P (eds): *Surgery of the Knee*, ed 2. New York, NY, Churchill Livingstone, 1993, pp 43–62.

Burstein AH, Wright TM (eds): Performance of implant systems, in *Fundamentals of Orthopaedic Biomechanics.* Baltimore, MD, Williams & Wilkins, 1994, pp 191–218.

Li S, Burstein AH: Ultra-high molecular weight polyethylene: The material and its use in total joint implants. *J Bone Joint Surg* 1994;76A:1080–1090.

Pappas MJ, Buechel FF: On the use of a constant radius femoral component in meniscal bearing knee replacement. *J Orthop Rheumatol* 1994;7:27–29.

Walker PS: Design of total knee arthroplasty, in Insall JN, Windsor RE, Scott WN, Kelly MA, Aglietti P (eds): *Surgery of the Knee*, ed 2. New York, NY, Churchill Livingstone, 1993, vol 2, pp 723–738.

Weaver JK, Derkash RS, Greenwald AS: Difficulties with bearing dislocation and breakage using a movable bearing total knee replacement system. *Clin Orthop* 1993;290:244–252.

Chapter 30
Fixation in Total Knee Replacement: Bone Ingrowth

Cement use in total knee arthroplasty (TKA) remains a controversial issue. Many cemented total knee replacement designs introduced over the years have failed and subsequently have been removed from the market. The few designs that remain have performed reasonably well because of specific characteristics, such as a well-fixed tibial component with an effective stem, multiple sizes of femoral components, a generous curvature on each femoral condyle, and a conforming polyethylene surface with a large articular contact surface area. With the advent of new instrumentation, these cemented implants, even in the hands of an inexperienced arthroplasty surgeon, have had a high rate of success. However, cement fixation remains a source of consternation for implant designers. Recent attempts to produce a cemented all-polyethylene tibial component resulted in a loosening rate of more than 20% after 5 years.

Implant Development Challenges

The instrumentation that has made cemented arthroplasty successful for most surgeons was developed primarily to ensure correct alignment for cementless knee replacement. Aside from instrumentation, many of the principles that resulted in successful cemented knee arthroplasty were not applied to the newer cementless components. Early in the process, developers often stated that implants designed for cemented installation could not be simply porous-coated and then used for cementless fixation to bone; later, it was found that the implants indeed could be used in this manner. Because established criteria of successful TKA design were not always taken into consideration in designing cementless knee components, short-term results were poor and long-term results catastrophic.

The early failure of cemented tibial components led to extensive research on fixation of the tibial component, and finally there was consensus in the published literature that the cancellous bone of the upper tibia was incapable of supporting the tibial component unless an effective stem was incorporated in the design. Nevertheless, the majority of the early cementless designs did not have a stem and failed to achieve adequate peripheral fixation of the tibial component to the cancellous-cortical structure of the upper tibia. Many of these tibial components loosened and required revision arthroplasty.

Attempts to produce a metal-backed, cementless patellar component led to further problems that were unrelated to a specific method of fixation but attributed to the absence of cement. Wear through the polyethylene to the metal backing followed by contamination of the articular surface with metal and polyethylene debris led to further damage of the already compromised tibial polyethylene components, and to large-scale osteolysis and loss of bone stock. Although often attributed to cementless fixation of the femoral and tibial components, these events really indicated that the design concepts and performance of the patellar component were poor. The patellar surface is difficult to replace with either a cemented or a cementless component, and use of metal backing on a thin polyethylene patellar component is a treacherous undertaking.

Although many cementless designs were unsuccessful even at early follow-up periods, some have been highly successful. In fact, the femoral component in almost all of the cementless designs reliably achieves fixation to bone, and is commonly used in hybrid TKA. The tibial component in both cementless and cemented TKA has been the greatest source of problems related to fixation because most designs are flawed from the onset because of inadequate fixation. Applying a rigid metal tray to a flat surface of cancellous bone does not provide adequate resistance to compressive failure of cancellous bone, liftoff of the opposite side, and toggling micromotion of the component. When early results showed problems with fixation, stems and peripheral screws began to be incorporated into new implant designs. Biomechanical studies clearly indicated that peripheral screws and stems on the tibial component were highly effective in enhancing fixation, and that micromotion of the tray was unacceptably high without these features. Preparation of the upper tibial surface is an important aspect of tibial component fixation that is commonly overlooked. Small surface irregularities and incongruities can have a devastating effect on fixation, but this aspect of fixation has not received much attention in most cementless tibial component designs.

Other features of cementless total knee replacement designs that are responsible for implant failure are flat polyethylene, heat-pressed polyethylene, and patch porous-coated surfaces. The combination of these features, along with poor quality assurance of polyethylene and gamma irradiation of this material, has caused considerable wear problems that have led to clinically significant osteolysis. The large amount of polyethylene debris generated by rapid destruction of the polyethylene component stimulates a florid inflammatory response in the synovial tissue of the knee. Subsequently, this tissue rapidly infiltrates all bone surfaces that are not protected by an effective fibrous tissue or bone ingrowth barrier. Smooth metal surfaces that separate pads of porous coating have been shown to produce metaphyseal and diaphyseal osteolytic lesions by conducting debris into areas of bone that are not protected by the mechanisms that capture wear debris and transfer it to the local lymphatic system. Although these osteolytic lesions have been ascribed to cementless fixation and to the use of screws, they are rare unless the tibial component design includes patch porous coating, inadequate fixation of the tibial component, and mechanisms that produce large amounts of particulate debris in the knee.

Clinical Results

Results of cementless total knee replacement during the past 15 years have proved to be highly dependent on design. In patients with excellent fixation of the tibial component, minimal constraint at the articular surface, or both, there have been very low rates of loosening, and these results have been reliable in all age groups and in the presence of inflammatory as well as degenerative arthritic conditions. Findings have shown that after 15 years from date of implant, the Ortholoc (Wright Medical Technology, Arlington, TN) total knee replacement (Fig. 1) and the Low Contact Stress (LCS, DePuy, Warsaw, IN) are similar in terms of loosening and wear. The Natural Knee (Sulzer Orthopaedics, Austin, TX) also has continued to deliver excellent clinical results when cementless fixation techniques are used. Recently, the Performance (Biomet, Warsaw, IN) total knee design and the Press-Fit Condylar (PFC, DePuy, Warsaw, IN) total knee design have been reported to perform similarly when fixed with cemented or osteointegrated techniques. These 5 knee systems have varying combinations of initial fixation, low articular surface constraint, and precise preparation of the upper tibial surface. A recent study of 10-year results with cemented and cementless technique using the Performance knee reported no difference in loosening, pain, or knee score.

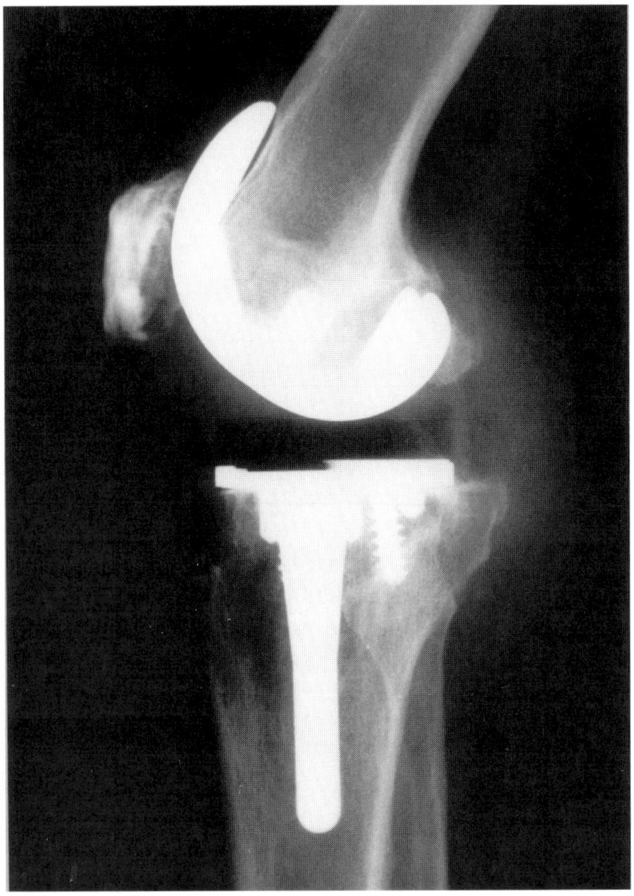

Figure 1

Lateral radiograph of a knee evaluated 14 years after surgery. An Ortholoc I knee replacement design was implanted with cementless technique, and remains stable with no evidence of loosening or migration. Minimal radiolucent lines are present where smooth metal surfaces are in contact with bone.

It is important to note in this study that the most demanding patients, that is, the young, active male patient, were all in the cementless group. In a randomized, prospective study comparing cemented and cementless fixation using the PFC knee design, clinical performance was virtually identical, but radiolucent lines were more likely to occur in cemented components. The present status of cementless TKA is the same as cemented TKA 10 to 15 years after its introduction. The design characteristics that consistently lead to success are now well known, and the surgical procedure is effective.

Cemented total knee replacement success rates have been fairly consistent, but the procedure itself has not yet become standardized. Some authors recommend superficial penetration of cement into the surface of the bone; others recommend deep penetration. Still others recommend cementing the tibial component only; some authors recommend that all components be cemented. Although there are many reports in the literature of excellent long-term results with cemented all-polyethylene tibial components, recent efforts to design an all-polyethylene tibial component that is reliable with a full cement technique have been fraught with fixation problems. One clinical review reported that 18% of the patients had revision or gross loosening at 1 year after surgery. Although this complication may be related to the articular surface design and to the flatness of the femoral component surface, a definite reason for this occurrence has not been established, and there may be other subtle features of cemented design that make it less than completely reliable.

Close evaluation of published long-term results indicates a rapid decrease in implant survival rate after 10 years. This is especially true in heavy, active individuals who begin to show radiographic evidence of failure as early as 4 years after surgery. One group reported a good 10-year survival rate, around 94%, when revision for loosening was considered the end point; however, when the end point was moderate pain, loosening, or revision, the survival rate dropped to 84% at 10 years. Worsening results over the 10-year period were caused by progressively increasing pain, instability, and deformity. This suggests that the implants gradually loosen and migrate. This explanation is supported in a study on motion of the tibial component of radiographically intact cemented Total Condylar (DePuy, Warsaw, IN) knee arthroplasties. In this study, 27 cemented knee arthroplasties were evaluated for motion between the tibial component and bone during varus-valgus stress testing. The least amount of motion was 0.2 mm and the greatest was 2.1 mm. All knees had detectable motion between the cement and bone. Because the bone-cement interface is subject to progressive osteolytic attack, which is especially rapid in cement interfaces with cancellous bone (such as with the acetabular component in total hip arthroplasty), it is not unlikely that the bone-cement interface in TKA is undermined during the first few years and develops a fibrous tissue interface without a surrounding sclerotic margin. Early studies comparing migration of cemented implants to that of cementless ones using the radiostereophotogrammetry technique found less migration in cemented components. As these studies progress and more effective cementless tibial component techniques are evaluated, it appears that progressive migration is minimized just as well with cementless technique when used with stem and screws. Recent reports comparing the current cementless technique to cemented fixation of the tibial component showed progressive migration of the cemented components over a 5-year observation period, whereas the cementless implants ceased to migrate during the first year.

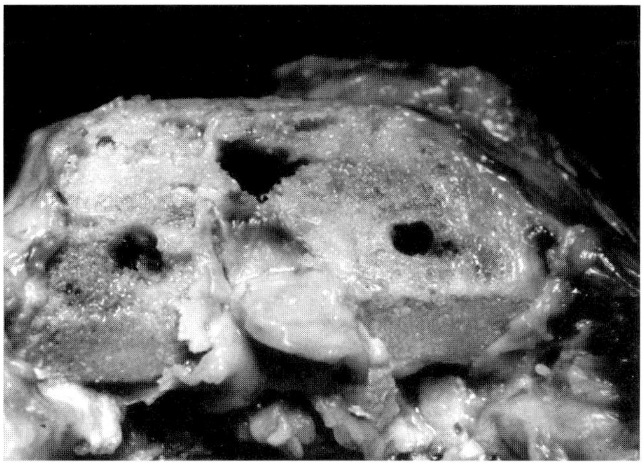

Figure 2

Intraoperative photograph of a femur at the time of revision for patellar failure. Bone stock and bone blood supply was well preserved and the knee was revised by using a cementless technique.

Osteolysis in cementless total knee replacement is clearly a function of the amount of particulate debris released and of the configuration of the porous coating. When the Ortholoc Modular tibial component, which has patches of porous coating separated by smooth metal bridges, was compared to the Ortholoc II tibial component, which has continuous porous coating on the undersurface, the rate of osteolysis was significantly greater in the design with patch porous coating. Another group also reviewed the effect of osteolytic attack in cementless TKA and found that smooth metal surfaces provided little resistance to progressive invasion of osteolytic tissue, whereas porous-coated metal interfaces with bone were highly resistant to osteolytic attack.

Of the few modern-design cementless implants that require revision, few require major bone grafting or cementing to restore bone stock and achieve stability. The bone-implant interface has been remarkably benign, even in cases with severe patellar wear and massive contamination of the joint by metal and particulate polyethylene debris (Fig. 2). After 20 years of clinical experience with cementless total knee replacement, the procedure can be recommended with confidence. It can be done quickly and effectively, the results are reliable and durable, and complications are relatively easy to handle.

Annotated Bibliography

Bassett RW: Results of 1,000 Performance knees: Cementless versus cemented fixation. *J Arthroplasty* 1998;13:409-413.

A retrospective review of 1,000 knees implanted with the Performance total knee prosthesis at a mean follow-up of 5.2 years is presented. There was no significant difference in clinical results between cemented and cementless implants. Cemented fixation was used for older, less active patients, and cementless fixation was used for younger, more active patients. Neither group had loosening or osteolysis.

Faris PM, Ritter MA, Meding JB, Bartel DL, Carr KD: Minimum 2 year clinical evaluation and finite element evaluation of a flat all polyethylene tibial component. *Orthop Trans* 1995;19:387.

This study describes the clinical results and finite element evaluation of a flat all-polyethylene tibial component and suggests that all-polyethylene tibial components are extremely design sensitive and may be unforgiving with regard to bonding mechanisms, stiffness, and load transfer.

McCaskie AW, Deehan DJ, Green TP, et al: Randomised, prospective study comparing cemented and cementless total knee replacement: Results of press-fit condylar total knee replacement at five years. *J Bone Joint Surg* 1998;80B:971-975.

This prospective study of total knee arthroplasty showed no significant difference between cemented and cementless fixation for pain, mobility, or movement; however, there was a notable disparity in the radiolucent line score. With cemented fixation there was a significantly greater number of radiolucent lines on anteroposterior radiographs of the tibial and lateral radiographs of the femur.

Tanner MG, Whiteside LA, White SE: Effect of polyethylene quality on wear in total knee arthroplasty. *Clin Orthop* 1995;317:83-88.

The results from this study suggest that improved quality control of polyethylene material would greatly decrease wear and delamination of TKA components.

White SE, Paxson RD, Tanner MG, Whiteside LA: Effects of sterilization on wear in total knee arthroplasty. *Clin Orthop* 1996;331:164-171.

The findings from this study suggest that ethylene oxide sterilization caused less microstructural damage to the polyethylene and resulted in significantly less wear than was found in those components sterilized with gamma radiation.

Whiteside LA: Clinical results of cementless total knee replacement at 12-15 year follow-up. *Orthop Trans* 1997;21:220.

This study reports the 12- to 15-year clinical results of a first-generation cementless total knee replacement design. Two studies showed that bone stock was preserved about the knee despite some early failures due to tibial polyethylene component and metal-backed patellar wear.

Whiteside LA: Effect of porous-coating configuration on tibial osteolysis after total knee arthroplasty. *Clin Orthop* 1995;321:92-97.

Retrospective review of patients implanted with a cementless total knee design whose tibial component contained patch porous coating with smooth metal bridges connecting the stem to the joint cavity. This tibial undersurface design resulted in a high rate of osteolysis when implanted without cement. Implants with full porous coating did not experience stem osteolysis.

Classic Bibliography

Bloebaum RD, Nelson K, Dorr LD, Hofmann AA, Lyman DJ: Investigation of early surface delamination observed in retrieved heat-pressed tibial inserts. *Clin Orthop* 1991;269:120-127.

Blunn GW, Walker PS, Joshi A, Hardinge K: The dominance of cyclic sliding in producing wear in total knee replacements. *Clin Orthop* 1991;273:253-260.

Buechel FF, Rosa RA, Pappas MJ: A metal-backed, rotating-bearing patellar prosthesis to lower contact stress: An 11-year clinical study. *Clin Orthop* 1989;248:34-49.

Engh GA, Dwyer KA, Hanes CK: Polyethylene wear of metal-backed tibial components in total and unicompartmental knee prostheses. *J Bone Joint Surg* 1992;74B:9-17.

Hofmann AA, Murdock LE, Wyatt RW, Alpert JP: Total knee arthroplasty: Two- to four-year experience using an asymmetric tibial tray and a deep trochlear-grooved femoral component. *Clin Orthop* 1991;269:78-88.

Hungerford DS, Kenna RV: Preliminary experience with a total knee prosthesis with porous coating used without cement. *Clin Orthop* 1983;176:95-107.

Insall J, Tria AJ, Scott WN: The total condylar knee prosthesis: The first 5 years. *Clin Orthop* 1979;145:68-77.

Kobs JK, Lachiewicz PF: Hybrid total knee arthroplasty: Two- to five-year results using the Miller-Galante prosthesis. *Clin Orthop* 1993;286:78-87.

Miura H, Whiteside LA, Easley JC, Amador DD: Effects of screws and a sleeve on initial fixation in uncemented total knee tibial components. *Clin Orthop* 1990;259:160-168.

Nelissen RG, Brand R, Rozing PM: Survivorship analysis in total condylar knee arthroplasty: A statistical review. *J Bone Joint Surg* 1992;74A:383-389.

Nilsson KG, Karrholm J: Increased varus-valgus tilting of screw-fixated knee prostheses: Stereoradiographic study of uncemented versus cemented tibial components. *J Arthroplasty* 1993;8: 529-540.

Ranawat CS, Flynn WF Jr, Saddler S, Hansraj KK, Maynard MJ: Long-term results of the total condylar knee arthroplasty: A 15-year survivorship study. *Clin Orthop* 1993;286:94-102.

Ryd L: The role of roentgen stereophotogrammetric analysis (RSA) in knee surgery. *Am J Knee Surg* 1992;5:44-54.

Ryd L, Lindstrand A, Rosenquist R, Selvik G: Micromotion of conventionally cemented all-polyethylene tibial components in total knee replacements: A roentgen stereophotogrammetric analysis of migration and inducible displacement. *Arch Orthop Trauma Surg* 1987;106:82-88.

Schmalzried TP, Kwong LM, Jasty M, et al: The mechanism of loosening of cemented acetabular components in total hip arthroplasty: Analysis of specimens retrieved at autopsy. *Clin Orthop* 1992;274:60-78.

Volz RG, Nisbet JK, Lee RW, McMurtry MG: The mechanical stability of various noncemented tibial components. *Clin Orthop* 1988;226:38-42.

Whiteside L, Summers RG: Anatomical landmarks for an intramedullary alignment system for total knee replacement. *Orthop Trans* 1983;7:546-547.

Chapter 31 Surgical Principles of Total Knee Replacement: Incisions, Extensor Mechanism, Ligament Balancing

Incisions

Total knee replacement (TKR) is commonly performed through a midline incision, which permits ready access. The midline approach permits ready access to either side of the knee joint and allows for further intervention into the knee without compromising the skin flaps. The flaps should be kept as minimal as possible to avoid skin compromise; however, it is critical to establish good surgical exposure to the joint, and the flaps may need to be extended to avoid poor exposure and a poor surgical result.

As TKRs age, there will be more revision surgery and more surgical exposures through old incisions. It is a good surgical principle to attempt to use the old incisions that may be present about the knee as often as possible. Although some authors believe that an incision about the knee can be ignored if it is 2 or more years old, this is not well-founded and requires careful examination. However, the surgeon may be faced with a transverse or lateral scar that does not permit easy exposure to the joint. In these circumstances it may be necessary to ignore the other incisions and use the midline approach with the best attempt to avoid skin compromise. Most authors recommend a 7-cm distance between incisions. It may be necessary to seek the help of a plastic surgeon in the most complicated situations, but the orthopaedic surgeon certainly should have a good grasp on the choices available for the surgery. Tissue expanders have been recommended for a knee that has skin compromise and may present a problem with the closure after the TKR is completed. Although this requires 2 surgical procedures, the placement of the subcutaneous expanders is relatively noninvasive and well worth the time to avoid later skin compromise, with possible loss of the TKR.

The only other standard incisions are the medial and lateral parapatellar. The medial parapatellar incision was the most popular before the 1970s and essentially mimicked the arthrotomy approach to the knee. The problem with this approach is that it limits exposure to the lateral side of the knee and makes the lateral skin flap larger than the medial flap. Because the skin on the lateral side of the knee has a poorer blood supply than the skin on the medial side, it makes more sense to try to limit the length of the lateral flap if at all possible. The lateral parapatellar approach to the knee, especially in the valgus knee, was recommended because it limited the lateral flap and brought the approach directly into the lateral compartment of the knee where most of the ligament balancing would take place. The problems with this approach are that it is less familiar to the surgeon, and that it limits the exposure on the medial side. Transverse, lateral, and medial oblique incisions had some use when open arthrotomies for meniscus surgery were standard. These approaches are now more historic than practical.

The skin incision is most important for the integrity of the skin flaps. The approach to the knee joint itself is determined more by the arthrotomy incision. The arthrotomy can begin on the medial or lateral side of the patella. With the midline approach to the knee, the arthrotomy begins over the middle to medial third of the patellar surface and peels the extensor mechanism from the anterior surface of the patella to enter the joint on the medial side of the patella. The parapatellar arthrotomies extend the incision proximally into the quadriceps tendon. The extensor mechanism is then everted medially or laterally. Once the quadriceps tendon is incised, there will be a certain degree of weakening of extension and possible quadriceps lag. The parapatellar incisions divide the superior geniculates on the same side as the arthrotomy. This does not significantly compromise the blood supply to the patella unless both of the superior vessels are divided. If, after a medial parapatellar incision, a lateral release of the patella is required for patellar tracking, the patellar bone becomes avascular for some months after the surgery and may be subject to fracture.

Several approaches have been devised to avoid compromise of the quadriceps mechanism that occurs with the parapatellar approaches. The subvastus arthrotomy proceeds beneath the vastus medialis and lifts the entire quadriceps mechanism laterally with eversion of the patella. Although this technique completely avoids any incision into the quadriceps tendon, there is danger of injuring the femoral artery in the adductor canal and a problem in exposing the lateral aspect of the joint, especially in the obese patient. This problem was recognized and the approach was modified by dividing the mid and distal third of the vastus medialis and everting the mechanism from that point laterally. It has been shown that the muscle is innervated from posterior and that the distal third does not become denervated if it is divided from the proximal portion. This technique lifts less muscle across the joint for the exposure and does not interfere with the quadriceps tendon.

In the trivector approach, the incision was along the medial aspect of the patella and proceeded vertically into the vastus muscle belly. This approach did not compromise the quadriceps tendon; however, it essentially isolated the medialis from the extensor mechanism and encouraged lateral subluxation of the patella.

Extensor Mechanism

All of the approaches described thus far are more vertical in nature and preserve the longitudinal integrity of the quadriceps mechanism. When the surgery becomes more complex, especially in the setting of revision TKR, it may be necessary to alter the extensor mechanism both to facilitate the exposure and change the motion of the knee after the operation. On the proximal side of the extensor mechanism, the quadriceps tendon can be lengthened in a "Z" fashion with multiple transverse incisions on the medial and lateral side to the tendon. This technique will lengthen the tendon, allow more range of motion, and improve the exposure of the joint; however, the knee may have a persistent lag after the surgery. Quadricepsplasty enters the quadriceps tendon with an inverted "V," then closes with a "Y" that permits lengthening of the tendon at the expense of a lag in the extensor mechanism. A quadriceps "snip" has been described that transects the quadriceps tendon far proximally and permits better eversion of the extensor mechanism without an additional lag (Fig. 1). This approach can also be extended distally on the lateral side of the quadriceps tendon in a similar fashion to the quadricepsplasty technique with less morbidity.

The extensor mechanism can also be modified distally at the tibial tubercle site. Several articles describe osteotomy of the tubercle with clear exposure of the joint and reattachment with a wire technique. This approach is not completely benign. There were 2 partial avulsions in 136 cases; however, there was no loss of extensor mechanism and no evidence of nonunion. The initial articles described a long tubercle osteotomy that has subsequently been shortened.

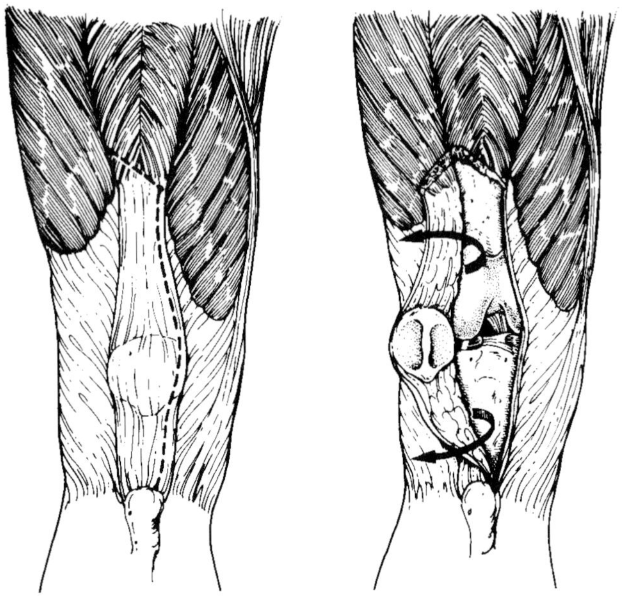

Figure 1

The quadriceps snip divides the tendon proximally, permits extended exposure, and does not weaken the extensor mechanism significantly. (Reproduced with permission from Garvin KL, Scuderi G, Insall JN: Evolution of the quadriceps snips. *Clin Orthop* 1995;321: 131–137.)

Ligament Balancing and Alignment of the Knee

The overall objective of total knee arthroplasty (TKA) is to establish a valgus aligned knee in the standing position with the tibial component perpendicular to the tibial shaft in the coronal plane and the valgus in the femoral component. The ideal replacement should have a full range of motion from zero to approximately 125°. The patella should track in the midline throughout the range. Finally, the knee should have good collateral ligament balance in full extension and at 90° of flexion.

The alignment of the TKA has become a fairly well understood concept with emphasis on the standing radiograph and the patient's anatomic landmarks seen in the operating room. The 2 primary types of instruments rely either on the intramedullary canal or on extramedullary references. On the tibial side, intramedullary and extramedullary instruments are equally accurate. In the valgus knee, the tibial shaft can be in valgus in up to 70% of the knees. In these knees, the intramedullary rods cannot be fully placed into the tibia, and extramedullary techniques are more successful. However, the accuracy of both approaches for tibial alignment is similar.

On the femoral side, intramedullary instruments are more

accurate because the femoral shaft is readily accessible and the landmarks for extramedullary alignment are often difficult to palpate on the pelvis. Radiographic markers can also be used to help with extramedullary referencing; however, these techniques require added time in the operating room and are not superior to the intramedullary systems.

If the tibial cut is perpendicular to the tibial axis and the femoral cut is in 4° to 6° of valgus, the knee should be aligned in 4° to 6° of valgus if the ligaments are properly balanced.

Ligament balancing remains controversial in TKA. All authors agree on the final goal with the replacement; however, the techniques for the balancing and the time of the releases during the surgery all vary. The surgeon must allow for proper fitting of the components on the surface of each bone and must also allow for proper ligament balance. At the present time, the balance of the collateral ligaments is referenced at full extension and 90° of flexion. If the ligaments are equally tight at these 2 points, the knee is thought to be "balanced". More authors are now evaluating the balance at 30°, 60°, and 120° of flexion to be sure that the knee is truly balanced throughout a full range of motion. Presently, instruments for evaluating the knee in these intermediate ranges of motion are inadequate.

There are 2 philosophies for the bone resections and 2 approaches to institution of the surgical procedure. The "measured resection" technique for the bone cuts removes the exact amount of bone necessary for the prosthetic device on the femoral and tibial sides. If the femoral component is 9 mm thick at the distal portion, the technique calls for a 9-mm resection of the distal femur. In a similar fashion, the amount of bone that is removed from the proximal tibia matches the thickness of the component to be inserted. Both sides are cut independently, and then the collateral ligaments are tested for proper balance in flexion and full extension. This technique requires precise cuts that reproduce the bone anatomy; however, the surgeon must be careful not to forget the balancing of the knee. Improper balance can lead to instability or to loss of full range of motion despite the fact that the components fit perfectly on the end of the femur and the tibia.

The second philosophy for bone resection incorporates ligament balancing with the cuts and is often referred to as the "flexion-extension gap" technique. This was popularized in the early 1970s. The initial bone cuts are made for the proximal tibia and the distal and posterior surfaces of the femur. Subsequently, the gap is measured in flexion and full extension. Resection of bone from the proximal tibia increases the gap in flexion and full extension equally. Resection of bone from the distal femur affects the extension gap only. Thus, if the gap in flexion is larger than the gap in full extension, more bone can be removed form the distal femur to equalize the gaps. If the gaps in flexion and full extension are both too small, more bone can be removed from the proximal tibia. If the gap in flexion is smaller than the gap in extension, more bone must be removed from the posterior femur. This can be accomplished by removing the posterior bone and "downsizing" the femoral component. The smaller femoral component is smaller both medial to lateral and anterior to posterior. The decreased anterior to posterior size will allow more space in the flexion gap. Once the gaps have been properly equalized, the finishing cuts can be made on both the femoral and tibial side to accommodate the precise components.

The surgical procedure can be performed with 2 basic approaches. The surgery can begin on the femoral side or on the tibial. Surgery on the femoral side usually begins with the bone cuts for a measured resection technique. As part of this resection, the rotation of the component must also be considered. The use of the femoral epicondyles for the reference point for the rotation (Fig. 2) has become popular. The anatomic centers of the medial and lateral epicondyles are clearly identified. Subsequently, a line is drawn across the distal femoral surface connecting the 2 epicondyles. The anterior and posterior femoral cuts are referenced from this line. This reference line is more accurate than the posterior condylar axis line and is independent of the flexion gap technique. The anteroposterior axis has shown similar accuracy to the epicondylar axis. Comparison of the epicondylar axis to the

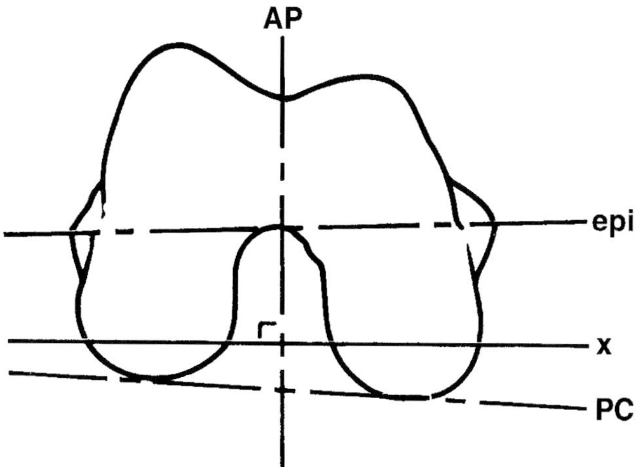

Figure 2

The anteroposterior (AP) axis, epicondylar axis (epi), posterior condylar axis (PC), and the resection line (x) on the distal femur. Note that the resection line drawn perpendicular to the AP axis and parallel to the epi axis is externally rotated with respect to the PC axis. (Reproduced with permission from Arima J, Whiteside LA, McCarthy DS, White SE: Femoral rotational alignment based on the anteroposterior axis, in total knee arthroplasty in a valgus knee: A technical note. *J Bone Joint Surg* 1995;77A:1331–1334.)

posterior condylar axis has shown a 3° to 8° variation between these axes with more reproducibility with the epicondylar reference. The remaining femoral cuts are referenced to the transepicondylar axis. After the femoral cuts are completed, the proximal tibia is resected perpendicular to the shaft of the bone in the coronal plane and angled from 0 to 7° with respect to the sagittal plane, depending on the individual design of the particular prosthesis. After the femoral and tibial cuts are finished, the balance of the knee from extension to flexion is corrected.

The second surgical technique begins on the tibial side and "builds" to the femoral side. After the tibial cut is completed, the first femoral cuts are set up to match the proximal tibial cut as in the flexion gap approach. The anterior and posterior femoral cuts are rotated to match the proximal tibia and produce a rectangular space. This step requires that the medial and lateral collateral ligaments are "relatively" balanced in flexion so that the cuts correlate with this balance and produce a rectangular space. The next cut for the distal femur is again matched to the tibia in full extension. Once the distal femoral cut is made, the knee is balanced in flexion and full extension, and the remaining femoral cuts can be completed. With this approach, the gaps and the ligament balance are both addressed throughout the surgical procedure. With the surgery beginning on the femoral side and with a more measured resection technique, the gaps and the ligament balance are approached later in the procedure, almost as a separate portion of the operation.

The rotation of the femoral component has been discussed above. The tibial rotation remains slightly less well-defined in the literature. The tubercle is a prominent landmark for referencing; however, it is subject to variation (external rotation) or previous surgery. Most authors use several references with the tubercle remaining the primary one. The tibial tray can be rotated and checked with the malleoli of the ankle. The tray can be checked with reference to the femoral component at 90° of flexion, or the tray can be positioned on the surface of the tibia and allowed to "seek" its own position of rotation versus the femoral component throughout the full range of motion of the knee.

The rotation of the femoral and tibial components is critical for proper articulation of the 2 primary components throughout the full range of motion and for the proper tracking of the patella. Internal rotation of either the femoral or tibial component can lead to patellar dislocation. Patellar dislocation in TKR is more commonly caused by internal rotation of the components than extensor mechanism malalignment.

The discussion thus far has centered on the flexion and extension gaps and the collateral ligament balancing. The collateral ligaments directly correlate with the varus and valgus alignment of the knee and the gap balancing. The cruciate ligaments must also be considered with the balancing and add another level of difficulty. Most knee replacements sacrifice the anterior cruciate ligament. There are 3 types of prostheses: posterior cruciate retaining, posterior cruciate sacrificing, and posterior cruciate substituting.

Retention of the posterior cruciate ligament (PCL) is most common in the United States. Tensioning of this ligament can sometimes be difficult, especially if there is considerable valgus or varus deformity. It is imperative that the tibial and femoral cuts are set properly so that the PCL is equally tight throughout the range of motion. One author has stated that it is difficult for the operating surgeon to tense the ligament properly and that 1 to 2 mm of bone resection can significantly affect the tension. If the PCL is too tight, the knee components will open up like a book in flexion; the tibial plastic insert will slide forward; the tibial insert will lift off of the underlying tray; and the trial femoral component will be pulled away from the underlying bone as the knee is flexed. If the PCL is too loose, there will be minimal posterior rollback in flexion and there will be flexion laxity.

The PCL cannot be tightened with techniques such as the Krackow approach, but it is possible to lengthen the ligament with releases on the femoral or tibial side. The releases are difficult to perform without completely sacrificing the ligament's integrity. The tibial side permits a more gradual release but requires more time to remove and replace the components with each step of the gradual release. The femoral side is easier to release because of its direct exposure; however, it is difficult to partially release the femoral side and the PCL often becomes an incompetent structure. If the PCL is inadvertently cut completely free from either the femoral or tibial side, the prosthesis should be changed to a PCL-substituting design.

The collateral ligaments often require balancing, either lengthening or tightening. Releasing the tight ligament is a gradual process and is much easier than tightening the loose ligament. Krackow has published the most material concerning tightening the loose ligament and has clearly illustrated the procedure. In his hands the procedure proves quite successful; however, this approach is more demanding than release and should be reserved for unusual cases. The suturing technique is well-described and should be followed strictly.

There are several popular releases, and each approach can be applied in a sequential fashion. In the varus knee, the medial structures are contracted and the lateral structures are stretched. If a tightening procedure is chosen, the lateral collateral ligament (LCL) would require tightening on the femoral side. More commonly, the surgeon will release the tight medial collateral ligament (MCL) from the tibial side. In a sequential fashion, the deep MCL, the posteromedial capsule, the semimembranosus insertion, the superficial MCL, and, finally, the reflection of the MCL over the soleus muscle are released. Once the reflection is released, the medial side of the knee becomes much more unstable and it may be necessary to support the arthroplasty with a more constrained prosthesis. The release is continued until the medial structures and the lateral structures are equally tight to distraction force in the operating room both in flexion and full extension.

The valgus knee requires either tightening of the loose MCL on the femoral side or release of the tight LCL structures on both the femoral and tibial sides. Once again, the tightening procedure requires the suture technique with the anchor screw.

The releases on the lateral side of the knee have been modified multiple times. The release can proceed from superficial structures to deep or from deep to superficial. The release from deep begins with the LCL from the femoral condyle and proceeds to the posterolateral capsule, the iliotibial band (from the tibial insertion, the joint line, or above the joint line), the popliteus tendon from the femur, and, finally, the biceps insertion on the fibular head. Release of the popliteus tendon increases the instability in flexion and may require additional constraint in the prosthesis. A multiple puncture technique for the posterolateral capsular structures has recently been described that gradually releases the structures without individually identifying each. This technique may permit greater release with less concern for the instability that results when the popliteus is released; however, the puncture technique adds an element of concern for possible injury of the peroneal nerve if the punctures are too aggressive. Currently, there are no reports of such a complication. Finally, an epicondylar osteotomy on either the medial or lateral side of the femur has been described that permits greater surgical exposure and allows for tensioning of the ligament at the time of the closure.

Summary

In the past 5 years, the surgical techniques for the approach to TKA have been continually modified with increasing success. The management of the soft tissues about the knee is of extreme importance to the outcome of the TKA. The extensor mechanism modifications are helpful and allow better exposure. The alignment instruments have been improved, and the ligament releases have been further subclassified to permit more gradual correction of deformity.

Annotated Bibliography

Arima J, Whiteside LA, McCarthy DS, White SE: Femoral rotational alignment, based on the anteroposterior axis, in total knee arthroplasty in a valgus knee: A technical note. *J Bone Joint Surg* 1995;77A:1331–1334.

The authors conclude that the anteroposterior axis is more accurate than the posterior condylar axis and easier to find than the epicondylar axis.

Engh GA, Parks NL: Surgical technique of the midvastus arthrotomy. *Clin Orthop* 1998;351:270–274.

The authors describe a midvastus arthrotomy to avoid splitting the quadriceps tendon as in the standard medial parapatellar approach. They report a quicker return of quadriceps muscle control as well as a more stable patellofemoral articulation.

Engh GA, Parks NL, Ammeen DJ: Influence of surgical approach on lateral retinacular releases in total knee arthroplasty. *Clin Orthop* 1996;331:56–63.

Two surgical approaches are studied in this article: medial parapatellar arthrotomy and midvastus splitting arthrotomy. Lateral retinacular release of the patella was done in 50% of the parapatellar approaches and in only 3% of the midvastus. The authors conclude that the midvastus approach leaves a portion of the vastus medialis intact and helps with patellar tracking.

Garvin KL, Scuderi G, Insall JN: Evolution of the quadriceps snip. *Clin Orthop* 1995;321:131–137.

The authors review 16 patients who underwent quadriceps snip as part of the surgical procedure. The range of motion was increased by an average of 30°, and the Cybex testing was no different than for the opposite total knee.

Gold DA, Scott SC, Scott WN: Soft tissue expansion prior to arthroplasty in the multiply-operated knee: A new method of preventing catastrophic skin problems. *J Arthroplasty* 1996;11:512–521.

The authors review 10 knees in 9 patients who underwent soft-tissue expansion prior to revision knee surgeries. An implantable tissue expander was placed in the soft-tissue bed and gradually inflated to increase available skin for subsequent closure after revision TKR. No wound complications were reported.

Greenfield MA, Insall JN, Case GC, Kelly MA: Instrumentation of the patellar osteotomy in total knee arthroplasty: The relationship of patellar thickness and lateral retinacular release. *Am J Knee Surg* 1996;9:129–132.

The authors show that a measured resection technique for the patellar resurfacing leads to a lower incidence of lateral retinacular release. They aimed for a thickness equal to or less than that of the original patella and produced better tracking results than with the "eyeball" technique.

Hirsch HS, Lotke PA, Morrison LD: The posterior cruciate ligament in total knee surgery: Save, sacrifice, or substitute? *Clin Orthop* 1994;309:64–68.

Two hundred forty-two patients were divided into 3 groups before undergoing TKA. In group 1, the PCL was released from the tibia; in group II, the PCL was retained; and in group III, the PCL was substituted. The authors found an increased range of motion in the group III knees.

Kleinbart FA, Bryk E, Evangelista J, Scott MN, Vigorita VJ: Histologic comparison of posterior cruciate ligaments from arthritic and age-matched knee specimens. *J Arthroplasty* 1996;11:726–731.

Twenty-four PCLs harvested at the time of knee arthroplasty were histologically compared to age-matched controls. The harvested ligaments showed more degenerative changes than the controls. The authors conclude that the retained PCL may be biomechanically abnormal. The authors support PCL sacrifice.

Poilvache PL, Insall JN, Scuderi GR, Font-Rodriguez DE: Rotational landmarks and sizing of the distal femur in total knee arthroplasty. *Clin Orthop* 1996;331:35–46.

The authors examined 100 knees undergoing TKA and concluded that the transepicondylar axis is more accurate than the anteroposterior axis and easier to find.

Whiteside LA: Exposure in difficult total knee arthroplasty using tibial tubercle osteotomy. *Clin Orthop* 1995;321:32–35.

One hundred thirty-six arthroplasties in which an extended tibial tubercle and tibial crest osteotomy was performed for exposure were studied from 1986 to 1994. Two or 3 wires were used for fixation. There were 2 partial avulsions, 2 fractures, and no nonunions. The results are excellent with an average range of motion of 94.

Classic Bibliography

Berger RA, Rubash HE, Seel MJ, Thompson WH, Crossett LS: Determining the rotational alignment of the femoral component in total knee arthroplasty using the epicondylar axis. *Clin Orthop* 1993;286:40–47.

Keblish PA: The lateral approach to the valgus knee: Surgical technique and analysis of 53 cases with over two-year follow-up evaluation. *Clin Orthop* 1991;271:52–62.

Krackow KA, Jones MM, Teeny SM, Hungerford DS: Primary total knee arthroplasty in patients with fixed valgus deformity. *Clin Orthop* 1991;273:9–18.

McMahon MS, Scuderi GR, Glashow JL, Scharf SC, Meltzer LP, Scott WN: Scintigraphic determination of patellar viability after excision of infrapatellar fat pad and/or lateral retinacular release in total knee arthroplasty. *Clin Orthop* 1990;260:10–16.

Stern SH, Moeckel BH, Insall JN: Total knee arthroplasty in valgus knees. *Clin Orthop* 1991;273:5–8.

Teeny SM, Krackow KA, Hungerford DS, Jones M: Primary total knee arthroplasty in patients with severe varus deformity: A comparative study. *Clin Orthop* 1991;273:19–31.

Chapter 32
The Knee: Rehabilitation

Pain Management

Pain control after total knee arthroplasty (TKA) remains a significant concern for both surgeon and patient. The anxiety is appropriate because TKA is a relatively painful procedure, especially in the immediate postoperative period. Commonly, patients undergoing total knee replacement surgery have significantly more pain than patients who have had a total hip arthroplasty. Successful pain management allows reasonable postoperative comfort, as well as aiding in successful completion of the rehabilitation process. Ambulation and bending exercises are easier to complete when patients are not focused on their discomfort. However, these same goals of early mobilization and early knee flexion make achieving adequate pain control more difficult during the initial postoperative period. Common methods of pain control include parenteral narcotics, patient-controlled analgesia (PCA), and epidural analgesia.

Parenteral Injections

For years the hallmark of pain control after a TKA has been the parenteral injection of narcotics. Administration of parenteral narcotics is normally either intramuscular or subcutaneous. Commonly, these injections are administered every 3 to 4 hours on an as-needed basis (prn). These medications still represent one of the most accepted methods of pain control used after TKA. Advantages of parenteral narcotics include their low cost, ease of use, and familiarity to most physicians and nurses. Dosages and side-effects are widely known and understood. However, the "as needed" dosing of parenteral narcotics has been viewed as a disadvantage in some studies. Theoretically, patients receiving parenteral narcotics have to request their medications when pain occurs. Therefore, there can be a significant time lag between pain onset and medication administration. Thus, many patients feel dependent on hospital personnel for the medication, which can lead to increased anxiety and feelings of loss of control. Side effects of parenteral narcotics include allergic reactions and respiratory depression. Physicians need to be especially careful with these medications in patients undergoing TKA because many of these patients are elderly and may be extremely sensitive or have idiopathic responses to their use.

Patient-Controlled Analgesia

Because of limitations with parenteral narcotics, there has been a recent trend allowing patients more control of their analgesia. This increased control can take many forms. However, the most common method of PCA involves the intravenous administration of narcotics through a patient-controlled pump. The pump is connected to the patient's intravenous (IV) tube and is controlled by a bedside button. By depressing the button, patients are able to immediately self-administer a controlled IV narcotic dose. The pump is calibrated to control both the magnitude and frequency of drug administration. PCA machines allow patients to receive analgesia within minutes of activating the button. The major advantage of this method of pain management is increased patient control. Patients have a more secure feeling and less anxiety knowing that they can instantaneously self-administer pain medication on an as-needed basis. Proponents of this technique believe that patients tolerate pain better with this technique. In addition, there is evidence that the overall dosage of pain medication injected tends to be less with use of a PCA machine, as compared with the more traditional prn method. Disadvantages with this technique include the increased complexity associated with the PCA machine and the mandatory increased vigilance associated with its use. This is especially important to ensure that the dosing and concentration of the narcotic administered are correct.

Epidural Analgesia

There has been recent emphasis on the use of epidural anesthesia for patients undergoing TKA. This has also led to a concurrent increase in the use of epidural analgesia in the postoperative period. When this technique is used, the epidural catheter is left in place after the arthroplasty procedure. Depending on the institution, common medications that may be injected into the epidural space include narcotics and/or anesthetics. One of the advantages of epidural analgesia is the degree of pain control that can be achieved. In general, successful epidural analgesia allows the most comprehensive degree of pain control while the catheter is functioning. Commonly, epidural catheters are left in place for 1 to 3 days after a TKA procedure. At least 1 report stated that patients receiving epidural analgesia had a shorter hospital stay and an earlier return of knee flexion than did patients with traditional pain management techniques.

However, there are clear difficulties with epidural analgesia. Many patients are unable to fully complete a course of epidural analgesia because of technical reasons. Catheters can twist, kink, or become dislodged from the appropriate epidural space. Successful epidural analgesia requires both anesthesia and nursing departments be familiar and comfortable with this technique. Yet even in the most experienced institutions, technical difficulties can prevent its full use in some patients. In addition, patients receiving epidural analgesia must continually be monitored for side effects. Specifically, these include nausea, hypotension, and respiratory depression. Furthermore, most patients require supplemental analgesia after the epidural catheter is removed, and thus also require either parenteral narcotics or PCA-controlled analgesia. Finally, there is concern that postoperative epidural analgesia may increase the risk of peroneal nerve palsy. This was examined in at least 1 study, in which the authors believed that epidural analgesia was not a significant risk factor for the development of nerve palsy. However, in their report, all cases of peroneal nerve palsy occurred in patients receiving postoperative epidural analgesia and were diagnosed after discontinuation of the epidural. The authors pointed out that a diagnosis of nerve palsy can be delayed in patients with postoperative epidural analgesia, and that these patients should be monitored closely, especially those with known risk factors. In addition, they suggested consideration of either a dilute local anesthetic or an opiated infusion in patients believed to be at increased risk.

Intra-Articular Narcotics

Intra-articular injections, although commonly used after arthroscopic knee procedures, are not widely used after TKA. In fact, 1 study found that the total amount of postoperative medication was not statistically different between patients receiving intra-articular medication and those injected with saline. This method is not in widespread use in the United States.

Antibiotics

Infection remains one of the most devastating complications that can occur after TKA. Perioperative antibiotics have emerged as one of the mainstays of infection prophylaxis, and it is now well accepted that intravenous antibiotics should be used to minimize the risk of infection. In general, most surgeons stress the importance of administering the first antibiotic dose before the commencement of surgery. Ideally, this dose should be given before tourniquet inflation. The duration of antibiotic administration in the postsurgical period is somewhat more controversial. Most institutions use a 1- to 3-day course of antibiotic coverage after routine TKA, although there does not seem to be any strong evidence favoring any of these regimens.

Because *Staphylococcus aureus* is the most common pathogen in sepsis after TKA, antibiotics should be chosen based on the sensitivities of this microbe. Therefore, many institutions use a first-generation cephalosporin for routine antibiotic prophylaxis after joint arthroplasty. These drugs have several advantages that make them particularly well suited for this indication. They are widely available, easy to administer, well tolerated, and not overly expensive. Most importantly, first-generation cephalosporins combine excellent *S aureus* coverage with reasonable gram-negative organism coverage. (Gram-negative organisms are common pathogens in urinary tract infections.) However, other antibiotics may be appropriate at some hospitals, depending on the institution's local bacterial flora. Some hospitals use second-generation cephalosporins for routine prophylaxis. Generally, these antibiotics offer increased effectiveness against gram-negative organisms, while sacrificing some gram-positive coverage. In institutions where there is concern about methicillin-resistant *S aureus*, vancomycin may be used. Vancomycin is effective against methicillin-resistant staphylococcus. However, it must be administered carefully, it is expensive, and it has more side effects than the cephalosporins. In addition, it offers relatively poor coverage against gram-negative bacteria, and thus may need to be supplemented with an aminoglycoside.

Physical Therapy

Specific aspects of physical therapy after TKA vary depending on each individual institution's protocol. However, several general concepts are used commonly at most facilities. The recent trend is to mobilize patients earlier than in the past. Currently, the basic goals of therapy after knee arthroplasty are optimizing ambulation and knee motion in a safe and expeditious fashion. This is in contrast with historic rehabilitation, which included extended bed rest and immobilization of the operated extremity.

Ambulation after TKA begins in a controlled setting. Customarily, patients use whatever assistive device (walker, cane, or crutch) is appropriate depending on their level of independence. After cemented TKA, many physicians allow their patients to progress to a cane for their assistive device and to bear weight as tolerated. The assistive device is used for approximately 4 to 6 weeks after arthroplasty. At that point, many patients are able to ambulate independently and wean themselves off any assistive device. For patients with uncemented prosthetic components, some physicians use a more extensive course of protected weightbearing. However, others allow these patients to bear weight as tolerated in a manner similar to those with cemented components. There does not appear to be any conclusive evidence that either protocol is more appropriate.

Currently, knee flexion is initiated relatively soon after knee arthroplasty. Most institutions use a combination of passive, active, and active-assisted flexion exercises coordinated by a physical therapist. These can be supplemented with a continuous passive motion (CPM) machine. CPM machines are used at many hospitals to augment other exercises in achieving knee flexion. Traditional CPM involves starting the machine's use with an initial arc of motion between full extension and approximately 30° to 40° of flexion. Flexion is increased approximately 10° per day. The machine can be used as many hours as possible and, if tolerated, patients can sleep in the machine. In general, CPM machines used in this manner are believed to be helpful in promoting early knee flexion. However, most CPM designs are less effective at flexion angles past approximately 80° to 90°. At these higher flexion angles, it is difficult for patients to keep their buttocks against the machine, and commonly the CPM can bend to 90° to 100° while the patient's knee flexes only about 75°. In addition, knees tend not to come to full extension while in the CPM despite the device straightening all the way to 0°. Thus, if a patient is having difficulty with extension or has a flexion deformity, CPM may not be useful. In these instances, use of a knee immobilizer should be considered.

Recently, an early flexion protocol using CPM has been instituted at several institutions. The goal is to rapidly achieve knee flexion and work backward towards extension. When used in this manner, the knee is placed immediately after surgery in a CPM machine cycling between 70° and 100°. The machine's extension is then increased over the first several postoperative days so the arc of motion is between 0° and 100°. Advocates of this technique believe that it more reliably achieves knee flexion and leads to less stiffness, pain, and manipulations. Several studies have shown equal or improved results with the CPM machine used in this manner. However, certain patients find this rapid flexion protocol painful and have difficulty tolerating it.

In any event, the long-term efficacy of CPM machines remains controversial. Theoretically, they may promote early knee flexion, but this has not convincingly been proven. In addition, multiple studies have shown that at longer follow-up, there are rarely differences in knees treated with or without CPM machines.

Early Discharge

Traditionally, TKA patients spent several weeks in the hospital recuperating from the surgery while undergoing a rehabilitation program that stressed knee flexion and ambulation. However, over the last several years the average length of stay after knee arthroplasty has decreased throughout the United States. Many institutions now have length of stays averaging 5 days or less after this procedure. In general, this decrease in the amount of time the average patient spends in the acute hospital setting has been achieved without compromising the results of the procedure. Many institutions have found that patients can be safely and effectively mobilized and discharged using an aggressive rehabilitation protocol and clinical pathways.

Clinical pathways are a simple tool to standardize patient activities in the postoperative period. Theoretically, the increased standardization leads to more predictable outcomes, while ensuring that important milestones are met in a timely fashion. It is important to remember that even with pathways and early mobilization, the basic medical, surgical, and rehabilitation goals must be achieved before discharge. It is important that the patient be assessed by physical therapy before discharge to ensure that adequate gait training has been achieved. In addition, the patient's medical status needs to be suitably evaluated before discharge. Finally, the patient's home situation also needs to be appropriate for a person who has recently undergone a TKA. In general, it is useful for discharge planning to begin before the patient's hospital admission. The patient and the family should be aware of the discharge goals and options. Arrangements for appropriate home help from family and friends should be encouraged. If possible, the home should be prepared to minimize excessive walking or stair climbing in the immediate postoperative period.

For certain patients, early discharge to home is inappropriate. In these cases, many patients are transferred from the acute inpatient hospital setting to a rehabilitation or skilled nursing facility. Used correctly, this technique allows appropriate rehabilitation in the postoperative period, while maintaining judicious use of the acute care hospital.

Deep Vein Thrombosis and Testing

Testing

The optimal manner of dealing with the issues associated with thrombophlebitis after total joint arthroplasty remains controversial. Contentions include the most appropriate prophylactic agent, the duration of treatment, the necessity for diagnostic testing, and, if present, the best treatment of established thrombophlebitis. The issues associated with deep vein thrombosis (DVT) are especially problematic because many clots are asymptomatic and resolve uneventfully. Conversely, DVT can also lead to pulmonary embolism with its concurrent morbidity and possible catastrophic mortality.

Diagnostic Testing As with most issues associated with thrombophlebitis, the need for and the best method of thrombophlebitis screening remains controversial. Common modalities for detection of DVT include physical examination, venography, and ultrasound.

Physical Examination Physical examination is commonly believed to be unreliable in testing for DVT. DVT can occur without any clinical signs or symptoms. In addition, the clinical signs of DVT, including calf swelling and calf pain, are extremely common in patients after TKA. Therefore, these clinical findings are neither reliable nor predictable. Accordingly, few institutions are willing to restrict prophylactic medication only to clinically symptomatic patients. Thus, most surgeons in the United States institute some form of DVT prophylaxis for TKA patients in the immediate postoperative period. Some physicians continue with routine prophylaxis and avoid regular DVT screening. Other surgeons proceed with routine screening and modify their prophylaxis depending on results of the diagnostic study.

Ultrasonography Duplex ultrasonography using B-mode ultrasound has become a standard diagnostic tool at many institutions to evaluate for DVT. This is a noninvasive test allowing the technician to evaluate the venous system for blood clots. In the presence of thrombus, the B-mode ultrasound may reveal either the thrombus or a noncompressible vein. In the hands of a skilled operator, it is believed to be extremely accurate in the diagnosis of acute or chronic DVT. However, the technology is limited by its complexity. It is not available at all institutions, and it is highly operator-dependent. In addition, duplex ultrasonography appears least reliable in evaluating isolated calf thrombi (clots distal to the popliteal region). However, the clinical significance, if any, of these distal clots remains controversial because proximal clots are traditionally viewed as the most prone to produce significant pulmonary emboli.

Many institutions still use Duplex ultrasonography as a screening tool. However, the results can be variable, and there is concern that it may lead to overtreatment of certain patients. Some studies have shown that routine screening of patients even with duplex ultrasound is not necessary.

Venography Venography is classically described as the "gold standard" for diagnosis of DVT. It is believed to be the most reliable and predictable diagnostic test for assessing the presence and extent of DVT. However, because it is an invasive study, there are inherent problems with its use. Specifically, venography can be uncomfortable and necessitates a dye load for the patient. In general, it has fallen out of favor as a routine screening test in patients who have had knee arthroplasty procedures. However, it remains the mode of choice at many institutions to diagnosis DVT in patients with a high clinical suspicion for thrombophlebitis, especially if the availability or experience with duplex ultrasonography is limited.

Summary At this time there is no consensus on whether routine screening for DVT after knee arthroplasty should be carried out. However, the current trend appears to be away from routine DVT screening after TKA. The current emphasis appears to be on instituting some form of DVT prophylaxis (pharmacologic, mechanical, or both) in all patients after knee replacement procedures. Diagnostic DVT studies are limited to patients with high clinical suspicion for thrombophlebitis and in whom a positive result would alter the routine prophylactic measures already in place.

Treatment

As with diagnosis, the actual treatment of established DVT remains controversial. Once again there is no specific consensus in regard to all the issues and options, and treatment must be individualized depending on the particular circumstances. In general, because large and proximal DVTs have a greater risk associated with embolization, these clots may require consideration of more aggressive treatment.

Benign Neglect It is not clear that all DVTs need treatment. Specifically, whether calf clots (those distal to the popliteal vein) require any specific therapy is controversial. The controversy exists because there is no consensus on the potential for propagation of these distal clots. Some physicians believe that the risks associated with pharmacologic treatment (ie, bleeding after anticoagulation) of these distal DVTs may be greater than the intrinsic risks posed by these clots if left untreated. Therefore, it may be possible in ambulatory patients who are doing well to treat distal DVTs with benign neglect, possibly supplemented with a repeat diagnostic study to rule out clot progression.

Warfarin Warfarin remains the prototypical long-term pharmacologic treatment of established DVT. It is an oral medication that inhibits the synthesis of vitamin K-dependent coagulation factors. It has a long track record of use, is inexpensive, and is commonly available. It acts to prevent propagation of established thrombophlebitis, although classically it has not been believed to dissolve established clot. However, there are clear limitations and difficulties associated with use of this medication. Warfarin has unpredictable pharmacokinetics, making regular blood monitoring (prothrombin time [PT] and/or international normalized ratio [INR] values) necessary throughout its use.

Further limitations include its slow mode of onset. Because warfarin inhibits the synthesis of new coagulation factors, it does not affect existing coagulation factors. Thus, in the clinical situation where rapid anticoagulation is desired, warfarin alone normally would not suffice. In these situations, many physicians supplement warfarin anticoagulation with an adjunctive anticoagulant that has a rapid onset of action (commonly heparin). Combined heparin and warfarin therapy can be continued until the anticoagulation effect from the warfarin, as manifested by the patient's PT or INR, is satisfactory. At that point, the heparin can be discontinued.

The duration of warfarin treatment for established DVT needs to be individualized, depending on the particular patient issues. Commonly, the length of treatment ranges from 3 and 6 months. In addition, the goal for the level of anticoagulation, as manifested by the patient's blood tests, tends to be slightly higher when treating established DVT, as compared with its use as a routine prophylactic agent.

Intravenous Heparin Historically, heparin, administered intravenously, has also been used in the treatment of established DVT. Heparin is a mixture of polysaccharide chains of varied molecular weights. It acts through mediation of other factors to inhibit the blood coagulation cascade. Because heparin administered intravenously has a rapid mode of onset, it is an ideal medication to achieve immediate anticoagulation. However, like warfarin, the pharmacokinetics of heparin are relatively unpredictable. Patients undergoing heparin therapy must be closely monitored, especially patients in the postoperative period, because of the bleeding risks associated with IV administration. At least 1 article has reported a significantly increased risk of bleeding when IV heparin is used within the first week after total joint arthroplasty.

While undergoing heparin treatment, the patient's partial thromboplastin time (PTT) must be followed closely. Because of heparin's narrow therapeutic zone, it is difficult to achieve adequate anticoagulation, while at the same time preventing bleeding complications. In addition, patients receiving heparin therapy should also have their platelet counts monitored because of the incidence of heparin-induced thrombocytopenia.

Low-Molecular-Weight Heparin Low-molecular-weight heparin (LMWH) has recently become available in the United States. Enoxaparin was the first LMWH approved for use by the Food and Drug Administration (FDA), although others are now available. While enoxaparin's initial FDA indication was prophylaxis after joint arthroplasty, some physicians have used it or other LMWHs as treatment for established DVT. This use is supported by some studies in the literature. However, at this time, LMWHs have not received FDA approval for use as treatment of established thrombophlebitis. Thus, use of LMWHs in this manner currently remains an "off-label" use of these medications and only should be employed if in the judgment of the treating physician such use is medically indicated to treat a patient's condition.

Theoretic advantages of LMWH include its ability to be given subcutaneously, and thus administered in an outpatient setting. Outpatient administration is a significant advantage, because it means the expense and inconvenience of hospital admission can be avoided. Finally, treatment with LMWH theoretically does not require the same intensive monitoring as required with intravenous heparin. However, if enoxaparin is used in the treatment of an established DVT, the dosing usually needs to be increased above the standard prophylactic regimen of 30 mg twice a day. The specific dosage and frequency used would need to be titrated depending on the patient's individual circumstances. Because LMWHs are relatively new medications, and their use in treatment of established DVT currently remains non-FDA approved (Class III), they are normally used for this indication by physicians who are familiar with them. The exact length of treatment with LMWH for established DVT is controversial.

Vena Cava Filters One further option for the treatment of established thrombophlebitis is the placement of a vena cava (Greenfield) filter. This treatment is normally used in patients with significant DVT or pulmonary embolism in whom anticoagulation therapy is either contraindicated or has been ineffective. Placement of the vena cava filter does not directly treat the DVT. However, the filter theoretically prevents embolisms from migrating to the pulmonary vasculature.

The major advantage of this technique is the theoretic prevention of further lung emboli without the inherent bleeding risks associated with most anticoagulation methods. Therefore, this method is especially useful early in the postoperative period when the risks of bleeding are the most profound. Disadvantages of vena cava filters center on the invasiveness and permanence of this technique. Placement of a vena cava filter requires an experienced interventional radiologist. In addition, because the filters do not act to dissolve clot, the risk of a "postphlebitic syndrome," in which patients have permanent increased swelling of the extremity, is unchanged after this treatment.

Annotated Bibliography

Pain Management

Horlocker TT, Cabanela ME, Wedel DJ: Does postoperative epidural analgesia increase the risk of peroneal nerve palsy after total knee arthroplasty? *Anesth Analg* 1994;79:495–500.

Eight peroneal palsies were identified after a chart review of 361 TKAs (2.2%). Postoperative epidural analgesia (used in 108 TKAs) was not believed to be a significant risk factor for development of a peroneal nerve palsy. However, all cases of nerve palsy occurred in patients receiving epidural analgesia and were diagnosed after discontinuation of the anesthetic. The authors recommended close monitoring of patients receiving epidural analgesia, as well as consideration of a dilute local anesthetic or an opioid infusion in patients at increased risk of nerve palsy.

Ilahi OA, Davidson JP, Tullos HS: Continuous epidural analgesia using fentanyl and bupivacaine after total knee arthroplasty. *Clin Orthop* 1994;299:44–52.

Eighty consecutive TKA patients received a continuous epidural infusion for postoperative analgesia. Of these, 19 were unable to complete the 3-day postoperative epidural treatment, two thirds for technical reasons and one third because of adverse affects. In patients who were able to complete the 3-day course of treatment, there was a shorter hospital stay and earlier return of flexion compared with patients who had the epidural removed sooner.

Love DR, Owen H, Ilsley AH, Plummer JL, Hawkins RM, Morrison A: A comparison of variable-dose patient-controlled analgesia with fixed-dose patient-controlled analgesia. *Anesth Analg* 1996;83:1060–1064.

The authors compare variable-dose patient-controlled analgesia (VDPCA) with conventional fixed-dose patient-controlled analgesia (FDPCA). The VDPCA was believed to be more complex, but did not offer any advantage over FDPCA.

Mauerhan DR, Campbell M, Miller JS, Mokris JG, Gregory A, Kiebzak GM: Intra-articular morphine and/or bupivacaine in the management of pain after total knee arthroplasty. *J Arthroplasty* 1997;12:546–552.

The authors report a prospective, double-blind, randomized study of 105 patients undergoing TKA who were divided into groups receiving intra-articular injections of saline, morphine sulfate, bupivacaine, or a combination of morphine and bupivacaine. The total amount of postoperative pain medications used in the first 24 hours after surgery was not statistically different in the 4 groups. The authors said "the results put into question the benefit of postoperative intra-articular administration of morphine or bupivacaine in patients undergoing TKA."

Antibiotics

Friedman RJ, Friedrich LV, White RL, Kays MB, Brundage DM, Graham J: Antibiotic prophylaxis and tourniquet inflation in total knee arthroplasty. *Clin Orthop* 1990;260:17–23.

Patients undergoing TKA were randomized into 3 groups based on tourniquet inflation 1, 2, or 5 minutes after receiving 1 g of cefazolin. A higher percentage of patients who had a 5-minute interval before tourniquet inflation achieved the desired cefazolin concentration.

Mauerhan DR, Nelson CL, Smith DL, et al: Prophylaxis against infection in total joint arthroplasty: One day of cefuroxime compared with three days of cefazolin. *J Bone Joint Surg* 1994;76A:39–45.

This prospective, double-blind, multicenter study compared 1 day of cefuroxime with 3 days of cefazolin. For patients who underwent primary TKA, the rate of deep wound infection was 0.6% (1 of 178) in patients receiving cefuroxime as compared with 1.4% (3 of 207) in patients treated with cefazolin.

Physical Therapy—Continuous Passive Motion

Kumar PJ, McPherson EJ, Dorr LD, Wan Z, Baldwin K: Rehabilitation after total knee arthroplasty: A comparison of 2 rehabilitation techniques. *Clin Orthop* 1996;331:93–101.

This randomized prospective study compared 46 TKAs in which a CPM machine was used with a second group of 37 TKAs in which early passive flexion (drop and dangle) was used. Postoperative physical therapy was otherwise the same for both groups. Patients in whom the drop and dangle technique was used were discharged from the hospital 1 day earlier and had statistically better extension (2.8° at 6 months). The authors believed that knee motion and hospital discharge could be achieved in a comparable manner with or without the CPM device, and they believed that this device was not required for postoperative TKA rehabilitation.

McInnes J, Larson MG, Daltroy LH, et al: A controlled evaluation of continuous passive motion in patients undergoing total knee arthroplasty. *JAMA* 1992;268:1423–1428.

A randomized controlled trial in 102 patients of CPM plus standard rehabilitation versus standard rehabilitation alone was performed. The authors found that CPM use increased active flexion and decreased swelling and need for manipulations, but did not significantly affect pain, active and passive extension, quadriceps strength, or length of hospital stay. At 6 weeks there was no difference in motion between the 2 groups.

Montgomery F, Eliasson M: Continuous passive motion compared to active physical therapy after knee arthroplasty: Similar hospitalization times in a randomized study of 68 patients. *Acta Orthop Scand* 1996;67:7–9.

The authors report a randomized study of 68 patients undergoing TKA who received either CPM and physical therapy or active physical therapy alone. The CPM group had less postoperative knee swelling and more rapid initial improvement in knee flexion. However, there was no difference in flexion at discharge nor was there any difference in pain or length of hospitalization.

Pope RO, Corcoran S, McCaul K, Howie DW: Continuous passive motion after primary total knee arthroplasty: Does it offer any benefits? *J Bone Joint Surg* 1997;79B:914–917.

In this prospective randomized study, 53 patients were grouped into 3 postoperative protocols. At 1 week, there was a statistical increase in knee flexion in the most aggressive CPM group compared with the no-CPM group. However, at 1 year there was no difference in the 3 groups in regard to knee flexion, range of motion, fixed flexion deformity, or functional results. Patients treated with the CPM required more analgesics. The authors believed "that CPM had no significant advantage in terms of improving function or range of movement, and that its use increased blood loss and analgesic requirements."

Ververeli PA, Sutton DC, Hearn SL, Booth RE Jr, Hozack WJ, Rothman RR: Continuous passive motion after total knee arthroplasty: Analysis of cost and benefits. *Clin Orthop* 1995;321:208–215.

A prospective study comparing daily CPM combined with physical therapy (51 patients) with physical therapy alone (52 patients) was done. At discharge, knees treated with CPM had significantly increased flexion. There was no difference in pain, wound healing, knee swelling, wound drainage, pulmonary embolism, or length of hospital stay. At 2 years, there was no difference in knee flexion or knee scores between the 2 groups. The authors believed that CPM was effective in increasing short-term knee flexion and decreasing knee manipulations without increasing costs.

Yashar AA, Venn-Watson E, Welsh T, Colwell CW Jr, Lotke P: Continuous passive motion with accelerated flexion after total knee arthroplasty. *Clin Orthop* 1997;345:38–43.

A randomized, prospective study of 210 consecutive total knee arthroplasties was performed. One group (control) started CPM at 0° to 30°, progressively increasing flexion. The accelerated flexion group started flexion in a CPM between 70° and 100° in the recovery room. The accelerated flexion group had statistically greater flexion at day 3 and at discharge. There was no statistical difference at longer follow-up intervals. The authors concluded that "continuous passive motion using accelerated flexion allows increased flexion during the hospital stay without increased risk of complications, pain or blood loss."

Early Discharge

Fisher DA, Trimble S, Clapp B, Dorsett K: Effect of a patient management system on outcomes of total hip and knee arthroplasty. *Clin Orthop* 1997;345:155–160.

Five hundred fifty-three patients undergoing total hip replacement and total knee replacement with a patient management system were compared with a retrospective group of 340 patients. The length of stay and hospital charges were significantly decreased after institution of the patient management system. There was no significant difference in complications between the 2 groups.

Mabrey JD, Toohey JS, Armstrong DA, Lavery L, Wammack LA: Clinical pathway management of total knee arthroplasty. *Clin Orthop* 1997;345:125–133.

This is the report of a retrospective cohort study examining 2 groups of atients with the same attending surgeon before and after initiation of clinical pathways and an outcomes management program. The program reduced length of stay by 57%. Hospital costs were reduced 11%. The authors believed that the implementation of appropriate clinical pathways at their institution resulted in significant length of stay reductions without compromising clinical outcome.

DVT Therapy and Testing

Ciccone WJ II, Fox PS, Neumyer M, Rubens D, Parrish WM, Pellegrini VD Jr: Ultrasound surveillance for asymptomatic deep venous thrombosis after total joint replacement. *J Bone Joint Surg* 1998;80A:1167–1174.

Prospective data on 123 total hip arthroplasty patients and 94 total knee arthroplasty patients from 2 university medical centers were analyzed. Routine surveillance with ascending contrast venography was compared with duplex ultrasonography complemented with color-flow Doppler imaging. Duplex ultrasonography with color-flow Doppler imaging identified 2 of 3 proximal thrombi and 5 of 52 (10%) calf thrombi. There were 2 false-positive ultrasounds. The authors conclude that "the interinstitutional variability and insensitivity of duplex ultrasonography with color-flow Doppler imaging for the detection of asymptomatic deep venous thrombi in the calf after total joint replacement make it unreliable as a routine surveillance after total hip or knee arthroplasty."

Hull RD, Raskob GE, Pineo GF, et al: Subcutaneous low-molecular-weight heparin compared with continuous intravenous heparin in the treatment of proximal-vein thrombosis. *N Engl J Med* 1992;326:975–982.

This multicenter, double-blind clinical trial compared fixed-dose LMWH (213 patients) with intravenous heparin (219 patients) for treatment of patients with proximal vein thrombosis. LMWH was at least as effective and safe as standard intravenous heparin treatment. The authors concluded that "the simplified therapy provided by low-molecular-weight-heparin may allow patients with uncomplicated proximal deep-vein thrombosis to be cared for in an outpatient setting."

Mosca PJ, Haas SB: Thromboembolic disease, in Fu FH, Harner CD, Vince KG (eds): *Knee Surgery*. Baltimore, MA, Williams & Wilkins, 1994, vol 2, 1493–1506.

This is an overview of thromboembolic disease including pathogenesis, risk factors, clinical presentation, diagnostic tests, prophylaxis, and treatment.

Robinson KS, Anderson DR, Gross M, et al: Ultrasonographic screening before hospital discharge for deep venous thrombosis after arthroplasty: The post-arthroplasty screening study. A randomized, controlled trial. *Ann Intern Med* 1997;127:439–445.

The authors report a double-blind randomized study of 1,024 patients undergoing either hip or knee arthroplasty. All patients received warfarin prophylaxis and were randomized either to bilateral compression ultrasonography or a sham procedure before hospital discharge. There was no statistical difference in outcomes between the 2 groups. The authors concluded that screening compression ultrasonography was not justified in this setting.

Chapter 33
Evaluation of Results of Total Knee Arthroplasty

Introduction

Total knee arthroplasty (TKA) has evolved over the past 3 decades into one of the most successful reconstructive procedures in orthopaedic surgery today. The success of any knee arthroplasty is dependent on many factors, including patient selection, type of implant, surgical techniques, and rehabilitation. One of the most important factors, which is also the most difficult to quantify, involves patient expectation and satisfaction. There has been no uniformity in reporting previous clinical and radiographic results. However, the success of TKA is unquestioned as reflected by a meta-analysis of nearly 10,000 patients in 130 published reports. Overall results were good to excellent in nearly 90% of patients at short- to medium-term follow-up. A high incidence of clinical satisfaction continues to be observed even with longer-term follow-up.

In the past, surgeons generally reported data gathered by assessing the clinical and radiographic results of a series of TKAs. Many such reports included operations performed by multiple surgeons with different experiences. Some reports also included many different implant designs and surgical techniques. Many surgeons over the past decade have advocated the need to draw data together so that it will present the success or failure of a TKA based on patient-oriented assessment. Moreover, evaluation of TKAs should ideally provide a basis for comparison among different series from different centers.

Knee Rating Systems

One of the most popular methods used over the past 20 years is to assign a score. Various end points are given points, which are then added together to provide a knee score. These scoring systems are generally based on a scale of 0 to 100. Despite the lack of uniformity and the crude nature of assigning arbitrary numbers to reflect the function of a knee joint, the scoring method has the virtue of clarity and is easy for the readers to understand.

The most popular and accepted rating system prior to the 1990s has been the Hospital for Special Surgery Knee Rating Scale. This scoring system consists of 6 categories, including pain relief, function, motion, muscle strength, flexion deformity, and stability. In addition, points are subtracted for the use of walking aids, extension lag, and excessive varus or valgus deformities. Patients are then assigned 1 of the 4 standard clinical categories: excellent (90 to 100 points), good (80 to 89 points), fair (70 to 79 points), and poor (less than 70). One of the major limitations of this system is that aging and deterioration of the patient's general health status may have an adverse effect on the knee score. As a solution to this concern, The Knee Society rating system was devised and proposed in 1989 (Table 1). This rating system has evolved into the most standard method used to report the clinical outcome of TKAs over the past decade. Knee rating and functional assessment are separated in this scoring system. It provides quantitative assessment of 3 main parameters: pain, stability, and range of motion. Functional assessment includes walking and stair climbing. In addition, the patients are divided into 3 categories according to other factors that may impair function, similar to the Charnley functional categories for assessment of hip arthroplasties. Patient category A is for unilateral TKA, or someone who has had a successful contralateral TKA. Patient category B is for unilateral TKA with a symptomatic contralateral knee. Patient category C is for multiple joint arthritis or medical infirmity.

Patient-Oriented Outcome Assessment

Outcomes assessment has become increasingly important over the past decade, especially as emphasis has shifted from technical advancement to accountability, partly because of financial and political considerations. Physician-defined measures of clinical outcome have been replaced with patient-reported measures of function and improvements in quality of life following TKAs. Any rating system for assessing knee function should be valid, reliable, and responsive. Responsiveness is especially important to distinguish those patients who benefited from an operation from those who did not.

Patient-reported measures of function can include general

Table 1
Knee Score

	Points
Patient category	
Unilateral or bilateral (opposite knee successfully replaced)	
Unilateral, other knee symptomatic	
Multiple arthritis or medical infirmity	
Pain	Points
None	50
Mild or occasional	45
Stairs only	40
Walking and stairs	30
Moderate	
Occasional	20
Continual	10
Severe	0
Range of Motion	
(5° = 1 point)	25
Stability (maximum movement in any position)	
Anteroposterior	
< 5 mm	10
5-10 mm	5
10 mm	0
Mediolateral	
< 5 mm	15
6°-9°	10
10°-14°	5
15°	0
Subtotal	
Deductions (minus)	
Flexion contracture	
5°-10°	2
10°-15°	5
16°-25°	10
> 20°	15
Extension lag	
5°-10°	5
10°-25°	10
> 20°	15
Alignment	
5°-10°	0
0°-4°	3 points each degree
11°-15°	3 points each degree
Other	20
Total deductions	
Knee score	
(If total is a minus number, score is 0).	
Function	
Walking	
Unlimited	50
> 10 blocks	40
5-10 blocks	30
< 5 blocks	20
Housebound	10
Unable	0
Stairs	
Normal up and down	50
Normal up; down with rail	40
Up and down with rail	30
Up with rail; unable down	15
Unable	0
Subtotal	
Deductions (minus)	
Cane	5
Two canes	10
Crutches or walker	20
Total deductions	
Function score	

(Reproduced with permission from Insall JN, Dorr LD, Scott RD, Scott WN: Rationale of the Knee Society Clinical Rating System. *Clin Orthop* 1989;248:13–14.)

and disease-specific measures of health status. General measures can be applied across different disease processes and demographic subgroups. Most common general health assessment methods used for patients with orthopaedic conditions include the Medical Outcomes Study Short Form-36 (SF-36), and the Sickness Impact Profile (SIP). These instruments do not offer any specific measure of knee function. One of the most popular disease-specific measures is the Western Ontario and McMaster Universities Osteoarthritis Index (WOMAC). This self-administered health status assessment measures clinical symptoms in 3 major areas: pain, stiffness, and physical function. There are other disease-specific outcomes measure instruments for the knee joint such as the Lysholm Knee Scale, and the Cincinnati Knee Scale, both of which are principally designed to evaluate symptoms and impairments related to ligamentous or meniscal injuries. The focused nature of some of these instruments has limited the assessment of patients who may have concomitant disease processes. An additional problem with existing methods is the lack of a rationale for the scaling systems used to assign a score. Some systems may assign 50% of the score in one category, which can potentially bias the overall outcome, especially if comparative analysis is done using other rating systems.

Outcomes measure instruments are considered valid if small observer variability within a given population is present, and if it controls for differences between study populations. Differences between study populations might include unrecognized risk factors that can become confounding variables. These variables may result in an increase in undesirable outcome or influence the choice of treatment. Thus, case-mix adjustment is used to minimize the effects of confounding variables (such as age or socioeconomic issues) that may affect outcome measures. A recent study was designed to specifically examine the effects of some clinically relevant factors on commonly used knee rating systems. The authors examined 200 volunteers who never had any symptoms or surgery of the knee joint. The 4 knee rating systems selected were all designed to evaluate the outcome of TKAs: The Hospital for Special Surgery system, The Knee Society system, system of Hungerford and Kenna, and the system of Hofmann and associates. The results demonstrated that certain demographic variables had a significant negative correlation with the knee rating of these patients: advanced age greater than 85 years, family income below the poverty level, and 2 or more major medical comorbidities. Moreover, the average normalized knee scores were lower than expected in these asymptomatic patients. Therefore the question is whether the existing scoring scales and categorization of clinical outcome based on these scores following TKAs are sufficiently valid.

In addition to reliability and validity, responsiveness of any outcomes measure instrument is of great importance to separate those patients who have received benefit from those who have not. A more responsive instrument, in theory, may be able to identify more subtle changes in patient status. A recent study conducted by Canadian investigators tested the responsiveness of 6 knee outcomes measures in patients undergoing TKAs. The study was based on consecutive series of 68 patients undergoing TKAs performed by 2 senior surgeons using similar surgical techniques and implant designs. The 6 instruments selected were: The Knee Society system, WOMAC, SF-36, 6-minute walk test, 30-second stair climb test, and quality of life time trade-off utility measure. These instruments were administered before surgery and at 3-month and 6-month postoperative intervals. The highest statistical significance in improvement of outcome following TKAs was found with The Knee Society system and the WOMAC index. In regard to responsiveness, The Knee Society system and the WOMAC again proved to be the best. The least useful instrument was the time trade-off utility measurement.

The usefulness of many of the existing knee rating systems is limited by the fact that these instruments often are designed for specific pathologic conditions and resulting functional limitations. These limitations make it difficult to select an instrument for the assessment of patients who may have concomitant multiple pathologies of the knee joint. A new knee evaluation method, The Knee Outcome Survey, has recently been proposed as an instrument for outcomes measure for the assessment of limitations experienced by patients who have various pathologic disorders. This patient-reported outcomes measure was developed at The University of Pittsburgh. It consists of 2 separate scales: The Activities of Daily Living Scale (ADLS), and the Sports Activity Scale. The ADLS is especially useful to assess functional disability related to conditions affecting the knee, including ligamentous and meniscal injuries, patellofemoral pain, degenerative arthritis, and posttraumatic symptoms related to previous fractures.

The symptoms included in the ADLS for this particular instrument are pain, stiffness, crepitus, swelling, instability, and weakness. The functional limitations as a result of these symptoms include walking on level surfaces or stairs, standing, kneeling, squatting, sitting, and rising from a chair. The responses to each of the 17 items included in this instrument are assigned a numerical value ranging from 0 (most limiting) to 5 (normal). A study was conducted to test the usefulness of this instrument in nearly 400 patients enrolled over a 1-year period. Sophisticated statistical analysis of the vast amount of data generated confirmed that ADLS is a valid, reliable, and responsive instrument for the assessment of functional limitations. One of the major limitations of this particular study in regard to assessment of TKAs was that less than 10% of the sample population was affected with osteoarthritis. Moreover, only 1.4% of the patients eventually underwent either an osteotomy or TKA for their osteoarthritis. The usefulness of the ADLS in assessing outcome following TKAs should be enhanced by additional studies with larger patient populations.

Gait Analysis

Assessment of functional improvement following TKAs using gait analysis has been reported by several authors. Gait analysis is an excellent way to evaluate the kinematics and biomechanics of any joint function. Early data generated using gait analysis following TKAs were initially reported over 15 years ago. The information may no longer be valid because the prosthetic designs evaluated are no longer used for clinical application. However, some very fundamentally important facts were demonstrated. Abnormal features of gait were present even in asymptomatic patients with excellent clinical ratings. Major findings included shorter than normal stride length, reduced knee flexion at midstance, and abnormal external flexion-extension moment. Differences from matched control population were even more pronounced in stair climbing. These early data also suggested that prosthetic designs with less constraint fared better than those with greater degrees of constraint.

In another study using relatively crude methods for gait analysis, the authors reported consistent improvement following unilateral or bilateral TKAs. Specific parameters of gait that were shown to be improved included shorter stance phase, shorter single-limb support time, greater stride length, and shorter double support time. All of these factors contributed to increased walking speed. The swing phase time was not significantly different after surgery. An important outcome of this analysis was that patients with bilateral TKAs demonstrated better gait parameters than those patients who had bilateral knee arthritis but only underwent unilateral TKA. Moreover, the absolute values of these different parameters of gait approximated more to normal control values in patients with bilateral TKAs than in those patients with only unilateral TKA, regardless of whether or not the contralateral knee was arthritic.

Gait analysis has become more refined over the past decade. Newer data have been generated in assessing the outcome of TKAs. These data especially have provided more insight into the differences between cruciate-retaining and cruciate-sacrificing designs. In one study, the authors evaluated 11 patients with bilateral TKAs at an average follow-up of 5 years. In each patient, a cruciate-retaining design was used on 1 knee, and a cruciate-sacrificing design on the other. There was no difference in patient satisfaction, radiographic examinations, or knee scores between sides. Both designs were shown to result in decreased stance phase and a stiff-leg stance phase with less flexion during this phase of gait. Patients with the cruciate-sacrificing design demonstrated more varus moment and thus greater medial joint reaction loading during level walking than those patients with the cruciate-retaining design. Muscle activities were also analyzed using fine-wire techniques. It was demonstrated that increased quadriceps and biceps femoris muscle activities resulted during level walking in patients with the cruciate-sacrificing design. Moreover, these patients also required more soleus muscle activities to assist in maintaining knee stability during stair climbing.

Conflicting data were reported in another study evaluating the effects of TKA on stair ascent and descent as compared with unoperated knees. Symmetrical kinematic patterns between the TKA and control populations were demonstrated. This was in contrast to previous reports that despite successful TKA, patients continued to demonstrate gait analysis parameters inferior to those of control subjects. The motion data were superior in those patients with cruciate-retaining design than previously reported data by the same authors on patients with cruciate-sacrificing design. Electromyographic data demonstrated greater duration of muscle activity on the TKA side. The muscle groups studied included the quadriceps, medial and lateral hamstrings, and the gastrocnemius-soleus.

Gait analysis has indeed provided useful information concerning differences in kinematics and biomechanics following TKA as compared with controls. The common limitations of the reported studies are small patient populations and different methodologies used for gait analysis. Although valuable quantitative outcomes assessment can be generated using gait analysis, it remains of limited practical value to many surgeons because of the lack of available gait laboratories and increased costs.

Radiographic Evaluation

Radiographic examination has become a standard part of the outcome assessment of any TKA because it can provide valuable information about fixation stability, wear, and osteolysis. Most importantly, certain radiographic findings have been demonstrated to have a high positive correlation with predictive value in assessing the longevity of a TKA. Radiographic examination is especially useful if there are standardized techniques, sequential time intervals, and uniform criteria for the interpretation of the radiographs. A high correlation between radiographic finding of suboptimal results and clinical rating has been documented. A radiolucency of more than 1 mm, progressive radiolucencies, and migration of any component have all been demonstrated to be significant features in predicting loss of fixation. Studies have also shown limitations of radiographic evaluations in regard to standardization of position and rotation of the knee while the radiographs are being obtained, and a tendency to underestimate the width and extent of radiolucencies.

Critical evaluation of radiographs is essential to determine subtle changes that may explain the patient's symptoms. The importance of standardizing techniques has been illustrated in an in vitro study in which position of the limb, in particular rotational position, significantly affected the final analysis of the alignment of the reconstruction. The overall alignment and position of the tibial component of a TKA can change completely, from varus to valgus based on variability associated with changes in rotation and flexion of the limb while the radiographs are being obtained.

The most widely accepted radiographic examination method currently is that proposed by The Knee Society (Fig. 1). This system includes assessment of overall alignment, position of the components in relation to the anatomic axes of the femur and the tibia, and presence and location of radiolucencies in the cement-bone and prosthesis-bone (for cementless fixation) interfaces. The zonal distribution has been standardized, thus providing the surgeons a tool to compare different series of TKAs performed by different surgical techniques and using different implant designs. Presence of radiolucencies in 10 or more zones around the components signifies impending loss of fixation.

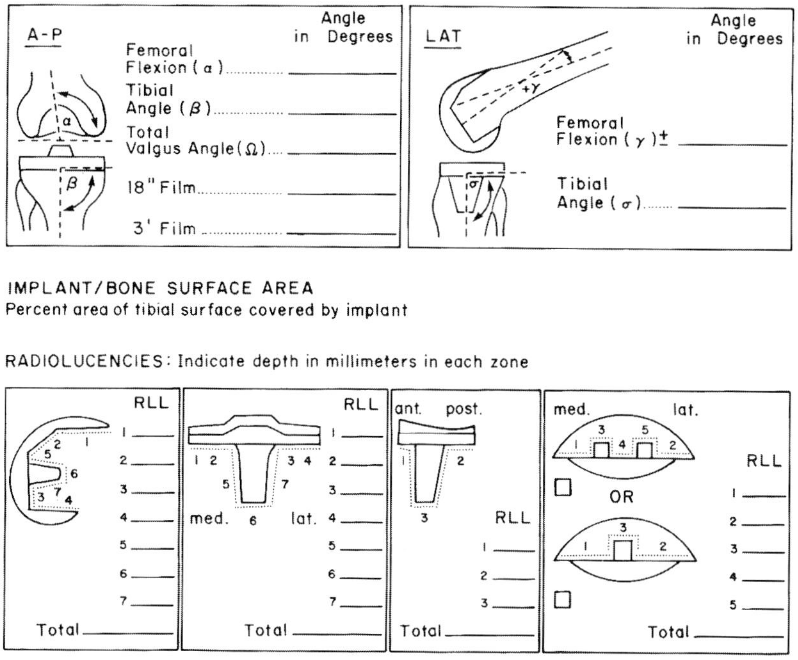

Figure 1

One-page Knee Society Roentgenographic Evaluation and Scoring System. Individual designers/developers should substitute their own prosthetic silhouette and assign zones at the bottom of the form. (Reproduced with permission from Ewald FC: The Knee Society Total Knee Arthroplasty Roentgenographic Evaluation and Scoring System. *Clin Orthop* 1989;248: 9–12.)

Several authors have proposed the additional value of using fluoroscopy to assess radiolucencies in TKAs. An earlier report nearly a decade ago demonstrated that fluoroscopically guided radiographs allowed accurate measurement of radiolucencies as small as 1 mm, and migration of 0.5 mm or less. Plain radiographs obtained during the same experiment failed to identify these changes. In another more recent study, 20 symptomatic TKAs were evaluated using fluoroscopic radiographs. Initial evaluation of these knees with standard established methodologies did not yield definitive findings. Aseptic loosening was determined to be the possible cause in 14 of 20 knees evaluated using fluoroscopic techniques. Loosening of fixation was confirmed at revision surgery in all 14 knees. The advantage of using this adjunct technique is that loosening can be excluded with greater confidence, and workup can subsequently be directed toward other sources.

Summary

Outcomes assessment is necessary in evaluating any TKA. Both physician-oriented and patient-oriented methodologies should be used routinely. Gait analysis currently has limited application beyond assisting the surgeons and engineers in determining the kinematics and biomechanics following TKAs. Plain radiographs supplemented with fluoroscopic techniques in specific situations can provide excellent evaluation of the causes of impending failure of a TKA.

Annotated Bibliography

Knee Rating Systems

Brinker MR, Lund PJ, Barrack RL: Demographic biases of scoring instruments for the results of total knee arthroplasty. *J Bone Joint Surg* 1997;79A:858–865.

Four knee rating systems were used to evaluate 200 healthy volunteers without knee joint symptoms. Demographic variables with a significant negative correlation with all knee rating systems included advanced age, lower income, and 2 or more major medical comorbid conditions. These differences may significantly affect the results of knee surgery if the patient populations are not matched for these factors.

Irrgang JJ, Snyder-Mackler L, Wainner RS, Fu FH, Harner CD: Development of a patient-reported measure of function of the knee. *J Bone Joint Surg* 1998;80A:1132–1145.

The authors reported a new outcomes measurement instrument developed to evaluate a variety of clinical conditions related to the knee joint. The Activities of Daily Living Scale (ADLS) specifically measures functional limitations imposed by pathologic disorders and impairment of the knee during daily living. Data from nearly 400 patients demonstrated that the ADLS was a reliable, valid, and responsive instrument.

Kreibich DN, Vaz M, Bourne RB, et al: What is the best way of assessing outcome after total knee replacement? *Clin Orthop* 1996;331:221–225.

The authors tested the responsiveness of 6 different rating instruments for outcome assessment following TKAs. The patients were tested before surgery and at the 3-month and 6-month postoperative intervals. The highest responsiveness was found with the WOMAC and The Knee Society clinical rating scale. The worst observations were seen with the SF-36 and time tradeoff, a utility method of measurement.

Radiographic Evaluation

Fehring TK, McAvoy G: Fluoroscopic evaluation of the painful total knee arthroplasty. *Clin Orthop* 1996;331:226–233.

Twenty patients with painful TKAs that had normal plain radiographs were evaluated using fluoroscopic techniques. Fourteen of 20 were determined to have probable loosening of fixation. All were proved to be loose at revision surgery. Clinical improvement occurred with all 14 knees after revision surgery. The other 6 knees were managed with other means besides revision surgery.

Lonner JH, Laird MT, Stuchin SA: Effect of rotation and knee flexion on radiographic alignment in total knee arthroplasties. *Clin Orthop* 1996;331:102–106.

The authors found significant differences in radiographic assessment of knee alignment when there was flexion or rotation greater than 10° associated with position of the limb.

Classic Bibliography

Andriacchi TP, Galante JO, Fermier RW: The influence of total knee-replacement design on walking and stair-climbing. *J Bone Joint Surg* 1982;64A:1328–1335.

Berman AT, Zarro VJ, Bosacco SJ, Israelite C: Quantitative gait analysis after unilateral or bilateral total knee replacement. *J Bone Joint Surg* 1987;69A:1340–1345.

Dorr LD, Ochsner JL, Gronley J, Perry J: Functional comparison of posterior cruciate-retained versus cruciate-sacrificed total knee arthroplasty. *Clin Orthop* 1988;236:36–43.

Ewald FC: The Knee Society total knee arthroplasty roentgenographic evaluation and a scoring system. *Clin Orthop* 1989; 248:9–12.

Insall JN, Dorr LD, Scott RD, Scott WN: Rationale of the Knee Society clinical rating system. *Clin Orthop* 1989;248:13–14.

Kelman GJ, Biden EN, Wyatt MP, Ritter MA, Colwell CW Jr: Gait laboratory analysis of a posterior cruciate-sparing total knee arthroplasty in stair ascent and descent. *Clin Orthop* 1989; 248:21–26.

Chapter 34
Long-Term Results of Total Knee Replacement

Unicompartmental Knee Arthroplasty

Unicompartmental knee arthroplasty (UKA) has been a controversial procedure since its introduction 3 decades ago. Early discouraging results led to questioning of the role of unicondylar arthroplasty in the treatment of knee arthritis. Over the ensuing years more favorable results have emerged both in terms of primary UKA as well as its conversion to total knee arthroplasty (TKA). This change in results has largely been the result of refinement of surgical techniques, narrowing of patient selection to those ideally suited for the procedure, and improvements in implant design.

Currently, UKA represents an alternative to high tibial osteotomy (HTO) and tricompartmental knee replacement in the elderly patient with unicompartmental noninflammatory disease. When compared to HTO, UKA has a higher initial success rate, allows a more rapid course of rehabilitation, and results in fewer early complications. Conversion to TKA, if necessary, may be accomplished more readily and with better expected results following UKA when compared to osteotomy.

When compared to TKA, UKA has the advantage of preservation of both cruciate ligaments, allowing for more normal kinematic function of the knee. UKA also allows preservation of bone stock of the patellofemoral joint and the opposite compartment, as well as decreased surgical blood loss and a more rapid rehabilitation. The long-term survivorship of UKA has not yet reached the 90% survival of TKA at 10 years or longer. This data, however, has been generated based on implants done at a time when patient selection, surgical technique, and implant design were still evolving. It is hoped that the survivorship of today's unicondylar knee replacements approach that of TKA.

In the last several years, there have been major advancements in the study of UKA, such as documentation of excellent results with long-term follow-up, examination of the role of UKA as an alternative to HTO in younger patients, and documentation of the results of conversion of modern UKA to TKA.

One or more of the authors or the departments with which they are affiliated have received something of value from a commercial or other party related directly or indirectly to the subject of this chapter.

Long-Term Results

In the past several years, UKA has proved to be a useful tool in the treatment of localized arthritic disease of the knee. Survivorship data of large series of patients followed for 10 years or longer show that UKA can be a successful and durable procedure. When done with proper patient selection, meticulous surgical technique, and modern implants, UKA can be expected to provide 10-year survivorship rate of 85% to 90%, based on recent series.

Long-term data have also shown that these patients retain continued excellent results in terms of pain relief, knee range of motion, and improved functional status. In fact, patients with 1 total knee replacement and 1 unicondylar replacement most often report a preference for the UKA because of better functional performance and range of motion. Theoretically, an advantage often claimed for UKA has been the preservation of the anterior cruciate ligament (ACL) and anticipated better maintenance of normal knee biomechanics and, therefore, function. In comparing gait analysis results of patients who have undergone UKA to those who have had tricompartmental replacement, quadriceps mechanics during level walking were normal in the UKA patients.

One major reason for the improved results seen with UKA may be related to alterations in component design. On the femoral side it has been found that many early failures were caused by inadequate capping of the distal femur because of narrow component width. Modern designs of UKA are usually available in multiple sizes to allow maximum medial to lateral bone coverage and stress distribution. Another reason for improved results is that the shape of the femoral prosthesis has been shown to impact implant durability. Biomechanical testing has shown that a femoral component with a sharply angled bone-prosthesis interface fails secondary to shear forces at the interface, with toggling of the implant and resultant loosening. Implants with this design have demonstrated early clinical failure as well. A design with a curved or spherical interface is preferred in order to avoid this situation. In addition, 2 fixation lugs or a fin ought to be present on the femoral component in order to maximize rotational stability. On the tibial side, adequate capping of the tibial plateau is again necessary to provide stable and durable fixation. The issue of using a metal-backed versus all-polyethylene component is unresolved. Each has been shown to produce excellent long-term results given proper patient selection and technique. An all-polyethylene tibial component does allow for maximization of plastic thickness for a given level of bone resection. A third reason is that with regard to articular surface topography, an implant with a relatively large radius of curvature allowing adequate metal to plastic contact without excessive constraint is preferred. Excessive constraint at the articular surface has been associated with early femoral loosening, whereas a flat articulation can result in point contact and accelerated wear. Therefore, an optimally designed UKA should thus sacrifice minimal bone at the time of implantation and provide maximal bone coverage and initial implant stability.

Patient Selection

Improper patient selection is still reported as a major reason for failure of UKA. In general, the selection criteria for UKA have been consistent: noninflammatory arthritis localized to a single compartment; patient age of 60 years or older; a patient who is neither obese nor a heavy laborer; a knee flexion arc greater than 90° with less than a 5° flexion contracture; angular deformity under 10°; and an intact ACL. Based on these criteria a patient can be designated as a candidate for unicondylar replacement, osteotomy, or tricompartmental replacement. Whether a patient age 60 or younger may be a better candidate for UKA rather than HTO is often difficult to determine. The main issues to examine in attempting to define the optimal procedure for such a patient are the success and durability of UKA versus HTO, as well as the difficulties associated with the conversion of each to TKA, and the subsequent results.

UKA has a higher initial success rate, a more rapid rehabilitation, and fewer early complications when compared to an HTO. In patients with bilateral disease, bilateral UKA can be performed with a single anesthetic and full recovery achieved within 3 months. Bilateral simultaneous HTOs are not common. When performed in a staged fashion, bilateral osteotomies require 2 surgeries separated by an interval of 3 to 6 months, and under such circumstances full recovery would not be expected for up to 1 year following the initial procedure.

Given the recently reported excellent long-term results of UKA, its use in younger patients (younger than age 60 years) has been investigated. Long-term survivorship data in these patients is not yet available. At 2 to 6 years of follow-up, however, results in terms of pain relief and function have been equal to those seen in older patient groups. This data is in contrast to HTO in similarly aged patients in whom postoperative activity levels generally are below preoperative levels and gradually decline with time. UKA also has the advantage of preservation of a normal limb mechanical axis rather than the creation of a secondary deformity as produced by HTO. When considering the results of conversion of a UKA to a TKA versus the conversion of an osteotomy to a TKA, unicondylar replacement may represent an alternative to HTO in carefully selected patients. UKA is especially attractive in a female patient, avoiding the secondary cosmetic deformity of osteotomy.

Conversion of a UKA to TKA

Before UKA is performed in younger patients, its eventual conversion to a TKA must be considered, especially in comparison to the conversion of an osteotomy to a TKA. Early reports of conversion of a UKA to a tricompartmental arthroplasty were disappointing in that the procedure was found to be similar to revision of a TKA because of the surgical difficulties encountered with regard to the restoration of bone loss. Postoperative results were also similar to those seen with revision TKA and were not comparable to the outcomes reported for primary TKA.

Recent reports on the conversion of UKA to TKA have not demonstrated such difficulties. Augmentation of bone defects, usually using metal wedges, has been required in about 20% of such procedures. With the use of modern revision total knee instrumentation systems augmentation in this manner should not be considered particularly difficult. It has also been shown that in the majority of cases, the posterior cruciate ligament (PCL) can be retained and a standard cruciate-preserving prosthesis implanted at the time of UKA conversion to a TKA. Finally, the results of conversion to a tricompartmental arthroplasty have been shown to be comparable to a primary TKA in terms of pain relief and restoration of function and superior to those following TKA revision.

In contrast to the results of conversion of a UKA to a TKA, the conversion of an HTO to a TKA has been shown to have several difficulties. These problems include altered patellofemoral mechanics because of patella infera, problems with joint exposure and hardware removal, decreased postoperative range of motion, and an increase in the rate of complications such as flexion contracture, wound infection, and peroneal nerve palsy. Therefore, recent data suggest that the conversion of a failed modern UKA to a TKA can be performed with less technical difficulty and be expected to yield better results than conversion of an HTO to a TKA.

Summary

UKA has been shown to be a successful and durable treatment option for localized noninflammatory arthritis of the knee. Proper patient selection, surgical technique, and implant design remain key in obtaining successful results. Using modern designs of UKA, conversion to a TKA can be expected to provide results similar to the results of primary TKA without significantly increased surgical difficulty. The use of UKA as an alternative to HTO in patients younger than age 60 has shown promise in the short term and deserves further study and consideration in the future.

Cruciate-Retaining TKA

TKA has been used to treat pain and restore function to patients with arthritis for over 25 years. Numerous successful implant designs are in use, including implants that sacrifice, retain, or substitute for the PCL. But just as importantly, many prostheses have been tried and abandoned because so-called design improvements have led to inferior outcomes. It is incumbent on the surgeon to select an implant that will provide both durability and good performance; long-term follow-up studies can help to guide this decision.

However, the continuous release of new devices and modifications of older designs make this process complex, and the sheer number of available implants is daunting. A recent survey in the United Kingdom identified a total of 37 commercially available TKA prosthesis designs; of these, only 5 have 10-year survival data and, more disturbingly, over half have no published series of follow-up results in peer-reviewed journals.

This chapter outlines results from long-term follow-up studies published in the last several years on cruciate-retaining (CR) TKAs. Salient design features of the implants are presented, along with results at greater than 10 years for cemented designs; and 5- to 10-year follow-up series on the newer cementless implants are also reviewed. Results obtained with devices that sacrifice and substitute for the PCL are covered elsewhere in this volume.

Nearly all studies covering the long-term follow-up of CR-TKA are retrospective case series that examine a single, cemented implant (Table 1). A smaller number are retrospectively controlled reviews of CR-TKA in specified subgroups of patients (eg, those with rheumatoid arthritis) using either a variety of CR implants, or comparing CR- to PCL-substituting TKAs (Table 2). Reviews of cementless or so-called "hybrid" TKAs (cemented tibial and patellar components, uncemented femoral component) are limited to follow-up of between 5 and 10 years. To date, there are no published prospective or randomized comparative studies of CR implants with intermediate- or long-term follow-up.

Most of the devices reviewed resemble the original Total Condylar prostheses (Howmedica, Rutherford, NJ), with provision made for preservation of the PCL.

Cemented Designs: Follow-Up at 10 Years and Beyond

Kinematic Condylar Knee

Among the best-studied implants is the Kinematic Condylar prosthesis (Howmedica, Rutherford, NJ). This is a resurfacing prosthesis that includes a metal-backed tibial component, an all-polyethylene patellar button, and femoral component geometry that resembles the distal femur more closely than that of the original Total Condylar device. Results beyond 10 years have been published in both the United States and England, with prosthesis survival ranging from 92% to 97.4% in trials ranging from 9 to 12 years mean follow-up. However, where revision or poor knee score were the failure criteria, clinical success was achieved in only 78% of patients in the 2 studies that stratified data in this manner. Ultimate range of motion (ROM) was typically satisfactory (between 100° and 105°), similar to that seen with posterior stabilized (PS) implants of this generation. Postoperative pain was in the none to mild range for greater than 90% of patients.

Despite fairly gratifying long-term clinical results, complications and reoperations were common with the Kinematic. Manipulation under anesthesia to achieve satisfactory ROM was needed in 7.7% of patients in one study, and open surgical quadricepsplasty was required in 4.5% of rheumatoid patients in a different series. Patellofemoral problems and polyethylene wear, which plagued many of the early Total Condylar-type implants, were the most common causes of failure of the Kinematic. Fracture of the tibial baseplate occurred in 2.5% in one study, and this complication was reported in another.

Posterior-Cruciate Condylar

The cruciate-sparing version of the Total Condylar prosthesis (Howmedica, Rutherford, NJ; and Johnson & Johnson Orthopaedics, New Brunswick, NJ) is nearly identical to the original Total Condylar prosthesis; the only difference is a cutout on the posterior aspect of the tibial component to allow for preservation of the PCL. All of these devices are bicondylar, with conforming tibial polyethylene and a dome-

Table 1
Long-term follow-up of cemented cruciate-retaining deigns

Device	Series	N†	Mean Follow-up (Range)	Survivorship	Comments
Kinematic	Weir, 1996	208 consecutive	12 (10-14)	92%*	3.3% loss to follow-up No knee scores/ranges of motion given Aseptic failures: polyethylene wear, fractured tibial baseplate, aseptic loosening Device no longer available
Kinematic	Malkani, 1995	168 consecutive	10 (6-12)	96%	1.2% loss to follow-up 7.7% manipulated for poor range of motion Most revisions: patellar loosening
Kinematic	Ansari, 1998	445	10 (??)	96%	4% loss to follow-up Most revisions: tibial > femoral loosening 18% of nonrevised patients with moderate-to-severe pain at last follow-up
CR-TC**	Ritter, 1994	278	8 (1-18)	96.8% @ 12 years	5.4% loss to follow-up 3.2% excluded for infection Most revisions: early tibial or late femoral loosening Device no longer available
CR-TC**	Rand,1993	78	10 (8-11.5)	96%	2.6% loss to clinical follow-up 29.4% loss to radiographic follow-up
CR-TC**	Dennis,1992	42	11 (9.3-13)	95.3%	6.3% loss to follow-up 9.5% reoperated for patellar or extensor mechanism complications
AGC***	Ritter,1995	71	> 10 years	See text	Loss to follow-up not given, probably substantial Excluded many patellar failures; patella redesigned during study Device still available

*All survivorship data in this table given with revision as the end point at mean follow-up unless otherwise noted
** Cruciate-retaining Total Condylar or Posterior-Cruciate Condylar; the same design was produced by 2 manufacturers
***Anatomic Graduated Component
† N = number of knees, not patients

shaped patella. Most series with follow-up beyond 10 years on this device used an all-polyethylene tibia, although in 1 study, the all-polyethylene tibias were compared to metal-backed components in a nonrandomized fashion.

Survivorship of these implants, defined as retention of the original device, ranged from 88% to 98% at 8 to 11 years. Overall success, based on radiographic criteria plus Hospital for Special Surgery (HSS) knee scores in the good to excellent range, was between 85% and 94% in the studies that provided these data. ROM was similar in all published series (100° to 106°). The most common causes of failure, as in more contemporary devices, were patellofemoral problems and tibial loosening. No differences were found between metal-backed tibial components and all-polyethylene bearings, although statistical power was not calculated for this relatively small study group. In summary, the results with the PCL-sparing

Table 2
Selected cohort studies of cruciate-retaining designs

Subcohort	Series	N†	Mean Follow-up, Years (Range)	Survivorship	Comments
Age < 55	Gill,1997	72	9.9 (5–18)	95.8%*	1.4% loss to follow-up, but 18% phone examinations 40% rheumatoid arthritis 100% good/excellent pain relief 71% good/excellent functional scores 11% manipulated for poor range of motion
Age < 45	Dalury, 1995	103	7.2 (5.5–13)	98.1%	15.5% loss to follow-up, but deaths may have been included in this 87% rheumatoid arthritis or juvenile rheumatoid arthritis No aseptic loosening tibia/femur
Rheumatoid arthritis	Hanyu,1997	88	Minimum 10	93%	No loss to follow-up; 51% died during study period 1/3 posterior stabilized because of absent/deficient posterior cruciate ligament Aseptic failures: supracondylar femur fracture, and aseptic loosening 4.5% quadricepsplasty for range of motion
Rheumatoid arthritis	Laskin,1997	116	8.2 (minimum 6)	88.8%	10.5% loss to follow-up 97.8% survival in control group (rheumatoid arthritis patients, posterior stabilized total knee arthroplasty) 85% of revisions for posterior instability
Fixed deformity	Laskin,1996	65 varus 46 normal	Minimum 10 Minimum 10	72% 90%**	3.1% loss to follow-up Range of motion worse in patients with fixed deformity given cruciate-retaining designs
Obesity	Mont,1996	50 obese 50 nonobese	7 (2–11)	92% 96%	Difference not statistically significant; power calculation not provided

* All survivorship data in this table given with revision as the end point at mean follow-up unless otherwise noted
** $p < 0.0001$; no difference seen between cruciate-retaining implants in patients without fixed varus, and posterior cruciate ligament-substituting implants in patients with fixed varus
† N = number of knees, not patients

Total Condylar device seem very comparable to the results at greater than 10 years using the original design, which sacrificed or substituted for the PCL, as can best be determined within the limitations of retrospective study design.

Anatomic Graduated Component

The Anatomic Graduated Component (AGC, Biomet, Warsaw, IN) has been used with PCL retention since the early 1980s. Of the devices covered thus far, it is the only one that remains available today, using substantially the same materials and geometry. The cobalt-chrome femoral component was available as either universal or anatomic (left and right components available), and it was available with porous coating. The tibial component was a nonmodular, compression-molded, nearly flat polyethylene bearing fixed to a cobalt-chrome baseplate and a central stem. Initially, the patellar component was metal-backed; in 1987, it was changed to all-polyethylene because of patellar failures and dissociation of the polyethylene from the metal backing.

Authors of the single long-term follow-up study of this device point to a 98% survival at greater than 10 years' follow-up; the AGC also demonstrated excellent durability in the Swedish Knee Arthroplasty Registry. The fact that this device continues to be sold in the United States and abroad attests to the continued demand for it. However, several problems severely limit the conclusions drawn by the follow-up study on the AGC. Loss to follow-up appears to have been significant, but was not quantified. Twenty-one hundred AGC knees were implanted at the 3 participating sites, but the results at 10 years present data on only 71, or 3.3%, of that cohort. The authors also excluded 27 known patellar failures attributed to polyethylene dissociation, and they did not include revisions for infection in their survival data. Given these problems, particularly the loss to follow-up, interpreting the published results of the AGC is somewhat difficult.

Long-Term Results of CR-TKA in Patient Subgroups or Specific Diagnoses

Young Patients

Two studies have investigated CR-TKA in young patients. Both reports included a variety of implant designs that had PCL preservation in common. In addition to the young age of the patients evaluated, these studies differed from the unselected cohorts already outlined in that the younger groups were heavily weighted towards a diagnosis of rheumatoid arthritis (RA). The follow-up interval in these studies was a mean of 10 and 7 years, respectively.

Despite the young age of the patients, the results of these trials were very satisfactory and support the use of these devices in younger individuals when TKA is clinically indicated. Survivorship was between 95% and 98%; loss to follow-up was not excessive. Pain relief and ultimate ROM were reliably good and comparable to series of unselected patients. There were more patients in these groups with bilateral TKAs, and functional knee scores did not improve as much as pain scores; these differences, as well as the surprisingly good implant survival, may reflect the higher proportion of patients with inflammatory arthritis—presumably a lower-demand cohort—within these groups.

Rheumatoid Arthritis

Two series specifically studied the intermediate- or long-term survivorship and results of CR-TKA in RA patients, but came to significantly different conclusions. Several differences between the studies help explain the discrepancies: One group performed a retrospective review of CR-TKA in RA patients and used a group of historical controls with RA who received a cruciate-substituting, PS-TKA design. That study did not indicate how the surgeon decided which implant was used in a given case, apart from stating that in the CR patients the PCL was "observed to be grossly intact." Also, the implants used were of significantly different designs in the CR and PS groups (CR: Tricon, Smith & Nephew Richards, Memphis, TN; PS: Insall-Burstein, Zimmer, Warsaw, IN). The other study in this patient population made a careful assessment of the PCL at the time of surgery. If the PCL was absent or nonfunctional, that group implanted a PS component; this was necessary in one third of the patients. The implant design used (Kinematic, Howmedica, Rutherford, NJ) was the same in all patients, apart from the difference in how the PCL was handled. Unfortunately, this study did not have a strictly defined control group, and it did not separate the results into CR and PS subcohorts.

For those reasons, it is somewhat difficult to compare the conclusions drawn in those reports. Nonetheless, the group that excluded patients from the CR subgroup because of an absent or nonfunctional PCL seemed to have better results. Many of the failures noted in the other reports were because of late instability. These findings highlight the importance of assessing the competence of the ligament, even when it is apparently present as a discrete anatomic structure. Other investigators have pointed out that in both RA and osteoarthritis patients, histologic study often reveals degeneration within the PCL. This also supports the importance of verifying that the PCL functions well if a CR-TKA is to be used successfully in patients with RA.

Fixed Varus Deformity

Some investigators feel that the PCL is intrinsic to arthritic deformity and may contribute to failure of the reconstruction in patients with fixed preoperative angular malalignment. One study tested this hypothesis in a clinical review of patients with combined fixed varus and flexion contractures measuring 15° or more. The authors retrospectively divided patients who received TKA into 3 subcohorts: one group with preoperative varus/flexion deformity undergoing CR-TKA, another group of CR-TKA in patients without such deformity, and a third group with fixed deformity who underwent PS-TKA during the study period. After 10 years, the CR group without fixed deformity had results (pain, ROM, aseptic loosening rates) comparable to the PS group, but despite correction of the initial gross deformity, the CR group with fixed deformity fared significantly worse. Kaplan-Meier survivorship was 20% lower in the CR group, and ROM was decreased by 20°; outcomes relating to knee pain were also poorer in the CR patients. Posterior instability, interestingly, was not identified as a problem in this group. Unfortunately, this study did not present its criteria for use of the CR or PS implants, and this significantly limits its generalizability. Also, the study did not indicate if the combined deformity that defined the inclusion criterion was due more to varus or to flexion.

Obese Patients

One small study examined the effect of obesity on patients undergoing cementless CR-TKA using the Porous-Coated Anatomic (PCA, Howmedica, Rutherford, NJ) prosthesis with a mean follow-up of 7 years (Table 2). Although there was a trend toward poorer results in the obese cohort (more fair and poor results, more revisions), statistical significance was not achieved in this study, and analysis of statistical power was not provided to determine the effect of ß-error on the results. Overall, the results with the PCA knee in this study were comparable to those achieved in other series using this knee at this length of follow-up (see below).

Cementless Designs: 5- to 10-Year Results

Cementless designs are newer, with the earliest commercial devices seeing service only in the early 1980s. Based on intermediate-term follow-up data (5 to 10 years), hybrid TKA appears equivalent to cemented TKA with respect to prosthesis revision and aseptic loosening rates; cementless TKA is generally inferior to both hybrid and cemented TKA. Long-term results (longer than 10 years) with any technique apart from fully cemented TKA have yet to be published.

Anatomic Modular Knee (DePuy, Warsaw, IN)

This CR-TKA may be used with or without cement; it is one of only a few that remains commercially available in its original design. The longest follow-up series describing results with this prosthesis used it predominantly as a hybrid implant, rather than completely cementless. This device uses a porous-coated CoCr femoral component with a raised lateral flange and a 7° laterally divergent sulcus for improved patellar tracking. The tibial baseplate is modular, made from porous-coated titanium alloy, and stem extensions are available. The patella is all-polyethylene.

One recent series documented very good results on 186 consecutive Anatomic Modular Knees with 5.3% loss to follow-up. Clinical outcomes were excellent, with 94% of patients achieving good or excellent results, ROM averaging 107°, and there were few complications. Osteolysis was not observed in this series. Nine patients (6.3%) required revision of one or more components at a mean of 6.9 years, although 7 of those were simple tibial polyethylene exchanges. Patellar complications were absent from this series; this was attributed to the wide, divergent patellar sulcus and the elliptical patellar component, which matches the femoral radii of curvature in flexion and extension.

Freeman-Samuelson (Protek AG, Bern, Switzerland)

This early device was available with either an uncemented all-polyethylene tibial component or a metal-backed tibial tray (the latter with or without a metal stem), a patellar sulcus in the femoral component, and a congruent single radius of curvature between the femur and tibia providing some constraint to the articulation. The all-polyethylene tibia achieved fixation with fins in the pegs to achieve a "macrointerlock."

Results with this device would not be considered satisfactory by contemporary standards, with revision for aseptic loosening of 13% to 21% of components anticipated at 10 years (the mean follow-up of the studies was about 7 years). In one study that used more stringent criteria for failure—revision, moderate-to-severe pain (clinical failure), or radiographic failure—only 33% of patients succeeded.

Miller-Galante I (Zimmer, Warsaw, IN)

The report of a small series of this cementless CR-TKA presents results at a minimum 5-year follow-up. The device incorporated a number of design features that are now generally agreed to be undesirable, including a metal-backed patellar component, a titanium femoral component with unfavorable patellofemoral tracking, and a carbon-fiber reinforced polyethylene tibial bearing. Over half of patients in this series required revision of one or more components, 10% developed osteolysis, and patellofemoral complications were common. This device is no longer available commercially except for revisions of it that are already in service.

Porous-Coated Anatomic (Howmedica, Rutherford, NJ)

Because this implant was among the first cementless TKA prostheses, it is among the most thoroughly studied of the cementless designs. The PCA used a flat articular bearing of heat-pressed polyethylene, a pegged tibial baseplate, and a metal-backed patella with asymmetric (so-called "anatomic") medial and lateral facets.

Results with this device were generally unsatisfactory. Osteolysis, particularly in the earlier generations of this device, was seen as a serious and common complication that could complicate revision surgery. In one series, a 90% incidence of osteolysis and a 50% incidence of patellar loosening were reported; patellar instability and subluxation were common in another report, as well. Two reports indicated survivorship rates of only 88% at 8 years, lower than the 10-year results of the cemented devices shown in Table 1. In addition, both of those studies were compromised by 15% to 25% loss to follow-up. Results of a third series at a mean follow-up of 5.8 years were similarly unsatisfactory compared to cemented results, with 8.6% of components already revised at that time.

Press-Fit Condylar (Johnson & Johnson, Raynham, MA)

One large study of this device at intermediate-term (mean, 6.5 years) follow-up has been published. The Press-Fit Condylar (PFC) is a fixed-bearing, condylar-type CR-TKA. Initially, the patella was metal-backed and cementless, but in 1987 it was changed to an all-polyethylene, cemented component; tibial and femoral components may be implanted with or without cement. The PFC is one of the few devices in this review that remains commercially available in nearly its original form.

The report covered 378 consecutive PFC TKAs, with 5% loss to follow-up at a mean of 6.5 years. Fourteen knees (3.8%) underwent revision for any reason; most for patellar failures related to the early metal-backed patellar component or for tibial polyethylene liner failure. That study included cemented, cementless, and hybrid knees, with excellent knee scores in all groups; unfortunately the radiographic results were not separated into cementless and cemented cohorts. Osteolysis was not observed in this series. Radiolucent lines under the tibia were common, but tended to be incomplete and nonprogressive.

Posterior-Stabilized TKA

Several prosthetic designs, including posterior cruciate-substituting, posterior cruciate-sacrificing, and posterior cruciate-retaining prostheses, have withstood the test of time and are associated with excellent long-term results. When accurately balanced, retaining the PCL in TKA allows for femoral rollback during flexion and affords stability throughout the full ROM. This, however, is not always the case, and the PCL may need to be lengthened or recessed to balance the knee. Errors in balancing the PCL can give rise to either a tight PCL with loss of motion and polyethylene wear or a loose PCL with associated flexion instability. Posterior cruciate-substituting designs provide more predictable kinematics along with long-term clinical success and great patient satisfaction.

Since the introduction of the Insall Burstein Posterior Stabilized (IBPS) Total Knee Prosthesis (Zimmer, Warsaw, IN) in 1978, the controversy regarding retention or substitution of the PCL has been ongoing. However, the popularity of the posterior-stabilized design continues to grow because of its continued excellent clinical outcome. In 1992, 8% of primary TKAs were PCL-substituting, while in 1997 it was estimated that this number had grown to 25%.

The original posterior-stabilized prosthesis was designed by Insall and Burstein to succeed the total condylar design, which was a PCL-sacrificing prosthesis. The intention was to improve stair climbing, increase ROM, and prevent posterior subluxation. The IBPS prosthesis was designed with bicondylar tibial wells that conform to the femoral articulation. The femorotibial articulation is dished in the frontal and sagittal planes to provide the maximum conformity and surface area compatible with a fixed bearing prosthesis. In the sagittal plane the articulation conforms in full extension but, because of the decreasing radius of the femoral component, has partial conformity in flexion, which allows 15° of internal and external rotation. To ensure that maximal conformity is maintained throughout 120° of flexion, the amount of rollback and movement of the femur on the tibia should be reproducible and predictable. To this end, the PCL is excised and its function assumed by a tibial post and femoral cam—a "mechanical PCL." The cam mechanism of the IBPS design contacts the tibial spine at 70° of flexion and maintains contact through further flexion, resisting posterior subluxation. The cam mechanism has no effect on knee stability in extension and does not substitute for the collateral ligaments.

Since its introduction in 1978, the IBPS prothesis with an all-polyethylene tibial component has undergone several modifications. In 1980, the tibial component was metal-backed when finite element analysis demonstrated enhanced load transfer to the underlying bone with metal-backed tibial components. The patellofemoral groove was deepened in 1983, and modularity was introduced in 1988. When the modular IB II was introduced, the tibial spine was shortened and moved posteriorly to enhance femoral rollback and increase flexion; unfortunately, this created a potentially unstable situation in flexion. Although infrequent, this situation was worrisome, so the tibial spine was moved anteriorly 2 mm and heightened 2 mm. This reestablished the spine cam mechanism to its originally successful and stable position.

Increasing popularity of the IBPS knee has stimulated many manufacturers to design other styles of posterior-stabilized knees. Proprietary rights resulted in variations in the cam mechanism, including different shapes, placements, and tibial spine heights. When these design parameters are changed, prostheses have different kinematics, different inherent anterior or medial-lateral stability, as well as dissimilar cam spine contact. There are several other contemporary designs. The NexGen Legacy Prosthesis (Zimmer, Warsaw, IN), in order to improve the patellofemoral articulation, lengthened the trochlea, causing the femoral cam to be moved more posteriorly. The spine cam mechanism, with this design, still engages at 70° of flexion and provides improved flexion stability. With the Legacy Prosthesis, the cam rides down the tibial spine as the knee goes into greater flexion, in contrast to the IBPS knee, in which it moves up the tibial spine. The Kinematic Stabilizer (Howmedica, Rutherford, NJ) has a cam mechanism designed to achieve both anterior and posterior constraint with the knee in extension, in contrast to the IBPS knee. The central tibial post and femoral housing restrain both anterior and posterior movement of the tibia from 0° to 30° of flexion. Beyond 30° of flexion, the intercondylar surface replaces the function of the PCL and is designed to smoothly guide posterior rollback. The Genesis Posterior Stabilized Knee (Smith & Nephew Richards, Memphis, TN) has a femoral conversion module for PCL substitution and a thinner and taller tibial spine that provides greater medial-lateral support, but the flatter tibial articular surface implies a smaller contact area. The Sigma (Johnson & Johnson, Raynham, MA), Exactect prosthesis, and Wright posterior-stabilized prosthesis have a cam mechanism similar to that of the IBPS knee. A unique variation is the Anatomic Graduated Components (Biomet, Warsaw, IN), which has no tibial post, but a recessed groove in the tibia with an anterior polyethylene buildup. The femoral component has a raised intercondylar ridge that articulates with the tibial recess as the knee flexes and acts to prevent posterior tibial subluxation. Theoretically, this mechanism engages more smoothly and gradually.

Kinematics

In the natural knee, movement is controlled by the ACL, the PCL, and collateral ligaments. In the prosthetic knee, the ACL is excised, the PCL and collateral ligaments are often pathologic, and the articular surface is altered by the prosthetic geometry. The 4-bar linkage is therefore disrupted, and TKA will only by chance reproduce normal knee motion.

By substituting for the PCL in TKA, designers can predictably control the in vivo kinematics of the knee. In contrast, while the intention of PCL retention is to create a natural knee, preserve femoral rollback, and increase ROM, the kinematics are less predictable. In most PCL-retaining knees, the PCL is either too tight resulting in excessive rollback or too loose causing uncontrolled skidding or, worse, posterior flexion instability.

Recent fluoroscopic studies suggest that the in vivo kinematics of PCL-retaining knee designs are unpredictable. These designs have demonstrated a femorotibial contact point, which is posterior in extension and anterior in flexion. This paradoxic anterior femoral translation, along with a discontinuous skidding motion, may promote premature polyethylene wear in cruciate-retaining designs. In contrast, the kinematics of the posterior stabilized knees were more predictable, reproducible, and governed by the interaction of the spine cam mechanism. While the PS design more closely reproduced normal knee kinematics, neither the PS nor cruciate-retaining designs fully displayed normal femoral rollback. Mahoney has shown that both the PS and cruciate-retaining designs result in less femoral rollback and less quadriceps efficiency than the normal knee. However, the PS knee did produce more femoral rollback and better quadriceps efficiency than the cruciate-retaining knee designs.

There has been some confusion regarding conformity and constraint in posterior-stabilized designs. Simply, conformity does not imply constraint. Conformity of design relates to the similarity of the femoral and tibial radii of curvature. In the frontal plane, a fully conforming articulation would have a ratio of 1 throughout the full ROM. This ratio between the femoral and tibial radii of curvature could be one with either a flat articulation or a dished surface. Biomechanical studies have shown that as the ratio of the contact surfaces increases, the contact stresses increase. To simulate knee kinematics in a fixed bearing prosthesis, the femoral component has at least 2 radii of curvature in the sagittal plane, 1 for extension and the other for flexion. Although it is not possible to achieve sagittal conformity in both flexion and extension, it is possible to achieve conformity in the frontal plane, unlike a flat-on-flat design. Another advantage of a conforming dished articular surface is that it prevents edge loading of the tibial polyethylene surface if there is component liftoff. In contrast, constraint restricts the rotational or translational movement of an implant and is determined by specific design features, such as those found in a constrained condylar prosthesis.

At the time of the introduction of posterior-stabilized designs, there was concern that the interaction of the spine cam mechanism would cause early component loosening. Clinically and radiographically this has not occurred. Interaction of the femoral cam with the tibial post results in a net compressive force directed down the shaft of the tibia and bone cement well-suited to withstand compressive forces. The durability of cemented posterior-stabilized knees has been reported, and there is no clinical evidence of bone-cement deterioration in long-term studies of these knees.

Clinical Results

Many new posterior cruciate-substituting designs have become available in recent years, but are yet unproven. Not all posterior-stabilized designs have published long-term reports; when interpreting published results it is important not to extrapolate successful results to all designs, because there are significant design differences.

The design that has been extensively studied and reported in the most publications is the IBPS knee. Insall initially reported the 2- to 4-year results of 118 IBPS knees in 1982. In that report, 88% of the knees were rated excellent, 9% good or fair, and 3% poor. In a long-term study of the IBPS prosthesis with a metal-backed tibial component, 74 patients (101 knees) were evaluated at a follow-up of 10 to 11 years. The mean Knee Society clinical score was 92, and the mean functional score was 71. There were 4 revisions: 2 for aseptic loosening of the femoral component, 1 for recurrent hemarthrosis, and 1 for recurvatum. No tibial components were clinically or radiographically loose, and there were no revisions because of polyethylene wear or osteolysis.

Survivorship analysis has also confirmed these clinical results with the IBPS prosthesis. In the largest series of IBPS prostheses, 2,301 knees were tracked, including 265 IBPS knees with an all-polyethylene tibial component and 2,036 with metal-backed tibial components (IB I and IB II). When failure was defined as a prosthesis revised for any reason or one for which a revision has been recommended, this prosthesis with an all-polyethylene tibial component had an average annual failure rate of 0.38% and a 16-year success rate of 94.1%. When considering the worst case scenario, in which cases lost to follow-up were considered failures, the cumulative success rate was 90.25%. In this group there were 14 failures: 5 infections; 3 loose tibias, and 6 loose femurs. The same prosthesis with a metal-backed tibial component (IB I and IB II) had an average annual failure rate of 0.14% and a 14-year success rate of 98.1%. In the worst case scenario, the overall success rate was 93.1%. There were 26 failures, including 13 infections, 7 loose femurs, 3 recurvatum, 2 recurrent hemarthrosis, and 1 loose tibia.

Other investigators have also reported successful clinical results. One group obtained similar results at 3 to 8 years of follow-up, with 90% excellent and good results. Another group demonstrated 98% excellent and good results with the IBPS knee at 2 to 8 years. The results confirmed the advantage of prosthetic conformity in minimizing polyethylene wear without compromising fixation. Cemented TKA with the IBPS design has also been shown to be an effective and durable surgical treatment for osteoarthritis in younger patients in whom other surgical procedures have failed.

While the majority of clinical and outcome studies have involved the IBPS prosthesis, there are several studies on other prosthetic designs. One group reviewed the 4- to 6-year results with the posterior cruciate-substituting design of the Press Fit Condylar Modular Total Knee System. Ninety-six patients with 125 knees were evaluated. The mean functional and clinical Knee Society scores were 78 and 93 points, respectively. The result was excellent for 103 knees, good for 13, fair for 3, and poor for 6. Of the knees with poor results, 2 were revised for infection, 1 was revised for instability, and 3 experienced flexion instability with dislocation of the cam spine mechanism. These investigators suggest that these cases of flexion instability were related to the early design, which had a tibial spine height of only 8 mm. Subsequent to that design, the tibial spine height was increased to 14.3 mm, and no other instances of instability occurred.

An early study of the Kinematic Stabilizer Prosthesis included both primary and revision arthroplasties. Of the 79 arthroplasties reviewed at a mean of 37 months (range, 24 to 74 months), 53 were for revision. Twenty-four of the 26 primary arthroplasties (92%) were rated excellent or good by the HSS knee rating system. These investigators found an 11% incidence of patellar complications with the posterior-stabilized condylar design. In a review of 109 primary Kinematic Stabilizer TKAs in 95 patients at a mean follow-up of 12.7 years (10 to 14 years) the end point was revision in survivorship analysis. The cumulative success rate was 95% at 10 years and 87% at 13 years. Most patients had RA, and it was noted at latest follow-up that nearly all the surviving patients had polyarticular RA. This is also reflected in the mean Knee Society function score of 27 (range, 0 to 90). The mean knee score was 84 (31 to 100). Nine revisions were reported: 4 for gross polyethylene wear, 3 for loosening without any evidence of wear or infection, 1 for infection, and 1 for traumatic rupture of the medial collateral ligament.

In a prospective study of the Genesis Knee System, no difference was found between the cruciate-retaining and posterior-stabilized designs with respect to clinical outcome, radiographic appearance, and complication rate. This average 4-year study was biased toward cruciate-retaining; of the 105 TKAs performed, only 11 were posterior-stabilized knees. The authors did state that toward the end of their study they began to use the posterior-stabilized design because of the encouraging results and the technical difficulties in balancing the PCL.

Proprioception and Gait Analysis

Although it has been suggested that preservation of the PCL maintains proprioception of the knee following TKA, recent studies have demonstrated marked neurologic degeneration of the PCL as part of the arthritic process. This fact may be one reason why there have been conflicting reports about patient preference.

Early gait studies suggested that patients with cruciate-retaining TKAs had more normal stair climbing ability than patients with posterior-stabilized knees. All patients with a TKA demonstrated gait abnormalities during normal walking including shorter stride length, reduced midstance flexion, and abnormal flexion and extension moments. Using comprehensive gait analysis and isokinetic muscle testing, one group of investigators found significant difference between posterior-stabilized TKAs and normal knees in regard to spatial temporal gait parameters. No difference was seen in knee ROM during stair climbing or in isokinetic muscle strength. When compared to historical controls, the posterior-stabilized TKA was judged to be equivalent to the cruciate-retaining designs and superior to the cruciate-sacrificing total condylar knee. A matched series of bilateral TKAs with a posterior-stabilized knee on one side and a cruciate-retaining knee on the opposite side found no difference in gait parameters or stair climbing ability between designs.

Complications

As the number of TKAs performed annually increases, so does the number of associated complications. Although some complications are physiologic and related to the general well-being of the patient, others are related to the surgical technique or the mechanical limitations of the prosthetic design. Along with the successful results of posterior-stabilized TKA, there have been reports of complications that tend to be related more to technique than to prosthetic flaws.

Patellar Clunk Although the patellar clunk has been associated with the posterior-stabilized prosthesis, it has also been reported with other prosthetic designs. This complication is related to the buildup of a suprapatellar fibrous nodule along the undersurface of the quadriceps tendon, which impinges on the anterior superior edge of the femoral intercondylar notch. As the knee extends from midflexion, this nodule snaps and may be painful. A short femoral trochlea with a sharp transition into the intercondylar notch may predispose an implant design to patellar clunk. When this complication was noted with the IBPS design, the femoral trochlea was deepened and the transition into the intercondylar notch was rounded. Similarly, the press-fit condylar trochlear groove was deepened and its congruency with the patellar component optimized to allow a broad surface of contact, intended to minimize soft-tissue impingement. To ensure a smoother patellofemoral articulation, the NexGen Legacy prosthesis elongated and deepened the trochlea, compared to its precursor, the IBPS prosthesis. The influence of surgical technique should not be neglected when considering patellar clunk. Fibrous tissue and hypertrophic synovium should be excised from the undersurface of the quadriceps tendon, the bone prosthetic patella composite should be reconstructed to the original patellar thickness, and the patellar tracking should be central to reduce the chances of patellar clunk.

Intercondylar Fracture Insall noted intraoperative distal femoral intercondylar fractures, but others brought attention to the issue of nondisplaced intraoperative intercondylar distal femoral fractures. In a comparative series, the incidence of fractures between the IBPS and the Maxim Posterior Stabilized Knee (Biomet, Warsaw, IN) was compared. Although a difference in the incidence of fracture with prosthetic design was reported, the complication is technique-specific. Correct sizing and orientation of this intercondylar bone resection, along with proper component to bone orientation during insertion and extraction of the femoral component will reduce the chances of this complication.

Flexion Instability The early studies of the IBPS prosthesis did not report any cases of posterior subluxation or dislocation, and it was not until 1988 that 2 cases of posterior dislocation were described in the report of a series of 832 IBPS TKAs. In that study, both patients had a severe preoperative valgus deformity requiring an extensive lateral soft-tissue release to correct the angular deformity. In another study, the investigators reported 15 dislocations in 3,032 TKAs using the same prosthesis. These authors, however, related the dislocations to the shorter and more posteriorly positioned tibial spine, which was introduced with the modular IB II prosthesis. Since the tibial component was modified as described above, these investigators had only 1 dislocation in a series of 656 IBPS TKA (0.15%).

Posterior dislocation is not restricted to the IBPS prosthesis. Three dislocations with the PFC Posterior Stabilized Prosthesis were reported in a series of 125 knees. These investigators attribute the dislocations to the early design, which had a tibial spine height of 8 mm. The subsequent design was modified, increasing the spine height to 14.3 mm. With the Kinematic Stabilizer Prosthesis, 2 sets of investigators have reported cases of posterior tibial subluxation or recurrent posterior dislocation.

Flexion instability is not isolated to posterior cruciate-substituting designs. This complication has also been reported with cruciate-retaining designs, and in fact, these designs appear to have a higher incidence because the PCL either becomes attenuated over time or is not balanced at the time of the index procedure. Regardless of design, balancing the flexion and extension spaces has been important to the success of TKA. Biomechanical studies have shown that it is difficult to reproduce the normal strain pattern in the PCL with a cruciate-retaining design. Recent clinical reports have suggested that late rupture of the PCL can result in flexion instability. This issue of flexion instability is easily addressed by PCL substitution. The interaction of the spine cam mechanism stabilizes the knee in flexion and reduces the chance of posterior subluxation.

Despite the presence of the spine cam mechanism, posterior instability is possible and is attributed to either ligamentous instability or a mismatch of the flexion and extension spaces. In this latter situation, if flexion space is larger than the extension space the cam can potentially jump over the tibial spine resulting in a dislocation. The way to avoid this complication is to equalize the flexion and extension spaces, with appropriate bone resection and meticulous balancing of the collateral ligaments. Another factor to consider is the design of the spine cam mechanism. The spine cam mechanism does vary from design to design. The distance that the cam has to travel to sublux over the tibial spine is termed the jump distance. A design like the NexGen Legacy prosthesis has a greater jump distance than other designs, particularly in full flexion, because as the knee flexes the cam travels down the tibial spine and seats deeper on the tibial polyethylene spine.

Conclusion

Posterior-stabilized TKA has demonstrated excellent success with predictable and durable results. Although the greatest clinical success has been reported with IBPS prosthesis, many other designs have been developed. Although the general philosophy may be similar, the prosthetic designs are different. It is important not to extrapolate the successful results of 1 prosthesis to a different design. Resection of the PCL and substitution with a mechanical PCL is becoming more popu-

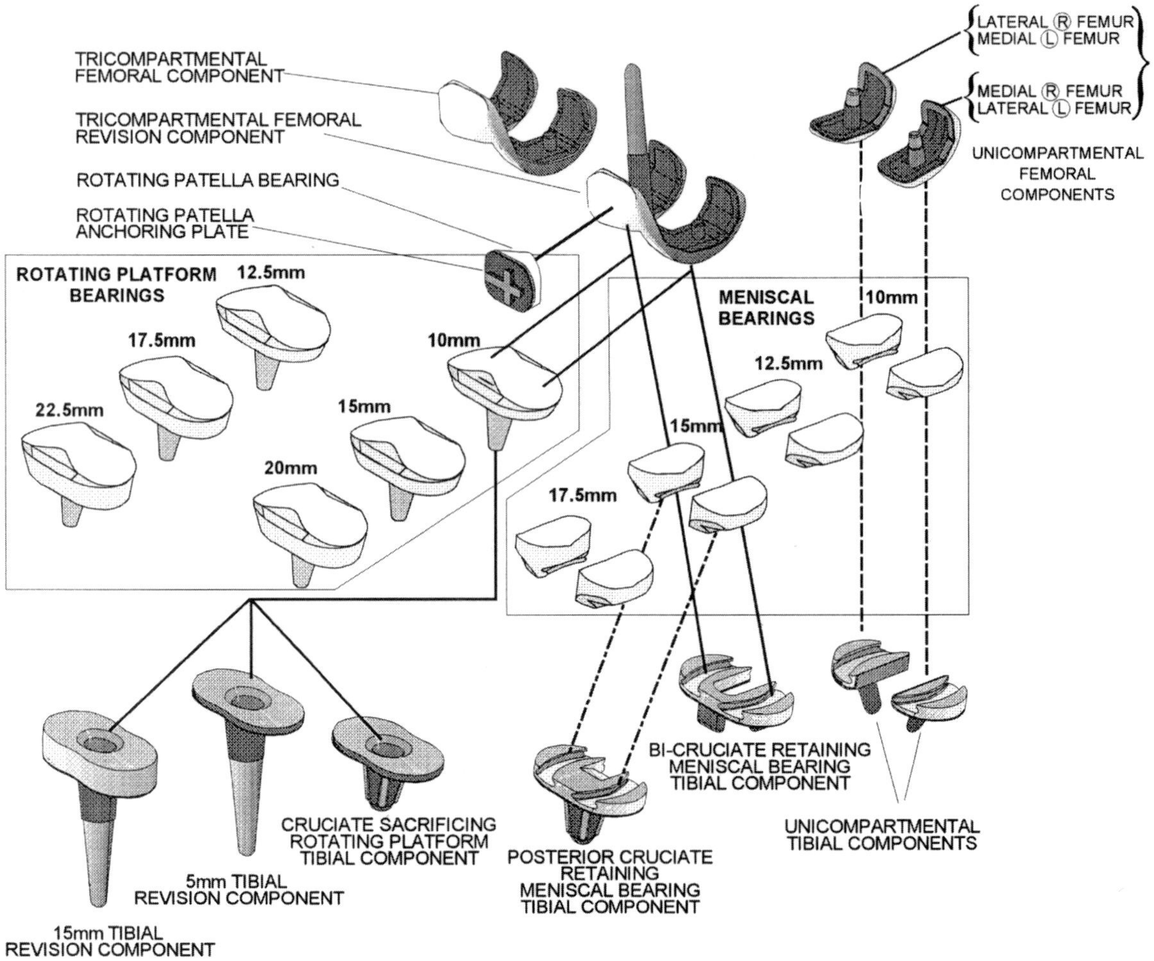

Figure 1

New Jersey Low Contact Stress knee replacement system.

lar because in vivo and in vitro studies have yielded long-term success with sound kinematics.

Mobile Bearing Total Knee Replacement

History and Development of Mobile Bearings

The first complete systems approach to total knee replacement (TKR) using meniscal bearings was developed in 1977 and reported in 1986. Unicompartmental, bicompartmental, and tricompartmental disease was managed with a variety of primary and revision components that allowed retention of both cruciate ligaments, only the posterior cruciate, or no cruciate ligaments. Additionally, the first metal-backed, rotating-bearing patellar replacement was developed in 1977 to provide mobility with congruity in patellofemoral articulation. This New Jersey Low-Contact-Stress (LCS) total knee system, initially used with cement in 1977, was expanded to noncemented use in 1981 with the availability of sintered-bead, porous coating and remains the only knee system in the United States to have undergone formal U.S. Food and Drug Administration-Investigational Device Exemption (FDA-IDE) clinical trials in both cemented and cementless applications before being released for general clinical use (Fig. 1).

The kinematic tibiofemoral motion requirements dictate the use of spherical upper tibial bearing surfaces and a flat undersurface to accommodate the variety of movements in the most congruent way. The Oxford meniscal knee uses matching spherical surfaces for the femoral component and the upper meniscal bearing surface and a flat surface to match a flat tibial component.

This preferred geometry appears to work well as a medial unicompartmental replacement, but has had dislocation problems in other applications. These problems most likely are caused by a larger than normal single radius of curvature of the femoral component, which under the pull of the PCL in flexion moves the bearing too far posteriorly.

A design solution to the Oxford problem in the presence of cruciate ligaments is seen in the LCS femoral component, which uses the same spherical surface of revolution in the medial-lateral plane but decreases the radius of curvature from extension to flexion, thus maintaining full-area contact on the upper meniscal bearing surface from 0 to 45°, where walking loads are encountered, and maintaining at least spherical line contact at deeper flexion angles. This surface geometry allows a more central femoral component position in flexion by reducing the PCL tension, which tends to pull the femur posteriorly when overstretched. Another design solution to prevent meniscal bearing dislocation is the use of radial tracks on the LCS tibial components. These tracks allow axial rotation and controlled anteroposterior translation, which impedes direct dislocation by means of the cruciate bone bridge posteriorly and the patellar tendon anteriorly. When combined with stable flexion and extension gaps at surgery, the LCS meniscal bearings can be safely used when both cruciate ligaments are intact or if only the PCL is intact.

In the event of a nonfunctional or absent PCL, central stability with the ability to axially rotate is essential. Long-term survivorship studies have demonstrated that a centrally stabilized total condylar knee replacement is predicted to last for 15 years in over 90% of cases, when used in elderly patients with low loading demands. These important studies prove that cruciate function is not essential for successful long-term fixation and function in low-demand situations.

Because wear increases as the loads and demands increase, it seems most appropriate to use the proven fixation and central stabilizing concepts of the total condylar device and provide a more wear-resistant and dislocation-resistant bearing surface to achieve better long-term survivorship and reduce wear-related failures. These concepts led to the development of a rotating platform total knee device that uses the same spherical surface geometry as the meniscal bearings.

The patellofemoral design process, like the tibiofemoral design process, seeks to provide proper motion and maintain contact stresses below the ideal 5 MPa during walking, stair climbing, and deep knee bending. Button or nonrotating anatomic type patellar replacements suffer from either point or line contact stresses or from overconstraint. High contact stress will cause early wear failure while overconstraint will cause early loosening failure. For these reasons, a rotating-bearing patellar replacement was developed to maintain spherical area contact on the medial and lateral facets while congruently matching the surface of revolution of the deep-sulcus femoral groove. Rotating-bearing patellar replacement of the LCS design greatly improves on the contact stress seen in other design configurations.

Wear Properties of Mobile Bearings and Fixed Bearings

Retrieval analysis of the tibiofemoral and patellofemoral bearing surfaces has demonstrated a high clinical wear rate in nonconforming fixed-bearing knee replacements, especially in combination with poor quality polyethylene and gamma sterilization. Similar retrieval analyses of meniscal bearings, rotating platform bearings, and rotating patellar bearings demonstrated significantly less wear than with fixed bearings. Although mobile bearings allow reduced contact stress, they can be overloaded to failure by excessive weight, excessive activity, malalignment, or a combination of these factors. However, by their nature, spherically surfaced mobile bearings accommodate malalignment without overload more easily than fixed bearings.

Fixation of Mobile Bearings Methylmethacrylate bone cement was the initial adjunctive method of bony attachment for the first LCS unicompartmental meniscal bearing device used in 1977 and for subsequent bicompartmental and tricompartmental devices.

The tibial fixation surface of the LCS unicompartmental knee replacement has a flat, tibial loading plate and a short angled stem to resist tipping and shear loads. Bicruciate retaining LCS tibial components use 3 short fixation fins for anchorage, while posterior cruciate retaining (PCR) LCS meniscal bearing and LCS rotating platform tibial components use a short, conical metaphyseal fixation stem centered in the proximal tibia. All femoral components use shallow cement locking pockets and centralized femoral fixation pegs.

The rotating-bearing patellar replacement uses a cruciform fin geometry for fixation. This geometry reinforces the thin metal plate against torsional failure and reinforces the patellar remnant against fractures while engaging the patellar bone stock sufficiently to prevent loosening.

Cementless fixation with sintered-bead Co-Cr-Mo porous coating on the Co-Cr-Mo substrate using the same articulating and fixation geometries was first used clinically in 1981. Bicruciate retaining and rotating platform tibial components were developed with 4 screw holes and spherical seats. These implants used 6.5-mm cancellous bone screws to augment fixation.

Concerns over fretting corrosion, screw breakage, osteolysis, and potential neurovascular injuries from screw penetration led the developers away from screw fixation later in the same year. These early concerns are now complications that have been documented by several authors in other cementless knee devices.

Press fit, nonscrew-fixed, mobile bearing knee replacements with porous coating have been in successful clinical use since late 1981. Ten-year studies have demonstrated a 96.5% overall survivorship using nonscrew-fixed, press-fit, porous-coated, cementless fixation, thereby justifying its continued use.

Clinical Application of Mobile Bearings

Unicompartmental Knee Replacement Unicompartmental meniscal bearings are well adapted for knee replacement, because they allow retention of both cruciate ligaments and allow the normal forward and backward translational movement of the femur on the tibia as well as axial rotation and varus-valgus movement with excellent congruity of the bearing surfaces. The Oxford meniscal bearing unicompartmental device has had excellent success when used as a medial unicompartmental replacement, but has functioned less consistently as a lateral compartment replacement because of significant dislocation problems.

The cementless LCS unicompartmental knee replacement was approved by the FDA Orthopaedic Advisory Panel in August 1991 and released for general use by the FDA in November 1992 after successful completion of an FDA-IDE clinical trial. Good or excellent results using a strict knee scoring scale were seen in 98.4% of 122 patients followed for 2 to 6 years (mean, 3.3 years). One bearing fractured after trauma, and one tibial component loosened in a patient with posttraumatic, osteoporotic bone deficiency. Progressive disease in the opposite knee compartment was an additional cause for revision. Such disorders represent current failure mechanisms for this device and are now considered contraindications.

Bicompartmental Knee Replacement The articulating geometry of the femoral component is critical to the success or failure of the patellar component. A bispherical, continuous-surface-of-revolution femoral groove matching a bispherical, congruently tracking patellar component will provide for a long service life for the patellar bearing. This same femoral groove can match the anatomic patellar geometry and can allow retention of the natural patella, with highly predictable results. No difference has been reported between bicompartmental (retention of natural patella) and tricompartmental (replaced patella) knee replacements, using the unique femoral groove of the LCS design, in a 10-year clinical series of 52 patients in whom one patella was replaced and the other patella was retained.

Such predictability can allow patellar retention in patients such as farmers or laborers who require repetitive squatting loads that may increase patellar component wear. Additionally, patellar retention in conditions such as patella infera, alta, or hypoplasia can facilitate central tracking without fear of early knee replacement failure. Finally, those patients with previous patellectomies can undergo a patellar tendon bone grafting and enjoy a well-functioning bicompartmental replacement with improvement in both quadriceps leverage and tibiofemoral dislocation resistance.

Tricompartmental Knee Replacement The concept of retaining both viable cruciate ligaments is appealing, because normal knee kinematics depend on the anterior-posterior translation of the femur on the tibia, which is under the direct control of these intact structures. Ligament loads greater than body weight have been recorded for all knee ligaments.

Thus, in theory at least, in the absence of each ligament structure these loads would need to be carried by the remaining ligaments and perhaps transferred to the prosthesis itself. As such, retention of all load-bearing ligaments would be ideal, if normal kinematic knee motion were allowed. Based on these concepts, the bicruciate-retaining, LCS meniscal bearing knee replacement was developed and successfully tested in FDA-IDE clinical trials.

The use of 3 fixation fins rather than a central conical peg has led to a greater incidence of tibial component loosening with this device than with central conical peg devices. Also, reports from Holland indicate that loosening of these trifinned components is increased in patients with previous HTOs or proximal tibial fractures. Such conditions appear to alter blood flow and impede osseointegration in cementless bicruciate-retaining knees and as such remain contraindications to their cementless use. Additionally, early or late rupture of the ACL degrades the arthroplasty to the level of an ACL-deficient knee in many cases and raises doubts as to whether ACL retention should be attempted in other than circumstances of youth, good bone stock, and a perfect ACL, which is a rare situation at best. Nevertheless, those knees with intact ACLs, excellent bone stock, and solid fixation of components represent the best possible TKRs because they function and act as normal knees.

The overall failure rate of bicruciate-retaining, meniscal bearing TKR as a result of fracture, dislocation, or bearing wear-through has been 3 out of 95 TKRs or 3.2% in a series of primary and multiply-operated knee replacements followed for 10 to 19 years (mean, 13 years). Only one undersized cemented tibial component loosened. The survivorship of these primary, cemented, bicruciate-retaining meniscal bearing TKRs using an end point of revision of any component is 88.8% at 18 years. The primary cementless bicruciate survivorship is 92.3% at 14 years.

Retention of the PCL has been reported to improve quadriceps leverage, increase extension torque, and improve flexion over cruciate-sacrificing designs. In fixed bearings, this increased motion and function is related to increased posterior roll-back or roll-forward on the incongruent tibial bearing surface, which increases wear over cruciate-sacrificing, fixed-bearing designs. A meniscal bearing device allows more congruent roll-back or roll-forward in flexion to improve wear resistance over fixed-bearing designs.

The Oxford meniscal knee, however, functioned poorly with only an intact PCL. Therefore, the Oxford knee developers did not recommend using the Oxford device in any ACL-deficient knee and cautioned against the use of any meniscal-bearing device in the absence of the ACL. The significant dislocation rate of 9.3% reported in 1990 for use of rotating platform and PCR LCS knee replacements would tend to support this concept. However, as was pointed out in rebuttal to that report, meniscal or rotating bearings require adequate control of the flexion and extension gaps during surgery to maintain contact stability of the prosthesis. Thus, failure to maintain flexion and extension gap stability will compromise the results of any mobile bearing knee replacement, whether both, one, or no cruciate ligaments are preserved.

The successful FDA-IDE cementless clinical trial of the PCR, meniscal bearing LCS knee replacement documented the ability to retain only the PCL and maintain long-term stability and function with a meniscal bearing device.

Tibial component subluxations and dislocations were seen in knees with poor flexion stability and were noted to be technique-related rather than implant-related. Early or late PCL instability remains a concern for this arthroplasty. Intraoperative diligence to avoid any release of this ligament attachment is desirable, and if PCL compromise is noted, then replacement to a centrally stabilized, rotating platform is advisable for long-term stability and function.

The overall failure rate of cementless PCR meniscal bearing TKR as a result of fracture, dislocation, or bearing wear-through has been 3 out of 178 TKRs or 1.7% in a series of primary and multiply-operated knee replacements followed for 7 to 14 years (mean, 10 years). No loosening of any component was seen. The survivorship of these primary cementless PCR meniscal-bearing knee replacements using revision as an end point is 96.2% at 14 years. A long-term radiograph of a right cementless PCR meniscal-bearing device is shown in an obese patient with bilateral knee replacements (Fig. 2).

Cruciate sacrifice is often desirable in certain conditions, such as fixed flexion, fixed valgus, and some severe fixed varus deformities. It is often unavoidable in conditions where significant trauma, RA, or inflammatory arthritis have destroyed these structures. In such cases, a centrally stabilized device with long-term fixation and excellent wear properties would be most desirable. The cemented total condylar knee replacement has been used in such cases of elderly patients over a 10- to 15-year period with exceptionally good results and reported 90% survivorship, using revision as an end point.

Considering these results to represent the standard for future design comparisons, any cemented or cementless cruciate-sacrificing design should demonstrate at least a 90% 10-year survivorship and have contact stresses less than the total condylar device to merit any attention. Additionally, since total condylar ROM was only considered to be fair (85° to 95°) and dislocations fairly frequent, any new design should improve upon motion and dislocation resistance.

The LCS rotating platform knee replacement represents an improvement over the total condylar device in concept and in clinical performance. Conceptually, the deeper engagement of the rotatable, spherically congruent surfaces allows lower contact stresses during normal walking, namely 25 MPa for total condylar and 4.9 MPa for LCS. This deeper engagement also improves dislocation resistance over the total condylar device. The LCS device uses a conical central tibial component stem that approximates the successful total condylar stem. Thus, similar fixation is achieved with rotational relief of shear stresses to tibial fixation with the rotating-platform design.

FDA-IDE clinical trials have demonstrated long-term safety and efficacy of the rotating-platform in a wide variety of primary and multiply-operated cases in both cemented and cementless applications. The FDA Orthopaedic Advisory Panel recommended approval of the cemented LCS rotating-platform device in 1984 and the cementless device in 1991, making the rotating-platform the first and, currently, the only total knee device in the United States to be approved for both cemented and cementless applications.

The overall failure rate of rotating platform TKRs as a result of bearing dislocation has been 2 out of 294 TKRs, or 0.6%, in a series of primary and multiply-operated knee replacements followed for 4 to 18 years (mean, 10 years). Two rotating-platform bearings (0.6%) developed severe wear, requiring revision in multiply-operated cases; no fractured bearings were seen. No component loosening was seen. One valgus knee with postoperative ligament laxity required revision to a larger bearing to gain stability. The survivorship of these primary cemented rotating-platform knee replacements using revision as an end point is 97.9% at 18 years. The primary cementless rotating-platform survivorship is 98.1% at 15 years. A long-term radiograph of a left cemented rotating-platform device in the same patient with a cementless PCR device in the opposite knee is also shown in Figure 2.

Failures of the rotating-bearing patella have been rare and usually associated with displaced patellar fractures, malposition, subluxation, or excessive, repetitive hyperflexion loads.

The overall complications of rotating-bearing patellar replacements that required revision surgery in 515 knees originally followed for 6 months to 11 years and now followed for 8 to 19 years (mean, 12.5 years) was 5 of 515 or 0.97%. Wear-through of the bearing on the lateral facet and transverse bearing fractures have been the dominant mechanisms of mechanical failure. These have been associated with unrecognized poor quality polyethylene and gamma-radiation oxidation, which has also negatively affected the tibial bearings of the past 2 decades.

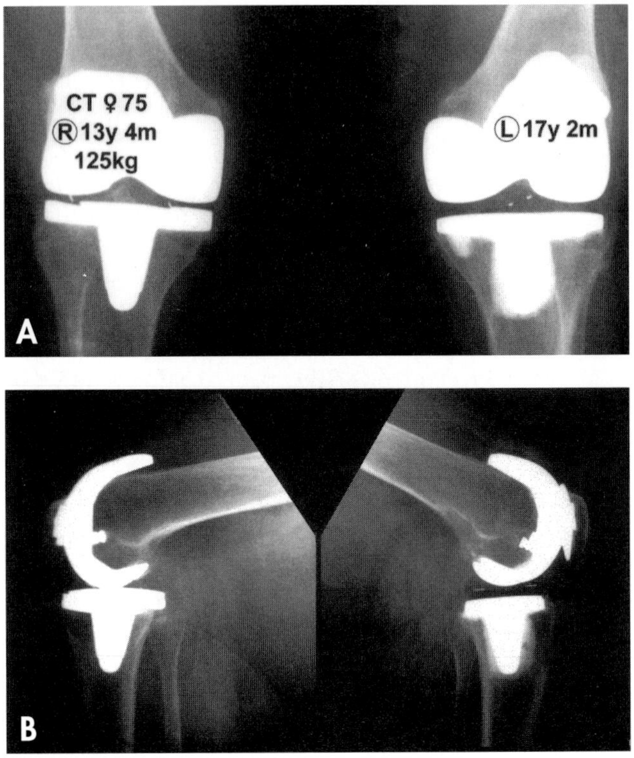

Figure 2

A, Standing anteroposterior radiographs of a 75-year-old, 125 kg (275 pound) osteoarthritic woman with a cementless posterior cruciate retaining (PCR) meniscal bearing right total knee replacement (TKR) at 13 years, 4 months after surgery and a left cemented rotating platform TKR at 17 years, 2 months after surgery. **B**, Lateral right knee radiograph, *left* (cementless PCR meniscal bearing TKR); lateral left knee radiograph, *right* (cemented rotating platform TKR).

Revision TKR

Aseptic, failed knee replacement surgery is usually accompanied by a loss of bone stock and a loss of the cruciate ligaments. In such cases, a centrally stabilized, rotating-platform device with intramedullary stems can be used to successfully salvage a wide variety of complex pathologies. These stems can be fixed to the femoral or tibial components or be modular constructs with the ability to increase or decrease diameter as well as length similar to that found in current revision hip replacements.

Attention to surgical technique, in regard to flexion-extension stability, as well as varus-valgus ligamentous balancing remains crucial to revision success. In 5.8% of 86 revision rotating platform cases, persistent instability continued to be a problem, requiring a thicker rotating bearing or the use of a Total Condylar III or rotating-hinge design to achieve acceptable stability.

Future Directions of Mobile Bearing Knee Replacement Meniscal bearings represent the logical approach for future development of human knee joint replacements. This fact is supported by long-term survivorship and contact-stress studies, which favor mobile bearings over fixed-bearings in a wide variety of clinical applications varying from unicompartmental to tricompartmental arthroplasty. As such, it is important to explore alternative bearing geometries and biomaterials, such as wear resistant titanium nitride ceramic coatings, to optimize future designs.

In the meantime, bearing exchange techniques are currently available to maintain well-fixed metallic components while replacing worn or broken bearings with improved polyethylene that has been gas sterilized to enhance future wear properties. Such techniques allow extended performance of currently available mobile-bearing devices with same-day or overnight-stay surgery. Patient acceptance of elective bearing exchange surgery over the past 4 years has been extremely favorable, with patients reporting less pain and faster recovery than they experienced after their original primary knee replacement procedure.

Future mobile-bearing knee designs should continue to provide these important features of wear resistance and bearing exchangeability to maintain optimal knee function for a maximum duration with a minimum of surgical intervention.

Acknowledgment

Dr. Buechel would like to acknowledge Linda A. Carter for her excellent technical assistance in the research for and preparation of portions of this manuscript.

Annotated Bibliography

Unicompartmental Knee Arthroplasty

Cartier P, Sanouiller JL, Grelsamer RP: Unicompartmental knee arthroplasty surgery: 10-year minimum follow-up period. *J Arthroplasty* 1996;11:782–788.

Sixty UKAs were followed for a minimum of 10 years (mean, 12 years). A 10-year survivorship of 93% was demonstrated.

Chakrabarty G, Newman JH, Ackroyd CE: Revision of unicompartmental arthroplasty of the knee: Clinical and technical considerations. *J Arthroplasty* 1998;13:191–196.

Seventy-three UKAs that underwent conversion to TKAs were reviewed. Forty-two percent of the procedures were considered the same as a primary arthroplasty, and only 22% required augmentation for the reconstruction of bone defects.

Chassin EP, Mikosz RP, Andriacchi TP, Rosenberg AG: Functional analysis of cemented medial unicompartmental knee arthroplasty. *J Arthroplasty* 1996;11:553–559.

Gait analysis was used to compare patients who had undergone a unicompartmental arthroplasty with those who had undergone a tricompartmental arthroplasty. During level gait, patients with a UKA and preservation of the ACL maintained normal quadriceps mechanics.

Levine WN, Ozuna RM, Scott RD, Thornhill TS: Conversion of failed modern unicompartmental arthroplasty to total knee arthroplasty. *J Arthroplasty* 1995;11:797–801.

Thirty-one failed UKAs that underwent conversion to TKA were reviewed. In all but 1 case the PCL was preserved, and augmentation of bone defects with metal wedges was necessary in only 6 cases. Results were similar to those for primary TKA.

Riebel GD, Werner FW, Ayers DC, Bromka J, Murray DG: Early failure of the femoral component in unicompartmental knee arthroplasty. *J Arthroplasty* 1995;10:615–621.

Biomechanical testing of the femoral component of a UKA was done following implantation in cadaver limbs. Early femoral component loosening was attributed to designs having an angled bone-implant interface caused by increased shear stresses at this interface. Use of a femoral component with a curved interface is recommended.

Schai PA, Suh JT, Thornhill TS, Scott RD: Unicompartmental knee arthroplasty in middle-aged patients: A 2- to 6-year follow-up evaluation. *J Arthroplasty* 1998;13:365–372.

Twenty-eight UKAs implanted in patients younger than 60 years (average age, 52 years) were reviewed after 2 to 6 years of follow-up. Early results in terms of pain relief and improved function were excellent and were found to be superior to those following osteotomy.

Tabor OB Jr, Tabor OB: Unicompartmental arthroplasty: A long-term follow-up study. *J Arthroplasty* 1998;13:373–379.

Sixty-three consecutive UKAs were followed for an average of 9.7 years (range, 5 to 20 years). Survivorship was 84% at 10 years and 79% at 15 years. Relief of pain and improved knee function was maintained with long-term follow-up.

Cruciate-Retaining TKA

Ansari S, Ackroyd CE, Newman JH: Kinematic posterior cruciate ligament-retaining total knee replacements: A 10-year survivorship study of 445 arthroplasties. *Am J Knee Surg* 1998;11: 9–14.

This is a thorough follow-up series of the Kinematic cemented CR-TKA. Ten-year survivorship was 96%, 78%, and 69%, depending on whether revision/recommended revision, revision or moderate to severe pain, or revision or loss to follow-up was used as the end point.

Bugbee WD, Ammeen DJ, Parks NL, Engh GA: 4- to 10-year results with the anatomic modular total knee. *Clin Orthop* 1998;348:158–165.

This large consecutive series evaluated the AMK, which is one of only a few implants still commercially available in its original design. The revision rate was 6.3% of 186 patients at 6.9 years, though most of those were simple polyethylene exchanges. The authors cited several features of implant design for the absence of patellar complications in this report.

Dalury DF, Ewald FC, Christie MJ, Scott RD: Total knee arthroplasty in a group of patients less than 45 years of age. *J Arthroplasty* 1995;10:598–602.

This study evaluated 67 patients who underwent CR-TKA before age 45, using a variety of implants, at an average follow-up of 7.2 years. Survivorship was 98.1% in a population consisting predominantly of inflammatory arthritis patients. There was 15% loss to follow-up, though the number of deaths was not quantified.

Fanning JW, Joseph J Jr, Kaufman EE: Follow up on uncemented total knee arthroplasty. *Orthopedics* 1996;19:933–939.

This small study of the cementless Miller-Galante I (MG-I)TKA found a revision rate of more than 50% at 5- to 7-year follow-up. The cementless MG-I was a first-generation device that incorporated a number of design features now known to be undesirable, including carbon-fiber polyethylene, a titanium femoral bearing surface, and unfavorable patellofemoral geometry.

Gill GS, Chan KC, Mills DM: 5- to 18-year follow-up study of cemented total knee arthroplasty for patients 55 years old or younger. *J Arthroplasty* 1997;12:49–54.

The authors report 10-year mean follow-up of CR-TKA in a young population using several different prosthesis designs. Loss to follow-up was minimal, and relief of pain was excellent. A large minority of patients in this series (40%) had rheumatoid arthritis, which may have contributed to somewhat lower knee scores for function.

Hanyu T, Murasawa A, Tojo T: Survivorship analysis of total knee arthroplasty with the Kinematic prosthesis in patients who have rheumatoid arthritis. *J Arthroplasty* 1997;12:913–919.

This article demonstrated that excellent long-term survivorship of CR-TKA can be obtained even in patients with rheumatoid arthritis. The authors made an intraoperative decision regarding whether to use a CR or a PS component based on the competence of the PCL at surgery. Using an intact PCL as the indication to use a CR knee, survivorship was 93% at 10 years, with no loss to follow-up.

Kim YH, Oh JH, Oh SH: Osteolysis around cementless porous-coated anatomic knee prostheses. *J Bone Joint Surg* 1995;77B:236–241.

This study of 60 consecutive cementless PC knees found a 90% incidence of tibial osteolysis and a 50% incidence of patellar loosening. Progression of osteolysis became more rapid with time; the authors emphasized the need for careful clinical and radiographic surveillance of patients with this type of implant.

Laskin RS: Total knee replacement with posterior cruciate ligament retention in patients with a fixed varus deformity. *Clin Orthop* 1996;331:29–34.

This article evaluates the effect on fixed varus/flexion deformity on results of CR-TKA at 10 years' follow-up. CR-TKA in patients with fixed varus/flexion deformity > 15° had worse results than PS-TKA in patients with similar deformity. No criteria were given on how the CR/PS decision was made in each case.

Liow RY, Murray DW: Which primary total knee replacement? A review of currently available TKR in the United Kingdom. *Ann R Coll Surg Engl* 1997;79:335–340.

This startling review highlights the lack of long-term follow-up available for contemporary designs of TKA in the United Kingdom. Over half of commercially available implants have no published survival figures at all, including 3 of the 4 most widely used devices.

Malkani AL, Rand JA, Bryan RS, Wallrichs SL: Total knee arthroplasty with the kinematic condylar prosthesis: A ten-year follow-up study. *J Bone Joint Surg* 1995;77A:423–431.

Excellent results were seen in this consecutive series of 168 Kinematic CR-TKAs at a mean of 10 years, and loss to follow-up was minimal. Most revisions were related to the metal-backed patellar component.

Martin SD, McManus JL, Scott RD, Thornhill TS: Press-fit condylar total knee arthroplasty: 5- to 9-year follow-up evaluation. *J Arthroplasty* 1997;12:603–614.

This large consecutive series evaluated the PFC, which may be implanted with or without cement, and is one of only a few devices still available in nearly its original form. The revision rate was 3.8%, and most of those were attributed to a metal-backed patellar design that has since been changed to all-polyethylene, with good results.

Mont MA, Mathur SK, Krackow KA, Loewy JW, Hungerford DS: Cementless total knee arthroplasty in obese patients: A comparison with a matched control group. *J Arthroplasty* 1996;11:153–156.

This study of 50 obese and 50 nonobese patients found no statistically significant differences between the two groups in terms of clinical results or radiographic loosening. However, there were trends toward poorer results in the obese cohort, and no calculations of statistical power were provided for this relatively small study.

Ritter MA, Worland R, Saliski J, et al: Flat-on-flat, nonconstrained, compression molded polyethylene total knee replacement. *Clin Orthop* 1995;321:79–85.

This article presents results using the AGC knee, which is one of a very few implants still commercially available with > 10-year published follow-up. This knee also fared very well in the Swedish Knee Arthroplasty Register. Unfortunately, the substantial loss to follow-up severely limits the interpretability of this article.

Weir DJ, Moran CG, Pinder IM: Kinematic Condylar total knee arthroplasty: 14-year survivorship analysis of 208 consecutive cases. *J Bone Joint Surg* 1996;78B:907–911.

This is a survivorship analysis at a mean of 12 years of a cemented CR-TKA with minimal loss to follow-up. The Kinematic Condylar device had a low revision rate in this and other series; this article did not present knee scores, radiographic end points, nor ROM data.

Posterior Stabilized TKA

Bolanos AA, Colizza WA, McCann PD, et al: A comparison of isokinetic strength testing and gait analysis in patients with posterior cruciate retaining and substituting knee arthroplasties. *J Arthroplasty* 1998;13:906–915.

Fourteen patients with a posterior-stabilized prosthesis in one knee and a posterior cruciate-retaining prosthesis in the other knee were evaluated by isokinetic muscle testing and comprehensive gait analysis at a mean follow-up of 8 years. No difference was found between designs with regard to gait, knee range of motion, and electromyographic findings. Both designs performed equally well with level walking and stair climbing.

Colizza WA, Insall JN, Scuderi GR: The posterior stabilized total knee prosthesis: Assessment of polyethylene damage and osteolysis after a ten-year-minimum follow-up. *J Bone Joint Surg* 1995;77A:1713–1720.

Seventy-four patients (101 knees) were evaluated with a minimum follow-up of 10 years. Ninety-six percent of knees had an excellent or good result. There were no revisions because of polyethylene wear or osteolysis. This prosthetic design included a metal-backed monoblock tibial component, which demonstrated no evidence of loosening.

Diduch DR, Insall JN, Scott WN, Scuderi GR, Font-Rodriguez D: Total knee replacement in young active patients: Long-term follow-up and functional outcome. *J Bone Joint Surg* 1997;79A: 575–582.

One hundred and three posterior cruciate substituting TKAs performed in patients with a preoperative diagnosis of osteoarthritis or posttraumatic arthritis and an average age of 51 years were analyzed at an average follow-up of 8 years (3 to 18 years). All but 2 patients improved their level of activity, with 24% indicating regular participation in such activities as tennis, skiing, cycling, or manual labor. Within this follow-up period, polyethylene wear, osteolysis, and loosening were not major problems in these younger active patients.

Emmerson KP, Moran CG, Pinder IM: Survivorship analysis of the Kinematic Stabilizer total knee replacement: A 10- to 14-year follow-up. *J Bone Joint Surg* 1996;78B:441–445.

In a long-term study of 109 cemented Kinematic Stabilizer total knee replacements, the 10-year survivorship was 95% and the 13-year survivorship was 87%. This confirms the value of posterior cruciate substituting designs.

Font-Rodriguez DE, Scuderi GR, Insall JN: Survivorship of cemented total knee arthroplasty. *Clin Orthop* 1997;345:79–86.

The survivorship method of analysis was used to compare the failure rate and overall success of 2,629 cemented primary total knee arthroplasties during a 22-year period. Long-term results have confirmed the advantage of prosthetic conformity in that it minimizes polyethylene wear without compromising fixation.

Laskin RS, O'Flynn HM: Total knee replacement with posterior cruciate ligament retention in rheumatoid arthritis: Problems and complications. *Clin Orthop* 1997;345:24–28.

When a cruciate-retaining prosthesis was implanted in patients with rheumatoid arthritis, there was an increased incidence of posterior flexion instability and recurvatum deformity, resulting in an increased revision rate. In these patients a posterior-stabilized prosthesis should be used.

Lattanzio PJ, Chess DG, MacDermid JC: Effect of the posterior cruciate ligament in knee-joint proprioception in total knee arthroplasty. *J Arthroplasty* 1998;13:580–585.

Knee joint proprioception was measured in 10 patients with a posterior-stabilized prosthesis and 10 with a cruciate-retaining prosthesis. The findings suggest that the preservation of the PCL in TKA may not improve knee joint proprioception and, subsequently, may not improve functional performance.

Lombardi AV Jr, Mallory TH, Waterman RA, Eberle RW: Intercondylar distal femoral fracture: An unreported complication of posterior-stabilized total knee arthroplasty. *J Arthroplasty* 1995;10:643–650.

Intraoperative distal femoral intercondylar fracture represents a potential complication of posterior stabilized TKA and can be avoided with careful bone resection, component size verification, and proper orientation during implantation.

Mokris JG, Smith SW, Anderson SE: Primary total knee arthroplasty using the Genesis Total Knee Arthroplasty System: 3- to 6-year follow-up study of 105 knees. *J Arthroplasty* 1997;12: 91–98.

When comparing cruciate-retaining and posterior-stabilized knees, there was no difference with respect to clinical results, radiolucencies, range of motion, alignment, or complication rate.

Ranawat CS, Luessenhop CP, Rodriguez JA: The press-fit condylar modular total knee system: Four- to six-year results with a posterior-cruciate-substituting design. *J Bone Joint Surg* 1997; 79A:342–348.

Ninety-six patients (125 knees) with press-fit condylar posterior stabilized prostheses were followed for an average of 4.8 years. The average Knee Society functional score was 78 and the clinical score was 93. The overall survival rate was 97% at 6 years. Although there were 3 revisions, 2 for infection and 1 for instability, there were an additional 3 cases of flexion instability that were not revised.

Stiehl JB, Komistek RD, Dennis DA, Paxson RD, Hoff WA: Fluoroscopic analysis of kinematics after posterior-cruciate-retaining knee arthroplasty. *J Bone Joint Surg* 1995;77B: 884–889.

Forty-seven cruciate retaining TKAs, including 5 different designs, were evaluated fluoroscopically. PCL retaining TKAs did not reproduce normal knee kinematics and physiologic rollback was not demonstrated. The femur started posterior on the tibia in extension and translated anteriorly with flexion. These findings were not design specific.

Wilson SA, McCann PD, Gotlin RS, Ramakrishnan HK, Wootten ME, Insall JN: Comprehensive gait analysis in posterior-stabilized knee arthroplasty. *J Arthroplasty* 1996;11:359–367.

Almost 4 years after an IBPS TKA, 16 patients and 32 age-matched controls underwent a comprehensive gait analysis. No difference was seen between groups in velocity, cadence, and stride length during level walking. No difference was noted in knee range of motion during stair ascent. Persistent gait abnormalities of patients with a posterior-stabilized knee are comparable to those of patients with cruciate-retaining knees and superior to those of patients with cruciate-sacrificing designs.

Mobile Bearing TKR: Fixation

Buechel FF: New Jersey Low-Contact Stress Knee Replacement System: 7 to 15 year clinical and survivorship outcomes, in Niwa S, Yoshino SI, Kurosaka M, Shino K, Yamamoto S (eds): *Reconstruction of the Knee Joint.* Tokyo, Japan, Springer, 1997, pp 176–185.

This study updates the LCS knee with 7- to 15-year follow-up of cemented and cementless knee replacements. Survivorship at 15 years was 86.7% of all components in the cemented group and was 95.1% of all components in the cementless group at 12 years.

Future Directions of Mobile-Bearing Knee Replacement

Pappas MJ, Makris G, Buechel FF: Titanium nitride ceramic film against polyethylene: A 48 million cycle wear test. *Clin Orthop* 1995;317:64–70.

This resurfacing hip replacement simulation study loads polished titanium nitride ceramic film (8-mm thick) against a metal-backed polyethylene bearing for 48 million walking cycles at a 2200 N fluctuating load at 5Hz in distilled water. Results demonstrated < 2 mm wear of the ceramic film and < 0.02 mm wear of GUR415 extruded rod polyethylene used for the bearing. A great potential as a lifetime bearing couple was noted.

Classic Bibliography

Unicompartmental Knee Arthroplasty

Barrett WP, Scott RD: Revision of failed unicondylar unicompartmental knee arthroplasty. *J Bone Joint Surg* 1987;69A: 1328–1335.

Broughton NS, Newman JH, Baily RA: Unicompartmental replacement and high tibial osteotomy for osteoarthritis of the knee: A comparative study after 5 to 10 years' follow-up. *J Bone Joint Surg* 1986;68B:447–452.

Jackson M, Sarangi PP, Newman JH: Revision total knee arthroplasty: Comparison of outcome following primary proximal tibial osteotomy or unicompartmental arthroplasty. *J Arthroplasty* 1994;9:539–542.

Laurencin CT, Zelicof SB, Scott RD, Ewald FC: Unicompartmental versus total knee arthroplasty in the same patient: A comparative study. *Clin Orthop* 1991;273:151–156.

Marmor L: Unicompartmental arthroplasty of the knee with a minimum ten-year follow-up period. *Clin Orthop* 1988;228: 171–177.

Mont MA, Antonaides S, Krackow KA Hungerford DS: Total knee arthroplasty after failed high tibial osteotomy: A comparison with a matched group. *Clin Orthop* 1994;299:125–130.

Scott RD, Cobb AG, McQueary FG, Thornhill TS: Unicompartmental knee arthroplasty: Eight- to 12-year follow-up evaluation with survivorship analysis. *Clin Orthop* 1991;271: 96–100.

Staeheli JW, Cass JR, Morrey BF: Condylar total knee arthroplasty after failed proximal tibial osteotomy. *J Bone Joint Surg* 1987;69A:28–31.

Windsor RE, Insall JN, Vince KG: Technical considerations of total knee arthroplasty after proximal tibial osteotomy. *J Bone Joint Surg* 1988;70A:547–555.

Weale AE, Newman JH: Unicompartmental arthroplasty and high tibial osteotomy for osteoarthrosis of the knee: A comparative study with a 12- to 17-year follow-up period. *Clin Orthop* 1994;302:134–137.

Cruciate-Retaining TKA

Dennis DA, Clayton ML, O'Donnell S, Mack RP, Stringer EA: Posterior cruciate condylar total knee arthroplasty: Average 11-year follow-up evaluation. *Clin Orthop* 1992;281:168–176.

Knutson K, Lewold S, Robertsson O, Lidgren L: The Swedish knee arthroplasty register: A nation-wide study of 30,003 knees 1976-1992. *Acta Orthop Scand* 1994;65:375–386.

Rand JA: Comparison of metal-backed and all-polyethylene tibial components in cruciate condylar total knee arthroplasty. *J Arthroplasty* 1993;8:307–313.

Ritter MA, Herbst SA, Keating EM, Faris PM, Meding JB: Long-term survival analysis of a posterior cruciate-retaining total condylar total knee arthroplasty. *Clin Orthop* 1994;309: 136–145.

Posterior Stabilized TKA

Aglietti P, Buzzi R, Gaudenzi A: Patellofemoral functional results and complications with the posterior stabilized total condylar knee prosthesis. *J Arthroplasty* 1988;3:17–25.

Galinat BJ, Vernace JV, Booth RE Jr, Rothman RH: Dislocation of the posterior stabilized total knee arthroplasty: A report of two cases. *J Arthroplasty* 1988;3:363–367.

Gebhard JS, Kilgus DJ: Dislocation of a posterior stabilized total knee prosthesis: A report of two cases. *Clin Orthop* 1990;254: 225–229.

Hanssen AD, Rand JA: A comparison of primary and revision total knee arthroplasty using the Kinematic Stabilizer prosthesis. *J Bone Joint Surg* 1988;70A:491–499.

Hozack WJ, Rothman RH, Booth RE Jr, Balderston RA: The patellar clunk syndrome: A complication of posterior stabilized total knee arthroplasty. *Clin Orthop* 1989;241:203–208.

Insall JN, Lachiewicz PF, Burstein AH: The posterior stabilized condylar prosthesis: A modification of the total condylar design. Two to four-year clinical experience. *J Bone Joint Surg* 1982; 64A:1317–1323.

Lombardi AV Jr, Mallory TH, Vaughn BK, et al: Dislocation following primary posterior-stabilized total knee arthroplasty. *J Arthroplasty* 1993;8:633–639.

Mahoney OM, Noble PC, Rhoads DD, Alexander JW, Tullos HS: Posterior cruciate function following total knee arthroplasty: A biomechanical study. *J Arthroplasty* 1994;9:569–578.

Scott WN, Rubinstein M, Scuderi G: Results after total knee replacement with a posterior cruciate-substituting prosthesis. *J Bone Joint Surg* 1988;70A:1163–1173.

Stern SH, Insall JN: Posterior stabilized prosthesis: Results after follow-up of nine to twelve years. *J Bone Joint Surg* 1992;74A: 980–986.

Mobile Bearing TKR

Buechel FF: Cemented and cementless revision arthroplasty using Rotating-Platform total knee Implants: A 12 year experience. *Orthop Rev Suppl* 1990;XIX:71–75.

Buechel FF: Meniscal bearing knee replacement: Development, long-term results, and future tchnology, in Scott WN (ed): *The Knee.* St. Louis, MO, Mosby, 1994, pp 1157–1177.

Buechel FF, Pappas MJ: The New Jersey Low-Contact-Stress Knee Replacement System: Biomechanical rationale and review of the first 123 cemented cases. *Arch Orthop Trauma Surg* 1986;105: 197–204.

Buechel FF, Pappas MJ: New Jersey Low Contact Stress Knee Replacement System: Ten-year evaluation of meniscal bearings. *Orthop Clin North Am* 1989;20:147–177.

Buechel FF, Pappas MJ: Long-term survivorship analysis of cruciate-sparing versus cruciate-sacrificing knee prostheses using meniscal bearings. *Clin Orthop* 1990;260:162–169.

Buechel FF, Pappas MJ, Makris G: Evaluation of contact stress in metal-backed patellar replacements: A predictor of survivorship. *Clin Orthop* 1991;273:190–197.

Buechel FF, Rosa RA, Pappas MJ: A metal-backed, rotating-bearing patellar prosthesis to lower contact stress: An 11-year clinical study. *Clin Orthop* 1989;248:34–49.

Collier JP, Mayor MB, McNamara JL, Surprenant VA, Jensen RE: Analysis of the failure of 122 polyethylene inserts from uncemented tibial knee components. *Clin Orthop* 1991;273: 232–242.

Engh GA, Dwyer KA, Hanes CK: Polyethylene wear of metal-backed tibial components in total and unicompartmental knee prostheses. *J Bone Joint Surg* 1992;74B:9–17.

Goodfellow JW, O'Connor J: Clinical results of the Oxford knee: Surface arthroplasty of the tibiofemoral joint with a meniscal bearing prosthesis. *Clin Orthop* 1986;205:21–42.

Peters PC Jr, Engh GA, Dwyer KA, Vinh TN: Osteolysis after total knee arthroplasty without cement. *J Bone Joint Surg* 1992;74A: 864–876.

Scuderi GR, Insall JN, Windsor RE, Moran MC: Survivorship of cemented knee replacements. *J Bone Joint Surg* 1989;71B: 798–803.

Ranawat CS, Flynn WF Jr, Saddler S, Hansraj KK, Maynard MJ: Long-term results of the Total Condylar knee arthroplasty: A 15-year survivorship study. *Clin Orthop* 1993;286:94–102.

Chapter 35 Complications Associated With Total Knee Arthroplasty

Infection

Infection is one of the most serious complications that can occur following total knee arthroplasty (TKA). Successful TKA can improve quality of life, but the presence of infection can be devastating to both patient and surgeon. Therefore, a thorough understanding of the concepts of infection, focusing on its prevention, prompt and accurate diagnosis, and sound management, is essential in minimizing associated morbidity. Because the risk of infection is always present in any surgical procedure and can never be fully eliminated, it is important to maximize preventive efforts and refine treatment methods.

The economic impact of treating infected TKAs is staggering. In the United States alone, over 200,000 TKAs are performed annually; this number is projected to double over the next decade. With a current incidence of infection of 1% to 2% and an average cost of $70,000 for individual treatment, a conservative estimate of annual costs for treatment of infected TKAs would be $140 to $280 million. In addition, the incidence of infection in the TKA revision setting has been reported to be as high as 5% to 6%. The number of cases can be expected to increase because of the rising number of TKAs used in younger patients, whose life expectancy exceeds the life of the implant. By studying the advances made in the field of total joint arthroplasty over the past 30 years, understanding and defining the principles associated with infection, evaluating current treatment protocols, and expanding on these concepts with further research and technology, the overall impact of this complication can be minimized.

Incidence and Predisposing Factors

A review of the literature has shown the overall incidence of infection in TKA to range from 0.5% to 23%. Contemporary measures implemented to reduce TKA infection, including the use of prophylactic antibiotics, improvements in the operating room (for example, proper surgical attire, limiting of personnel/traffic, clean air systems), and the use of less constrained implants, have been successful in lowering the incidence of infection to its current level of 1% to 2%. According to numerous reports, these rates have been constant over the past several years and may be due in part to the inherent anatomic risk factors, which include the joint's relatively superficial position and thin fascial and muscular envelope. Other factors that may play a role in this lowered incidence include host factors, wound issues, operating room environment, implant choices, and surgical technique.

In a recent review evaluating the rate of infection from 1969 to 1996, an incidence of 2.5% was found in 18,749 TKAs. Further analysis of the data showed that after primary operations, the incidence of infection was 2%, or 320 of 16,036 cases, and the risk of infection after revision surgery was found to be 5.6%, or 152 of 2,714 cases. These findings confirm previously documented data showing an association between an increased risk of infection and patents with multiple previous operations. Impaired circulation and compromise of the soft-tissue envelope in patients with previous surgery increase the risk of infection and make eradication of infection more difficult, with lower overall success rates. Moreover, a subset of these revision cases represent low grade cryptogenic infection that is present before revision but is not clinically manifested until after surgery.

Several predisposing factors of infection have been identified. The inability of the host to prevent infection may be one of the most significant, as evidenced by the increased risk of infection in immunocompromised patients. In patients with rheumatoid arthritis, especially in males, the rate of infection has been 2 to 3 times higher compared to that of patients diagnosed with osteoarthritis. Studies show that patients with diabetes are also at an increased risk of infection, with the rate ranging from 3% to 7%. Moreover, patients with malnutrition, who experience frequent skin breakdown and wound complications, are predisposed to deep sepsis.

Other factors, such as obesity, oral steroid use, urinary tract infection, and concurrent infection at other sites, have been associated with increased rates of infection. Advanced age, an extended period of postoperative hospitalization, debilitation, and malignancy may also play a role in infection. Nonrheumatoid medical conditions have not been associated with increased risk. The type of implant used is also known to increase the risk of infection. Hinged and highly constrained implants have been associated with rates of infection of up to 16%, even with the use of contemporary prophylactic measures. The overall operating room environment with its numerous variables, including number of personnel, type of clothing worn, use of airflow systems, surgical technique, and operating time, all interact to have an impact on the overall incidence of infection.

Definition and Classification

Infection can be defined as superficial or deep. Superficial infection is confined to the skin and subcutaneous tissues. Although superficial infection can lead to deep prosthetic infection, its prognosis is more favorable. Prompt diagnosis and aggressive surgical intervention in dealing with wound drainage, erythema, or hematoma should prevent the occurrence of deep infection. Deep sepsis is defined as the presence of infection deep to the fascial layer with intra-articular involvement. Differentiating between superficial and deep infection can be challenging, although a complete patient history and risk factor assessment, along with a physical examination, radiographs, laboratory tests, aspiration, and nuclear imaging can help to make an accurate diagnosis. Generally, any chronic superficial infection strongly suggests deep involvement, and a draining sinus tract is indicative of subfascial involvement.

In order to determine the etiology of the infection and provide a guideline for treatment, classification is based on the timing of infection in relation to when the arthroplasty was performed. Generally, early infections are the result of surgical contamination or wound healing problems, and late infections usually represent hematogenous seeding. Some authors have classified infections as early or late with the subdivisions acute, subacute, or chronic. Others have described a 3-tiered classification system based on the time of onset of infection. However, there is wide variation in defining these terms; some authorities have described early infection as occurring within the first 6 weeks while others have described this period to be as late as 6 months after surgery. Greater emphasis has been placed on the duration of infection because it has important implications in regard to treatment and prognosis, with earlier infection being more amenable to prosthetic retention. Seventy-six infections in 74 patients were evaluated in a recent study. Based on duration of symptoms, the infections were classified as acute (less than 2 weeks) or chronic (2 weeks or longer), and the follow-up period was 2 to 10 years. The initial treatment modality chosen was successful in 69 of 76 patients (90%). The authors recommended that treatment selection based on duration of infection can result in predictable and successful results most of the time.

Diagnosis

The patient's clinical history, physical examination, and radiographic and laboratory studies, combined with the physician's suspicion, are usually adequate to make a diagnosis. Accurate and early diagnosis are important because a delay in diagnosis may decrease the likelihood of successful eradication of infection and limit potential treatment options. Because the most consistent finding associated with infection is pain, the possibility of infection should be considered when evaluating a patient with a painful TKA, especially if risk factors are present. Although the onset of pain in a TKA is alarming and easily identified, it may be difficult to differentiate normal postoperative pain from early infection. Poor postoperative rehabilitation, changes in pain intensity or character, or pain of a persistent, relentless nature are factors more likely to be associated with infection. Furthermore, rest or nighttime pain are more likely due to an infectious etiology compared to startup or activity-related pain associated with aseptic loosening. Physical examination findings typically include a warm, swollen, erythematous, stiff joint that is tender with range of motion. In addition, wound problems, including drainage, skin necrosis, cellulitis, or sinus tract formation, should heighten suspicion for the likelihood of infection.

Laboratory tests that can be performed include peripheral white cell count, erythrocyte sedimentation rate (ESR), and C-reactive protein (CRP) level. Because of the poor correlation of peripheral white cell count with infection, reliance on this test in establishing a diagnosis should be discouraged. The ESR may be elevated in cases of deep infection, although in a series of 72 infected arthroplasties, a sedimentation rate greater than 30 was reported to have a sensitivity of only 60% and a specificity of 65%. CRP levels may be more specific for infection because they are not likely to be elevated in cases of aseptic loosening and also have the benefit of returning to a normal level within a few weeks after surgery. The use of acute phase reactants may be of value in the diagnosis of infection, although their real benefit may be in assessing a response to and monitoring treatment once a diagnosis is made.

Radiographs will sometimes show minimal findings initially, and should be evaluated for component loosening, osseous resorption around the prosthetic margins, and other reasons for TKA failure. Bone scans, including those using technetium Tc 99m, gallium Ga 111, and indium-labeled white blood cells and antibodies, are used regularly and have varying levels of sensitivity and specificity in the diagnosis of infected TKAs. Their use may be best suited for cases in which the diagnosis is not clear.

Although joint aspiration has been questionable based on poor sensitivity and false negative rates of 15% to 20%, it remains an essential component in the diagnosis of infection in TKA. Based on intraoperative cultures, a recent study has shown a 100% sensitivity, specificity, and accuracy in diagnosis of infection in preoperative aspiration of 43 knees prior to undergoing revision arthroplasty. Because other variables, including white cell count, acute phase reactants, symptoms, and radiographs, correlate poorly with infection, aspiration was recommended as the most helpful approach to confirm or rule out the presence of infection in TKA. It is important that systemic antibiotics be discontinued for 10 to 14 days prior to aspiration to make sure that sensitive organisms are not suppressed.

Recently, polymerase chain reaction (PCR) has been used to help in the diagnosis of infection by detecting and amplifying bacterial DNA in aspirates. Benefits of this new technology include early and accurate diagnosis of synovial fluid for infection, which serves as an adjunct, or possible alternative, to current diagnostic modalities. Questions have been raised over a potentially high false positive rate and the detection of noninfectious or nonbacterial sequences. However, recent studies show that this may be less of a concern as new diagnostic protocols are introduced and current methods continue to be refined. Intraoperative frozen section also remains a valuable and reliable diagnostic method. A recent study showed that greater than 10 polymorphonuclear leukocytes per high power field was suggestive of infection, with a sensitivity of 84% and specificity of 99%. The authors reported that cell counts of less than 10 per high power field were not indicative of active infection despite previous reports in the literature.

Prevention

When discussing ways to prevent infection in TKA, it is important to consider the interaction of several factors, including the host, implant, and specific characteristics of the infecting organisms. The presence of an immunoincompetent zone surrounding implants, the affinity of certain organisms for binding to polyethylene or cement, or the ability of specific organisms to produce a protective mucopolysaccharide glycocalyx are all examples of local factors that may contribute to an orthopaedic infection. A thorough understanding of the biology of implant-related infections is essential to maximize the benefit that can be obtained when appropriate preventive measures are used.

Outline 1 lists organisms commonly associated with infected TKA. Although the literature shows that the prevalence of each organism varies, *Staphylococcus aureus* is predominant, followed by *S epidermidis* for prosthetic infections. The emergence of methicillin- and vancomycin-resistant organisms is of much concern as this limits possible treatment options, making certain infections more difficult or impossible to eradicate. Gram negative infections, while less common, can be difficult to eradicate because they are often refractory to treatment. Also reported in the literature are various cases of

Outline 1
Organisms involved in infected TKA

Predominant
- *Staphylococcus aureus* (coagulase +)
- *S epidermidis* (coagulase -)
- *Streptococci*

Emerging
- Methicillin-resistant *S aureus*
- Methicillin-resistant *S epidermidis*
- Vancomycin-resistant *Enterococcus faecium*
- *Enterococcus*

Other
- Gram negative: *Escherichia coli*, *Pseudomonas*, *Proteus*, *Bacteroides*, *Serratia*
- Fungal: *Candida albicans*
- Mycobacterial: *Mycobacterium fortuitum*, *Mycobacterium tuberculosis*
- Anaerobic
- Polymicrobial

fungal and mycobacterial infections, which require individualized treatment considerations. In addition, the possibility of polymicrobial contamination may present diagnostic and treatment dilemmas that require special attention.

Outline 2 reviews the methods available for the prevention of infection in TKA. Of all possible methods, administration of prophylactic perioperative antibiotics has been the most significant in reducing infection rates. Current recommendations for systemic intravenous antibiotics are listed in Outline 3. There are data that support the use of a first-generation cephalosporin to adequately cover the most common organisms related to TKA infection. The first dose is most important and should be administered 5 to 30 minutes prior to surgery to ensure adequate levels of antibiotics in the postoperative hematoma, and should be continued for 24 to 48 hours postoperatively. Specific modifications at individual institutions may be necessary because of hospital environment and specific infectious patterns. With an increase in cephalosporin-tolerant and -resistant organisms there is a tendency to consider vancomycin or the aminoglycosides as prophylaxis. Unless there is a cluster of infections with these organisms, routine prophylaxis with vancomycin or gentamicin should be avoided to prevent the emergence of organisms resistant to these agents.

Currently, there is no consensus on the use of antibiotics in cement at the time of implantation, although their use is warranted in certain clinical situations. In dealing with the immunocompromised host with systemic illness, or patients with significant risk factors, previous sepsis, or in the revision setting, the addition of antibiotics to cement appears to be beneficial. Commonly used antibiotic regimens include tobramycin 600 mg or gentamicin 0.5 to 1.0 g per 40 g of cement. The strength of the cement is not adversely affected when antibiotics are used in these doses. Significantly higher doses are used in cases of revision surgery, up to 4.8 g of tobramycin per 40 g of cement, where the cement serves as a temporary antibiotic depot when the structural properties are not a concern. Furthermore, the addition of more than 1 drug to the cement has been shown to improve elution and increase the intra-articular concentrations.

People are the main source of bacteria in an operating room. Limiting personnel and minimizing traffic in and out as well as around the operating room is beneficial. Variables such as good skin preparation and draping, surgical technique, antibiotic irrigation, and execution of a well-planned procedure in a timely fashion will also lower the risk of infection. Data also support the use of ultraviolet light to reduce airborne bacterial counts. Although their benefit has been questioned recently, closed air exhaust suits have historically been shown to reduce infection rates and provide the surgical team protection from patient contamination. Horizontal laminar airflow systems should probably not be used in TKA

Outline 2
Methods for infection prevention in TKA

Perioperative antibiotics

Surgical technique

Operating room environment

Ultraviolet light

Closed air exhaust suits

Vertical laminar airflow systems

Horizontal laminar airflow systems

Antibiotic irrigation

Antibiotic-impregnated cement

Late antibiotic prophylaxis

Outline 3
Prophylactic antibiotic regimens for TKA prevention

Cefazolin

- 1 g at surgery
- 1 g every 8 hours for 24 to 48 hours

Cefuroxime

- 1.5 g at surgery
- 750 mg every 8 hours for 24 to 48 hours

Vancomycin*

- 1 g at surgery
- 500 mg every 12 hours for 24 to 48 hours

*Use if allergic to penicillin or cephalosporin

because of documented increased rates of infection; therefore, vertical systems are recommended.

Finally, there has been debate over the use of late antibiotic prophylaxis for routine dental procedures. Although routine prophylaxis has been reported to be unnecessary in the dental literature, the potential risks and documented cases of infection create controversy. Current recommendations suggest a compromise that includes prophylaxis for all patients for 2 years following arthroplasty and then only for high-risk patients after this period, or in any case in which extensive dental procedures are to be performed. Outline 4 lists the recommended medications and doses for late antibiotic prophylaxis.

Treatment

Treatment options that are available for the management of infected TKA are reviewed in Outline 5. Although it is often appealing to attempt to eradicate infection using less aggressive methods, the basic premise that infected TKA is surgical disease that requires prompt and thorough surgical treatment is paramount. Consideration of several factors, including host factors, timing of diagnosis, infecting organism, and skin and soft-tissue concerns, is important in determining the best treatment plan. Differentiating superficial from deep sepsis is also important in selecting treatment and in determining overall prognosis, but aggressive surgical management along with intravenous antibiotics are required to prevent the occurrence of deep sepsis.

Retention of the prosthesis and treatment with repeated aspirations and antibiotics generally is thought to be inadequate. Because of the inability of the antibiotics to penetrate bacteria located deep within a glycocalyx, eradication rates are very low, often around 10% to 15%. In addition, spread of the infection to the interfaces between the implant and the bone make it inaccessible, rendering this form of treatment a method of suppression at best. Use of this method should be limited to cases in which very early diagnosis is made, usually within 48 hours, in which a penicillin-sensitive streptococcal organism is identified or in the patient who cannot tolerate the demands of more aggressive surgical management. If this option is chosen it is essential to have close follow-up of clinical and laboratory examinations to ensure a favorable clinical course. In addition, some recent reports have suggested that multiple drug combinations may further improve the overall efficacy of this regimen, and should be considered.

Outline 4
Late antibiotic prophylaxis recommendations

Clindamycin*
- 600 mg 1 tablet 1 hour prior to procedure

Cephalexin
- 500 mg 4 tablets 1 hour prior to procedure

*Alternative selection if allergic to penicillin

Outline 5
Treatment options

Prosthesis retention
- Long-term antibiotic suppression
- Multiple aspiration
- Debridement
- Arthroscopy
- Open arthrotomy

Prosthesis exchange
- 1-stage reimplantation
- 2-stage reimplantation (with or without articulating spacer)

Salvage procedures
- Arthrodesis
- Resection arthroplasty
- Amputation

The role of arthroscopy in the treatment of infected TKA remains unclear. Added benefits over aspiration include irrigation, debridement, and sampling of tissue to aid in culture and diagnosis. A few reports of success with this method have been reported; however, when compared to an open procedure, an incomplete synovectomy can be performed at best. In addition, although a modular polyethylene insert can be lifted to irrigate its undersurface, insert exchange cannot be achieved.

Open irrigation and debridement with retention of the components offers potential benefits that include a more thorough debridement and synovectomy, polyethylene exchange, and a lower morbidity associated with fewer and less aggressive surgical procedures. Historically, this treatment method has also been associated with higher failure rates of up to 75%. In a recent prospective study using strict criteria to select this treatment in 24 infected TKAs, all 10 of the immediate postsurgical infections and 10 of 14 late hematogenously infected knees remained infection-free at 48 months' follow-up. Diagnosis had to be made within 30 days after implantation or the patient had to have less than 30 days of symptoms in the late infection group. Radiographically there had to be a stable implant with sealed interfaces with no radiographic evidence of loosening or osteitis. Identified organisms had to be sensitive to standard antibiotics and the patients occasionally had to have multiple debridements. Another recent study had a success rate of 75% using this method with treatment selection based on symptom duration and patient class. Therefore, in a select group of patients in which a strict set of selection criteria are applied, debridement with retention may be a viable method of eradicating infection. Furthermore, data show that failure of this method does not compromise results obtained should subsequent 2-stage exchange need to be done.

Prosthesis exchange allows the added benefit of component and cement removal coupled with thorough debridement of bone and soft tissues. However, reported results are not as favorable with immediate exchange as they are in staged reimplantation protocols. Success rates from 30% to 80%, depending on organism virulence and other factors, have been reported. At the present time, immediate exchange is best considered when the infected patient presents with a loose or malaligned TKA that would otherwise fulfill the criteria for aspiration alone.

While optimum treatment of infected TKA continues to be debated, it appears that a 2-stage procedure with an interval period of antibiotics continues to be the most effective method to eradicate infection. Removal of the components and all cement, aggressive debridement of soft tissue and bone, addition of a local antibiotic depot, and a period of parenteral antibiotics (followed by subsequent reimplantation) is a typical protocol that is used. A recent study published the clinical results and survivorship in 64 cases using this technique with an average follow-up of 7.5 years. The reinfection rate was 9% with a 10-year survivorship of 77.4%; 78% of patients were satisfied with their overall result. The authors found this procedure to be an effective means of treatment and equated the results to that of revision of failed aseptic TKA. Another recent series reported a success rate of 87.2% in obtaining an infection-free and functionally satisfactory knee in 55 patients (average follow-up, 61.9 months). Based on these data, it appears that a 2-stage procedure still represents the standard of care in the treatment of infected TKA.

Discussion over the ideal duration for which intravenous antibiotics should be administered and the best time for reimplantation of components continues. A period of 6 weeks has been arbitrarily used in many protocols with success rates over 90%. It has been suggested that antibiotic penetration in the knee is negligible after 3 weeks because of significant scar tissue formation, and therefore the time to reimplantation can be shortened. Proponents of this method of treatment also recommend repeated debridements rather than prolonged antibiotics for this reason as well. Repeated debridements may also be required in certain cases of highly virulent organisms or polymicrobial infections to improve the overall success.

The recent use of articulating spacers loaded with high doses of antibiotics in cement in the interval period between component removal and reimplantation has been reported to have several advantages. Because movement and partial weightbearing are allowed, wound healing is enhanced, easier reimplantation is facilitated, and bone and soft-tissue quality and eventual functional range of motion are improved. A recent study reviewed 26 cases in which an articulating spacer was fashioned with high doses of antibiotics, tobramycin 4.8 g per 40 g of cement, in a 2-stage protocol with no recurrences of infection at average 30 months' follow-up. Another report using the Prosthesis of Antibiotic Loaded Acrylic Cement (PROSTALAC) system has shown successful results in a series of 37 infections with a cure rate of 92%. These reports suggest that use of a spacer has favorable effects on the soft tissues and improves the functional outcome while decreasing the risk of reinfection.

Refractory cases with resistant organisms, immunocompetent hosts, failure of previous methods of treatment, and inadequate skin and soft tissues are the main indications for a salvage procedure. Arthrodesis can reliably provide eradication of infection and solid fusion in a good position in about 90% of cases, although patients may be dissatisfied with a stiff limb. Resection arthroplasty is usually reserved for patients with significantly limited activity or the nonambulator, because functional results are predictably poor. Finally, amputation should be considered in those cases of life-threatening sepsis or as a last resort after failure of all other treatment options.

There is concern that economic factors may influence the choice of options in the treatment of an infected TKA. Hospital reimbursement is structured such that significant losses occur in the management of an infected TKA by delayed exchange. The potential financial loss coupled with the fear of colonizing the institution may discourage certain centers from accepting transfer of patients with an infected

TKA. Moreover, if less costly immediate exchange can expect 80% success compared with 90% from delayed exchange, will a 10% improvement in results justify the increased expenses as payers increasingly become the gatekeepers of care?

Reinfection of TKA

Although the occurrence of reinfection of previously treated infected TKA is low, especially with the use of a 2-staged protocol, it presents a significant challenge to the surgeon. The decision to undergo a subsequent 2-stage procedure or perform a salvage procedure is difficult. The Mayo Clinic reported on 24 cases of reinfection that were treated with numerous salvage procedures. Based on the successful results, nonarthroplasty options were strongly recommended in these cases. A more recent report has recommended reimplantation as the procedure of choice over resection arthroplasty or fusion based on their results in 12 patients with reinfections. Although it is an early report with a limited number of patients, the results are encouraging, allowing salvage of the knee while maintaining adequate functional outcome. Specific guidelines should be met before undertaking this treatment method and include the presence of a susceptible organism, immunocompetent host, adequate soft-tissue coverage, and an intact extensor mechanism. In addition, careful consideration of the patients' expectations and a detailed discussion with them prior to the reimplantation of another prosthesis is critical for a successful outcome.

Summary

The unique host, organism, and mechanical variables in each infected TKA limits rigorous adherence to a single treatment paradigm. Multiple factors, including the timing of the diagnosis, duration of symptoms, organism characteristics, antibiotic sensitivities, host factors, and bone and soft-tissue quality, all should be taken into account when formulating the individual treatment plan. It is critical, however, to collate these data and create a treatment plan with viable alternative contingencies in order to direct appropriate therapy for this complication. The goals of eradicating infection while optimizing functional outcome and maximizing patient satisfaction are among the many challenges the surgeon faces.

Patellofemoral Complications

The incidence of patellofemoral complications following TKA has been reported to range from 2% to 10%. Additionally, these complications account for a large percentage of revision total knee procedures. Patellofemoral complications are often related to component design and errors in surgical technique.

Early total knee prosthetic designs did not include patellofemoral resurfacing, resulting in residual patellofemoral symptoms in up to 30% of patients. More recent prosthetic designs allow for resurfacing of the patellofemoral compartment. While routine patellar resurfacing remains controversial, most would resurface patellae in patients with advanced Outerbridge III or IV articular changes, patellofemoral arthritis, and inflammatory arthritis of the knee. Obesity is associated with an increased incidence of anterior knee pain following TKA regardless of patellar management. Improvements in prosthetic design and in surgical techniques have led to a recent decrease in the incidence of patellofemoral complications. This section will review complications of the extensor mechanism following TKA including soft-tissue impingement, patellar component loosening and wear, fracture, disruption of either the quadriceps or patellar tendon, and instability.

Soft-Tissue Impingement

A fibrous module may develop on the undersurface of the distal quadriceps tendon following TKA. A painful clunking sensation occurs in these knees with active extension from approximately 60° to 30°. The pathogenesis of this nodule is not clear. Contributing factors may include a large patellar component with proximal patellar overhang, as well as abrupt changes in the radius of curvature of the femoral component, with irritation of the quadriceps tendon. Recent femoral component design changes, with deepening and elongation of the femoral groove as well as excision of synovial tissue in this location at initial surgery, have led to a marked reduction in the incidence of patellar clunk syndrome.

If this soft-tissue impingement is diagnosed early, exercise such as on a stationary bike with repetitive knee flexion and extension, may resolve the problem. Patients who remain symptomatic may be successfully managed with arthroscopic debridement of the nodule. Recurrence of soft-tissue impingement following arthroscopic debridement is uncommon.

Patellar Component Failure

A number of factors have been associated with an increased incidence of patellar component failure. These include increased thickness of the patellar-implant composite, oversizing of the femoral component, obesity, increased postoperative knee flexion, and increased patient activities. Patellar component failure has been more frequently associated with metal-backed implant designs. The advantage of metal backing is to minimize deformity of the overlying polyethylene, allowing more uniform distribution of load transmission as well as providing a mechanism for cementless fixation. The addition of metal backing results in reduction in polyethylene thickness, particularly at the periphery of the implant.

Failure modes reported with metal-backed designs include poor ingrowth into porous designs, with loosening polyethylene wear and fracture, peg failure secondary to high sheer stresses at this interface, dissociation of both the polyethylene and the metal plate, and component fracture. Polyethylene wear and dissociation complications expose the femoral component to the metal of the patellar component, resulting in audible grating, synovitis, and pain. This converts the patellar problem into a potential global joint problem secondary to metal-on-metal wear and rapid joint failure. In some situations, patellar component revision may require revision of all 3 components. Regardless, isolated patellar component revision is associated with a higher expected complication rate.

Loosening of cemented patellar components is infrequent with an incidence of less than 2%. Multiple predisposing factors have been reported (Outline 6). Management options vary. Patients who have minimal symptoms may be observed, but the majority will require surgical intervention. Isolated arthroscopic or open component removal may be used, or a femoral component revision can be done if the remaining patellar bone composite is adequate. With inadequate remnant of patellar bone, either a patelloplasty or patellectomy may be performed.

Presently, the majority of implant designs have an all-polyethylene patellar component using 2 or 3 peripheral pegs with cemented fixation. The use of polyethylene in these designs does not appear to be problematic, and component failures are infrequent.

Outline 6
Patellar component loosening

Predisposing factor

- Avascular necrosis of the patella
- Patellar fracture
- Patellar subluxation
- Osteoporosis
- Component(s) malposition
- Asymmetric patellar resection
- Cementing into deficient bone
- Failure of bone ingrowth

Patellar Fractures

Patellar fractures following TKA are uncommon, although one study reported a 21% incidence. A variety of causative factors have been implicated. These include mechanical compromise secondary to improper patellar resection, peg fixation, and cementation; patellar maltracking; avascularity of the patella; prosthetic design; obesity; increased knee flexion; excessive patient activity; and trauma.

An excessively thin or thick patella or an asymmetric resection may predispose to fracture. Although in vivo experiments suggest minimum patellar thickness of 15 mm, long-term clinical success without increased incidence of patellar fracture has been demonstrated with residual thickness of 12 to 13 mm. Excessively large femoral components in the anteroposterior diameter may increase the risk of patellar fracture.

Avascularity of the patella may occur during routine surgical exposure with a medial parapatellar incision and lateral retinacular release. The complex intraosseous and extraosseous patellar blood supply may be significantly compromised, contributing to an increased incidence of fracture. The importance of preserving the superior lateral geniculate artery during the release remains controversial. However, proper patellar tracking is critical to a successful arthroplasty. Maltracking can contribute to the development of "shear" type fractures of the patella.

Additional, large central patellar fixation lugs may require removal of a significant amount of bone, which can contribute to patellar fractures. Use of 3 peripheral fixation lugs is preferred in most present designs.

Patellar fracture patterns and their influence on clinical outcome have been classified. Fractures that do not involve loosening of the patellar component, disruption of the extensor mechanism, or major component malalignment may be treated nonsurgically with good clinical success. Surgical treatment of patellar fractures has been associated with poor results and is reserved typically for cases of implant loosening or severely displaced or comminuted fractures with significant extensor lags. Loose patellar components may be removed and the patellar resurfaced if 10 to 12 mm of bone remains. If not, a patelloplasty is preferred. Elaborate open reduction and internal fixation techniques are associated with significant complication rates and should be avoided. A partial patellectomy with extensor mechanism repair may be a more successful alternative.

Extensor Mechanism Rupture

Extensor mechanism rupture is an uncommon but devastating complication of TKA. Patellar tendon rupture occurs more frequently than quadriceps rupture, with a reported incidence of .17% to 2.3%. Causes of rupture are multifactorial, involving mechanical, vascular, and surgical technique factors.

While nonsurgical treatment is reported, rupture of the extensor mechanism requires surgical repair in most cases. Clinical results of acute repair are superior to delayed repairs. Augmentation of the repair with the semitendinosus tendon or allograft material may be preferred. Regardless of surgical technique, the clinical results are often disappointing, with persistent tendon rupture and extensor lag. Chronic patellar tendon ruptures may be salvaged with an extensor mechanical allograft. Prevention of extensor mechanism rupture by use of meticulous surgical technique and alternative exposure techniques during TKA is critical.

Patellofemoral Instability

The reported incidence of symptomatic patellar instability following TKA ranges from 1% to 20%. Patellar instability as recurrent patellar subluxation occurs more commonly than frank patellar dislocations. Patellofemoral instability may be related to trauma or prosthetic design. However, the majority of cases are secondary to errors in surgical technique and largely avoidable (see technique).

The reoperation rate for patellar instability is reported to be less than 1%. The specific mechanism of failure should be ascertained in each case. Standard radiographs, including proper patellar axial views, are mandatory. Computed tomography may be used to determine proper rotation of the femoral component with reference to the transepicondylar axis of the femur. Nonsurgical treatment is typically unsuccessful.

Isolated lateral retinacular release may be sufficient for patellar subluxation with normally aligned components. Proximal realignment may be used for recurrent dislocation-subluxation, especially secondary to quadriceps imbalance. Some surgeons have advocated distal realignment procedures, including a modified Roux-Goldthwait procedure, medial transfer of the medial half of the patellar tendon, and medial transfer of the tibial tubercle. An increased incidence of patellar tendon rupture and local hematoma have been reported with distal realignment procedures. If significant errors in femoral or tibial component positioning are present, especially internal rotation of the components, revision of the component(s) is the preferred solution. Critical to the successful management of patellar instability following TKA is proper identification of the etiology of maltracking.

Surgical Technique

The vast majority of patellofemoral complications are related to errors in surgical technique and can be avoided. Adequate surgical exposure is required to perform successful TKA. Good clinical success has been reported with a standard paramedian arthrotomy as well as a midvastus or subvastus approach. In stiff knees with limited motion, great care should be taken to preserve the integrity of the patellar tendons. Alternative exposure techniques such as the quadriceps snip, modified V-Y quadriceps turndown, or tibial tubercle osteotomy should be used.

Femoral component size will influence patellofemoral mechanics. Selecting an oversized component will lead to "overstuffing" the patellofemoral compartment and decrease knee flexion. Proper femoral component rotation is critical to achieve proper patellar tracking. The femoral component is positioned in line with the midepicondylar axis. The surgical techniques used to achieve this vary somewhat. The femoral component should be positioned laterally, in the mediolateral plane if possible, and excessive axial valgus alignment should be avoided.

Correct rotation of the tibial component is necessary for proper patellofemoral biomechanics. The tibial component should be positioned in external rotation with respect to the tibial surface. Internal rotation should be avoided. Useful anatomic landmarks include the anterior tibial cortex, the tibial tubercle, and the ankle joint. Proper rotary position typically necessitates slight uncovering of the tibial surface. Again, lateralization of the tibial component is preferred when possible.

Restoration of patellar bony thickness is desired. Similar composite thickness or slightly less may be achieved with either calibrated cutting or reaming guides or "eyeball" patellar osteotomy using calipers. The patellar osteotomy should begin at the chondro-osseous junction of the patella and typically removes more bone medially than laterally. One should avoid an oblique patellar cut with placement of the component primarily on the lateral facet, which can contribute to tracking. Medialization of the patellar component improves tracking. Cemented all-polyethylene components, using smaller peripheral peg fixation, are preferred. Poor results have been reported with metal-backed patellar components despite theoretical advantages. Use of all-polyethylene cemented components is recommended.

Tracking

Careful evaluation of patellofemoral tracking is performed using the modified "no thumbs" technique. We apply longitudinal traction to the extensor mechanism to maintain tension on the quadriceps during both flexion and extension. If lateral tracking or tilting is observed, a lateral retinacular release is performed from inside-out, preserving the superior lateral genicular artery. If maltracking persists, it is necessary to reevaluate the femoral and tibial component position. Occasionally, proximal and/or distal realignment procedures may be necessary to correct patellar tracking.

Excellent clinical results can be obtained with patellar resurfacing in TKA. The majority of complications are secondary to errors in surgical technique and are largely avoidable.

Periprosthetic Fracture

Distal Femur Fracture

The reported incidence of fracture of the distal femur proximal to TKA is 0.3% to 2.5%. Reported risk factors associated with this fracture include osteopenia, rheumatoid arthritis, chronic steroid use, revision arthroplasty, neuromuscular disorders, osteolysis, stiff knee, poor flexion arc, and anterior femoral notching in patients with osteopenia or anterior femoral notches greater than 3 mm in depth.

Fractures of the distal femur proximal to TKA are generally associated with low velocity trauma. However, minor injury is frequently associated with major damage to the knee. Condylar type femoral implants increase stress at the proximal end of the anterior femoral flange. Stemmed femoral components may transfer load to the proximal tip of the stem and predispose to more proximal fractures at the junction of the metaphysis and diaphysis of the distal femur.

The goal of treatment of these fractures is a painless, stable, mobile knee that permits a patient to return to prefracture activity. Clinical investigators have not been able to determine any method of treatment of these fractures that is superior. A meta-analysis reviewed 195 cases of fractures reported in 12 articles. Successful outcome was achieved in 83% of patients with nondisplaced fractures who were treated without surgery. In sharp contrast, 64% of patients with displaced fractures achieved successful outcomes regardless of surgical or nonsurgical treatment. Among the patients with displaced fractures, surgical treatment yielded 67% satisfactory outcomes, and nonsurgical treatment yielded 61% satisfactory outcomes. Considerations in choosing a method of treatment include fracture characteristics (displacement, alignment, rotation, comminution) and the integrity of the fixation of the femoral component to bone.

Nonsurgical treatment of these fractures is indicated for nondisplaced and minimally displaced fractures in a stable position with satisfactory alignment and rotation that are amenable to functional treatment with cast or cast brace. Surgical treatment of these fractures is indicated for displaced, malaligned, malrotated, and comminuted fractures that cannot be reduced satisfactorily. Methods of surgical treatment include osteosynthesis with blade plates, condylar screw plates, or condylar buttress plates; antegrade intramedullary rods; retrograde intramedullary rods with or without locking; and external fixation. Surgical treatment also includes revision knee replacement surgery with intramedullary stems with or without allograft augmentation. Surgical treatment of these fractures can be technically demanding. Surgeons who choose to treat these fractures should be expert with fracture reconstruction techniques and revision knee replacement techniques. These fractures may best be referred to specialized centers for knee reconstruction.

Evaluation and treatment of these fractures require satisfactory radiographic images. Oblique views may be required to obtain true anteroposterior and lateral views of the distal femoral condylar segment, which define the fracture characteristics and the integrity of the fracture implant fixation. Inadequate bone stock secondary to osteopenia or comminution can compromise a surgeon's ability to achieve fracture fixation. Methods for augmenting fixation in the distal condylar segment include intramedullary bone graft, polymethylmethacrylate bone cement, interfragmentary compression screws, and extramedullary allograft struts secured with cerclage wires. The approach to these fractures can be anterior or lateral. When retrograde intramedullary fixation is chosen, the design of the femoral component must permit sufficient intercondylar distance for introduction of the intramedullary nail. Postoperative mobilization of surgically repaired fractures aids rehabilitation, but it must be prescribed judiciously, depending on the stability of the reconstruction.

Nonsurgical treatment of these fractures reduces the possibility of infection and wound problems. However, immobility resulting from traction or splinting has been associated with muscle wasting, stiffness, bedsores, thromboembolic disease, urinary tract disorders, and psychologic deterioration. Surgical treatment of these fractures has the potential to create an anatomic distal femoral reconstruction with a stable, mobile knee, but is associated with increased infection and nonunion rates compared with nonsurgical treatment.

Proximal Tibia Fractures

Proximal tibia fractures below TKA are uncommon. No specific incidence has been reported. Stress fracture of the proximal tibia has been associated with malalignment and component loosening. Treatment of tibial fractures below TKA depends on the fracture characteristics and the integrity of the tibial implant fixation to the tibia. When the tibial implant is well fixed to bone, functional fracture treatment can be used to restore limb alignment and knee function. When the tibial implant is loose, fracture treatment must include revision arthroplasty. Stemmed tibial components are very useful in managing these fractures. The stem can bypass a proximal tibial reconstruction with or without allograft augmentation, and the stem can provide distal intramedullary fixation.

Patella Fractures

This topic is covered in the section on patellofemoral complications.

Wound Healing

Risk factors for wound problems following TKA include prior incisions about the knee; history of direct compressive trauma to the anterior knee; history of prior infection of the knee; history of burns or radiation to the anterior knee; use of azathioprine and short-acting antirheumatic drugs for treatment of rheumatoid arthritis; immunosuppression due to disease or medications; obesity; malrotation; extensive dissection associated with complex TKA; subcuticular skin closure with polydioxanone sutures; and associated conditions that may alter microcirculation, including diabetes mellitus, rheumatoid arthritis, and prolonged corticosteroid use that may be dose-related. Correction of severe deformity may also be associated with compromise of skin vascularity when the former concave side is stretched during realignment. Vascular studies of skin flap viability document lower transcutaneous oxygen tension on the edges of lateral skin flaps compared with medial skin flaps for several incisions. The more medial the incision, the lower the lateral flap oxygen tension. This information supports anterior midline incisions for TKA.

Prevention is the best treatment for wound problems following TKA. History of sepsis should be evaluated aggressively before surgery. Prophylactic antibiotics should be used. Prior incisions about the knee can be problematic during TKA. The surgical approach should be performed through existing incisions if possible. If this is not possible, skin bridges of at least 7 cm should be maintained. Smaller strips of skin that lie between 2 incisions risk skin necrosis, skin slough, and subsequent sepsis.

Wound problems from multiple incision, prior trauma, or prior infection may be averted by soft-tissue reconstruction before TKA. Soft-tissue expansion of contracted tissue about the knee with balloon skin expansion has been reported to be successful in preventing wound healing problems. Excision of abnormal skin and coverage with gastrocnemius flaps, soleus flaps, and free vascular flaps have provided satisfactory soft-tissue coverage prior to TKA and when treating soft-tissue defects postoperatively.

Lateral patellofemoral retinacular release is associated with an increased incidence of wound discoloration, superficial wound infection, and decreased skin oxygen tension. Although lateral release is effective in balancing the extensor mechanism, this technique should be used judiciously.

Wound problems following TKA should be treated aggressively. Persistent drainage, progressive and painful erythema, and marginal skin necrosis may be early signs of infection. The joint should be aspirated to document the presence or absence of deep infection. Antibiotic therapy should not be used until satisfactory deep and superficial cultures have been obtained. Early debridement, irrigation, and secondary closure may prevent deep sepsis and the prolonged sequelae of infection. After a TKA implant has been exposed because of tissue loss, aggressive reconstructive techniques, such as soft-tissue flaps, are required.

Neurovascular Compromise

Vascular Complications

Vascular compromise following TKA is uncommon. No specific incidence has been reported. Members of the British Association for Surgery of the Knee reported 14 arterial complications following TKA. Of these, 3 were the result of direct trauma to the popliteal artery or its branches, and 11 were due to thrombosis in the femoral popliteal system. In the 3 instances of direct injury to the artery, good recovery followed vascular surgery. Of the 11 instances of thrombosis, 2 patients died soon after surgery, 6 patients required amputation, 1 patient had persistent vascular symptoms and died 2 years later, and 2 patients recovered completely after vascular surgery.

The role of a tourniquet in arterial complications associated with TKA has been questioned. The tourniquet problem may be accentuated in patients who have diseased arteries that are not compressible and in patients who have a hypercoagulable state. There have been no reported cases of thrombosis of the vascular tree following TKA in which a tourniquet has not been used. Surgeons may give consideration to performing TKA without a tourniquet in patients with a history of vascular compromise.

Neural Complications

The most common neurologic injury following TKA is peroneal nerve palsy, which has a reported incidence of 0.3% to 4.0%. Peroneal nerve palsy is associated with correction of severe valgus and severe flexion deformity. The mechanism of peroneal injury following TKA has been reported to be traction on the nerve due to realignment of the limb. Direct compression of the nerve has also been suggested as a mechanism of injury. Reported risk factors for peroneal nerve palsy following TKA include severe valgus deformity, severe flexion deformity, use of epidural anesthesia, previous lumbar laminectomy, and previous proximal tibial valgus osteotomy.

Treatment of peroneal palsy following TKA should include preoperative recognition of risk factors and early recognition of nerve palsy. The physician should remove all dressings around the leg down to the skin, flex the knee, and reassure the patient at the time of diagnosis that full recovery is possible. It is not clear whether there is benefit associated with exploration of the nerve or removal of the wound hematoma.

Outcome following peroneal palsy associated with TKA is variable. Partial palsies generally lead to full recovery, and full palsies are associated with variable recovery.

Annotated Bibliography

Infection

Ayers DC, Dennis DA, Johanson NA, Pellegrini VD Jr: Common complications of total knee arthroplasty. *J Bone Joint Surg* 1997; 79A:278–311.

This article reviews the common complications associated with total knee arthroplasty, including infection, and concentrates on methods of prevention and offers recommendations for treatment of the infected total knee.

Backe HA Jr, Wolff DA, Windsor RE: Total knee replacement infection after 2-stage reimplantation: Results of subsequent 2-stage reimplantation. *Clin Orthop* 1996;331:125–131.

This study addresses the difficult situation of reinfection of total knee arthroplasty after initial successful 2-stage reimplantation. Early, although encouraging, results are obtained with reimplantation and the authors recommend this technique over arthrodesis or resection as long as appropriate guidelines are followed.

Duff GP, Lachiewicz PF, Kelley SS: Aspiration of the knee joint before revision arthroplasty. *Clin Orthop* 1996;331:132–139.

This study reviews the effectiveness of aspiration in the diagnosis of infection and compares it to other methods. The authors conclude that preoperative aspiration is the most useful study for the diagnosis or exclusion of infection in knee arthroplasty.

Goldman RT, Scuderi GR, Insall JN: 2-stage reimplantation for infected total knee replacement. *Clin Orthop* 1996;331: 118–124.

The study evaluates the long-term results of 2-stage reimplantation of infected total knee arthroplasty. Sixty-four cases in 60 patients were treated with an average follow up of 7.5 years. The authors report a 10-year predicted survivorship of 77.4%, which is comparable to revision of aseptic knee arthroplasty.

Hanssen AD, Rand JA: Evaluation and treatment of infection at the site of a total hip or knee arthroplasty. *J Bone Joint Surg* 1998;80A:910–922.

This comprehensive report reviews the prevalence, etiology, diagnosis, and prevention of infection at the site of total hip and knee arthroplasty.

Hirakawa K, Stulberg BN, Wilde AH, Bauer TW, Secic M: Results of 2-stage reimplantation for infected total knee arthroplasty. *J Arthroplasty* 1998;13:22–28.

The authors report the results of 2-stage reimplantation at an average follow-up of 5 years for infected total knee arthroplasty. They emphasize the importance of organism virulence, diagnosis, and previous surgery in determining overall success and describe their protocol for management.

Hofmann AA, Kane KR, Tkach TK, Plaster RL, Camargo MP: Treatment of infected total knee arthroplasty using an articulating spacer. *Clin Orthop* 1995;321:45–54.

Twenty-six patients with late infected total knee arthroplasty were treated using a method of staged reimplantation with an articulating spacer loaded with high doses of antibiotics. There have been no recurrences of infection at average follow-up of 30 months. The authors believe this technique decreases the risk of reinfection and optimizes functional outcome.

Lonner JH, Desai P, Dicesare PE, Steiner G, Zuckerman JD: The reliability of analysis of intraoperative frozen sections for identifying active infection during revision hip or knee arthroplasty. *J Bone Joint Surg* 1996;78A:1553–1558.

This article presents a prospective study demonstrating the reliability of frozen section to establish a diagnosis of active infection in revision arthroplasty. The authors state that at least 10 polymorphonuclear leukocytes per high power field is highly suggestive of infection.

Mariani BD, Martin DS, Levine MJ, Booth RE Jr, Tuan RS: Polymerase chain reaction detection of bacterial infection in total knee arthroplasty. *Clin Orthop* 1996;331:11–22.

The results of this study show the excellent sensitivity and accuracy of polymerase chain reaction to assist in the diagnosis of bacterial infection in patients with symptomatic knee arthroplasty. The authors conclude that this method should provide an additional, or possible alternative, assay in the diagnosis of infection when compared to standard microbiologic techniques.

Mont MA, Waldman B, Banerjee C, Pacheco IH, Hungerford DS: Multiple irrigation, debridement, and retention of components in infected total knee arthroplasty. *J Arthroplasty* 1997;12: 426–433.

This prospective study used specific criteria for selection of patients with infected knee arthroplasty for debridement and retention of components. There were 24 cases, 10 immediate postsurgical and 14 late hematogenously infections. All 10 of the acute and 10 of the 14 late cases were infection-free at final follow up of 48 months.

Wasielewski RC, Barden RM, Rosenberg AG: Results of different surgical procedures on total knee arthroplasty infections. *J Arthroplasty* 1996;11:931–938.

The authors evaluate the importance of basing treatment selection on duration of infection and the musculoskeletal condition of the patient. Seventy-six infected knee athroplasties were managed with the initial treatment modality being successful in eliminating infection in 90% of cases.

Patellofemoral Complications

Patellar Resurfacing

Barrack RL, Wolfe MW, Waldman DA, Milicic M, Bertot AJ, Myers L: Resurfacing of the patella in total knee arthroplasty: A prospective, randomized, double-blind study. *J Bone Joint Surg* 1997;79A:1121–1131.

One hundred eighteen total knee arthroplasties (58 with patellar resurfacing and 60 with patellar retention), utilizing a posterior cruciate ligament retaining design were evaluated at a mean 30 months. Total knee arthroscopy with retention of the patella yielded clinical results comparable with those of total knee arthroplasty with patellar resurfacing but was associated with a 10% need for subsequent resurfacing due to anterior knee pain.

Feller JA, Bartlett RJ, Lang DM: Patellar resurfacing versus retention in total knee arthroplasty. *J Bone Joint Surg* 1996;78B: 226–228

Comparative evaluation at 3 years of 40 patients randomized to either patellar retention or patellar resurfacing during total knee arthroplasty was performed. Evaluation included a specific patellar score. Results were comparable with both groups having lower scores in women and obese patients.

Soft-Tissue Impingement

Diduch DR, Scuderi GR, Scott WN, Insall JN, Kelly MA: The efficacy of arthroscopy following total knee replacement. *Arthroscopy* 1997;13:166–171.

Forty arthroscopic procedures performed on 38 patients with problematic total knee arthroplasties were evaluated following extensive nonoperative treatment. Arthroscopy successfully identified all cases of soft-tissue impingement, prosthetic loosening or wear, and successfully treated 73% of patients without recurrence. Patients were treated with 24 hours of perioperative antibiotics. No complications were reported.

Patellar Component-Design and Failures

Andriacchi TP, Yoder D, Conley A, Rosenberg A, Sum J, Galante JO: Patellofemoral design influences function following total knee arthroplasty. *J Arthroplasty* 1997;12:243–249.

The functional influence of patellofemoral design was evaluated testing two cohorts of patients following total knee arthroplasty while walking, climbing stairs, or arising from a chair. The designs differed primarily in the curvature of the femoral trochlea. There was no difference during walking or arising from a chair. However, the more anatomic femoral trochlear design demonstrated a significant functional advantage during stair climbing.

Feinstein WK, Noble PC, Kamaric E, Tullos HS: Anatomic alignment of the patellar groove. *Clin Orthop* 1996;331:64–73.

The variability in alignment of the natural patellar groove was determined about various anatomic axes of the femur using 3-plane radiographs and electronic digitization. The average orientation most closely approximated perpendicular to the transepicondylar axis in the coronal plane. However, the range varied extensively with no absolute reliable reference axis.

Healy WL, Wasilewski SA, Takei R, Oberlander M: Patellofemoral complications following total knee arthroplasty: Correlation with implant design and patient risk factors. *J Arthroplasty* 1995;10:197–201.

Two hundred eleven total knee arthroplasties were reviewed retrospectively regarding patellofemoral complications. Patellofemoral complications occurred in 27 knees (12.8%). Significantly higher rates of complications were noted in metal-backed patellar implants and those with cementless fixation. Less rate of patellar complications occurred in cemented all-polyethylene dome components.

Patellar Fractures

Ritter MA, Herbst SA, Keating EM, Faris PM, Meding JB: Patellofemoral complications following total knee arthroplasty: Effect of a lateral release and sacrifice of the superior lateral geniculate artery. *J Arthroplasty* 1996;11:368–372.

Four hundred twenty-eight out of 1,205 total knee arthroplasties performed between 1987-1989 underwent lateral release at surgery. In 107 knees the superior lateral geniculate artery was preserved. Preservation of this artery had no effect on patellar dislocation, radiolucency, loosening, or fracture. Lateral release was associated with significantly more patellar fractures.

Patellofemoral Instability

Whiteside LA: Distal realignment of the patellar tendon to correct abnormal patellar tracking. *Clin Orthop* 1997;344:284–289.

Thirty-one knees requiring distal realignment of the extensor mechanism to treat lateral patellar subluxation following total knee arthroplasty were reviewed at 2 to 16 years followup. Medial tibial tubercle transfer (18), modified Roux-Goldthwait (10), as well as medial transfer of the patellar tendon (31) were utilized. No late patellar subluxation or dislocations have occurred in these cases. Hematomas developed in three medial tubercle transfers.

Surgical Technique

Hsu H-C, Luo Z-P, Rand JA, An KN: Influence of patellar thickness onpatellar tracking and patellofemoral contact characteristics after total knee arthroplasty. *J Arthroplasty* 1996;11:69–80.

The influence of patellar thickness on patellofemoral kinematics and contact characteristics was investigated. Patellar thickness did not influence patellar flexion, rotation, or proximal distal shift significantly. A 2 mm thicker patella had a medial shift and remained laterally tilted during most of the knee flexion angles contributing to maltracking. Either a thicker or thinner patella had a smaller contact area. The authors recommend reproducing the original patellar thickness during patellar resurfacing in TKA.

Lewonowski K, Dorr LD, McPherson EJ, Huber G, Wan Z: Medialization of the patella in total knee arthroplasty. *J Arthroplasty* 1997;12:161–167.

Sixty-two knees were randomized into total knee arthroplasties with a centrally placed patellar component (31) or a patellar component placed on the medial two thirds of the patella (31). After 1 year, there was no difference with respect to either clinical or radiographic results. However, there was a reduction in the incidence of lateral release with medialization of the patellar component.

Periprosthetic Fracture, Wound Healing, Neurovascular Compromise

General

Ayers DC, Dennis DA, Johanson NA, Pellegrini VD Jr: Common complications of total knee arthroplasty. *J Bone Joint Surg* 1997; 79A:278–311.

This article is a good review of the diagnosis and treatment of complications following total knee arthroplasty.

Fractures: Distal Femur

Chandler HP, Tigges RG: The role of allografts in the treatment of periprosthetic femoral fractures. *J Bone Joint Surg* 1997;79A: 1422–1432.

This review article describes specific methods for using allografts to treat distal femur fractures proximal to TKA.

Ritter MA, Keating EM, Faris PM, Meding JB: Rush rod fixation of supracondylar fractures above total knee arthroplasties. *J Arthroplasty* 1995;10:213–216.

The authors present 22 displaced distal femur fractures of minimally constrained TKAs treated with Rush rod fixation. All fractures healed with a functional outcome. At follow-up, there was an increase in the valgus tibiofemoral angle following treatment. This method of surgical treatment is less invasive than plate osteosynthesis. However, fixation is less stable, and this method of fixation is not amenable for all distal femur fractures above TKA treated surgically.

Rolston LR, Christ DJ, Halpern A, O'Connor PL, Ryan TG, Uggen WM: Treatment of supracondylar fractures of the femur proximal to a total knee arthroplasty: A report of four cases. *J Bone Joint Surg* 1995;77A:924–931.

The authors report four cases of distal femur fractures proximal to TKA treated with a locked retrograde intramedullary nail. Indications for treatment and technical considerations are discussed. The authors highlight the importance of knowing the intercondylar geometry of the femoral condylar implant.

Sochart DH, Hardinge K: Nonsurgical management of supracondylar fracture above total knee arthroplasty: Still the nineties option. *J Arthroplasty* 1997;12:830–834.

These authors review principles of treating distal femur fractures proximal to TKA. In evaluating treatment options, they recommend nonsurgical treatment.

Fracture: Proximal Tibia

Felix NA, Stuart MJ, Hanssen AD: Periprosthetic fractures of the tibia associated with total knee arthroplasty. *Clin Orthop* 1997; 345:113–124.

The authors review 102 periprosthetic fractures of tibia and present a classification system: Type I = tibial plateau; type II = adjacent to implant stem; type III = distal to implant stem; type IV = tibial tubercle. Subclassifications were as follows: A = well-fixed implant; B = loose implant; C = intraoperative fracture.

Healy WL: Tibial fractures below total knee arthroplasty, in Insall JN, Scott WN, Scuderi GR, (eds): *Current Concepts in Primary and Revision Total Knee Arthroplasty.* Philadelphia, PA, Lippincott-Raven, 1996, pp 163–167.

Treatment of these fractures depends on fracture location, fracture characteristics, and tibial implant fixation. Surgical treatment requires fracture reconstruction struts and revision TKA expertise.

Wound Healing

Casha JN, Hadden WA: Suture reaction following skin closure with subcuticular polydioxanone in total knee arthroplasty. *J Arthroplasty* 1996;11:859–861.

The authors document a 20% incidence of suture reaction following TKA in wounds closed with subcuticular polydioxanone sutures.

Escalante A, Beardmore TD: Risk factors for early wound complications after orthopedic surgery for rheumatoid arthritis. *J Rheumatol* 1995;22:1844–1851.

Of 367 orthopaedic operations on patients with rheumatoid arthritis, 57 wound complications were reported, 26 of which were considered major. Factors significantly related to the occurrence of complications included Hispanic ethnicity and preoperative use of azathioprine. A nonstatistically significant increase in complications was noted in patients with diabetes mellitus, patients taking slow-acting antirheumatic drugs, and patients taking corticosteroids.

Gold DA, Scott SC, Scott WN: Soft tissue expansion prior to arthroplasty in the multiply-operated knee: A new method of preventing catastrophic skin problems. *J Arthroplasty* 1996;11: 512–521.

The authors report 10 knees in nine patients who had gradual soft-tissue expansion prior to knee surgery with balloon expanders. All patients had multiple prior surgical procedures around the knee. Subsequent major knee surgery requiring an arthrotomy was performed following removal of the tissue expander. All wounds healed without any complications.

Vascular Complications

Kumar SN, Chapman JA, Rawlins I: Vascular injuries in total knee arthroplasty: A review of the problem with special reference to the possible effects of the tourniquet. *J Arthroplasty* 1998;13: 211–216.

The authors report 14 arterial complications following TKA obtained by a survey of 147 members and associate members of the British Association for Surgery of the Knee. Three were due to direct trauma, 11 were due to thrombosis. The outcome following treatment for direct vascular injury is good. The outcome for vascular injury due to thrombosis is poor. The majority of surgeons used a tourniquet for TKA unless specific contraindications to a tourniquet existed.

Neural Complications

Idusuyi OB, Morrey BF: Peroneal nerve palsy after total knee arthroplasty: Assessment of predisposing and prognostic factors. *J Bone Joint Surg* 1996;78A:177–184.

Thirty-two peroneal nerve palsies in 30 patients were documented in a retrospective review of 10,361 consecutive TKA operations. Risk factors for peroneal nerve palsy included valgus knees, epidural anesthesia, previous laminectomy, and previous proximal tibial osteotomy. The authors highlight the high frequency of delayed presentation of this complication.

Classic Bibliography

Patellofemoral Complications

Patellar Resurfacing

Emerson RH Jr, Head WC, Malinin TI: Reconstruction of patellar tendon rupture after total knee arthroplasty with an extensor mechanism allograft. *Clin Orthop* 1990;260:154–161.

Engh GA, Parks NL, Ammeen DJ: Influence of surgical approach on lateral retinacular releases in total knee arthroplasty. *Clin Orthop* 1996;331:56–63.

Figgie HE III, Goldberg VM, Figgie MP, Inglis AE, Kelly M, Sobel M: The effect of alignment of the implant on fractures of the patella after condylar total knee arthroplasty. *J Bone Joint Surg* 1989; 71A:1031–1039.

Arthroscopy (Soft-Tissue Impingement)

Berry DJ, Rand JA: Isolated patellar component revision of total knee arthroplasty. *Clin Orthop* 1993;286:110–115.

Patellar Component Failure

Rosenberg AG, Andraicchi TP, Barden R, Galante JO: Patellar component failure in cementless total knee arthroplasty. *Clin Orthop* 1988;236:106–114.

Theiss SM, Kitziger KJ, Lotke PS, Lotke PA: Component design affecting patellofemoral complications after total knee arthroplasty. *Clin Orthop* 1996;326:183–187.

Tria AJ Jr, Harwood DA, Alicea JA, Cody RP: Patellar fractures in posterior stabilized knee arthroplasties. *Clin Orthop* 1994; 299:131–138.

Patellofemoral Instability

Grace JN, Rand JA: Patellar instability after total knee arthroplasty. *Clin Orthop* 1988;237:184–189.

Hofmann AA, Tkach TK, Evanich CJ, Camargo MP, Zhang Y: Patellar component medialization in total knee arthroplasty. *J Arthroplasty* 1997;12:155–160.

Lynch AF, Rorabeck CH, Bourne RB: Extensor mechanism complications following total knee arthroplasty. *J Arthroplasty* 1987; 2:135–140.

Periprosthetic Fracture, Wound Healing, Neurovascular Compromise

Chen F, Mont MA, Bachner RS: Management of ipsilateral supracondylar femur fractures following total knee arthroplasty. *J Arthroplasty* 1994;9:521–526.

Gerwin M, Rothaus KO, Windsor RE, Brause BD, Insall JN: Gastrocnemius muscle flap coverage of exposed or infected knee prostheses. *Clin Orthop* 1993;286:64–70.

Healy WL, Siliski JM, Incavo SJ: Operative treatment of distal femoral fractures proximal to total knee replacements. *J Bone Joint Surg* 1993;75A:27–34.

Johnson DP: Midline or parapatellar incision for knee arthroplasty: A comparative study of wound viability. *J Bone Joint Surg* 1988;70B:656–658.

Johnson DP, Eastwood DM: Lateral patellar release in knee arthroplasty: Effect on wound healing. *J Arthroplasty* 1992; 7(suppl):427–431.

Klein NE, Cox CV: Wound problems in total knee arthroplasty, in Fu FH, Harner CD, Vince KG, Miller MD (eds): *Knee Surgery.* Baltimore, MD, Williams & Wilkins, 1994, vol 2, pp 1539–1552.

Krackow KA, Maar DC, Mont MA, Carroll C IV: Surgical decompression for peroneal nerve palsy after total knee arthroplasty. *Clin Orthop* 1993;292:223–228.

Rush JH, Vidovich JD, Johnson MA: Arterial complications of total knee replacement: The Australian experience. *J Bone Joint Surg* 1987;69B:400–402.

Weiss AP, Krackow KA: Persistent wound drainage after primary total knee arthroplasty. *J Arthroplasty* 1993;8:285–289.

Chapter 36 Revision Total Knee Replacement

Modes of Failure

Failure of a total knee arthroplasty (TKA) is often a subjective determination to be made by both the patient and the surgeon involved. Although the need for revision has been considered the definition of failure, each patient needs to be assessed separately in the context of that patient's preoperative condition and general functional status. A knee arthroplasty that is painful, unstable, or functions poorly may also be considered a failure. The surgeon's assessment of the knee's status may not match that of the patient, and the expectations of the patient both preoperatively and postoperatively must be taken into account. A frank discussion before primary surgery of the possible outcomes will help to align patient expectations with the eventual result.

Evaluation of Failure

A thorough evaluation of the painful or failed total knee replacement begins with a careful history. Detailed questioning as to the primary problem is important. Patients may complain of pain, instability, stiffness, poor function, or a combination of symptoms. The time course of the complaint and whether it has been present since the time of surgery should be determined. The duration of the pain, radiating pain, if present, and any association with position or activity should be noted. The patient should also be asked about possible signs of infection, such as fevers or chills. The patient's ability to walk and perform daily activities, including stair climbing, are also important. The need for assistive aids, such as a cane or walker, should be recorded.

Physical examination usually begins with inspection concentrating on the status of the incision and any skin lesions or vascular changes that are present. Range of motion is recorded, with special attention paid to the extensor mechanism. Quadriceps lag and fixed flexion contractures may be present. Patellar clunking, patellar subluxation, and poor patellar tracking are all common forms of failure that can be detected through physical examination. Palpation of the patella while the knee is taken through a range of motion can help to reveal these findings. The knee should then be carefully palpated, and painful areas noted. Stability should be evaluated in varus/valgus, anterior/posterior, and rotational planes. Overall alignment of the limb and rotational deformity, if noted, should be carefully evaluated to determine the source of the deformity. Finally, the neurologic and vascular status of the limb should be assessed and compared to that of the contralateral limb.

Examination of the hip, spine, and abdomen may elicit other sources of pain, which may not be the result of knee arthroplasty. Lumbar radiculopathy, especially in the L4 distribution, can cause pain localized to the knee and can be diagnosed by careful physical examination and appropriate radiographic studies. Bursitis of the iliotibial or pes anserinus bursa may cause localized pain and respond to anesthetic and steroid injection. The pain of an arthritic hip may radiate to the knee. Finally, the patient's psychiatric health and employment situation may be contributing factors to a poor outcome and should be evaluated. A disparity between the patient's subjective level of symptoms and the physical findings may be due to referred pain or may be magnified for secondary gain. Any legal issues involved should also be noted.

Radiographic Examination Radiographs of the affected knee should be performed, preferably in a weightbearing position. They should consist of an anteroposterior view, a lateral view, and a Merchant view of the patella. If necessary, tracking of the patella can be evaluated by repeating the Merchant view in multiple degrees of flexion. Radiographs will provide important information about position of the components, loosening, ligamentous laxity, and any bone loss that may have occurred. If ligamentous laxity is suspected, stress views are occasionally helpful. Comparison with older radiographs will help define migration or loosening. Evaluation of the joint line can be made more accurately by comparison to the contralateral limb. Finally, failure of the polyethylene spacer or excessive wear can usually be detected on plain radiographs. In some cases, fluoroscopically guided films may be necessary to detect radiolucent lines or rotational malalignment.

Other studies may be indicated in selected patients. Bone scan may be helpful in confirming the presence of loosening or infection. Computed tomography (CT) scans and magnetic resonance imaging are seldom useful, because of artifact, but they can detect fractures or mass lesions around the knee. Arthrography is rarely indicated.

Laboratory Test All painful TKAs should be aspirated to rule out infection. Fluid should be sent for aerobic, anaerobic, fungal, and mycologic cultures. White cell count with differential cell count should also be performed on aspirated fluid. Routine blood tests should include white cell count and erythrocyte sedimentation rate. These tests are then evaluated in conjunction with the physical examination and radiographic studies to correctly diagnose an infected prosthesis.

Preoperative Considerations

Certain patient factors are associated with a higher rate of failure. Diabetes mellitus, rheumatoid arthritis, and prolonged steroid treatment have all been associated with a higher incidence of infection. Obese patients have an increased risk of postoperative patellar pain but have not been shown to have increased risk compared to median weight individuals.

Previous surgery may predispose the patient to higher rates of infection and failure of the implant. Bone loss and deformity following high tibial osteotomy or unicompartmental replacement may also reduce the expected rate of success. These patients often have patella baja as a result of their previous surgery. Past results after these procedures have more closely resembled revision surgery than primary surgery. Preoperative stiffness, which often limits range of motion postoperatively, should be discussed with the patient as a potential problem.

Implant Selection Implant selection may help to prevent early failure. Some designs have been especially prone to certain forms of failure. When considering revision of an implant, familiarity with the specific modes of failure will help with both evaluation and planning for surgery. For example, implants with a metal-backed patella have demonstrated higher rates of failure and should be noted if present. A boxy anteroposterior profile has been associated with development of quadriceps tendon scarring and the clinical syndrome of "patellar clunk." A flat, nonconforming tibial spacer has also been shown to result in early delamination of the polyethylene spacer and possible failure. Breakage of a component or failure of the interface between the tibial base plate and the polyethylene can also occur and result in instability, wear, and synovitis.

Pain

Pain following TKA must be carefully evaluated to identify the likely cause. Pain may be caused by mechanical failure of the implant or it may have a biologic source. Mechanical failure is characterized by pain with activity and, usually, a small effusion. Loosening of the implant, the most common mechanical cause of pain, is most easily diagnosed by tangential radiograph. Despite the common finding of loosening, knees that remain painful after the postoperative period must always be suspected of infection. Localization of pain to the patellofemoral joint or the tibiofemoral joint, especially with range of motion, may help to identify mechanical causes of pain. Biologic causes of pain include infection, neurogenic pain, and muscle weakness. Patients with unexplained pain who undergo revision surgery have a poor prognosis.

Superficial pain, which can be detected by careful examination and selective anesthetic injection, may be caused by a neuroma or by nerve injury following primary surgery. Some authors have reported successful treatment following superficial neurolysis.

Instability

Postoperative instability of the knee can manifest as locking, pain with activity, or limited function. Instability may be the result of poor placement of the components, migration of the components, excessive polyethylene wear, or ligament rupture. The direction of instability may help to pinpoint the underlying mechanical or biologic failure. Varus/valgus instability or anterior/posterior instability may cause pain with weightbearing and require the need for a cane or walker. Posterior cruciate ligament (PCL) rupture after PCL-retaining knee replacement may cause excessive anterior/posterior subluxation. PCL-sacrificing systems may suffer from the same problem if the polyethylene insert is too thin. Flexion instability may also allow the femoral component to "jump" over the tibial post, resulting in dislocation. Many systems offer a more conforming polyethylene insert that may reduce anterior/posterior instability. Stability may be restored by revision to a more constrained component or insert. The use of a thicker insert may also restore stability.

Anterior knee pain is one of the most common complaints after TKA. Poor tracking of the patella or a nonresurfaced patella may be the cause of anterior symptoms. Patellar subluxation can be caused by a tight lateral retinaculum, malalignment of the components, or failure of the medial capsular closure. Muscle weakness or early fatiguing may manifest as instability and will respond to a course of exercise therapy. Continuing symptoms may require soft-tissue realignment or revision of the components.

Restricted Range of Motion

The most common cause of stiffness is a poor preoperative range of motion. Despite careful attention to motion during primary surgery, stiffness may recur postoperatively. Flexion contracture of the contralateral knee may force the patient to equalize leg lengths by holding the operative knee equally flexed. Poor attention to rehabilitation following primary surgery can also limit attainment of normal motion. Functional range of motion differs for each patient and depends on the desired activity. In most instances, walking requires about 66° of flexion. Stair climbing requires at least 90° of flexion and rising from a chair approximately 100°.

Implant selection may cause a decreased range of motion. A femoral component that is too large in the anteroposterior plane will limit flexion. A too large spacer will limit full extension. Finally, a tight PCL after PCL-retaining knee replacement may limit full flexion.

Treatment can be problematic. Manipulation under anesthesia may be effective in the first 3 postoperative months. Persistent flexion contracture can sometimes be addressed by dynamic extension knee bracing. A tight PCL can often be treated by arthroscopic lengthening or release. More recalcitrant cases may require revision in an attempt to remove scar tissue and release any contractures that have formed inside the knee capsule.

Malalignment

Malalignment of the components at the time of primary surgery can cause early failure. The femoral component can be malaligned in 1 of 8 different directions or a combination of more than 1, leading to instability, pain, and early component failure. Flexion or extension of the component can limit range of motion or lead to anterior pain. Varus or valgus malalignment can lead to point loading of the spacer and early polyethylene failure. Elevation or depression of the joint line of more than 8 mm can also lead to limited range of motion or instability of the joint. Internal rotation of the femoral component can increase the likelihood of patellar dislocation, most often in the lateral direction. Finally, excessive internal rotation of the femoral component can adversely affect patellar tracking.

The tibial component can also be maligned in a number of directions. The component can be internally rotated, adversely affecting patellar tracking. Excessive external rotation may lead to tibiofemoral malrotation and posteromedial polyethylene wear. Varus and valgus malalignment can also cause point loading of the polyethylene and early failure. Too much posterior slope can cause anterior/posterior instability and instability in flexion, and too little posterior slope can limit flexion.

Poor placement of the patella can result in patella alta or baja, which may limit range of motion and lead to anterior pain. Excessive lateral or medial placement may adversely affect patellar tracking. An oversized component may lead to stuffing of the joint, poor range of motion, and anterior knee pain. While mild malalignment of 1 component in 1 plane may be tolerated, a combination of malalignments in 1 or more components has been shown to predispose an implant to failure.

Trauma

Fracture may be caused by almost any traumatic event, from very high to very low energy. Osteoporotic bone may be more prone to fracture. Supracondylar femur fractures are the most commonly seen. Notching of the anterior femur during bone preparation, rheumatoid arthritis, and osteoporosis are all associated with supracondylar femur fracture. Open reduction and internal fixation with a plate or an intramedullary nail has become the most commonly advocated treatment. Patella fracture may be caused by direct trauma or by failure of weak bone exposed to the strong pull of the quadriceps mechanism. Sacrifice of the lateral geniculate artery or an overly aggressive patella bone cut (leaving less than 12 mm) have been associated with patellar fracture. Nondisplaced fractures may heal well after immobilization. Displaced fractures require open reduction and internal fixation or revision. Extensor mechanism rupture can occur after trauma of even a minor nature and requires surgical repair if the patient cannot actively extend the knee. Collateral ligament rupture can also follow trauma and can sometimes be treated with immobilization followed by early range of motion in a hinged brace. Persistent instability may require the insertion of a more constrained component or insert.

Aseptic Loosening

Malposition of components can lead to higher contact stresses in polyethylene, resulting in delamination, pitting, and large volumes of debris. The ensuing inflammatory reaction can lead to resorption of bone and eventual component loosening. Tibial inserts with areas less than 6 mm thick have also been associated with early failure and accelerated osteolysis. Loose polyethylene components are associated with accelerated loss of bone. Screw fixation of uncemented tibial components has shown to accelerate osteolysis in some cases. Chronic instability may also lead to accelerated polyethylene wear.

Any loosening evident on radiographs less than 2 years after the index arthroplasty should raise suspicion of infection. Finally, at the time of revision, the surgeon should be prepared to find more extensive bone loss than may be apparent on preoperative radiographs.

Infection

Infection can occur at any time after knee arthroplasty. Infections that occur less than 1 month after the primary procedure can be assumed to have become infected at the time of surgery. Later infections are more likely to be hematogenous in origin and have been reported many years after primary arthroplasty. Careful questioning may reveal a recent medical procedure, such as dental work, or a distant infection that may have been the source of the infection.

The most common symptom of infection is pain in the affected joint. Fever, chills, or erythema may be present, but their absence does not rule out infection. Erythrocyte sedimentation rate or creatine phosphate, if elevated, are good indicators of the presence of infection but are not specific enough for a definitive diagnosis. Aspiration has been the most reliable indicator of infection if the subsequent culture is positive. Differential cell count of the aspirated fluid can be very reliable if the white cell count is greater than 50,000 and the percentage of polymorphonuclear leukocytes is greater than 90%. Bone scan and indium-labeled scan may be helpful in a limited number of cases but are less specific.

The most successful treatment for infection has been 2-stage exchange revision arthroplasty. Other treatment options include irrigation and debridement, 1-stage exchange, and antibiotic suppression. There is some evidence that early infections, those occurring less than 1 month following primary arthroplasty, may be treated successfully by open irrigation and debridement until the tissues are grossly free of infection, followed by 6 weeks of intravenous antibiotics.

Other Causes of Failure

Reflex sympathetic dystrophy (RSD) is a syndrome of pain out of proportion to the clinical findings. Erythema, warmth, stiffness, and cutaneous hypersensitivity are often present. RSD is characterized by a slow postoperative course and poor function. Bone scan may demonstrate diffuse increased uptake in the affected area. RSD is a diagnosis of exclusion. The syndrome may respond to a concerted exercise program and sympathetic blockade.

Summary

Failure of TKA can be a frustrating and difficult problem for both the patient and the surgeon. Careful physical examination, appropriate diagnostic tests, and, in some cases, revision surgery may be able to improve an arthroplasty that has not performed up to expectations. A specific diagnosis should be made before any surgical intervention is contemplated.

Bone Defect Classification

Frequency of Bone Defects

Bone loss is commonly encountered in revision TKA. At the Anderson Orthopaedic Research Institute (AORI) in Alexandria, VA, 289 of 393 revision procedures (74%) involved knees with significant bone loss that required special management. Most of the severe bone damage in these cases was caused by debris-generated osteolysis or by septic or aseptic component loosening. Intraoperatively, even more bone may be lost when a well-fixed component is removed. Because this bone loss compromises the stability of the new components, bone grafts with stemmed components and salvage prostheses are needed in some situations to restore durable revision component fixation and knee stability.

Defect Classification as a Management Tool

A bone defect classification system is a useful tool when a revision knee arthroplasty is being planned. By defining the extent of bone damage from preoperative radiographs, the surgeon is able to select an appropriate revision knee system to properly reconstruct the knee. In most instances bone damage can be successfully managed by the modular augments available with a revision knee system. However, custom devices, rotating hinges, and allograft reconstruction with long-stemmed components are necessary when bone loss is severe. Special equipment such as high-speed burrs and mounting platforms used to prepare allograft bone must be prearranged and available in the operating room for the revision surgery.

Evaluation of Different Treatment Modalities

A variety of prosthetic options are available for managing bone defects at the time of revision surgery. The relative merit of these options has not been determined. When the extent of bone loss has been appropriately categorized, the surgeon is able to compare different revision prostheses and bone defect management techniques. For instance, rotating hinge implants are often used when bone loss is severe. Another option would be to repair the defect with an allograft and a long-stemmed revision component. With a bone defect classification system, the surgeon could determine the efficacy of such methods relative to the extent of bone damage. The clinical results of revision TKA are valid when the severity of bone damage is documented by an adequate percentage of cases in each category.

The AORI Bone Defect Classification

The AORI bone defect classification was developed to provide a rational and easily remembered description of bone loss to be used in revision knee arthroplasty. Bone loss that occurs with failed arthroplasty involves similar metaphyseal segment of bone on both the tibial and femoral side. Therefore, the same categories can be used to describe both femoral and tibial defects. Terms such as cortical versus cancellous, contained and uncontained, and central or peripheral are not used because bone defects often fall intermediate to such categories. Patellar bone defects are not classified because revision patellar prostheses are not available to manage such defects.

Three Types of Metaphyseal Bone Loss

The AORI bone defect classification defines 3 levels of bone loss. The cancellous bone of the metaphyseal segment of the distal femur or proximal tibia can be relatively intact, damaged, or deficient (Figs. 1 and 2). A type 1 defect (intact bone) is defined as relatively healthy metaphyseal bone with good cancellous structure present at a reasonably normal joint line level. It is appropriate to use primary style components in the revision of a type 1 defect. A type 2 defect (damaged bone) is defined as bone loss that includes some loss of cancellous structure for component fixation. Without repair of the bone damage, the joint line is altered. Component fixation would be precarious without the addition of a stem to the component. Modular and stemmed revision components are gener-

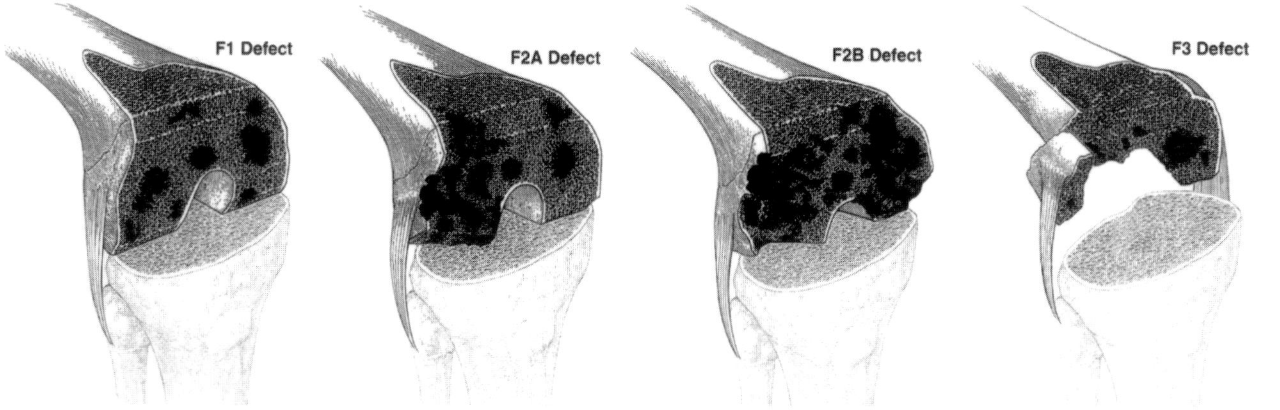

Figure 1

Anderson Orthopaedic Research Institute femoral bone defect classification. (Reproduced with permission from Engh GA: Bone defect classification, in Engh GA, Rorabeck CH (eds): *Revision Total Knee Arthroplasty*. Baltimore, MD, Williams & Wilkins, 1997, pp 63-120.)

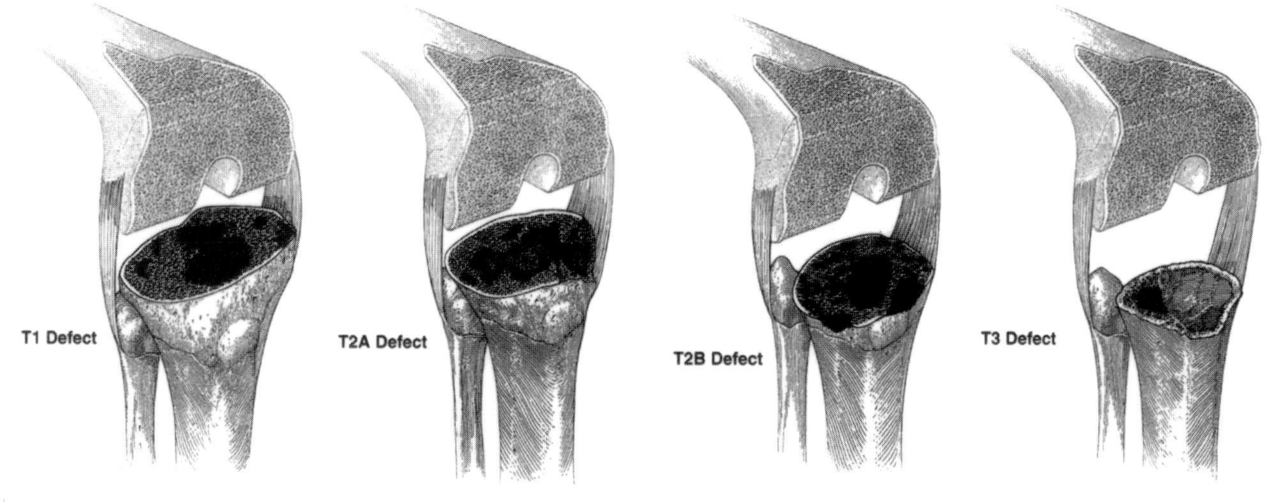

Figure 2

Anderson Orthopaedic Research Institute tibial bone defect classification. (Reproduced with permission from Engh GA: Bone defect classification, in Engh GA, Rorabeck CH (eds): *Revision Total Knee Arthroplasty*. Baltimore, MD, Williams & Wilkins, 1997, pp 63-120.)

ally recommended to manage type 2 defects. A type 3 defect (deficient bone) is defined as bone loss such that the cancellous structure will not provide adequate support for a condylar-shaped revision component. The cancellous structure will need to be reconstructed with an allograft, or sacrificed and replaced with a rotating hinge or custom component that provides prosthetic stability through intramedullary component fixation.

Type 1 Bone Defects The preoperative radiographs of type 1 femoral and tibial (F1 and T1) bone defects demonstrate a correctly aligned component, no evidence of osteolysis, no component migration, and a relatively normal joint line level. The metaphyseal segment appears full on anteroposterior (AP) radiographs with an intact segment of bone distal to the epicondyles (femoral defects) and proximal to the fibular head (tibial defects). The lateral radiographs demonstrate relatively normal AP dimensions of the femur, and the bone of the posterior femoral condyles is preserved (that is, the sagittal profile of the femur is intact).

With type 1 bone defects, healthy cancellous bone that will support either a primary or revision component should be present at the time of revision surgery. Small bone defects are managed either with cement fill or a small amount of morcellized bone graft. Augments are not necessary; therefore, revision components are usually not needed. The decision to use a primary component or a stemmed revision component is made based on the need for knee stability, not on quality of bone.

The postoperative radiographs of type 1 bone defects demonstrate full bone segments as would be seen on the postoperative radiographs of a primary knee arthroplasty. The flare of the metaphyseal bone is evident on the AP radiograph. On radiographs of an F1 defect, cancellous bone is visible between the epicondyles and the femoral implant. Likewise, on radiographs of a T1 defect, bone is present above the tibial tubercle and fibular head to the tibial component.

Type 2 Bone Defects The preoperative radiographs may demonstrate subsidence with circumferential radiolucency at the margins of a component. The component often subsides and migrates into an incorrect varus or valgus position in relation to the anatomic axis of the corresponding bone. The tibial component most commonly migrates into a varus position. Small areas of osteolysis may be visible at the margins of the component. These lesions usually have a scalloped border of sclerotic bone. Type 2 bone defects are commonly seen when a primary arthroplasty fails by component loosening.

Angular subsidence of a knee implant usually results in a bone defect in only one condyle or plateau. In this instance, the defect is classified as either an F2A or T2A defect (the A indicating that only one condyle or plateau is involved). Bone in the opposite condyle or plateau is present at a relatively normal joint line level.

Type F2 and type T2 bone defects are commonly encountered with revisions of failed stemmed implants. When a stemmed revision component loosens, the stem of the implant controls subsidence and prevents angulation of the component. Symmetrical bone loss usually occurs in both condyles or plateaus and the fullness of the metaphyseal bone segment is reduced. When both condyles or plateaus are involved, the corresponding defects are F2B and T2B.

Modular augments are usually used to reconstruct a type 2 bone defect. F2A bone defects are best managed by retaining the bone in the relatively undamaged femoral condyle and repairing the damaged condyle with modular distal and posterior augments. T2A bone defects are managed by repairing the damaged plateau with either wedge-shaped or step-wedge augments.

In some situations, it is contraindicated to restore the joint line through component augmentation. Joint line elevation is indicated when a large preoperative flexion contracture cannot be corrected by posterior capsular release alone. The surgeon may decide to resect bone at a more proximal level, converting an F2A defect to an F2B category.

The augments used to repair the corresponding defect are apparent on postoperative radiographs of a type 2 defect. The joint line has been restored with the augment filling the space between the damaged bone segment and the component. Cement fill, occasionally reinforced with bone screws, may have been used to replace lost bone. Small femoral bone grafts are usually not visible. On the lateral postoperative radiographs, the grafts are hidden by the box of a posterior stabilized femoral component.

If an augment is not used in the revision surgery, a type 2 defect would appear as component elevation from the normal joint line position. Patella baja and proximal overhang of the posterior femoral condyles of the component are radiographic features of a type F2B bone defect managed without femoral component augmentation.

Type 3 Bone Defects The prerevision radiographs of type 3 bone defects usually demonstrate either large osteolytic lesions, severe component migration, large areas of bone loss filled with cement from an earlier revision procedure, or the failure of a hinged component. When a component subsides and the epicondyles flare away from the femur, the bone loss is classified as an F3 defect. T3 defects are identified by loss of the trumpet-shaped proximal expansion of the tibia.

In many cases, the severity of bone loss secondary to osteolysis is not apparent on the preoperative radiographs. Femoral osteolysis is usually most severe adjacent to the posterior femoral condyles. On the AP radiograph, severe osteolytic bone destruction appears as a radiolucency, often with a sclerotic border expanding toward the cortical margins of the metaphyseal bone. On the lateral radiograph, these lesions are often demarcated by a sclerotic rim of bone. It is important to realize that even though the lesion may appear small, far greater areas of bone loss may be present. The appropriate components and graft material to manage severe type 3 defects should be available.

The surgical reconstruction of type 3 defects is a salvage type procedure requiring either substitution for lost bone with a hinged or custom component, or a repair of the metaphyseal segment with an allograft and long-stemmed implant. The bone may be deficient in one or both condyles or plateaus. Femoral head allografts may be used to fill defects in one condyle or plateau. Hemispherical reamers are used to prepare the allografts and the defect to matching shapes. Defects that involve the entire metaphyseal segment can be repaired using a distal femoral or proximal tibial allograft that substitutes for a deficient segment of bone. The epicondyles of the host bone are osteotomized and reattached to the allograft to achieve varus-valgus stability. Step cuts of the allograft and host bone provide rotational stability to the reconstruction.

When the deficient metaphyseal segment of a type 3 defect is managed with allograft reconstruction, the differing bone density of the allograft and host bone is visible on postoperative radiographs. With an allograft reconstruction, a polyethylene insert of nominal thickness can be used to restore a relatively normal joint line, also apparent on postoperative radiographs. All revision cases managed with hinged devices and tumor replacement prostheses are classified as F3/T3 bone defects because they replace much of the metaphyseal bone segment. Fixed and rotating hinge components are identified by the linkage that joins the components.

Using a Bone Defect Classification System

Learning to use a bone defect classification system requires practice. In most cases the defects are obvious and easy to classify. For cases that fall on the borderline, the preoperative and postoperative radiographs, along with the intraoperative findings and the type of implant used in the reconstruction, can be reviewed in order to confirm the type of defect. If the bone defect classification system was used correctly, the method of reconstruction should be appropriate.

Surgical Technique and Principles

Epidemiology

Approximately 100,000 Medicare patients per year undergo knee arthroplasty in the United States. Despite the demonstrated success at over a decade of follow-up, inevitably a small percentage of these patients will require revision surgery. Younger patients, who place a higher demand on their knees than Medicare patients, may also require revision knee arthroplasty. The probability of revision knee surgery 2 years after primary knee arthroplasty has been reported to be less than 3%. The likelihood of revision is related to several factors: (1) male gender, (2) younger age, (3) longer length of hospital stay for the primary knee replacement, (4) more diagnoses at the time of hospitalization for primary knee replacement, (5) unspecified arthritis type, (6) surgical complications during hospitalization for primary knee replacement, and (7) primary knee replacement performed at an urban hospital.

It can be concluded that younger, more active, male patients are likely to develop difficulties with knee replacement, as well as patients who are either infirm and medically predisposed to complications or who suffer technical problems that lead to complications with their arthroplasty. Revision knee arthroplasty does not resemble primary knee arthroplasty in either the technical demands placed on the surgeon or the depletion of resources experienced by the health care system. A 41% increase in surgery time has been reported for revision TKAs over primary surgeries without commensurate compensation. This increase provides little incentive for experienced surgeons to deal with problems that may have been generated outside their own practices. In addition, greater blood loss, increased length of hospital stay, and a much higher complication rate than primary knee arthroplasty are other factors related to revision knee arthroplasty that increase the surgeons' liability. It has been estimated that infected knee arthroplasties that required revision surgery used 3 to 4 times more hospital and surgeon resources than primary knee arthroplasty, and that infection approximately doubled the resource consumption when septic revisions were compared with nonseptic revision knee arthroplasty. The same report estimated that a hospital experienced a net loss of approximately $15,000 per case, and $30,000 per Medicare case, for the surgical treatment of an infected knee arthroplasty.

Basic Science

Most basic science evaluation of knee arthroplasty surgery is pertinent specifically to primary and not revision procedures and prosthetic devices. Some work, however, has been published on the pathophysiology of arthroplasty failure, specifically related to the production of wear debris and the biologic response to it. Interleukin-1β levels from synovial aspirates of knee joints have been quantified. In a comparison of osteoarthritic knees with failed arthroplasties involving titanium alloy prostheses and failed chrome cobalt arthroplasties, the greatest concentration of interleukin-1β appeared in the failed titanium prosthesis; the concentration was lowest in the osteoarthritic knee. This difference was attributed to the synovial response resulting from inflammatory wear debris produced by titanium prosthetic devices.

In a comparison of 65 cemented and 36 cementless knee and hip arthroplasties that had failed, 3 groups were identified: (1) loose implants with ballooning radiologic osteolysis, (2) loose implants without osteolysis, and (3) well-fixed implants. T-lymphocyte counts and interleukin-1 and interleukin-6 assays were performed, leading to the conclusion that different biologic mechanisms for loosening and osteolysis are present for cemented and uncemented implants. T-lymphocyte modulation of macrophage function, largely in response to wear debris, may be an important interaction at the prosthetic fixation interface.

Concern over generation of particle debris led to a study that evaluated the interface between the nonarticular polyethylene surface and the modular base plate in tibial components. More severe degrees of wear on the tibial insert undersurface correlated directly with tibial metaphyseal osteolysis or osteolysis around fixation screws, which suggests that the surface finish of these 2 materials, as well as the locking mechanisms, may need to be enhanced so that the cost of modularity does not outweigh its benefits.

Mobile bearing arthroplasties promise reduced wear because of increased articular surface contact area. These designs, however, may not ensure against generation of wear debris. Meniscal bearing thickness, malpositioning of the metal tibial tray, inability of mobile patellar bearings to rotate, and degradation of the subsurface of the polyethylene led to severe symptomatic polyethylene failure in a minority (8 of 276) of meniscal bearing implants. There seems to be a distinction, however, between the range of particle sizes generated by failed total hip replacements and those generated by failed knee arthroplasties. A larger range of particle sizes has been identified in failed knee arthroplasties; however, very small particles are common to both groups. This finding has been postulated to explain the more extensive osteolysis frequently observed in hips as opposed to knees despite the generally greater subsurface stresses that polyethylene experiences in knee prostheses.

Classification of Revision Knee Arthroplasty Failures

Failed revision knee arthroplasty embraces a wide range of diagnoses, each with specific implications for surgical treatment and prognosis. The first series of revision knee arthroplasties to acknowledge this difference reported the results of revision knee arthroplasty by reason of failure, and established 4 causes of failure: loosening, instability, malrotation and patellar instability, and undiagnosed pain.

Two important principles emerged from these causes. The first was that patients with undiagnosed pain rarely benefited from revision surgery. This principle establishes the absolute importance of determining precisely why the primary arthroplasty failed before planning revision. The second principle describes the inextricable relationship between patellofemoral instability and femoral and tibial component malposition. Following a later series of revision knee arthroplasties, 4 more causes of primary knee arthroplasty failure were added: breakage, sepsis, extensor mechanism rupture, and stiffness. Subsequently, a ninth cause, fracture of the femur or tibia as an indication for revision knee arthroplasty, completes the list of possible causes of failure. It is incumbent on the surgeon to establish a diagnosis, facilitated by this list (Table 1), before embarking on revision knee arthroplasty.

Preoperative and Intraoperative Evaluation of Failed Primary Knee Arthroplasty

Evaluation of the painful or failed knee arthroplasty must begin with a thorough history and physical examination. Three patterns of pain can be recognized: (1) The patient who describes the same pain, unaffected by the knee arthroplasty surgery, may well be experiencing pain from a referred source. The spine should be evaluated, and consideration of ipsilateral hip pathology is essential. (2) Pains that have persisted since the time of arthroplasty, but which differ in nature or intensity, suggest infection, a tight painful reconstruction, failure of bone ingrowth in uncemented prosthetic devices, or reflex sympathetic dystrophy. (3) New pains that occur months to years after the time of primary knee arthroplasty again suggest infection, but could also be caused by loosening, breakage, or fracture. The knee that has failed with instability, whether tibiofemoral or patellofemoral, will present with distinct symptoms and physical examination.

Imaging and CT Scanning

Conventional radiographs, usually performed during weight-bearing, that include anteroposterior, lateral, and patellofemoral views are essential. Radiographic evaluation

Table 1
Indications for revision knee arthroplasty

Type	Diagnosis	Percent of good or excellent results
I	Loosening	76%
II	Instability	100%
III	Malrotation and patellar instability	100%
IV	Undiagnosed pain	0%
V	Breakage	0%
VI	Sepsis	0%
VII	Extensor Rupture	0%
VIII	Stiffness	0%
IX	Fracture	0%

of the ipsilateral hip joint should be considered in the presence of a painful knee arthroplasty. A simple and effective method of fluoroscopic evaluation of painful knees can establish a diagnosis of aseptic loosening with a radiograph guided by fluoroscopy. These radiographs should include lateral views of each of the 3 important femoral component interfaces. This method can be of particular use in the evaluation of the uncemented femoral component, very commonly included in hybrid fixation techniques. Other researchers evaluated ^{99m}Tc methylene diphosphonate (TcMDP) scintigrams, as well as gallium (^{67}Ga) citrate scintigrams, on patients who have TKAs. These researchers identified patients with asymptomatic knees who were undergoing scans for other pathology, those with aseptic or septic loosening, and those with pain without radiologic evidence of loosening. Technetium and gallium scintigrams can be used to demonstrate aseptic or septic loosening in knee prostheses. Pain with a normal scan is probably not caused by loosening or infection. Our understanding of the painful knee arthroplasty has been increased by 3-dimensional imaging that reveals rotational positioning of femoral and tibial components. This imaging can be accomplished using CT. The internally rotated femoral component can cause many complications, including patellar tracking; there is reason to believe it may be responsible for pain, especially in the presence of poor motion. Tibiofemoral instability may be exacerbated by component malrotation.

Aspiration

Preoperative aspiration of synovial fluid prior to knee arthroplasty revision surgery represents the standard of care in the diagnosis of sepsis. In 1997, researchers reported an overall sensitivity of 55%, specificity of 96%, and accuracy of 84%. These figures were improved, however, when aspirations were performed after ensuring that the patient was not concurrently on antibiotic therapy, and subsequent researchers reported a sensitivity, specificity, and accuracy of 100% with aspirations off of antibiotics. Furthermore, the Westergren erythrocyte sedimentation rate, peripheral leukocyte count, and presenting symptoms correlated poorly with the diagnosis of infection. The accuracy of aspirations may be associated with quantitative evaluations of polymorphonuclear leukocyte (PMN) concentrations in the synovial fluid.

Intraoperative Evaluation

Quantitative microscopic evaluation of frozen sections procured at the time of the revision knee arthroplasty may be of great benefit in identifying infection. The sensitivity of an intraoperative frozen section was 43% with a specificity of 97% when the criteria of greater than 5 PMNs per high-powered field was established in at least 5 separate microscopic fields. A second study (in a community hospital) with a threshold of greater than 5 PMNs per high-powered field present in at least 3 fields had a 2% sensitivity and 93% specificity. An evaluation of revision hip and knee replacements ascribed little advantage to a criteria of greater than 10 PMNs per high-powered field. Other researchers concluded, however, that intraoperative microscopy of frozen sections was a much less sensitive study, although it still yielded very useful levels of specificity.

Surgical Exposure

Surgical exposure in revision knee arthroplasty is rendered more difficult by the presence of previous incisions, tightness, and loss of motion, as well as the inherent stiffness of scarring. Several recent review articles have cataloged the current knowledge of surgical techniques for safe exposure of the revision knee arthroplasty. The important issues are to ensure problem-free wound healing, to provide the surgeon with adequate exposure to perform the difficult revision knee arthroplasty, and to avoid damage to the all-important extensor mechanism, specifically the patella and patellar tendon. Removal of failed components requires greater exposure than primary arthroplasty. A review in 1997 covered all the principles of exposure in revision knee arthroplasty and focused on an osteotomy technique, which involves removal of the tibial tubercle with the extensor mechanism. In 136 TKAs studied, there was a low incidence of complications. Some surgeons may believe that many of these surgeries, although difficult, could be managed with soft-tissue procedures exclusively. An early soft-tissue maneuver, the V-Y quadricepsplasty, was evaluated in 14 patients. Postoperative results remained highly satisfactory despite a nonsignificant weakening of the extensor mechanism after the V-Y arthrotomy. This more aggressive soft-tissue approach has been modified by most revision arthroplasty surgeons to the "quadriceps snip." Careful attention to the details of soft-tissue handling during exposure, including maneuvers such as a lateral patellar retinacular release, quadriceps snip, and reestablishment of gutters on the medial and lateral sides of the femur as a means of exposing the majority of revision knee cases, are preferred. Osteotomy is an option, but some surgeons have ruled it out because of such complications as tibial shaft fractures.

Soft-Tissue Problems

Some catastrophic complications after revision knee arthroplasty can be avoided by identifying patients at risk prior to surgery. Extensive scarring, scars that adhere to underlying bone, and generally compromised soft tissue can be handled with the use of tissue expanders in some cases. In a case report, adherent scar tissue on the anterior proximal tibia resulting from multiple previous debridements and skin grafting of an infected primary TKA was enhanced with a tissue expander prior to revision knee arthroplasty. This procedure has been performed in several patients and reported by other surgeons. The ultimate soft-tissue complication, exposure of a prosthesis, is a dire situation synonymous with sepsis. In Denmark, 18 cases followed for 1 to 17 years were treated with myocutaneous muscle flaps and split-thickness skin grafts. Revision was ultimately necessary in 6 of these cases, with only 5 patients retaining a prosthesis, 3 of whom had considerable pain, poor mobility, and, presumably, persistent infection. Six of the patients died, 2 had a low femur amputation, and 5 had an arthrodesis. The general recommendation would be a 2-stage reimplantation protocol, if feasible, with extensive soft-tissue reconstruction using muscle transfer techniques.

In addition to loss of soft-tissue coverage, disruption of the extensor mechanism is a disabling complication for the patient with a revision knee arthroplasty. Tendon transfers from semitendinosus and extensor mechanism allograft techniques have been used to treat this complication.

Technique

It is difficult, but not impossible, to describe a coherent technique appropriate for all revision knee arthroplasty. Many such techniques can be conceived. Different surgeons have described the techniques with an emphasis at different times on fixation, reconstitution of bone defects, or reestablishment of the joint line. A 3-step technique has been described that is appropriate to all revision knee arthroplasties no matter which of the 9 types of failure is present. The reconstructive sequence begins with reestablishment of the tibial platform as a means of creating a foundation on which the revision can be built. This reference is established because the tibial articular surface is always in contact with the femur, irrespective of the position of the knee. This differs from the femur, where the distal component is in contact in extension only and the posterior articular surface is functioning in flexion.

The second step focuses on reconstruction of the flexion gap with the tibia and femur positioned at 90° to each other. The 3 goals described in this phase are reestablishment of the correct femoral component rotational position; selection of the appropriate component size, such that soft-tissue tension is reestablished; and coupling a given femoral component size with the appropriate thickness of articular polyethylene to stabilize the knee in flexion. At this time, there may be such great failure of collateral substance that recourse to constrained implants and/or ligament reconstructive procedures will be necessary.

The third and final phase of revision knee arthroplasty, stabilization of the knee in the position of extension, is accomplished by selecting the level of femoral component position either more distally to decrease the size of the extension gap so it matches the flexion space or more proximally (unusual except in cases of profound flexion contracture). The use of augments and bone grafts will be very important. Conventional ligament releases are essential in the correction of deformity, particularly when they have not been performed previously. Two indications for constraint or soft-tissue enhancement are flexion gaps of such dimensions that they cannot be stabilized by the selection of the appropriate femoral component size and varus/valgus instability resulting from failure of collateral ligaments.

The appreciation of rotational component positioning in the failure of primary knee arthroplasties and its tremendous importance in ensuring success of revision is newer and valuable information. The morphology of the transepicondylar axis and its application in primary and revision TKA have been evaluated in a detailed study that focused on cadaver specimens and examined the anterior intercondylar groove, compared the transepicondylar axis to the mechanical axis, and examined the posterior articular surface of the condyle.

In another study, which evaluated 75 embalmed anatomic specimens, it was concluded that the epicondylar axis provided a better indication of correct femoral component rotational positioning than the posterior condylar angle. Another report provides a thorough quantitative evaluation of the relationship between the transepicondylar axis and other indicators, based on intraoperative measurements that are very useful guides, not only for the rotational positioning of the femoral component, but also for reestablishment of a functional joint line.

Results

Earlier studies of revision knee arthroplasty contributed greatly to progress. However, the lack of uniformity in the types of implants that were used, as well as inconsistencies in identifying the causes of failure, leave these with largely historic value. Three recent series have used modular knee implant systems, with options for variable levels of constraint, and employ intramedullary stem extensions when appropriate to enhance fixation.

One study followed 44 revision knee arthroplasties for 2 to 6 years. This report was prompted by concern over the fixation techniques with uncemented stems in the presence of constrained implants. Thirteen patients had constrained condylar articulations and 21 had posterior stabilized (semiconstrained) prostheses. Three of 13 constrained implants and none of the 21 posterior stabilized prostheses experienced loosening.

In a follow-up series of 100 revision knee arthroplasties, which included the original 44, some intramedullary stems were treated by full cement fixation when constrained articulations were used in patients with poor quality bone, and there were no further cases of loosening. The development of newer soft-tissue techniques for revision stabilization resulted in several cases of instability, but with less of a dependence on mechanical constraint. The early series had been characterized by selection of large diameter modular intramedullary stems with excellent cortical contact. Because of the asymmetry of tibia and femoral bones, however, this technique sometimes compromised alignment, which may have contributed to the cases in which loosening was observed.

A similar modular prosthetic system was used in another study of 76 revision knee arthroplasties. Results with 2-stage reimplantations of infected devices were not included. Five knees (7%) had a fair or poor result and 6 knees (8%) experienced failure, necessitating another revision. The technique employed by this group often used more narrow diameter modular stems that appear to "dangle" in the intramedullary canal. Cortical contact may not have been achieved reliably, but alignment was less likely to be compromised by stem position.

In another study, 57 revision TKAs were evaluated at 36 to 120 months using a similar modular prosthetic system, but with a higher percentage of constrained articulations. Of 4 clinical failures, 3 were related to residual instability in patients with a posterior stabilized prosthesis. Complications in 3 knees were related to the extensor mechanism.

Further clinical series are anticipated, with careful identification of the causes for failure, and detailed information regarding the extent of constraint employed in the prosthesis. Outside of the United States, there has traditionally been a dependence on more constrained and even linked prosthetic devices for the purposes of revision knee arthroplasty. In 36 patients followed an average of 7 years, use of a hinged prosthesis was regarded as unavoidable in 6 knees (16.7%). Early complication rates, as in most revision series, were high, at 25%. Eighty percent of patients experienced an improved knee score, and in 73.3% the outcome was graded as good or excellent.

A large series from the United States identified 46 revision knee arthroplasties with no prior history of infection, which required 60 reoperations after revision surgery. These cases were part of a larger group of 655 revision knee arthroplasties performed over a 10-year period. In these reoperations, the extensor mechanism was the site of problems in 19 of the 46 (41%). Component loosening, deep infection, wound problems, tibiofemoral instability, poor motion, and debris synovitis were also cited as causes of reoperation. Given the more recent appreciation of the importance of femoral component rotational positioning and the relationship between rotational positioning and patellar complications, it seems probable that current enhanced understanding may help to decrease the incidence of extensor mechanism complications in future revision surgeries.

Revision of the Unicompartmental Replacement

Whether the unicompartmental primary knee arthroplasty represents a lesser intervention and an easier revision, should it fail, has been a source of controversy. This question becomes especially important when unicompartmental replacement is considered as an alternative to high tibial osteotomy in younger patients, for whom ultimate failure is regarded as inevitable. In a study from the United Kingdom, 73 failed unicompartmental replacements were revised, most of them because of progression of arthritis and implant failure. Of these, 88% were revised with a variety of condylar nonconstrained type prosthetic devices. Twenty osseous defects were described as either large, contained, or peripheral, and required reconstruction. Fifteen knees were lost because the patient died, 2 were lost to follow-up, and 3 required a second revision surgery. Of the remainder of the knees, 79% had excellent or good results at an average follow-up of 56 months. In another study, 29 patients with failed Robert Brigham metal-backed unicompartmental replacements underwent revision to TKA. The PCL was spared after revision in 30 of 31 knees, and 7 knees required bone graft for contained defects, 4 required tibial wedges, and 2 required femoral wedges. No defects required structural allograft, and it was concluded that conversion of unicompartmental TKA was an easier and more successful surgery than revision of tricompartmental replacements. This conclusion is in contrast to another study in which it appeared that failed unicompartmental replacements were as difficult to revise as failed tricompartmental ones.

Sepsis

Infection remains one of the most dreaded complications in arthroplasty surgery. Two-stage reimplantation protocols prevailed as the gold standard in the United States for the treatment of infected knee replacements. Attempts at arthroscopic treatment, open debridement, primary exchange, and chronic suppressive antibiotic therapy have not been comparably successful, nor have comparably large series been reported in the literature using these methods. Some series of 2-stage reimplantation protocols have reported the results in selected patients. This means, it should be remembered, that some patients were not believed to be appropriate candidates for inclusion in a 2-stage reimplantation protocol, either because of medical infirmity or extensive local destruction by sepsis. Accordingly, these patients may have been left with resection arthroplasties, or treated with arthrodesis. In a recent study of 2-stage reimplantation, with 66 total knees, 55 knees were evaluated at an average follow-up of 62 months (28 to 146 months). The implantation was successful in 80% of knees with low virulence organisms (coagulation negative staphylococcus or streptococcus), but the results were not as good in other circumstances. The rate of success was 71.4% in knees with polymicrobial infections. Those with high virulence organisms, such as methicillin-resistant *Staphylococcus aureus*, had good results in 66.7%. Patients with an original diagnosis of osteoarthritis had successful 2-stage reimplantation results in 82% of cases, but if the original diagnosis had been rheumatoid arthritis only 54% were successful. The success rate of 92% after an infected primary knee arthroplasty alone compares with 41% success if an infected knee replacement followed multiple previous knee operations such as arthroscopy, osteotomy, or prior revision TKA.

Another study evaluated 64 infected knee replacements treated between 1977 and 1983 with a 2-stage protocol. The results were reported with an average follow-up of 7.5 years (2 to 17 years). Reinfection had occurred in 6 knees (9%), but only in 2 with the same organisms. Four knees required a rerevision, 3 for aseptic loosening, and 1 for a periprosthetic fracture. The 10-year predicted survivorship of 2-stage reimplantation after infection in this study was 77.4%. In another study, 26 patients with late infected TKA were treated with a 2-stage protocol that included interposition of a polymethylmethacrylate articulating spacer, but allowed partial weight-bearing and some knee range of motion during rehabilitation. It was believed that this did not compromise the efficacy of eradication of infection, but did enhance functional results of 92% good to excellent. Researchers in Denmark evaluated 44 cases of deep infection after total knee arthroplasty that were treated by a variety of procedures. One received antibiotics only, 27 were treated with surgical debridement and antibiotics, and 16 had immediate removal of the prosthesis. In 21 of 27 cases, failed debridement was followed by removal of the prosthesis. Reimplantation surgery was attempted in 15 of the 37 cases in which the prosthesis had been removed, and sepsis was cured in 11 of these. In 25 cases that underwent removal of the prosthesis and arthrodesis, 4 ultimately underwent amputation. In no case in which osteitis was present was debridement and antibiotic therapy alone successful.

Fixation

Although uncemented techniques have begun to prevail in revision hip arthroplasty, there have been only limited reports in the literature of uncemented revision knee arthroplasty, and there were no new large series from 1994 until 1998. A report in 1993 described 56 cementless TKAs in 56 patients, using long-stemmed components and morcellized allograft. Two years after surgery, 54% of patients described no pain, 30% had mild pain, 9% had moderate pain, and 7% described severe pain. Another study described 16 patients with 17 revision TKAs, which used porous-coated tibial or femoral components, or both, without cement. Two revision tibial components were revised, one for proximal tibial fracture below the prosthesis and the other for prosthetic loosening and breakage. Both of these uncemented revision knee arthroplasty series concluded that the technique was promising. In general, uncemented revision knee arthroplasty has not displaced the use of methacrylate fixation for revision surgery in the United States.

As noted above, limited cement use with the introduction of modular intramedullary stems that are press fit has been popular. In contrast to this approach, however, some surgeons favor the technique of full cementation of extended intramedullary stems, with the technique resembling that used in hip arthroplasty. Of 40 revision TKAs with kinematic stabilized revision prostheses, at 24 to 111 months, 25 had long-stemmed tibial components and 38 had long-stemmed femoral components that were implanted with full cement fixation. No cases experienced loosening. The challenge that remains, however, is the extrication of all of the cement if revision becomes necessary because of septic failure.

Bone Defect Reconstruction

Several excellent classification systems have been described for bone defects in failed TKAs. Pragmatically, bone defects may be considered as contained, noncontained, or massive. There is an appropriate technique for reconstitution for each of these (Table 2).

Guidelines are available that describe new techniques required to reconstruct missing tibial or femoral bone for revision knee arthroplasty in the face of significant bone defects. Small defects can often be reconstructed using modular prosthetic systems. Fixation seems to have been successful with a wide variety of prosthetic devices, and the modes of attaching modular augments to their prosthetic counterparts have been reliable. In a study that evaluated 28 knees 2.3 years following surgery, clinical results were good. The only exception was a knee that required 2 revision procedures, the first for failure of the metal-backed patellar button and the second for aseptic loosening of the femoral component. Some radiolucent lines appeared in the bone-cement interface beneath a metal wedge in 13 knees, but none of these lines were progressive. Metal wedge augmentation was believed to be a useful option in knee arthroplasty surgery. Bulk allografts have been employed in a variety of defects. Results have varied, however, with allografts used to reconstruct contained defects and massive structural allografts used to replace large segments of the patient's metaphysis. One review describes 30 knees in 28 patients with revision TKA who required allograft to reconstruct massive bone defects. At an average of 50 months (24 to 132) postsurgery, 23 knees had improved. Seven knees were failures, caused by infection in 3, loosening of the tibial component in 2, fracture of the graft in 1, and nonunion of the allograft/host junction in 1. Another study described treatment of major defects of bone with bulk allograft in 30 patients with revision knee arthroplasty. Twenty-nine were femoral heads, 5 were distal femurs, and 1 was a proximal tibial allograft. Long-stemmed implants were used. Of the 30 patients, 87% had a good or excellent result, and no revisions were required at 24 to 120 months. It was recommended that components be cemented in all arthroplasty where graft is required. Although 3 components had subsided, none had proceeded to revision, and 2 of the 3 had a good clinical result. In another 15 patients, structural allograft was used as part of revision TKA. There were 7 distal femurs and 12 proximal tibias. Three patients had died and all of the 15 allografts had healed to host bone. One patient had a tibial component fracture over a proximal tibial allograft 3 years following surgery, 1 patient with a distal femoral allograft had tibial component loosening, another had a proximal tibial fracture after distal femoral allograft, and a third had an intraoperative patellar tendon avulsion. One of the earliest descriptions of tibial allograft applications to revision knee arthroplasty surgery described 12 knees in 10 patients with allografts for large tibial defects. Constrained condylar prostheses were used for all revisions, and the patients were followed an average of 32 months (25 to 51). At this early follow-up, 1 knee, which required a second revision because of painful nonunion of the medial structural graft, was considered a failure. There were no infections, and no grafts showed evidence of fracture or collapse.

Table 2
Classification of bone defects in failed total knee arthroplasties

Type	Treatment
Contained defect	Particulate bone graft or cement
Noncontained defect	Prosthetic modular augments
Massive bone loss	Structural allograft

Large structural allografts, although useful in reconstruction of difficult defects, are not yet fully understood. Progress in this area was established in a study of the histology of 9 structural bone grafts that had been used in the arthroplasty procedure. This study included autograft and allograft material. All allografts remained intact, but they had not revascularized. The autograft, by comparison, remained as viable bone. Stemmed components were believed to be important in bone graft reconstruction, because they protected the grafts from fatigue failure. A different approach to the reconstitution of large, but contained, defects, reported from Sweden, adapted the technique of impaction allografting of morcelized allograft with the use of cement fixation for revision TKA in 3 cases. Follow-up from 18 to 28 months showed good clinical and radiographic results. This procedure is most likely to be applicable in the failed stemmed component of either a hinged or constrained condylar design when intramedullary loosening and cortical expansion are experienced.

Summary

Revision knee arthroplasty surgery differs fundamentally from primary surgery. Progress has been slow because of the difficulties of the surgery, the relatively fewer numbers, and an incomplete understanding of the reasons for failure. It is a fascinating and challenging area of new information.

Several important principles have been established. No revision should be performed without a diagnosis in place, and a specific mechanical plan is required to address problems associated with the primary procedure. Results should be reported in the literature with a breakdown by cause of failure. There is no single prosthesis that should be applied to every failed arthroplasty. Modular systems are widely available that provide surgeons with the options to deal with the specific problem in a failed arthroplasty.

Completely uncemented revision knee arthroplasties do not yet seem to have found a place in revision knee surgery. The need for augmented fixation can sometimes be satisfied by uncemented press fit modular intramedullary stem extensions. Whether these should be fixed with full cementation in some or all cases is controversial.

Use of a constrained prosthesis is at times necessary, although they carry a greater risk of loosening. Bone defects can sometimes be reconstructed with modular prosthetic augments. The results of structural allograft reconstruction are promising, but no truly long-term results have yet been published.

Management of Bone Loss

Management of bone loss in revision total knee replacement (TKR) poses one of the more complicated technical considerations in the array of problems that can arise during surgery. Bone defects must be approached in a logical and consistent manner, using the available materials in view of the type and amount of bone loss and the age, size, and activity level of the patient. The surgeon's experience and comfort levels also should play a role in determining the method of reconstruction.

The materials available for reconstructing bone defects include polymethylmethacrylate (PMMA), PMMA with screw reinforcement, autogenous bone graft (local and remote), allogeneic bone graft (morcellized or structural), custom designed and manufactured prostheses, and modular prostheses with augments, wedges, and intramedullary rods. Any or all of these techniques may be used in a given revision construct.

PMMA alone should be restricted for use in small, contained defects less than 5 mm in depth. Only extremely small peripheral defects may be filled with PMMA, as PMMA extrusion and construct failure will occur if significant stress is applied to peripherally unsupported PMMA.

PMMA with screw reinforcement is applicable to somewhat larger defects, both contained and segmental, if the patient is elderly, less active, and preferably, of small stature. However, this construct should not be expected to support a prosthesis in which no supportive native bone is present in a femoral condyle or tibial plateau.

Autogenous bone has the greatest osteoinductive potential; however, structural graft for large defects is not easily accessible and local graft is sparse in the revision setting. When converting from a posterior cruciate-sparing to a posterior cruciate-sacrificing revision design, the femoral notch bone can provide local autogeneic bone for morcellized or small structural grafts. Remote donor sites such as the iliac crest provide inconsistent quality and quantity of bone and increase surgical morbidity.

Custom prostheses, as designed from x-ray or CT templates, have met with varied results. Cost, availability, and intraoperative difficulties led to the use of modular prostheses. These prostheses use wedges and augments of various angles and thickness and are most applicable to segmental defects of either the tibia or femur. Although some small augments or half wedges may be used with standard femoral or tibial components, most wedges and augments should be supported with intramedullary fixation. Biomechanically, augments appear to transfer compression load through PMMA and create less interface shear stress than wedges; however, no clinical differences have been noted. Conversely, wedges may allow reconstruction with less native bone sacrifice. Both techniques rely on adequate bone support and surface area for cement interdigitation and satisfactory long-term function. Neither technique, unless combined with bone graft, will enhance bone stock should further revision be required.

Wedges and augments are attached to the prostheses with screws or cement. Screws appear to be the most popular; however, the best method is unknown. Inherent in metal/metal abutment and screw attachment is the possibility of creating a metal debris machine that could lead to osteolysis. These concerns are speculative; however, these forms of revision constructs are the most versatile and easily applied and when used appropriately, are successful in the midterm follow-up period.

An extension of this construct for massive defects would include tumor prostheses as designed to replace the entire distal femur, proximal tibia, or both. These prostheses have rare TKR revision surgery indications.

Preservation and/or reconstitution of large areas that are bone-deficient can be accomplished only with bone grafting techniques. Impacted cancellous and structural allografts have provided satisfactory, stable constructs in a majority of patients. Incorporation of morcellized cancellous allografts with or without cement fixation appears to be excellent if adequate construct stabilizing is obtained via long (≥ 150 mm) press fit intramedullary rods and adequate native bony support for prosthesis seating. Biopsy of 14 cancellous allografts between 3 and 140 weeks revealed active new bone formations early followed by progressive maturation with entombed dead trabeculae. Early results are promising but longer follow-up and biomechanical testing of constructs for stability is required.

Structural allografts also aid in bone reconstitution and may be fashioned to fit major defects. Femoral head allografts may be fashioned to fit contained defects and for large tibial trumpet type defects, may be skewered with the intramedullary rod and impacted into the defect. It is generally believed that structural allografts should be fit to or fashioned to reconstruct the normal anatomy and seated on firm normal bone stock to maximize stability and compressive loading. The allograft, prosthesis, and host construct must be rigid. This can usually be achieved with press-fit intramedullary rods and a good graft/host fit; however, additional screw or plate fixation may be required. With this construct, host-allograft union can be obtained in greater than 90% of patients. Long-term follow-up is still lacking to determine survival rates and rates of graft collapse, resorption, or incorporation. Thoughtful preoperative planning and surgical experience is necessary in achieving successful revisions of this magnitude.

Modularity: Intramedullary Stems, Wedges, and Tibial Interface

Implant Modularity

Revision TKA is a complex procedure that requires special surgical skills. To ensure its success, several components are required. A detailed preoperative analysis of mechanisms of failure should be done to rule out infection and address bone loss and instability. To allow reconstruction of the joint line (frequently without reference to bony landmarks) and accurate soft-tissue balancing, revision instrumentation should be used. Modularity of the intended prosthesis is necessary to allow biomechanical stability without excessive use of cement, structural allograft, or customized implants. Intraoperative assessment is needed to ensure adequate exposure. Careful removal of the implant, cement, and membrane will ensure minimal bone loss, restoration of the joint line, soft-tissue balancing in flexion and extension, and correct extensor mechanism alignment.

Approximately 200,000 primary knee replacements and 20,000 revision knee arthroplasties are performed annually in North America. With a trend toward TKA in younger patients, the number of revision procedures will increase as patients outlive their implants. Failure of the primary implant is often associated with bone loss, which may increase when the prosthesis, cement, and membrane are removed. A careful preoperative assessment of the bone loss may anticipate the need for prosthetic modularity at the time of surgery. The AORI bone defect classification is the most commonly used and is summarized with indications for prosthetic modularity for each stage in Table 3.

With the implant positioned correctly to restore the joint line and balance the soft tissues, areas of bone loss may be so great as to leave large voids. These voids can be filled using cement, which is easy and cheap, but short-term results are poor and longer-term results are disastrous. The voids also can be filled using cement and screws; custom implants, which are expensive and difficult to manufacture but have obtainable good long-term results; or structural allografts, which are expensive and not always readily available. With these allografts, there is a steep surgical learning curve, and the risk of infection is increased. Postoperatively the patient's activities are usually limited until union has occurred. Structural allografts should be considered in defects greater than 2 cm. Modular implants offer a cheaper alternative to custom implants and structural allografts and allow minimal bone cement volume. Once the surgeon is familiar with the techniques of joint line restoration and soft-tissue balancing, modular implants should be considered to be the method of choice, particularly for defects up to 15 mm.

Bone loss presents challenging technical difficulties for the surgeon revising failed TKA. It is recommended that the joint line be restored to its correct level and that soft-tissue balance be achieved in both extension and flexion. Implant modularity makes it easier to achieve these goals without the need for expensive custom-made prostheses.

Intramedullary Stems Intramedullary stems allow fixation of the prosthesis to better quality bone stock in the metaphysis and diaphysis. Their design allows a variety of options, including variable length and width and the ability to use cemented or cementless fixation. The literature reflects no clinical difference at short-term follow-up between cemented or cementless tibial stems in revision TKA. Stress shielding may occur along the length of the stem; the longer the stem, the less proximal load transfer, which can lead to increased bone resorption at the prosthesis/bone interface and produce

Table 3
Anderson Orthopaedic Research Institute (AORI) bone defect classification and reconstruction considerations

AORI Classification	Description	Modularity Considerations
Femur		
F1	Minor bone defects following removal of implant, cement, and membrane. Intact metaphysis. Normal joint line.	Defects may be filled with allograft or cement. Implant will be stable without any modularity. Altering tibial insert thickness restores joint line.
F2A M-Medial condyle L-Lateral condyle	Varus/valgus malalignment of previous prosthesis. Metaphyseal bone loss of medial or lateral condyle following removal of implant, cement, and membrane.	Defect requires significant cement infill, allograft, or augments to restore joint line. An intramedullary stem is required.
F2B Both condyles	Metaphyseal bone loss of both condyles (may be unequal) following implant, cement, and membrane removal.	Defect requires significant cement fill, allograft, or augments to restore joint line. A long intramedullary stem is required.
F3	Extensive bone loss from medial or lateral or both condyles following removal of implant, cement, and membrane. Marked primary implant migration with knee instability. Loss of collateral ligament attachment. Supracondylar fracture.	Large defect requires allograft with or without augments and a long intramedullary stem to restore the joint line and stabilize the prosthesis.
Tibia		
T1	Minor bone defects following removal of the primary implant, cement, and membrane.	Defects may be filled with autograft or cement. Implant will be stable without any modularity. Altering the tibial insert thickness restores joint line.
T2A M-Medial condyle (common) L- Lateral condyle	Metaphyseal bone loss of either condyle. Tibial component loosening or loss of distance between the implant and fibular head.	Joint line restored using wedges or blocks with or without structural graft and prosthesis stabilized with a short or long intramedullary stem.
T2B Both condyles	Bone loss of both condyles, one of which extends to the level of the fibular head.	Joint line restored using structural graft, wedges, blocks, or extra-thick tibial insert. Prosthesis stabilized with a long intramedullary stem.
T3	Extensive metaphyseal cancellous and cortical bone loss.	Joint line difficult to restore. Structural graft and long intramedullary stem required.

a stress riser at the tip of the stem because of distal stress transfer. At present there are no reports concerning the clinical effects of these theoretical problems.

In addition, intramedullary stems prevent movement of the prosthesis. This factor is of particular importance when using semiconstrained (posterior stabilized or varus/valgus constrained) tibial inserts or constrained hinge type prostheses. With these implants the force transmitted across the joint onto the tibial component produces varus/valgus movements that can be counteracted by the stem. Taper stems are used with cement; however, press-fit stems with surface flutes or fins, which reduce rotation in the axial plane and the potential for subsidence, are used when further revision is anticipated.

The length of the stem is a controversial topic. Short stems are usually used in F2A and T2A bone defects (Table 3). Longer stems (Fig. 3) may be used in F2A and T2A bone defects at the surgeon's discretion but must always be used in type F2B, F3, T2B, and T3 bone defects. Press-fit long-stem designs have been associated with shin or thigh pain, which has been reduced by changing the metal of manufacture (most stems are now titanium) or the design (prostheses have flutes and notched stem tips, the so-called clothes peg design) to reduce implant rigidity and the stem tip stress riser.

Cemented stems should be used when bone stock or canal diameter makes cementless stems impractical. In most cases no contraindication exist for the use of either press-fit or cemented designs but when a second revision surgery is anticipated it is advisable that cementless stems be used because they preserve bone stock. Good results at 4.8 years and 8 years have been reported for prostheses with cementless intramedullary stems. However, in a study of cemented versus press fit stems, cement allowed better early stability of the tibial component. Generally, long stems (140 mm or greater) are less likely to result in a varus position of the tibial component and therefore are recommended.

Augments, Femoral Side Bone loss experienced with primary implants usually originates from the posterior and distal aspect of the condyles and is sometimes difficult to see on preoperative radiographs because of the overlying femoral component. Augments, which may be block- or wedge-shaped, are applied to the internal surface of the correctly sized femoral component and allow it to be positioned in the anatomically correct anteroposterior and sagittal planes (Fig. 4). Augments are attached to the femoral component by snap-fit, screws, or lugs, and in some designs by cement. Concern over fretting between augment and implant has been allayed by placing a layer of cement between the 2 substances; however, this increases the possibility of cement erosion with subsequent micro and macro third body wear particles. The newer mechanisms of attachment rarely fail, and to date only 1 separation of implant and augment has been reported. Femoral augments may be applied posteriorly or distally, separately or as a combined unit. This increased modularity allows greater options to augment bone loss. They are available in a variety of sizes up to 15 mm, and augments of different thickness may be placed medially or laterally on the same femoral implant.

Distal augments advance the femoral prosthesis distally, correcting the length of the femur and allowing the joint line to be placed at the correct level. Posterior augments allow the anatomically correct femoral implant to be used to restore correct anteroposterior dimensions. Without such implants the correct anatomically sized femoral component would be placed anteriorly or a smaller implant would have to be used. Both instances would result in poor soft-tissue balancing.

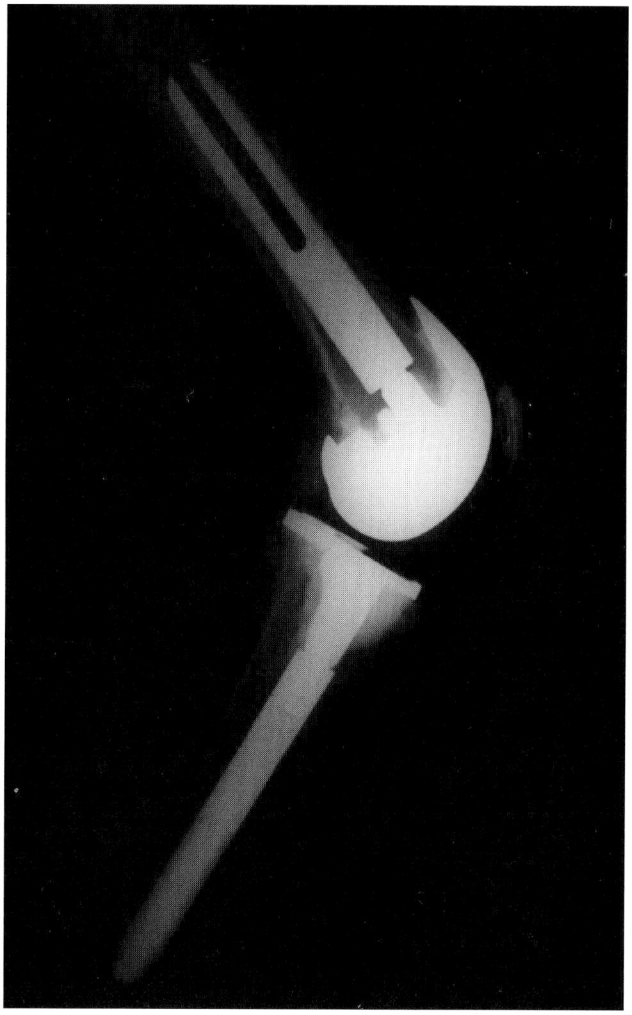

Figure 3

Contemporary design of revision total knee arthroplasty showing both femoral and tibial long stems.

Augments, Tibial Side Bone loss of the proximal tibia may be central or peripheral. In the former case, autologous bone graft should be used to fill the defect. In the latter case, the situation is more complex because the stability and fixation of the implant depend on good implant/cortex contact. By replacing the irregular bone edge of the area of bone loss by a smooth osteotomy cut obliquely or horizontally, wedges or blocks may be attached to the tibial tray so as to fill the bone defect. With accurate osteotomies, excellent implant/cortex

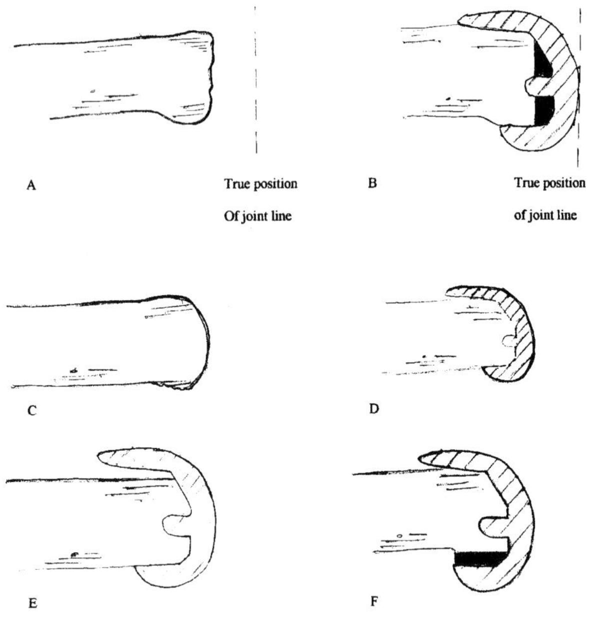

Figure 4

A, Lateral view of the distal femur with distal bone loss. **B**, Application of distal augments. **C**, Lateral view of the distal femur with posterior bone loss. **D**, Incorrect use of a small implant. **E**, Incorrect use of correct anatomically-sized implant with displacement anteriorly. **F**, Correct use of posterior augments and correctly-sized femoral component. Augments are shown shaded.

contact can be obtained.

Tibial augments attach to the undersurface of the tibial tray in a manner similar to augment attachment to the femur, with all components cemented onto the proximal tibia. In some designs the augment (full or half) is manufactured as a 1-piece tibial tray. Rectangular blocks attached to the medial and/or lateral halves of the tibial implant undersurface have a theoretical stability advantage over wedges, but this has not been shown clinically. Wedges may be placed below the medial or lateral surface of the tibial implant (half wedges) or extend across the whole of the tibial tray undersurface (full wedge), allowing irregular bone defects to be filled. The clinical implications of wedges versus blocks have not been recorded, but to date there appears to be no clinical advantage to either augment type. At present there is no long-term follow-up in the literature concerning tibial augments, but reports of up to 5.8 years show encouraging results.

Augments are very helpful in making up bone deficits of less than 15 mm. When making the tibial cuts, it is important to remember that the tibial augment will determine the rotation of the implant.

Summary

The frequency of revision knee arthroplasty will continue to increase. Advances in primary knee implant design and materials used, as well as advances in the treatment of osteolysis, will reduce the amount of bone loss encountered during revision surgery. New alloys will reduce rigidity of the femoral intramedullary stems; it is hoped that this will reduce thigh pain without compromising stem strength. Accurate preoperative assessment, a comprehensive revision arthroplasty implant system, and a surgeon well versed in its use remain the most important factors in revision surgery.

Prosthetic Design and Fusion of the Knee

Revision TKA requires balanced collateral ligaments, valgus alignment, equal flexion and extension gaps, full range of motion, and a centralized extensor mechanism. Throughout the entire surgical procedure, the stability of the knee replacement must be evaluated continuously. As the soft-tissue releases increase, it may be necessary to increase the constraint of the prosthetic design to augment the soft-tissue instability. Along with the soft-tissue considerations, bone defects and patellar tracking must also be included in the overall equation for knee revision.

In the early 1970s, some total knee designs attempted to spare both the anterior cruciate ligament (ACL) and the PCL, but they were not very successful and the concept of saving both of the cruciates was dropped. The designers decided to sacrifice the ACL and work with the PCL. Thus, two major schools developed. One school saved the PCL and designed the total knee around the ligament. The other school removed the PCL and designed the prosthetic knee with a substitution for the PCL. The results of the primary knee replacements from both schools have been very similar. However, the revision setting presents the surgeon with a different set of problems.

Definitions

The concepts of constraint and conformity are basic to total knee design. Conformity is often confused with constraint. Conformity is an indication of the degree of contact between 2 surfaces. Conformity can be measured by comparing the radius of curvature of the 2 articulating surfaces. As the radii approach each other, the ratio approaches one to one, the conformity increases, and the surface area of contact is maximized. With an increase in the contact area, the forces across the surface are decreased and the polyethylene is subject to less wear. However, as the surface area is increased, the range of motion of the knee may be compromised.

Constraint refers to the amount of mechanical stability that is designed into the implant. The degree of mechanical linkage between the femoral and tibial component represents the constraint. If the constraint between the components is increased, the knee replacement is more inherently stable by itself with less dependence upon the surrounding soft tissues. However, with the increase in the constraint, the surface immediately underlying the components is also subject to increased forces. The increased force can lead to loosening at the interface between the prosthesis and the bone or between the cement layer and the bone depending upon the implant design (cementless or cemented).

The Prosthetic Choices

In the revision setting the surgeon can choose between cruciate-sparing, cruciate-substituting, and hinged designs. The cruciate-sparing designs are the least constrained and the hinged knees are the most constrained, with the cruciate-substituting prostheses in the middle. In the primary knee setting, the most popular knee design presently used in the United States is the cruciate-sparing design. However, the substituting knees are rapidly gaining popularity.

Most surgeons will plan to use the least constrained device for the revision and try to implant a cruciate-sparing design. This type of design can be augmented with metal wedges, blocks, and intramedullary stems to allow for bone loss and some collateral laxity. However, even in the preoperative planning phase, it may be evident from the physical examination of the knee and from the standard radiographs that the PCL is no longer intact. If this is the case, a posterior cruciate-substituting design will have to be used without a choice involved.

During revision surgery, releases and soft-tissue balancing may lead to compromise of the collateral ligament integrity. The revision may, then, require a posterior cruciate-substituting design, which can also be augmented with blocks, wedges, and intramedullary stems. In the most unusual of circumstances, there may be minimal collateral ligament support and a hinged device may be warranted. The author has had only 1 case in 400 revision surgeries that required a hinged knee appliance.

It is difficult to indicate precisely when the soft-tissue stability of the knee decreases enough to require an increase in the level of constraint. The soft tissues and the prosthetic constraint are balanced together; similar to an equation that must always add up to the same 100 points.

Most surgeons release the tight ligament about the knee (as opposed to tightening the loose side). As the release of each structure proceeds, the laxity is increased on that side. There is a sequential release for the tight medial side of the varus knee, for the tight lateral side of the valgus knee, for the tight posterior capsule in the flexion contracture, and for the tight extensor mechanism in the extension contracture. Some authors believe that the entire medial side of the varus knee can be released without the need for additional constraint, but I believe that any complete release of either the lateral or medial side of the knee should be augmented with more constraint in the prosthesis. The additional constraint requires the use of a posterior stabilized knee design, ie, a constrained condylar knee.

When a revision knee replacement is scheduled, the surgeon must know his individual hospital and ascertain if all the required components will be available. Because it is often difficult to predict exactly how much instability will be present in the knee through the course of the revision surgery, it is in the surgeon's best interest to have all of the basic revision designs available at the time of the surgery.

The Surgical Procedure

The revision surgery begins with the establishment of a perpendicular tibial surface (as outlined in chapter 30). The next step balances the collateral ligaments in flexion, evaluates the integrity of the ligaments, and estimates the size of the flexion gap. At this point the surgeon should begin to think about the prosthetic constraint. If both collateral structures are intact and functional, a typical primary implant can be used. However, it is more common that the medial collateral structure is partially loose. If there is minimal or no end point to valgus stress of the knee in flexion, the surgeon should be prepared for a posterior stabilized or a constrained condylar knee design.

The extension gap is the next part of the surgical procedure. The surgeon must equalize the extension and flexion spaces. Usually, the extension gap will be larger than the flexion space and the femoral component will need to be advanced distally from the end of the remaining femoral bone surface. When the component is advanced with blocks beneath the femoral flanges, it is necessary to add an intramedullary stem for stability and support. Then, the ligamentous balance must be checked in full extension and the overall valgus alignment of the knee confirmed. Once again, releases may become necessary in full extension to create proper balance. Complete collateral releases should be supported with further constraint in the form of a constrained condylar knee.

On occasion it may be difficult to equalize the two gaps and obtain proper valgus alignment. If this difficulty should arise, a constrained condylar knee will often take up the laxity in one or the other position (ie, in either 90° of flexion or in full extension). While this is not a standard approach to the problem of gap inequalities, it does offer a good compromise solution when a hinged knee would be the only other alternative.

The hinged knee replacement is the most constrained of all of the designs. Hinges were some of the earliest knee replacements and were used in the 1950s. At that point in time, methylmethacrylate was not yet available and the soft-tissue procedures for ligament imbalance had not yet been described. The hinges had early loosening and caused a significant loss of bone substance when they failed. After the PCL-retaining and -substituting designs were well established in the late 1970s and early 1980s, the original hinged knee designs were modified for use in unusual circumstances, such as tumor resection and revision of a knee with absent medial or lateral soft-tissue structures. The femoral component includes a hinge with an attached polyethylene surface that inserts into a tibial base plate, allowing unrestricted rotation. This type of design helps to decrease some of the high forces that are imparted to the underlying bone in a true hinge. While these designs are unusual for a "standard" revision surgery, the modern hinges can be helpful in very difficult situations.

Knee Fusion

Knee fusion is an uncommon procedure in total knee surgery. In 1984, John Insall wrote in his textbook, *Surgery of the Knee*, that "arthrodesis of the knee is seldom performed." Today, fusion of the knee may still be necessary in failed knee infections, failed TKRs, and in tumor cases. Very few articles in the literature concerning this have been published in the past 10 years. The alternatives for fixation include external fixation, dual plate fixation, and intramedullary nails. The intramedullary techniques appear to be more appropriate; however, most series have reported success rates only in the 80% to 90% range. Even when knee fusion is chosen as a last resort, it may require more than one surgical procedure to successfully fuse the knee.

Annotated Bibliography

Modes of Failure

Dellon AL, Mont MA, Krackow KA, Hungerford DS: Partial denervation for persistent neuroma pain after total knee arthroplasty. *Clin Orthop* 1995;316:145–150.

The neural anatomy of the anterior knee is described and provides a rationale for denervation for postsurgical pain. Fifteen patients were identified who had persistent or worse knee pain after total knee arthroplasty. In each patient, component loosening, malalignment, knee instability, and infection had been excluded systematically as a source of pain. Each patient was tested with selective nerve blocks before surgery. All 15 patients had at least 1 of the nerves to the knee selectively denervated. All patients reported improvement.

Haas SB, Insall JN, Montgomery W III, Windsor RE: Revision total knee arthroplasty with use of modular components with stems inserted without cement. *J Bone Joint Surg* 1995;77A:1700–1707.

Seventy-six revision cemented total knee replacements were analyzed. Survivorship analysis was performed for all patients. Fluted rods were used in all patients and metal wedges were used as necessary. The average preoperative knee score was 49 points. Postoperatively, the knee score improved to an average of 76 points. In 6 (8%) of the 76 knees, the prosthesis failed, necessitating another revision.

Ritter MA, Worland R, Saliski J, et al: Flat-on-flat, nonconstrained, compression molded polyethylene total knee replacement. *Clin Orthop* 1995;321:79–85.

This study, which examines wear characteristics in the posterior cruciate ligament-sparing total knee with flat-on-flat articulations and compression molded polyethylene, included 2,001 arthroplasties from 3 institutions. There were 8 failures secondary to revision (5 tibial failures; 2 secondary to metallosis from patellar polyethylene dissociation; and 3 femoral failures) resulting in a 98% survival rate at 10 years.

Waldman BJ, Mont MA, Hungerford DS: Total knee arthroplasty infections associated with dental procedures. *Clin Orthop* 1997;343:164–172.

The authors describe 9 patients whose total knee arthroplasty infections were associated with a dental procedure. They found that 11% of all infected total knee arthroplasties are the result of hematogenous infection from the oral cavity.

Bone Defect Classification

Engh GA: Bone defect classification, in Engh GA, Rorabeck CH (eds): *Revision Total Knee Arthroplasty.* Baltimore, MD, Williams & Wilkins, 1997, pp 63–120.

This chapter presents the rationale and background development of the Anderson Orthopaedic Research Institution Bone Defect Classification System.

Engh GA, Ammeen DJ: Classification and preoperative radiographic evaluation: Knee. *Orthop Clin North Am* 1998;29:205–217.

This article demonstrates the use of a bone defect classification in the preoperative planning for revision knee arthroplasty.

Surgical Techniques and Principles

Epidemiology

Barrack RL, Hoffman GJ, et al: Surgeon work input and risk in primary versus revision total joint arthroplasty. *J Arthroplasty* 1995;10:281-286.

Based on a study of the complete financial and clinical data of 120 non-selected primary and revision total knee arthroplasty cases, revision surgery involved significantly more surgical time, greater blood loss, increased length of stay, and a much higher complication rate. Physician reimbursement constituted 18% of the total fees collected compared with 24% for the actual prosthesis cost. Surgeons performing revision surgery devote significantly more time and are at a higher liability than when performing primary total joint arthroplasty.

Heck DA, Melfi CA, et al: Revision rates after knee replacement in the United States. *Med Care* 1998;36:661-669.

In this study, there were more than 200,000 hospitalizations for primary knee replacements, with fewer than 3% of them requiring revision within 2 years. The following factors increase the chance of revision within 2 years of primary knee replacement: (1) male gender, (2) younger age, (3) longer length of hospital stay for the primary knee replacement, (4) more diagnoses at the primary knee replacement hospitalization, (5) unspecified arthritis type, (6) surgical complications during the primary knee replacement hospitalization, and (7) primary knee replacement performed at an urban hospital. This study was based on a comparison on ICD 9 codes for primary and revision knee arthroplasty surgery.

Hebert CK, Williams RE, et al: Cost of treating an infected total knee replacement. *Clin Orthop* 1996;331:140-145.

Twenty consecutive infected knee arthroplasty cases that were treated surgically required 3 to 4 times the resources of the hospital and the surgeon compared with a primary total knee implant, and approximately twice the resources of a nonseptic revision total knee implant. The reimbursement received resulted in an estimated net loss of approximately $15,000 per case to the hospital for the group as a whole, but approximately $30,000 per case per Medicare patient.

Ritter MA, Carr KD, et al: Revision total joint arthroplasty: Does Medicare reimbursement justify time spent? *Orthopedics* 1996;19:137-139.

Five different orthopaedic surgeons in a single group performed a total of 337 primary total knee replacements and 25 revision total knee arthroplasties. There was a 41% increase in the time it took to perform revision surgery. Allowable charges by Medicare in 1993 for a primary knee were $1,298. Revision total knee replacement increased 24.3% ($1,613) in the state of Indiana. These surgeons have concluded that there is little incentive for experienced surgeons to assume responsibility for difficult revision cases that may originate in other institutions.

Basic Science

Goodman SB, Huie P, et al: Cellular profile and cytokine production at prosthetic interfaces: Study of tissues retrieved from revised hip and knee replacements. *J Bone Joint Surg* 1998;80B: 531-539.

In this study, 65 cemented and 36 uncemented arthroplasties undergoing revision surgery were separated into 3 groups based on the results of tissue studies: loose implants with ballooning osteolysis, loose implants without osteolysis, and well-fixed implants. Tissue studies included numbers of macrophages, T-lymphocytes, and interleukins (IL-1 and IL-6). These results suggest that there may be different biologic mechanisms for loosening in cemented and uncemented arthroplasties, perhaps based on T-lymphocyte modulation of macrophage function.

Huang CH, Young TH, et al: Polyethylene failure in New Jersey low-contact stress total knee arthroplasty. *J Biomed Mater Res* 1998;39:153-160.

Eight of 276 meniscal bearing New Jersey Low Contact stress total knee arthroplasties were revised within 8 years of implantation because of severe polyethylene wear. There were 4 probable failure mechanisms associated with the catastrophic polyethylene wear: insufficient thickness of the meniscal bearing, malpositioning of the metal tibial tray in the transverse plane (resulting in the breaking of the meniscal bearing), and the inability of the patella to rotate because of tissue ingrowth and yellowing of the subsurface of the meniscal bearing (a sign of polyethylene failure).

Hirakawa K, Bauer TW, et al: Comparison and quantitation of wear debris of failed total hip and total knee arthroplasty. *J Biomed Mater Res* 1996;31:257-263.

Wear debris was characterized electronically from synovial samples of 32 knee arthroplasties undergoing revision surgery and compared with 21 samples from hip arthroplasties undergoing revision. Very small particles are common to both groups, but a larger range of particle sizes is present adjacent to failed knee arthroplasties, reflecting the perceived higher rate of failure because of delamination and fragmentation in the knee.

Kovacik MW, Gradisar IA, et al: A comparison of interleukin-1 beta in human synovial fluid of osteoarthritic and revision total knee arthroplasty. *Biomed Sci Instrum* 1997;33:519-523.

Interleukin-1β levels (IL-1β) were measured in synovial fluid from 3 groups of knees: osteoarthritic, titanium arthroplasties, and chrome cobalt arthroplasties. There was a significant difference with the titanium arthroplasties for revision with the highest levels of IL-1β and the osteoarthritic knees the lowest. The IL-1β levels may be a useful indicator of increased synovial activity and inflammation.

Wasielewski RC, Parks N, et al: Tibial insert undersurface as a contributing source of polyethylene wear debris. *Clin Orthop* 1997;345:53-59.

The polyethylene articular surface was retrieved from 67 failed knee arthroplasties at the time of revision and the nonarticular undersurface was scored for severity of wear. These scores correlated with the extent of osteolysis apparent radiographically, drawing attention to the locking mechanism of modular polyethylene inserts in the tibias of total knee arthroplasties.

Classification of Revision Knee Arthroplasty

Vince KG, Long W: Revision knee arthroplasty: The limits of press fit medullary fixation. *Clin Orthop* 317:172-177.

The classification system of Jacobs, Hungerford, and Krackow was expanded to include failure caused by breakage, sepsis, extensor mechanism rupture, stiffness, and fracture. There was a higher rate of mechanical failure caused by loosening when nonlinked constrained implants were used with limited cement technique and nonporous coated, uncemented intramedullary stem extensions. When posterior stabilized implants were used with the same fixation technique, no loosening was observed in 31 arthroplasties.

Imaging and CT Scans

Fehring TK, McAvoy G: Fluoroscopic evaluation of the painful total knee arthroplasty. *Clin Orthop* 1996;331:226-233.

Twenty patients with painful total knee arthroplasties, despite excellent radiographs, were evaluated with studies including fluoroscopically guided radiographs. Loosening was found in 14 patients and was confirmed in each at revision surgery. Each patient experienced relief after surgery. Fluoroscopically guided lateral radiographs may be the only way to diagnose loosening or, in most cases, failed bone ingrowth.

Henderson JJ, Bamford DJ, et al: The value of skeletal scintigraphy in predicting the need for revision surgery in total knee replacement. *Orthopedics* 1996;19:295-299.

Twenty-nine patients were evaluated with 99m technetium methylene diphosphonate (99mTc-MDP) and 67 gallium (67 Ga) citrate scintigrams. Three groups were identified clinically: asymptomatic knees (undergoing scans for other reasons), those with aseptic or septic loosening, and those with pain without radiologic evidence of loosening. These groups could be distinguished with the isotope studies, leading to the conclusions that sequential 99mTc-MDP and 67 Ga citrate scintigrams are useful for demonstrating the presence of aseptic and septic loosening in knee prostheses, and pain with a normal scan appearance is probably not caused by loosening or infection.

Aspiration

Barrack RL, Jennings RW, et al: The Coventry Award: The value of preoperative aspiration before total knee revision. *Clin Orthop* 1997;345:8-16.

In this study, 69 knee arthroplasties were aspirated prior to revision surgery. Infection was diagnosed in 20. Preoperative aspiration had an overall sensitivity of 55%, specificity of 96%, accuracy of 84%, positive predictive value of 85%, and negative predictive value of 84%. When the results of the reaspirations are included, the overall aspiration results improved to a sensitivity of 75%, specificity of 96%, and accuracy of 90%. The results of the study support the use of routine preoperative aspiration before total knee revision. Previous antibiotic use increases the risk of a false negative result, and reaspiration at a later date can be expected to significantly improve the value of this test in such cases.

Duff GP, Lachiewicz PF, et al: Aspiration of the knee joint before revision arthroplasty. *Clin Orthop* 1996;331:132-139.

The authors performed aspiration in 43 of 54 knee arthroplasties about to undergo revision surgery. In 19 knees, the aspiration showed growth on solid media, and in 18 of these knees the diagnosis of infection was confirmed by the intraoperative cultures. Preoperative aspiration is believed to be more reliable than any other laboratory test for the detection of infection in a knee arthroplasty.

Intraoperative Evaluation

Abdul Karim FW, McGinnis MG, et al: (1998). Frozen section biopsy assessment for the presence of polymorphonuclear leukocytes in patients undergoing revision of arthroplasties. *Mod Pathol* 1998;11:427-431.

Intraoperative frozen section with quantification of the number of polymorphonuclear leukocytes (PMNs) was performed on the tissue from 64 knee arthroplasties undergoing revision. A histologic examination was considered positive for infection if more than 5 PMNs per high-power field are present in at least 5 separate microscopic fields.

Lonner JH, Desai P, et al: The reliability of analysis of intraoperative frozen sections for identifying active infection during revision hip or knee arthroplasty. *J Bone Joint Surg Am* 1996;78: 1553-1558.

Intraoperative frozen sections were performed in 175 consecutive revision total joint arthroplasties (142 hip and 33 knee). Twenty-three had at least 5 polymorphonuclear leukocytes (PMNs) per high-power field on analysis and were considered to have an infection. Of these 23, 5 had 5 to 9 PMNs per high-power field and 18 had at least 10 PMNs per high-power field. At least 10 PMNs per high-power field was predictive of infection, while 5 to 9 PMNs per high-power field was not necessarily consistent with infection. Less than 5 PMNs per high-power field reliably indicated the absence of infection.

Pace TB, Jeray KJ, et al: Synovial tissue examination by frozen section as an indicator of infection in hip and knee arthroplasty in community hospitals. *J Arthroplasty* 1997;12: 64-69.

In a community hospital, frozen section examination was a reasonably specific predictor of deep infection in revision hip and knee arthroplasty.

Surgical Exposure

Ritter MA, Carr K, et al: Tibial shaft fracture following tibial tubercle osteotomy. *J Arthroplasty* 1996;11:117-119.

Tibial tubercle osteotomy was used in 9 out of 657 primary and 16 revision knee arthroplasties. Because of 2 tibial shaft fractures, this group of surgeons has curtailed their use of the osteotomy.

Whiteside LA: Exposure in difficult total knee arthroplasty using tibial tubercle osteotomy. *Clin Orthop* 1995;321:32-35.

Exposure with an extended tibial tubercle and tibial crest osteotomy was done for 136 total knee arthroplasties (26 primary arthroplasties, 76 revision, 10 repeated revision, 19 infected, and 5 repeated revision for infection). Adequate exposure was achieved and further release of the quadriceps mechanism was not necessary. Two or 3 wires were passed through the lateral edge of the tibial tubercle and through the medial tibial cortex to reattach the bone fragment and patellar tendon. Mean range of motion in these cases at 2 years after surgery was 93.7° (range, 15° to 140°). Two knees had extension lag, unchanged from their preoperative condition. Two tibial tubercles had partial proximal avulsion fracture, but did not separate widely. Two tibial fractures occurred in 1 patient with diabetic Charcot arthropathy, and another after manipulation.

Younger AS, Duncan CP, et al: Surgical exposures in revision total knee arthroplasty. *J Am Acad Orthop Surg* 1998;6:55-64.

This excellent review article catalogues the available strategies for safe exposure of difficult revision surgery. Likely complications have been described, along with techniques for avoidance and methods to deal with problems if they occur.

Soft-Tissue Problems

Santore RF, Kaufman D, et al: Tissue expansion prior to revision total knee arthroplasty. *J Arthroplasty* 1997;12:475-478.

A tissue expander was used prior to revision knee arthroplasty in a 76-year-old woman with extremely adherent scar tissue on the anterior aspect of the knee. Three-year follow-up reveals that the surgery has been successful.

Surgical Technique

Stiehl JB, Abbott BD: Morphology of the transepicondylar axis and its application in primary and revision total knee arthroplasty. *J Arthroplasty* 1995;10:785-789.

The transepicondylar axis (TEA) was evaluated in 13 cadaveric specimens. Multiple relationships can be defined. The TEA is an important landmark that, from this study, is virtually perpendicular to the mechanical axis of the lower extremity and parallels the knee flexion axis. Femoral component rotation and joint line positioning in total knee arthroplasty can be determined using the TEA.

Results

Haas SB, Insall JN, et al: Revision total knee arthroplasty with use of modular components with stems inserted without cement. *J Bone Joint Surg Am* 1995;77:1700-1707.

Of 76 revision total knee arthroplasties performed at the Hospital for Special Surgery, 88% had a complete clinical evaluation at 2 to 9 years. The original technique of cement fixation to the cut bone surfaces with introduction of an uncemented, nonporous coated intramedullary stem was evaluated. Postoperatively, the knee score improved to an average of 76 points (range, 0 to 97 points). Of the 67 knees that had complete follow-up, 56 (84%) had an excellent or good result, and 5 (7%) had a fair or poor result. In 6 (8%) of the 76 knees, the prosthesis failed, necessitating another revision.

Peters CL, Hennessey R, et al: Revision total knee arthroplasty with a cemented posterior-stabilized or constrained condylar prosthesis: A minimum 3-year and average 5-year follow-up study. *J Arthroplasty* 1997;12:896-903.

Revision total knee arthroplasties were performed for aseptic with a cemented posterior- stabilized or constrained condylar prosthesis and reevaluated at an average of 62 months (range, 36 to 120 months). The reason for revision was aseptic loosening of 1 or both components in 32 knees (56%), instability in 16 knees (28%), polyethylene wear and osteolysis in 4 knees (7%), supracondylar femur fracture in 2 knees (4%), and a failed allograft, pain, and arthrofibrosis in 1 knee each.

Vince KM, Mark; Kharrazi, D; Vermillion, D.; and Spitzer AI (1998). Revision Total Knee Arthroplasty with a Modular Prosthesis and a Three Step Reconstruction Technique: 2 to 10-Year Follow Up. 10th Combined Orthopedic Associations of the English Speaking World Meeting, Auckland, New Zealand.

In this study, 113 revision knee arthroplasties were evaluated at 2 to 10 years, including revisions for septic failure. The causes of failure include loosening, instability, malrotation and patellar instability, and inexplicable pain. This was the second revision in 10 patients; 3 patients had bilateral surgery. Nonlinked constrained implants were used in 19 knees and posterior stabilized in 79. Medullary fixation was required in 90 knee and structural allografts were required in 12. Modular augments were applied to 52 knees. A collateral ligament was reconstructed in 7 cases, avoiding constraint. Reoperations were required because of loosening in 4 cases, sepsis in 2, and instability in 1. All 7 were successfully revised. Good and excellent results were noted in 79% of cases.

Revision of the Unicompartmental Replacement

Chakrabarty G, Newman JH, et al: Revision of unicompartmental arthroplasty of the knee. Clinical and technical considerations. *J Arthroplasty* 1998;13:191-196.

Seventy-three unicompartmental knee arthroplasties were revised, usually because of progression of arthritis or implant failure. Forty-seven bone defects were small and contained, presenting little problem. Twenty defects were either large, contained, or peripheral, requiring reconstruction. Fifteen knees were lost as a result of death of the patient (but there had been satisfactory knee function); 2 were lost to follow-up evaluation, and 3 have required further revision. Seventy-nine percent of the remaining knees had excellent or good knee function at an average follow-up period of 56 months.

Levine WN, Ozuna RM, et al: Conversion of failed modern unicompartmental arthroplasty to total knee arthroplasty. *J Arthroplasty* 1996;11:797-801.

Thirty-one knees with a failed unicompartmental arthroplasty underwent revision to a total knee arthroplasty (TKA). The primary mechanism of failure was tibial polyethylene wear in 21 knees and opposite compartment progression of arthritis in 10 knees. Sixteen knees had particulate synovitis with dense metallic staining of the synovium. At revision, the posterior cruciate ligament was spared in 30 knees and substituted in 1 knee. Restoration of bony deficiency at revision required cancellous bone graft for contained defects in 7 knees, tibial wedges in 4, and femoral wedges in 2. No defects received structural allografts. The data suggest that failed, modern unicompartmental knee arthroplasty can successfully be converted to TKA. Moreover, the results of revision of failed unicompartmental knee arthroplasty are superior to those of failed TKA and failed high tibial osteotomy and comparable to the authors' results of primary TKA with similar-length follow-up periods.

Sepsis

Goldman RT, Scuderi GR, et al: 2-stage reimplantation for infected total knee replacement. *Clin Orthop*1996;331:118-124.

Between 1977 and 1983, 64 infected total knee replacements in 60 patients were treated with a 2-stage protocol for reimplantation. The clinical results and survivorship were determined at an average follow-up of 7.5 years (range, 2 to 17 years). At follow-up, 6 knees (9%) had become reinfected, but only 2 with the same organism. Four knees had been revised: 3 for aseptic loosening and 1 for a periprosthetic femur fracture. Two other knees were impending failures due to aseptic loosening. The 10-year predicted survivorship of 2-stage reimplantation is 77.4%.

Hirakawa K, Stulberg BN, et al: Results of 2-stage reimplantation for infected total knee arthroplasty. *J Arthroplasty* 1998;13:22-28.

In this study, 66 infected total knee arthroplasties had been treated with

2-stage reimplantation total knee arthroplasty between September 1980 and October 1993. Of these, 55 knees were available for follow-up at an average of 61.9 months (range, 28 to 146 months) Reimplantation was successful in 80% of knees with low-virulence organisms (coagulase-negative *Staphylococcus, Streptococcus*), 71.4% with polymicrobial organisms, and 66.7% with high-virulence organisms (methicillin-resistant *Staphylococcus aureus*). Reimplantation was successful in 82% of patients with osteoarthritis and in 54% of patients with rheumatoid arthritis ($p = .024$). The success rate was 92% if infection occurred after primary arthroplasty but only 41% if after multiple previous knee surgeries (arthroscopy, osteotomy, or revision total knee arthroplasty) ($p = .001$).

Hofmann AA, Kane KR, et al: Treatment of infected total knee arthroplasty using an articulating spacer. *Clin Orthop* 1995;321:45-54.

Twenty-six patients with infected total knee arthroplasties were treated by debridement, removal of components and cement with the interposition of an antibiotic impregnated methacrylate spacer block that permitted. All patients except 1 had reimplantation; this patient died of unrelated causes before revision. Range of motion before revision was 10° to 95°. Range of motion after reimplantation was 5° to 106°. There have been no recurrences of infection.

Bone Defect Reconstruction

Engh GA, Herzwurm PJ, et al: Treatment of major defects of bone with bulk allografts and stemmed components during total knee arthroplasty. *J Bone Joint Surg Am* 1997;79:1030-1039.

Thirty-five allograft reconstructions were evaluated at 2 to 10 years after revision surgery. Twenty-nine femoral head allografts, 5 distal femoral allografts, and 1 proximal tibial allograft were used in conjunction with a long-stemmed implant to reconstruct large osseous defects. None of the patients had collapse of the graft, subsidence of the implant, or revision. Twenty-six of the 30 patients (87%) had a good or excellent clinical result, and no revisions were necessary.

Ghazavi MT, Stockley I, et al: Reconstruction of massive bone defects with allograft in revision total knee arthroplasty. *J Bone Joint Surg Am* 1997;79:17-25.

Allograft bone was used to reconstruct a defect in the proximal aspect of the tibia or the distal aspect of the femur, or both, in 30 revision total knee arthroplasties. At an average of 50 months (range, 24 to 132 months; median, 36 months) postoperatively, the score for 23 knees (21 patients) had increased by at least 20 points, and these knees did not need additional surgery. Thus, the rate of success was 77%. The procedure was considered a failure for the remaining 7 knees because of infection in 3, loosening of the tibial component in 2, fracture of the graft in 1, and nonunion at the allograft-host junction in 1.

Mow CS, Wiedel JD: Structural allografting in revision total knee arthroplasty. *J Arthroplasty* 1996;11:235-241.

Structural allograft reconstruction was performed during revision knee arthroplasty in 15. All patients had large segmental, cavitary, or combination defects of the femur and/or tibia. Seven distal femurs and 12 proximal tibias required allografting. All but 1 patient, had improvement of pain and stability. All of the 15 allografts healed to host bone and 13 showed evidence of incorporation. There were no infections or fractures of the allografts. There was 1 complication directly related to the allograft; that patient had a tibial component fracture over a proximal tibial allograft 3 years after surgery. Component loosening, fracture, and extensor mechanism rupture occurred in 3 other cases.

Pagnano MW, Trousdale RT, et al: Tibial wedge augmentation for bone deficiency in total knee arthroplasty: A follow-up study. *Clin Orthop* 1995;321:151-155.

Metal wedge augmentation was used in 28 knees for tibial bone deficiency. Clinical results were excellent in 67%, good in 29%, and poor in 4%. The only poor result was in 1 knee that required 2 revision procedures: the first for failure of a metal-backed patellar component and the second for aseptic loosening of the femoral component. No deterioration of the wedge-prosthesis or wedge-cement-bone interface was seen at midterm follow-up.

Rand JA: Modularity in total knee arthroplasty. *Acta Orthop Belg* 1996;62(suppl 1):180-186.

In this study, 41 consecutive revisions were performed with a modular knee arthroplasty prosthesis. Incomplete radiolucent lines were seen adjacent to 61% of the components, but not adjacent to the long stems. The results were similar with either pressed fit or cemented long stems or posterior cruciate-retaining or posterior-stabilized articulations of the prosthetic design.

Rand JA: Modular augments in revision total knee arthroplasty. *Orthop Clin North Am* 1998;29:347-353.

This article presents a review of the usefulness of the modular knee arthroplasty system in restoring bone defects as well as stabilizing knees that have suffered instability as a result of defective bone stock. Intramedullary stem extensions can enhance fixation, and may be either press-fit or cemented.

Rorabeck CH, Smith PN: Results of revision total knee arthroplasty in the face of significant bone deficiency. *Orthop Clin North Am* 1998;29:361-371.

This article presents a general review of guidelines for the reconstruction of bone defects in revision knee arthroplasty.

Ullmark G, Hovelius L: Impacted morselized allograft and cement for revision total knee arthroplasty: A preliminary report of 3 cases. *Acta Orthop Scand* 1996;67:10-12.

Intramedullary impaction of morcellized allograft similar to the technique described for the hip has been used in 3 revision knee arthroplasties. Follow-up after 18, 21, and 28 months showed good clinical and radiographic results.

Management of Bone Loss

Engh GA, Herzwurm PJ, Parks NL: Treatment of major defects of bone with bulk allografts and stemmed components during total knee arthroplasty. *J Bone Joint Surg* 1997;79A:1030-1039.

Thirty patients with 35 allografts were followed for 50 months. In 87%, results were good or excellent. No re-revisions occurred with femoral head allografts. Four uncemented components on structural allografts yielded 3 with subsidence-no revisions. There were 8 complications in 7 patients (2 possible infections).

Haas SB, Insall JN, Montgomery W III, Windsor RE: Revision total knee arthroplasty with use of modular components with stems inserted without cement. *J Bone Joint Surg* 1995;77A: 1700-1707.

In this study, 74 revision total knee arthroplasties were performed on 76 patients. Average follow-up was 42 months. Both posterior stabilized and constrained polyethylene inserts were used. Results were good or excellent in 83%. Six failures occurred: 3 for infection, 2 with loosening, and 1 with instability.

Harris AI, Poddar S, Gitelis S, Sheinkop MB, Rosenberg AG: Arthroplasty with a composite of an allograft and a prosthesis for knees with severe deficiency of bone. *J Bone Joint Surg* 1995; 77A:373-386.

Fourteen patients with extensive structural grafts were followed for an average of 43 months. Results were good or excellent in 13. Two reconstructions in 1 knee failed. The junction healed in all but 1 patient. Six complications occurred with 4 patients (1 infection, 1 dislocation).

Mow CS, Wiedel JD: Structural allografting in revision total knee arthroplasty. *J Arthroplasty* 1996;11:235-241.

Fifteen patients underwent structural allografting for large segmental, cavitary, or combination defects. All 15 achieved host graft union. Average follow-up was 47 months. One complication included tibial component fracture over an area of graft resorption.

Modularity

Chen F, Krackow KA: Management of tibial defects in total knee arthroplasty. *Clin Orthop* 1994;305:249-257.

Osteotomy was performed on 12 bovine tibias with a medial plateau fashioned defect to produce oblique, horizontal, and vertical surfaces and to allow positioning of wedges or block augments attached to the tibial tray and cemented in situ. The construct was then assessed for rigidity, which was markedly better in block than in wedge augmentation.

Fehring TK, Peindl RD, Humble RS, Harrow ME, Frick SL: Modular tibial augmentation in total knee arthroplasty. *Clin Orthop* 1996;327:207-217.

In this cadaveric study, the way load strains are distributed for wedge and block tibial augments was assessed, and little difference was found between the 2 methods. It was suggested that the augment with the best fit should be used, with minimal proximal tibial bone resection. These results may not be the same in vivo because cadaveric bone has inferior subchondral architecture.

Murray PB, Rand JA, Hanssen AD: Cemented long stem revision total knee arthroplasty. *Clin Orthop* 1994;309:116-123.

Twenty-five tibial and 38 femoral cemented long stems in 35 patients were studied after 58.2 months; there was a 32% incidence of tibial radiolucencies of less than 1 mm that were nonprogressive. There was a 12% femoral incidence of radiolucency, with 1 case (3%) being progressive and resulting in aseptic failure.

Pagnano MW, Trousdale RT, Rand JA: Tibial wedge augmentation for bone deficiency in total knee arthroplasty. *Clin Orthop* 1995;321:151-155.

Twenty-eight total knee arthroplasties using wedge tibial augmentation were studied in 25 patients. Initial report at 2.3 years demonstrated 79% excellent and 21% good results. At 5.6 years, only 24 knees were available for clinical assessment. Results were excellent in 67% and good in 29%; there had been 1 revision for metal-backed patella failure. Beneath the metal wedge, there were 11 radiolucencies less than 1 mm and 2 radiolucencies 1 to 3 mm in width, none of which was progressive.

Prosthetic Design and Fusion of the Knee

Revision Knee Arthroplasty

Bourne RB, Crawford HA: Principles of revision total knee arthroplasty. *Orthop Clin North Am* 1998;29:331-337.

A summary of the principles for revision knee surgery and the indications for constrained total knee replacements.

Cuckler JM: Revision total knee arthroplasty: How much constraint is necessary? *Orthopedics* 1995;18:932-933, 936.

The article indicates that additional constraint may be necessary if the collateral ligaments are compromised.

Hartford JM, Goodman SB, Schurman DJ, Knoblick G: Complex primary and revision total knee arthroplasty using the condylar constrained prosthesis: An average 5-year follow-up. *J Arthroplasty* 1998;13:380-387.

The article reviews 33 knees that underwent constrained condylar replacements. Sixteen knees were for revisions and 17 knees were primary replacements with severe deformity. Three knees required another revision: one for recurrent infection, one for periprosthetic fracture, and one for tibial loosening. The article discusses the indications for constrained replacements and reports good results with the implant.

Heck DA, Melfi CA, Mamlin LA, et al: Revision rates after knee replacement in the United States. *Med Care* 1998;36:661-669.

A summary of the statistics concerning revision surgery within 2 years of the primary knee replacement. The incidence of reoperation is 3% and the factors that correlated with the revision are male gender, younger age, longer hospital stay for the primary knee replacement, more diagnoses at the time of admission, surgical complications during the primary knee replacement, and surgery at an urban hospital.

Lachiewicz PF, Falatyn SP: Clinical and radiographic results of the Total Condylar III and Constrained Condylar total knee arthroplasty. *J Arthroplasty* 1996;11:916-922.

The authors report no mechanical failures of the knees implanted in a primary setting and 2 loosenings in revision total knees. They conclude the prosthesis is a good implant in complex knee reconstructions.

Rosenberg AG, Verner JJ, Galante JO: Clinical results of total knee revision using the Total Condylar III prosthesis. *Clin Orthop* 1991;273:83-90.

The article reports 36 knees treated with the total condylar III prosthesis, 15 for infection and 21 for loosening. Twenty-five knees were excellent or good, 10 fair or poor, and 1 failure. The authors conclude that less constrained devices should be used; however, 50% of the tibias were cut in slight varus and 73% of the femurs were in slight flexion. The results may be prejudiced by the surgical technique and may not reflect the true results of a constrained condylar knee.

Vince KG, Long W: Revision knee arthroplasty: The limits of press fit medullary fixation. *Clin Orthop* 1995;317:172-177.

A review of the constrained condylar knee (CCK) in a press fit environment. The article indicates that the CCK should not be used with a press fit technology.

Knee Fusion

Cheng SL, Gross AE: Knee arthrodesis using a short locked intramedullary nail: A new technique. *Am J Knee Surg* 1995;8: 56-59.

A technique report concerning knee arthrodesis that favors intramedullary techniques and summarizes the various techniques available.

Windsor RE: Knee arthrodesis, in Insall JN, Windsor RE, Scott WN, Kelly MA, Aglietti P (eds): *Surgery of the Knee,* ed 2. New York, NY, Churchill Livingstone, 1993, pp 1103-1116.

This is a summary of the present state of knee fusion through the early 1990s. There have not been any significant changes since this article.

Classic Bibliography

Modes of Failure

Bargren JH, Blaha JD, Freeman MA: Alignment in total knee arthroplasty: Correlated biomechanical and clinical observations. *Clin Orthop* 1983;173:178-183.

Cameron HU, Hunter GA: Failure in total knee arthroplasty: Mechanisms, revisions, and results. *Clin Orthop* 1982;170:141-146.

Figgie HE III, Goldberg VM, Heiple KG, Moller HS III, Gordon NH: The influence of tibial-patellofemoral location on function of the knee in patients with the posterior stabilized condylar knee prosthesis. *J Bone Joint Surg* 1986;68A:1035-1040.

Moreland JR: Mechanisms of failure in total knee arthroplasty. *Clin Orthop* 1988;226:49-64.

Sisto DJ, Lachiewicz PF, Insall JN: Treatment of supracondylar fractures following prosthetic arthroplasty of the knee. *Clin Orthop* 1985;196:265-272.

Sledge CB, Ewald FC: Total knee arthroplasty experience at the Robert Breck Brigham Hospital. *Clin Orthop* 1979;145:78-84.

Stuart MJ, Larson JE, Morrey BF: Reoperation after condylar revision total knee arthroplasty. *Clin Orthop* 1993;286:168-173.

Vernace JV, Rothman RH, Booth RE Jr, Balderston RA: Arthroscopic management of the patellar clunk syndrome following posterior stabilized total knee arthroplasty. *J Arthroplasty* 1989;4:179-182.

Surgical Techniques and Principles

Berger RA, Rubash HE, et al: Determining the rotational alignment of the femoral component in total knee arthroplasty using the epicondylar axis. *Clin Orthop* 1993;286:40-47.

Briard JH: Patellofemoral instability in total knee arthroplasty. *J Arthroplasty* 1989;4(suppl):87-97.

Emerson RH Jr, Head WC: Extensor mechanism reconstruction with an allograft after total knee arthroplasty. *Clin Orthop* 1994;303:79-85.

Fehring TK, McAlister JA Jr: Frozen histologic section as a guide to sepsis in revision joint arthroplasty. *Clin Orthop* 1994;304: 229-237.

Jacobs MA, Hungerford DS, Krackow KA, Lennox DW: Revision total knee arthroplasty for aseptic failure. *Clin Orthop* 1988;226:78-85.

Kramhoft M, Bodtker S, Carlsen A: Outcome of infected total knee arthroplasty. *J Arthroplasty* 1994;9:617-621.

Mow CS, Wiedel JD: Noncemented revision total knee arthroplasty. *Clin Orthop* 1994;309:110-115.

Murray PB, Rand JA,: Cemented long-stem revision total knee arthroplasty. *Clin Orthop* 1994;309:116-123.

Padgett DE, Stern SH, et al: Revision total knee arthroplasty for failed unicompartmental replacement. *J Bone Joint Surg* 1991;73A:186-190.

Trousdale RT, Hanssen AD, et al: V-Y quadricepsplasty in total knee arthroplasty. *Clin Orthop* 1993;286:48-55.

Vince KG: Revision knee arthroplasty technique, in Heckman JD (ed): *Instructional Course Lectures* 42. Rosemont, IL, American Academy of Orthopaedic Surgeons, 1993; pp 325-339.

von Foerster G, Kluber D: Mid- to long-term results after treatment of 118 cases of periprosthetic infections after knee joint replacement using one-stage exchange surgery. *Orthopade* 1991;20:244-252.

Whiteside LA: Cementless revision total knee arthroplasty. *Clin Orthop* 1993;286:160-167.

Wilde AH, Schickendantz MS, et al: The incorporation of tibial allografts in total knee arthroplasty. *J Bone Joint Surg* 1990;72A:815-824.

Management of Bone Loss

Ritter MA, Keating EM, Faris PM: Screw and cement fixation of large defects in total knee arthroplasty: A sequel. *J Arthroplasty* 1993;8:63-65.

Whiteside LA: Cementless revision total knee arthroplasty. *Clin Orthop* 1993;286:160-167.

Modularity

Bourne RB, Finlay JB: The influence of tibial component intramedullary stems and implant-cortex contact on the strain distribution of the proximal tibia following total knee arthroplasty. *Clin Orthop* 1986;208:95-99.

Brooks PJ, Walker PS, Scott RS: Tibial component fixation in deficient Tibial bone stock. *Clin Orthop* 1984;184:302-308.

Index

A

AAOS MODEMS Project, 85–86
Abrasion (implant materials), 167
Acetabular components, 113–114
  cemented total hip replacement (THA) and, 186–190
  failure, 189
  revision THR and, 222–225
  socket survival in cemented THA and, 187–188
Acetabular rim syndrome, 105
Activities of Daily Living Scale (ADLS), 297
Activity
  after subchondral bone microfracture, 262
  arthritic knee scoring techniques and, 252
  arthritic knees and, 249
  cemented femoral components and, 183
  clinical care pathway, 54–55
  collateral knee ligaments and, 245
  cruciate ligaments and, 242–243
  high tibial osteotomy (HTO) and, 260
  patellofemoral mechanics and, 244
  posterior-stabilized total knee arthroplasty (TKA), 310–311
  TKA scoring systems and, 295–297
  uncemented TKA designs and, 276
  valgus bracing and, 257
Acute hematogenous infection (AHI), 140–141, 145
Acute normovolemic hemodilution (ANH), 62–65
Adhesion (implant materials), 167. *See also* Implant materials
Advisory Statements (AAOS), 139–140
Alcoholism
  dislocation and, 149, 152
  osteonecrosis and, 127–128, 131
Alignment. *See* Range of motion
Allergic reactions/side effects, 57
  antibiotics and, 140
  nonsteroidal anti-inflammatory drugs (NSAIDs) and, 255
  steroid injections, 255–256
  synovectomy and, 257
Allogeneic blood, 57–59. *See also* Allogeneic transfusion alternatives
Allogeneic transfusion alternatives
  acute normovolemic hemodilution (ANH), 62–63
  blood substitutes, 63
  directed donation, 59
  erythropoietin, 61–62
  experimental, 63
  hypotensive anesthesia, 62
  insurance and, 62
  intraoperative salvage, 63
  legal considerations, 63–64
  postoperative salvage, 63
  preoperative autologous donation (PAD), 59–61
Allografts
  biology of, 35–36
  bone defect reconstruction and, 351, 354
  bone defects and, 342, 345
  immunology of, 36–37
  infection and, 147
  particulate debris and, 176
  revision THR and, 222, 225, 231
  in THA, 37–38
  in TKA, 37–38
American Society of Anesthesiology, 51
Amikacin, 144
Ampicillin, 140
Amputation, 146, 327, 350
Analgesia after TKA, 287–288
Anatomic considerations. *See also* Patients; Surgical approaches
  hip kinematics/kinetics and, 97–98
  tibiofemoral joint and, 239–240
Anatomic Graduated Component (AGC), 304–306
Anatomic Modular Knee implant, 307
Anderson Orthopaedic Research Institute (AORI), 342–343, 353–354
Anemia
  medical management and, 54
  physiology of, 56
Anesthesia
  achievement of rigid implant fixation and, 188
  hip reconstruction and, 70–71
  hypotensive, 62
  knee reconstruction and, 71–72
  pain management and, 72–73
  patient-controlled, 71–72
  postoperative care and, 72
  preanesthetic evaluation, 67–68
  pulmonary disease and, 53
  techniques, 68–69
  thrombogenesis during, 15–16
Angina. *See* Cardiovascular disease
Ankylosis
  heterotopic ossification, 159
  spondylitis, 5
Anterior cruciate ligament (ACL), 240–243
  mobile bearing designs and, 314–316
  revision TKA and, 316–317, 356
  unicompartmental knee arthroplasty (UKA) and, 301–303
Anterior surgical approach (Iliofemoral/Smith-Petersen), 91, 149
Anterolateral surgical approach (Watson-Jones), 91
Antibiotics. *See also* Infection
  after TKA, 288
  during exchange arthroplasty, 146
  infection and, 138–140

infection treatments and, 327–328
PROSTALAC and, 146–147
suppression of, 144
wound healing and, 333
Anticoagulants
deep vein thrombosis (DVT) and, 290–291
guidelines for, 158–159
postoperative care and, 72
venous thromboembolic disease (VTED) and, 13–16, 17–22
Antigens. *See* Immunology
Aprotinin, 63
Arrhythmias. *See* Cardiovascular disease
Arthritis
heterotopic ossification and, 159
inflammatory, 3–5
of the knee
physical examination, 249–252
scoring techniques, 252–253
long-term TKA results and, 306–307
nonarthroplasty alternatives
arthroscopic lavage/debridement, 257–258
chondrocyte transplantation, 262–263
marrow stimulation techniques, 261–262
osteotomy, 258–260
steroid injections, 255–256
synovectomy, 256–257
valgus bracing, 257
osteotomy and, 103
psoriatic, 5
revision TKA and, 345
Arthrodesis
infection and, 146
infection treatments and, 327
synovitis and, 3
Arthrogram, 142
Arthrography, 76
Arthroplasty
algorithm for blood conservation, 64–65
allografts in THA, 37–38
allografts in TKA, 38–39
demineralized bone matrix (DBM) and, 43–44
exchanges/reimplantations, 145–146
hemisurface replacement, 134
hypovolemia and, 55–56
metal implant materials, 25–29
modified cup, 134
polyethylene implant materials, 30–33
polymethylmethacrylate (PMMA) implant materials, 33–34
postoperative care and, 71
postoperative pain management and, 70–72
resection, 135, 146
surface replacement, 134–135
synovitis and, 3
Arthroscopy, 327
Articulation
antibiotic in spacers and, 328
hip contact stresses and, 98–99
metal-on-metal implants, 29–30
metal-on-polyethylene implants, 27–29
polyethylene implant materials, 30–33
polymethylmethacrylate (PMMA), 33–34
Aseptic necrosis. *See* Osteonecrosis (ON)
Aspiration/arthrogram, 142
osteolysis and, 176
revision TKA and, 347
Aspirin
surgery and, 4
venous thromboembolic disease (VTED) and, 18–19
Assessment. *See* Outcomes assessment
Asthma, 53
Augments (revision TKA), 355–356
Autogenous chondrocyte transplantation, 262–263
Autografts
biology of, 35–36
bone defect reconstruction and, 351
immunology of, 36–37
Autologous blood. *See* Preoperative autologous donation (PAD)
Autolysed, antigen extracted, allogeneic bone (AAA) bone, 36–37
Avascular necrosis. *See* Osteonecrosis (ON)
Azathioprine, 4

B

Bacterial infections. *See* Gram positive/negative organisms; Infection
Bernese periacetabular osteotomy, 104–105
Bicompartmental knee replacement, 314
Biomechanics
cemented total hip replacement (THA) and, 185
fixation of TKA and, 275
gait observation/analysis and, 249, 257, 298
hip design
articular contact stresses and, 98–99
bone stresses and, 99
kinematics/kinetics, 97–98
loosening and, 167
of osteotomy, 103, 258–259
patellofemoral, 243–244
tibiofemoral joint and, 239–240
total knee design
fixation, 268
function, 265–266
load transfer, 266–268
wear, 268–270
uncemented femoral components and, 123–124
valgus bracing and, 257
wear studies and, 171
Bioresorption, 45
Biosynthetics. *See* Grafts
Blood loss. *See also* Transfusions
allogeneic transfusion alternatives, 59–64
arthroplasty and, 55–56
blood substitutes, 63
nonsteroidal anti-inflammatory drugs (NSAIDs) and, 255
obesity and, 203
reduction due to salvage, 63
transfusion indications, 56–57
trochanteric nonunion, 160–162
Blood urea nitrogen, 68
Bone cement. *See* Polymethylmethacrylate (PMMA)
Bone defect classifications
description, 342–345
reconstruction and, 351

Bone grafts. *See also* Grafts
  autogenous cancellous, 43
  bone defect reconstruction and, 351
  bone marrow/stem cells and, 44
  ceramics and, 44–46
  Collagraft and, 46
  demineralized bone matrix (DBM) and, 43–44
  Grafton gel and, 44
  muscle pedicle (osteonecrotic), 133
  revision THR surgical approaches and, 225
  types, 35–36
Bone ingrowth
  of cemented total knee arthroplasty, 275–277
  patellar component loosening and, 330
Bone loss. *See* Bone grafts
  bone defect classifications, 342–345, 353–354
  detection via computed tomography (CT), 76
  exchange arthroplasty and, 145–146
  osteolysis and, 177
  periprosthetic, 121–122
  revision THR and, 221–222
  revision TKA and, 352–353
Bone morphogenetic protein (BMP)
  bone healing enhancement and, 49
  osteoinduction and, 46–48
  as osteoinductive agent, 35–36, 42–44
Bone resorption, 177–178
  cemented acetabular components and, 189
  cemented femoral components and, 183
Bone scintigraphy, 76–78, 347
Bone stresses, 99–100. *See also* Stresses

C

C-reactive protein (CRP), 141, 324
Cancellous grafts (osteonecrotic), 133
Capacitive coupling (CC), 131–132
Cardiovascular disease
  medical management and, 51–52
  osteonecrosis and, 127
Cartilage
  chondrocyte transplantation and, 262–263
  lesion treatment, 261
  osteoarthritis and, 8–10
Cefaxolin, 140, 326
Cefuroxime, 326
Cement disease. *See* Osteolysis
Cement fatigue/stress. *See* Stresses
Cemented femoral components, 207–210, 213
Cemented total hip replacement (THR)
  acetabular components
    cementing techniques, 188–189
    corrosion/wear of implant devices, 187–189
    failure, 189
    hypotensive anesthesia and, 188
    modularity and, 187–188
    osteolysis and, 187
    radiostereometric analysis (RSA) and, 188
    socket survival, 187–188
  antibiotics and, 139
  centralizers and, 113
  debonding of, 167
  design evolution rationale for, 109–110
  femoral components
    cement technique, 208–209
    cementing techniques, 181
    centralizers and, 184
    design characteristics/failure mechanisms, 207–208
    design features of, 110–111, 185
    failure, 181–183
    generational techniques, 181
    modularity and, 185
    osteolysis and, 182–184
    porosity reduction in, 184–185
    radiologic evaluation, 208
    surface finish/precoat of, 185–186
    surgical technique, 209–210
  implant geometry for, 111–112
  internal collar of, 112
  material, 110–113
  osteolysis and, 177
  revision THR and, 222, 229–231
  surface finish of, 112–113
Cemented total knee arthroplasty (TKA)
  bone ingrowth and, 275–277
  long-term results, 303–306
  physical therapy after, 288–289
Cementing techniques
  acetabular components, 188–189
  femoral components, 181
Cementless total hip arthroplasty (THA). *See* Uncemented total hip arthroplasty
Cementless total knee arthroplasty (TKA). *See* Uncemented total knee arthroplasty
Centralizers
  and cemented femoral components, 113, 184
  hybrid THA femoral components and, 209
Centrifugation. *See* Porosity reduction
Cephalexin, 327
Cephalosporing, 288
Cephalothin, 144
Ceramics
  debonding of, 48
  hybrid THA acetabular components and, 212
  as osteoconductive material, 44–47
Cerebrovascular disease
  joint reconstruction and, 67
  medical management and, 52
Charnley flatback design, 109
  description, 111–113
  stem failure and, 165
  surface finish/precoat of, 185
Chondrocyte transplantation, 262–263
Chromium orthophosphate, 176
Chronic obstructive pulmonary disease (COPD)
  joint reconstruction and, 67
  medical management and, 53
Cincinnati Knee Scale, 297
Clindamycin, 140, 327
Clinical care pathway (THA), 54–55
Clinical care pathway (TKA), 289
Coating. *See also* Surface finish
  cemented femoral components and, 185–186
  countersurface roughness, 169
  dislocation and, 149
  of hybrid THA acetabular

components, 211
of hybrid THA femoral components, 207–208
osteolysis and, 177
polymethylmethacrylate (PMMA), 167–168
revision THR and, 217
stem failure and, 165
uncemented acetabular components, 201
uncemented femoral components, 198–199
uncemented femoral reconstruction and, 231–232
uncemented TKA designs and, 307–308
Cobalt-chromium implant material. *See* Metals; Polyethylene
Collagen
blood loss reduction and, 63
Collagraft, 46
as osteoconductive material, 43
supracondylar femoral osteotomy and, 259
Collagraft, 46
Collar of femoral design, 112, 207–208
Collateral knee ligaments
balancing of, 244–245, 282–285
revision TKA balancing, 356
Combined spinal epidural (CSE), 67
Complications. *See also* Allergic reactions/side effects; Infection
dislocation, 149–152, 162–164
heterotopic ossification, 159
of high tibial osteotomy (HTO), 259
infection after TKA, 323–329
intraoperative fracture, 160
nerve/vascular injuries, 165–166
neurovascular, 333–334
osteolysis, 175–179
patellofemoral, 329–332
periprosthetic fractures, 332–333
posterior-stabilized total knee arthroplasty (TKA), 311–312
revision THR and, 227–229
thromboembolism, 156–159
trochanteric nonunion, 160–162
wound healing, 333
Compressive dressings, 63
Computed tomography (CT)
arthritic knees and, 251
bone loss detection via, 76
revision THR and, 220, 228
revision TKA and, 346–347
Condyles of knee
cemented designs, 303–306
passive motion and, 239–242
Conformity, 356–357
Constraint, 356–357
Contact stresses (hip), 98–99
Continuous passive motion (CPM) machine, 289
Coralline calcium phosphate implants, 44–45
Core decompression (CD), 132
Coronary artery disease (CAD), 67
Corrosion/wear of implant devices, 25–27. *See also* Mechanical failure; Stresses
acetabular components, 113–114
acetabular socket survival in THA, 187–188
of cemented femoral components, 181–183, 186
cemented (TKA) and, 275–276
future trends, 190
of hybrid THA acetabular components, 212–213
mobile bearing designs and, 313–314
osteoconductive coatings and, 48–49
particulate debris and, 175–176
patient activity and, 171, 174
radiographic signs of, 76, 141
revision TKA and, 346
total knee design and, 268–270
ultrasound detection of, 78
in vivo assessment, 169–170
in vivo studies, 170–174
Cortical strut grafts (osteonecrotic), 132–133
Corticosteroids
inflammatory arthritis surgery and, 4
nonarthroplasty alternatives and, 255–256
osteonecrosis and, 127–128, 131
Costs
of complications, 137
of infected TKA, 323
outcomes assessment and, 253
revision TKA and, 345
Coumadin. *See also* Warfarin
inflammatory arthritis surgery and, 4
thromboembolism and, 158–159
Countersurface, 169, 176. *See also* Coating
Creep, 185
Cruciate ligaments
arthritic knees and, 251
balancing of, 284
gait observation/analysis and, 298
mobile bearing designs and, 314–316
passive motion and, 240–243
revision TKA and, 356
revision TKR and, 316–317
unicompartmental knee arthroplasty (UKA) and, 301–303, 314
unicondylar knees and, 265
Cyclooxygenase (COX), 255

D

Databases
AAOS MODEMS project, 85–86
aggregation of, 84
Hip and Knee Registry, 85
TKA scoring and, 253
"Dead leg" sensation, 105
Debonding. *See* Loosening (implant materials)
Debridement
infection and, 145
nonarthroplasty alternatives, 257–258
Deep vein thrombosis (DVT)
diagnosis of, 16–17
extended risk of, 21–22
Factor V Leiden and, 15
following surgery, 13
high tibial osteotomy (HTO) and, 259
magnetic resonance venography (MRV) and, 79–80
surgery duration and, 69
testing, 289–290
thromboembolism and, 156–159
treatment, 290–292

Deformities, 249–250
Demineralized bone matrix (DBM), 43–44
  as bone graft substitute, 47–48
Demographics
  osteoarthritis and, 7
  osteonecrosis and, 132
  outcomes assessment and, 83–85
  population studies, 8
  TKA outcomes assessment and, 297
  venous thromboembolic disease (VTED) and, 15
Dental patients, 139–140, 327
Design features. *See* Implant materials
  hybrid THA acetabular components and, 210–211
  of hybrid THA femoral components, 207–208
  uncemented acetabular components, 199–200
  uncemented femoral components, 195–196
Desmopressin, 63
Diabetes
  antibiotics prophylaxis and, 140
  infection and, 155
  joint reconstruction and, 67
  medical management and, 52–53
Diagnostic studies
  deep vein thrombosis (DVT), 289–290
  gait observation/analysis, 249, 257, 298
  infection and, 140–143
  laboratory tests, 54–55
Diclofenac, 255
Direct current (DC), 131–132
Direct lateral surgical approach (Modified Hardinge surgical approach), 91–92
Dislocation
  general description, 162–164
  mobile bearing designs and, 270
  osteoporosis and, 228
  patellar, 284, 331
  patient-related factors and, 149
  prevalence, 149
  prevention, 152
  prognosis, 152
  recurrent, 152, 164
  surgical factors, 150–151
  treatment, 151–152
Dislocation rate
  direct lateral (Modified Hardinge) and, 92
  posterior (Langenbeck/Moore) and, 93
  revision THR and, 228–229
Doxycycline, 144
Dripps' stratification system, 51
Dysplasia, 104–105

E

Early postoperative infection (EPOI), 140–141, 144, 145
Education
  dislocation and, 152
  of surgical patient, 3
Electrical stimulation, 131–132
Electrocardiogram (EKG)
  in pre/perioperative evaluation, 54–55
  as preoperative evaluation, 68
Endocrine disease, 54
Endoprosthetic replacement, 134
Enoxaparin, 20–21
Enterococcus feacalis, 137
Enteropathic arthritis, 5
Epidural analgesia/anesthesia, 287–288
Epidural anesthesia, 68–70, 334. *See also* Anesthesia
Erythrocyte sedimentation rate (ESR), 141, 324
Erythropoietin
  algorithm for blood conservation and, 64–65
  allogeneic transfusion alternatives and, 61–62
  use in hematologic/endocrine diseases, 54
Exeter femoral component, 111–112, 186
Experimental/future methods
  infection treatments and, 140, 147
  mobile bearing designs and, 317
  osteoarthritis and, 10
  osteolysis and, 179
  with polyethylene components, 190
  with polymethylmethacrylate (PMMA), 34
  uncemented THR and, 204
Extended trochanteric osteotomy, 94–95
Extensor mechanism
  quadriceps snip and, 282
  revision TKA and, 341, 348

F

Factor V Leiden, 14–15
Familial thrombophilia, 14–15
Fatigue (implant materials), 167. *See also* Stresses
Femur. *See also* Cemented total hip replacement (THR); Knee joint; Surface finish; Uncemented femoral components
  allografts of, 38
  biomechanics of, 123–124
  bone defect classifications and, 343–345
  bone marrow and, 44
  cemented femoral components, 181–186
  collateral knee ligaments and, 244–245
  distal fracture, 332
  intraoperative fracture, 160
  osteonecrosis and, 129–130
  patellofemoral mechanics and, 243–244
  periprosthetic fracture and, 218–219
  revision THR and, 221–222, 226–227
  revisions with osteotomy, 94–95
  THA after osteotomy of, 106
  uncemented THA, 117–124, 195–199
Fibrin glue, 63
Fluoroscopy
  arthritic knees and, 251
  revision TKA and, 347
  TKA evaluations and, 299
Forestier's disease, 159
Fracture healing
  electrical stimulation and, 131–132
  intraoperative, 160
  osteoinduction and, 46–47
  osteonecrosis and, 127, 129
  of patella, 341
  periprosthetic, 218–219, 228, 332–333

Free vascularized fibular grafts (FVFG), 133
Freeman-Samuelson implant, 307
Freezing/freeze-drying bone grafts, 35–37
Friction/frictional torque (implant materials), 168
Fungal infections, 138, 325–326

G

Gait observation/analysis, 249, 257, 297
Gallium scanning, 77–78
Gamma-radiation effect, 30–31
Gaucher's disease, 127–128
Gender as risk factor
  cemented femoral components and, 183
  dislocation and, 149
  infection and, 155
  osteolysis and, 178
  revision TKA and, 345
  wear studies and, 171
Gene technology, 46–47
Gentamicin, 144
Geographic variation. *See* Demographics
Geometry of uncemented femoral components, 117–119, 122–124
Glucocorticoids
  inflammatory arthritis surgery and, 3–5
  nonarthroplasty alternatives and, 255–256
Glucose, 68
Glycocalyx, 138, 145
Gonipora, 45
Grafts. *See also* Bone grafts
  biosynthetic materials and, 44–46
  cartilage transplantations, 261
  graft-versus-host disease (GVHD), 58
  one-stage exchange arthroplasty and, 145
  procedures, 132–134
Gram positive/negative organisms, 137
  after TKA, 288, 325–326
  infection and, 142–143, 220
Greenfield filters, 158
Gruen zonal analysis, 208

H

Heart disease, 67
Heberden's nodes, 7
Hematologic disease, 54
Hemisurface replacement arthroplasty, 134
Hemoglobin/hematocrit
  hematologic/endocrine diseases and, 54
  as preoperative evaluation, 55–57, 61, 68
Hemophilia
  antibiotics prophylaxis and, 140
  medical management and, 54
Heparin
  deep vein thrombosis (DVT) and, 291
  fractionated, 19–21
  thromboembolism and, 159
  venous thromboembolic disease (VTED) and, 15–17
Hepatitis
  allogeneic blood and, 57–58
  transfusions and, 60
Heterotopic ossification
  description, 159
  revision THR and, 229
  trochanteric nonunion and, 160
Hexacetide, 255
High tibial osteotomy (HTO), 258–259, 260–261, 301–303
Hinged knee replacement, 354, 358
Hip and Knee Registry, 85
Hip fusion, 135
Hip kinematics/kinetics, 97–98
  after total hip reconstruction, 99–100
Hip-locking, 105
Homan's sign, 157
Hospital for Special Surgery (HSS) Knee Score, 252, 260, 295, 297, 304
Hospital Infection Control Practice Advisory Committee, 137
Hospital Service Areas, 83–84
Human immunodeficiency virus (HIV), 57–58
Human T-cell lymphoma virus (HTLV), 57–58
Hyalgan, 256
Hybrid total hip replacement (THR)
  cemented femoral components
    cement technique, 208–209
    design characteristics/failure mechanisms, 207–208
    radiologic evaluation, 208
    surgical technique, 209–210
    results, 213
  uncemented acetabular components and
    design characteristics, 210–211
    radiologic evaluation, 212
    surgical technique, 211–212
    wear/osteolysis, 212–213
Hydroxyapatite (HA)
  in ceramic osteoconduction, 44–46
  dislocation and, 149
  as osteoconductive coating, 48–49
  as osteoconductive material, 43
  in uncemented femoral components, 198
Hylamer M, 213
Hypertension
  joint reconstruction and, 67
  medical management and, 52
Hypofibrinolysis, 128
Hypotension. *See* Hypovolemia
Hypotensive anesthesia
  acetabular cemented sockets and, 188
  algorithm for blood conservation and, 64–65
  as alternative therapy, 62
Hypovolemia, 56–57

I

IBPS prosthesis. *See* Posterior-stabilized total knee arthroplasty (TKA)
Iliofemoral/Smith-Petersen surgical approach, 91
Imaging. *See also* Radiographs; Scanning
  of arthritic knees, 251–252
  arthrography, 76
  bone scintigraphy, 76–78
  computed tomography (CT), 76
  magnetic resonance imaging (MRI), 78–79
  THA/TKA radiographs, 75–76
  ultrasound, 78
Imipenem, 144
Immunology
  allogeneic blood and, 58

of autografts/allografts, 36–37
immunoglobulin (Ig) scans, 78
Implant bone osteolysis, 176–177
Implant materials. *See also* Coating; Prosthesis
acetabular components, 113–114
biomechanics of, 123–124
biosynthetic grafts and, 44–46
for cemented total hip replacement (THA), 110–113
coatings of, 120–121
computed tomography (CT) of arthritic knees and, 251
effect on magnetic resonance imaging (MRI), 78–79
fracture of, 181–182
geometry of, 111–112, 117–119, 123–124
infections after TKA and, 323–324
initial stability, 117–119, 123
load transfer and, 266–268
long-term stability, 119–121, 123
loosening, 167
metal, 25–29
migration of, 100
mobile bearing designs and, 269–270
modularity and revision TKA, 353
osteoconductive coatings, 48–49
osteoinductive coatings, 49
polyethylene, 30–33
polyethylene implant materials, 113–114, 168–169
polymethylmethacrylate (PMMA), 33–34, 268
revision THR and, 217, 221, 232
revision TKA and, 340
revision TKA range of motion and, 341
rigid fixation of, 188
sizes, 118
stem failure, 164–165
sterilization of, 30–31
ultrahigh molecular weight polyethylene (UHMWPE) and, 265, 267–270
uncemented acetabular components, 199–200
uncemented femoral components, 197
uncemented TKA designs and, 307–308
unicondylar knees and, 265
Incisions, 281–282, 333
revision TKA and, 347–348
Indium, 78, 142, 220
Infection
allogeneic transfusion alternatives and, 60
biomaterial hypersensitivity, 138
definition/classification, 324
dental patients and, 139–140
detection via aspiration arthrography, 76
detection via bone scintigraphy, 77–78
detection via ultrasound, 78
diagnosis, 140–143, 324–325
future treatment trends, 140, 147
general treatment, 143–144
glycocalyx and, 138
gram negative organisms, 137
gram positive organisms, 137
incidence after THA, 137, 155
incidence/predisposing factors, 323–324
intravenous antibiotics and, 288
magnetic resonance imaging (MRI) and, 79
microbial adherence and, 138
microbial flora evolution, 137
mycobacterial/fungal, 138
osteolysis and, 176
prevention, 325–327
prophylaxis of, 138–140
psoriatic arthritis and, 5
radiographic signs of, 75–76
reinfection, 329
revision THR and, 218
revision TKA and, 340, 342, 350
rheumatoid arthritis and, 4
treatment, 327–329
treatment research, 147
vancomycin resistance and, 137
Inflammatory arthritis
enteropathic arthropathy and, 5
preoperative evaluation, 3–4
rheumatoid arthritis with, 3
treatment, 4–5
Inflammatory bowel disease, 128
Infrared spectroscopy, 30–31
Injury. *See* Trauma
Instrument validation, 84
Intra-articular narcotics, 288
Intraoperative cell salvage. *See* Salvage (RBC)
Ischemic necrosis. *See* Osteonecrosis (ON)
Isograft, 35

J

Judet oblique view (revision THR), 219–220
Juvenile inflammatory arthritis, 202–203
Juvenile rheumatoid arthritis, 5

K

Kellgren and Lawrence osteoarthritis criteria, 7
Kinematic Condylar prosthesis, 303
Kinematics. *See also* Activity; Biomechanics
gait observation/analysis and, 298
posterior-stabilized TKA and, 308–312
Knee fusion, 358
Knee joint
arthritic evaluation of, 249–253
collateral ligaments of, 244–245
cruciate ligaments of, 240–243
meniscal function, 240
passive motion of, 239–240
patellofemoral mechanics of, 243–244
rating systems, 295–299
Knee Society (KS) Score, 252, 260, 295, 297, 299
Krackow ligament approach, 284–285

L

Laboratory test. *See* Diagnostic studies
Langenbeck/Moore surgical approach, 92–93
Late chronic infection (LCI), 140–141, 144–145
Lateral collateral ligament (LCL)
arthritic knees and, 250–251
balancing/tightening of, 282–285
description, 244–245
Lateral parapatellar incision, 281

Leg length inequality, 228
Legal considerations of transfusions, 63–64
Lesions. *See* Osteonecrosis
Ligament balancing, 282–285
Ligaments
  arthritic knees and, 250
  outcomes assessment for, 297
  TKA and, 38
Loosening (implant materials)
  cemented versus uncemented versus hybrid TKA designs, 307–308
  description, 167
  of patellar component, 329–330
  revision THR and, 217, 219
  revision TKA and, 341
  uncemented THA results and, 202–203
Low Contact Stress (LCS), 276
Lower Extremity Instrument, 85
Lupus. *See* Systemic lupus erythematosus
Lysholm Knee Scale, 297

M

Magnetic resonance imaging (MRI)
  arthritic knees and, 252
  for infection, 141
  osteonecrosis and, 128–129, 131
  revision THR and, 220
  for THA/TKA, 78–79
Magnetic resonance venography (MRV), 79–80
Major histocompatibility complex (MHC), 37
Mallory classification of bone deficiency, 221
Malpractice suits (and transfusions), 64
Marrow stimulation techniques, 261–262
Materials. *See* Implant materials
Maxim Posterior Stabilized Knee, 311
McKee prosthesis, 109, 112
Mechanical failure. *See also* Loosening
  mechanisms of, 189, 207–208
  wear modes and, 167–168
Mechanical modalities
  and cemented THA, 109–110
  osteonecrosis and, 127–128
  venous thromboembolic disease (VTED) and, 19
Medial collateral ligament (MCL)
  arthritic knees and, 250
  balancing/tightening of, 282–285
  description, 244–245
Medial parapatellar incision, 281
Medical management
  cardiovascular disease and, 51–52
  cerebrovascular disease and, 52
  diabetes and, 52–53
  hypertension and, 52
  morbid obesity and, 53–54
  morbidity and, 51–52
  mortality and, 51–52
  myocardial infarction (MI) and, 51–52
  osteonecrosis and, 131
  preoperative evaluations and, 51–55
  transient ischemic attack (TIA) and, 52
Medical Outcomes Study, 84, 296
Medications. *See also specific medication*
  after TKA, 287–288
  clinical care pathway, 54–55
  for infection, 140
  inflammatory arthritis surgery and, 4
  joint reconstruction and, 67
  nonsteroidal anti-inflammatory drugs (NSAIDs), 255
  osteonecrosis and, 127
Meloxicam, 255
Meniscal knee functions
  description, 240
  outcomes assessment for, 297
  revision TKA and, 346
Mental health component summary (MCS) scales, 84
Metals. *See also* Implant materials
  implant corrosion/wear processes, 25–27
  metal-on-metal implants, 29–30
  metal-on-polyethylene implants, 27–29
Methotrexate, 4
Methylprednisolone, 255
Microbial adherence, 138
Microbial flora evolution, 137
Microfracture of subchondral bone, 261–262
Migration (settling), 100
Miller-Galante I implant, 307
Mobile bearing designs
  clinical application of, 314–316
  description, 269–270
  future trends, 317
  history/development of, 313
  revision TKR and, 316–317
  wear properties/fixation of, 313–314
MODEMS project, 85–86
Modified cup arthroplasty, 134
Modified Hardinge surgical approach, 91–92
Modularity
  cemented femoral stems and, 185
  cemented sockets and, 187–188
  dislocation and, 151
  uncemented acetabular components, 201–202
  uncemented femoral components and, 199
  in vivo wear assessment and, 169–170
Molecular diagnostic tools, 142–143
Morbidity, 327–328
  anemia and, 56–57
  bone marrow and, 44
  of graft-versus-host disease (GVHD), 58–59
  medical management and, 51–52
  thromboembolism and, 156–159
Mortality
  following surgery, 13–14, 16
  intraoperative salvage and, 63
  medical management and, 51–52
  nonsteroidal anti-inflammatory drugs (NSAIDs) and, 255
  osteonecrosis and, 127
  preoperative autologous donation (PAD) and, 61
Mosaicplasty, 262
Mueller prosthesis, 109, 111–112
Muscle flaps, 249–250
Muscle interaction with cruciate ligaments, 242–243
Muscle pedicle bone grafts (osteonecrotic), 133
Muscle relaxation importance, 69

Mycobacterial infections, 138, 325–326. *See also* Infection
Myocardial infarction (MI), 51–52

N

National Institutes of Health Consensus Conferences, 83–84
Natural Knee, 276
Necrosis. *See* Osteonecrosis (ON)
Negligence suits. *See* Malpractice suits
Nerve palsy, 165–166, 259, 333–334
Neural complications after TKA, 333–334
New Jersey Low-Contact Stress, 313
Nonsteroidal anti-inflammatory drugs (NSAIDs), 255
Nonarthroplasty arthritis alternatives
  arthroscopic lavage/debridement, 257–258
  chondrocyte transplantation, 262–263
  high tibial osteotomy (HTO), 258–259
  marrow stimulation techniques, 261–262
  steroid injections, 255–256
  supracondylar femoral osteotomy, 259–260
  synovectomy, 256–257
  valgus bracing, 257
Nonunions, trochanteric, 160–162
Nuclear medicine, 251

O

Obesity
  dislocation and, 149
  infections after TKA and, 323
  long-term TKA results and, 307
  medical management and, 53–54
  osteolysis and, 178
  uncemented THA results and, 203
Obstetrics. *See* Pregnancy
Ofloxacin, 144
Ogee injection cup design, 114
Oral glucosamine, 255
Ortholoc total knee replacement, 276–277
Ossification, heterotopic, 159
Osteoarthritis, 131
  aging and, 7
  arthritic changes/pathology, 8–9
  cartilage repair, 9–10
  diagnostic evaluation/ epidemiology, 7–8
  inflammatory arthritis, 3–5
  nonsteroidal anti-inflammatory drugs (NSAIDs) and, 255
  surgical treatment, 10
  TKA scoring systems and, 297
  versus rheumatoid arthritis, 3–4
  Western Ontario and McMaster University Osteoarthritis Index (WOMAC), 84–85
Osteochondral allografts (osteonecrotic), 133–134
Osteoconduction
  bone graft substitution and, 42–43
  ceramics and, 44–46
  coatings on THA, 48
  coatings on TKA, 48–49
  definition, 35
Osteogenesis, 35
Osteoinduction
  autolysed, antigen extracted, allogeneic bone (AAA) bone and, 36–37
  bone graft substitution and, 43
  coatings of, 49
  definition, 35
  growth factors of, 46–47
Osteolysis
  acetabular socket survival in THA and, 187
  arthritic knees and, 251
  biology of, 177–178
  bone defects and, 344–345
  cemented femoral components and, 182–184
  clinical presentation of, 176
  detection via computed tomography (CT), 76
  distal femur fracture and, 332
  future trends, 179
  hybrid THA acetabular components and, 212–213
  implant bone access and, 176–177
  management of, 178–179
  osteoconductive coatings and, 48–49
  particulate debris and, 175–176
  periprosthetic fracture and, 218–219
  sickle-cell disease and, 128, 203
  uncemented femoral components and, 121
  uncemented TKA designs and, 276
Osteonecrosis (ON), 127–133
  bone stresses in, 99
  cartilaginous lesions and, 261
  cemented femoral components and, 183
  conditions associated with, 127–128
  core depression (CD) and, 132
  etiology, 127–128
  fusion and, 135
  grafting procedures for, 132–134
  hip reconstruction and, 134–135
  magnetic resonance imaging (MRI) and, 128–129, 131
  nonsurgical treatment, 131–132
  osteotomies and, 105, 134
  pathophysiology, 128–131
  resection arthroplasty and, 135
  uncemented THA results and, 203
  vascularized fibula grafts and, 36
  wound healing and, 333
Osteoporosis
  osteoinductive coatings and, 49
  patellar component loosening and, 330
  periprosthetic fracture and, 218–219, 228
  revision TKA and, 341
Osteotomy
  articular contact stresses and, 98
  debridement and, 145
  dysplasia and, 104–105
  extended trochanteric, 94–95
  femoral head retrieval after, 105
  high tibial osteotomy (HTO), 258–259
  hip kinetics and, 98
  nerve palsy and, 334
  nonarthroplasty alternatives and, 258–260
  osteonecrosis and, 105, 134
  principles/goals of, 103–104
  revision TKA and, 347–348
  supracondylar femoral, 259–260
  THA after, 106
  TKA after, 260–261
  trochanteric nonunion and, 161–163

Outcomes assessment
arthritic knees and, 252
data aggregation, 84
general health status (SF-36), 84–85
Hip and Knee Registry, 85
instrument validation and, 84

P

Pain
after subchondral bone microfracture, 262
after TKA, 287–288
anesthesia and, 72–73
arthritic knee scoring techniques and, 252
arthritic knees and, 249
due to infection, 155–156
of dysplasia, 105
heterotopic ossification and, 159
high tibial osteotomy (HTO) and, 260
hip versus knee replacement, 4
infections after TKA and, 324
osteoarthritis and, 10
preemptive analgesia and, 69
revision THR and, 219
revision TKA and, 340–341
synovectomy and, 256
TKA scoring systems and, 296
of tourniquets, 70
uncemented femoral components and, 117, 123
valgus bracing and, 257
Paprosky classification of bone deficiency, 222–223
Plasminogen activator inhibitor (PAI), 128
Patellar clunk
revision TKA and, 340
as TKA complication, 311, 329
Patellar tendon
cruciate ligaments and, 242–243
rupture, 331
Patellofemoral complications
extensor mechanism rupture, 331
instability, 331
patellar component failure, 329–330
patellar fractures, 330
revision TKA infection, 340
soft-tissue inpingement, 329
surgical technique and, 331
tracking and, 331–332
Patellofemoral design, 271–272
Patient surgical postitioning. *See* Surgical approaches
Patients. *See also* Pain; *specific existing conditions*; Surgical approaches
activity level of, 171, 174, 176
cemented femoral components and, 183
control of analgesia by, 287
control of anesthesia by, 71–72
dental, 139–140, 327
disease-/region-specific questionnaires and, 84–85
dislocation risk factors, 149
early discharge (TKA), 289
education, 54–55, 63–64, 106
gait observation/analysis, 249, 257, 298
infection treatments and, 143–144
kinematics/kinetics after total hip reconstruction, 99–100
long-term results by subgroups, 306–307
osteonecrosis and, 131
outcomes assessment by, 295–297
predonation of blood, 59–60
preoperative evaluation, 51–55
surgical goals and, 3
uncemented THA results and, 202–203
wear studies and, 171
Penicillin, 140
Performance total knee design, 276
Periacetabular osteotomy. *See* Osteotomy
Periprosthetic fracture, 332–333
Peroneal nerve palsy, 259
Physical component summary (PCS), 84
Physical therapy after TKA, 288–289
Plasma flame spraying, 48
Polio, 259
Polyethylene components
acetabular cemented sockets and, 187–188
aseptic loosening (revision TKA) and, 341
countersurface roughness and, 169
description, 30–33, 113–114
friction/frictional torque and, 168
future trends, 190
hybrid THA acetabular components and, 212–213
infection and, 327–328
infection prevention and, 325–326
particulate debris and, 175–176, 178
for revision THR, 217
TKA and, 252
ultrahigh molecular weight polyethylene (UHMWPE), 265, 267–270
uncemented acetabular components and, 189
in vivo wear assessment, 169–170
in vivo wear studies, 170–174
Polymerase chain reaction (PCR), 142–143
Polymethylmethacrylate (PMMA)
bone defect reconstruction and, 352
description, 167–168, 178
hybrid THA femoral components and, 208–209
implant materials, 33–34
knee design fixation and, 268
porosity reduction and, 184–185
revision THR and, 217–218, 226–227
Population studies. *See* Demographics
Porites, 45
Porosity reduction
cemented femoral components and, 184–185
hybrid THA femoral components and, 208–209
Porous-Coated Anatomic implant, 307–308
Positive intraoperative cultures (PIOC), 140–141
Posterior-Cruciate Condylar. *See* Total Condylar prosthesis
Posterior cruciate ligament (PCL)
arthritic knees and, 251
balancing and, 284
description, 241–243
long-term TKA results and, 303
mobile bearing designs and, 314–316
revision TKA and, 340, 356–357

revision TKR and, 316–317
UKA conversion to TKA, 302–303
unicondylar knees and, 265
Posterior-stabilized total knee arthroplasty (TKA)
clinical results, 309–310
complications of, 311–312
description, 308–309
kinematics, 309
proprioception/gait analysis, 310–311
Posterior surgical approaches (Langenbeck/Moore)
description, 92–93
dislocation and, 149, 152
Postoperative care
allogeneic transfusion alternatives and, 63
anesthesia and, 72
antibiotics after TKA, 288
anticoagulants and, 72
blood loss and, 55–56
bone scans, 100
clinical care pathway (THA), 54–55
dislocation and, 152
dysplasia and, 104–105
early discharge and, 289
electrical stimulation and, 131–132
knee pain and, 70–72
obesity and, 53–54
pain management after TKA, 287–288
physical therapy after TKA, 288–289
trochanteric nonunion and, 163–164
Postoperative cell salvage. *See* Salvage (RBC)
Predonation of blood, 59–60
Preemptive analgesia, 69
Pregnancy
deep vein thrombosis (DVT) during, 15
osteonecrosis and, 128
as preoperative evaluation, 68
Preoperative autologous donation (PAD)
acute normovolemic hemodilution (ANH) and, 63
algorithm for blood conservation and, 64–65
allogeneic transfusion alternatives, 59–61
Preoperative evaluations
anesthesia and, 67–68
clinical care pathway, 54–55
dislocation and, 149, 152
and extended trochanteric osteotomy, 94–95
hybrid THA femoral components and, 209–210
imaging of arthritic knees, 251
inflammatory arthritis surgery and, 3–4
medical management and, 51–55
obesity and, 203
osteotomy and, 258
revision THR and, 227–228
for revision TKA, 339–340, 346
test recommendations, 68
Preservation systems, 35–37
Press-Fit Condylar (PFC), 276, 308
Pro Osteon, 45
Prophylaxis
antibiotic, 138–140
deep vein thrombosis (DVT) and, 259
existing diseases/conditions and, 139–140
future trends, 140, 147
infection treatments and, 327–328
PROSTALAC, 146–147, 328
Prosthesis. *See also* Dislocation; Implant materials
Anatomic Graduated Component (AGC), 304–306
of antibiotic loaded acrylic cement (PROSTALAC), 146–147
bone defect reconstruction and, 351–352
bone defects and, 342
cemented total hip replacement (THA) and, 111–112
flexion instability, 311–312
implant fixation and, 117–119
infection options regarding, 327–328
Kinematic Condylar prosthesis, 303
positive intraoperative cultures (PIOC) and, 140–141, 144
Posterior-Cruciate Condylar, 303
posterior-stabilized TKA, 308–312
revision TKA and, 342, 351–352, 358
stress transfer from, 113
wear modes of, 167–168
Prosthesis of Antibiotic Loaded Acrylic Cement (PROSTALAC), 146–147, 328
Proteoglycans (PGs), 8–9
Pseudomonas aeruginosa, 140
Psoriatic arthritis, 5
Pulmonary disease, 53
Pulmonary embolism (PE)
diagnosis of, 17
following surgery, 13, 156–159
Pulsing electromagnetic fields (PEMF), 131–132

Q

Quadriceps muscle
and collateral knee ligaments, 245
and cruciate ligaments, 242–243
Quadriceps tendon, 281–282
Questionnaires, 84–85

R

Radiographs
acetabular sockets and, 188
arthritic knees and, 251
bone defects and, 343–345
of cemented total hip replacement (THA), 110
digitized three-dimensional, 169–170
of dysplasia, 104
of femoral head after osteotomy, 105
gamma radiation, 30–31
of hybrid THA acetabular components, 212
of hybrid THA femoral components, 208
infection detection and, 141
infections after TKA and, 324
osteoarthritis and, 7–8
osteolysis and, 176, 251
osteonecrosis and, 130, 132
in pre/perioperative evaluation, 54–55
revision THR and, 219
revision TKA and, 339–340, 346–347

for THA/TKA, 75–76
thromboembolism and, 157–158
TKA evaluations and, 298–299
trochanteric nonunion and, 161
uncemented femoral components and, 196–197
uncemented THA results and, 203
Radionuclide scanning, 141–142. *See also* Bone scintigraphy
Radiostereometric analysis (RSA), 188
Range of motion
arthritic knees and, 250
biomechanics of knee design and, 265–266
dislocation and, 150–151
heterotopic ossification and, 159
ideal TKA, 282
inflammatory arthritis surgery and, 4–5
with Kinematic Condylar prosthesis, 303
osteotomy and, 106
revision TKA and, 341
trochanteric nonunion and, 164
Recombinant human bone morphogenetic protein (rh-BMP). *See* Bone morphogenetic protein (BMP)
Red blood cell salvage, 63
Reflex sympathetic dystrophy, 342
Reinfection, 329
Rejection. *See* Immunology; Rejection
Replamineform (ceramic osteoconduction), 44–45
Resection arthroplasty, 135
Resistance
antibiotic suppression and, 144
antibiotics and, 137, 139, 140, 350
to methicillin/vancomycin, 325
Revision total hip replacement (THR)
cemented THR results and, 229–231
complications of, 227–229
component instability, 218
femoral deficiency classifications, 221
femoral reconstruciton, 226–227
incidence, 217
infection and, 218
mechanical failure, 218
periprosthetic fracture and, 218–219
preoperative assessment, 219–220
surgery considerations, 220
surgery equipment, 220
surgical acetabulum technique, 225
surgical approaches, 224–225
surgical treatment
acetabular side, 222–224
femoral side, 221–222
uncemented acetabular reconstruction, 231
uncemented femoral reconstruction, 231–232
wear debris and, 218
Revision total knee arthroplasty (TKA)
aseptic loosening and, 341
bone defect classifications, 342–345
bone defect reconstruction, 351
bone loss management and, 352–353
constraint, 271
epidemiology, 345
fixation, 270–272, 350–351, 353–354
implant modularity and, 353–356
incisions and, 281
infection, 340, 342
2-stage reimplantation, 350
instability and, 340
knee fusion, 358
malalignment and, 341
mobile bearing designs and, 316–317
pain and, 340
prosthetic design, 356–358
range of motion and, 341
reflex sympathetic dystrophy (RSD), 342
results of studies, 349
surgical technique, 348–349, 357–358
trauma and, 341
uncemented designs and, 277
Revision total knee replacement (TKA)
failure evaluation, 339–340, 346
preoperative considerations, 339–340, 346
Rheumatoid arthritis (RA)
antibiotics prophylaxis and, 140
cemented femoral components and, 183
cemented sockets and, 188
distal femur fracture and, 332
infection and, 155, 323
inflammatory arthritis, 3–5
juvenile, 5
long-term TKA results and, 306
medical management and, 53
osteoarthritis and, 7
revision TKA and, 341
supracondylar femoral osteotomy and, 259
synovectomy and, 256–257
treatment, 4–5
wound healing and, 333
Ribotyping, 142–143
Rifampin, 144
Rotating platform knee replacement, 316
Roughness. *See* Surface finish

S

S-ROM, 152, 226
Salvage (RBC)
algorithm for blood conservation and, 64–65
as allogeneic transfusion alternatives, 63
Scanning. *See also* Radiographs
gallium, 77–78
magnetic resonance imaging (MRI) and, 141
osteonecrosis and, 128–129
pulmonary embolism (PE) diagnosis using, 17
radionuclide, 141–142
revision THR and, 220
thromboembolism and, 157–158
trochanteric nonunion and, 163
use in implant wear process determination, 27–28
white blood cell, 78
Scars
arthritic knees and, 249
high tibial osteotomy (HTO) and, 259
infection treatments and, 328
TKA incisions and, 281
Scintigraphy. *See* Bone scintigraphy
Scoring systems
gait observation/analysis, 298
patient-oriented outcome assessment, 295–297

Screw-home movement, 239–240
Sedimentation rates, 141
Segmental cement extraction system, 226
Sickle-cell disease
  medical management and, 54
  osteonecrosis and, 128
  uncemented THA results and, 203
Sickness Impact Profile (SIP), 296
Skin expansion devices, 249–250
Socket fixation. *See* Acetabular components
Soft tissue
  arthritic knees and, 249–250, 252
  impingement after TKA, 329
  infection detection in, 78
  infection treatments and, 327–328
  magnetic resonance imaging (MRI) and, 79
  revision TKA and, 340, 348, 356–357
  TKA extensor mechanism, 282
  TKA ligament balancing/ tightening, 282–285
Spinal anesthesia, 68–69. *See also* Anesthesia
Spondylitis. *See* Ankylosis
Sports Activity Scale, 297
SRS (for ceramic osteoconduction), 45
Stability
  arthritic knees and, 249
  collateral knee ligaments and, 245
  cruciate ligaments and, 240–243
  description, 122–123
  flexion instability, 311–312
  of patella, 243–244
  radiographic (TKA) signs of, 298
  revision THR and, 218
  revision TKA and, 339–340
Standards. *See* Outcomes assessment
Staphylococcus aureus, 325
Staphylococcus epidermidis, 325
Staphylococcus albus, 155
Staphylococcus aureus, 137, 139, 140, 145, 147, 155, 288
Staphylococcus epidermidis, 139, 144, 145, 155
Stem cells
  and bone grafts, 44
  ceramic hydroxyapatite (HA) and, 46
Sterilization of implant material, 30–31
Steroids
  as arthroplasty alternative, 255–256
  distal femur fracture and, 332
  infections after TKA and, 323
  side effects, 255–256
Strains. *See* Stresses
Stresses
  of bone, 99–100
  cemented femoral design materials and, 110–111
  conformity changes and, 269–270
  creep and, 185
  revision THR and, 217–218
  transfer from prosthesis, 113
  ultrahigh molecular weight polyethylene (UHMWPE) and, 267–270
  uncemented femoral components and, 121–122, 196
Strut grafts, 132–133
Subchondral bone microfracture, 261–262
Supracondylar femoral osteotomy (SFO), 259–260
Surface finish, 112–113, 119–120. *See also* Coating
Surface replacement arthroplasty, 134–135
Surgical approaches
  anterior (Iliofemoral/Smith-Peterson), 91
  anterolateral (Watson-Jones), 91, 224
  direct lateral (Modified Hardinge), 91–92
  extended trochanteric osteotomy, 94–95
  to osteolysis, 178–179
  osteonecrosis and, 132–135
  posterior (Langenbeck/Moore), 92–93, 224
  revision THR and, 220–225
  revision TKA and, 231
  to TKA ligament balancing, 282–285
  trochanteric slide, 93, 224
  uncemented femoral components and, 118
  vastus slide, 93–94
  wear studies and, 171
Surgical approaches/techniques
  hybrid THA acetabular components and, 211–212
  hybrid THA femoral components and, 209–210
Surgical techniques
  importance of muscle relaxation, 69
  infections after TKA and, 325–326
  revision TKA and, 348–349, 357–358
  as TKA complication, 331
  TKA extensor mechanism, 282
  TKA incisions for, 281–282
  TKA ligament balancing, 282–285
Synovitis
  osteolysis and, 176
  preoperative evaluation and, 3
Synvisc, 256
Systemic lupus erythematosus
  antibiotics prophylaxis and, 140
  osteonecrosis and, 128
  treatment, 5

T

Technetium phosphate, 142
  use in bone scintigraphy, 76–78
Tetracycline, 144
The New England Baptist Hospital, 158–159
Thrombin inhibitors, 21
Thromboembolism. *See* Pulmonary embolism (PE)
Thrombophilia, 128
Thrombosis. *See* Venous thromboembolic disease (VTED)
Tibia
  bone defect classifications and, 343–345
  ceramic osteoconduction and, 46
  proximal fractures, 332–333
Tibiofemoral joint
  anatomy, 239–240
  revision TKA and, 340
Total Condylar prosthesis, 303
Total hip arthroplasty (THA). *See also* Arthroplasty; Cemented total hip replacement (THR); Hybrid total hip replacement (THR)
  acetabular deficiency classification and, 222

after previous osteotomy, 106
allografts in, 37–38
anesthesia and, 70–71
bone stresses and, 99–100
clinical care pathway, 54–55
dislocation and, 149–152
femoral deficiency classification (AAOS), 221
incidence, 217
kinematics/kinetics and, 99–100
magnetic resonance imaging (MRI) of, 78–79
osteoconductive coatings on, 48
osteonecrosis and, 127
postoperative care and, 71
radiographs of, 75–76
Total hip replacement (THR)
osteonecrosis and, 134
Total joint reconstruction
bone availability for harvest and, 43
osteoinductive growth factors and, 46–47
Total knee arthroplasty (TKA). *See also* Arthroplasty; Knee joint; Revision total knee arthroplasty (TKA)
after osteotomy, 260–261
allografts in, 38–39
anesthesia and, 71–72
antibiotics after, 288
arthritis and
physical examination, 249–253
cement fixation and, 275–277
deep vein thrombosis (DVT) after, 289–292
early discharge, 289
infection
diagnosis, 324
incidence, 323–324
prevention, 325–327
reinfection, 329
treatment, 327–329
infection and
organisms involved, 325
knee rating systems, 295–299
long-term results
cemented designs, 303–306
cruciate-retaining, 303
mobile bearing designs and, 313–317
by patient subgroups, 306–307
posterior-stabilized, 308–313
uncemented designs, 307–308
magnetic resonance imaging (MRI) of, 78–79
osteoconductive coatings on, 48–49
pain control after, 287–288
patellofemoral design and, 271–272
physical therapy after, 288–289
postoperative pain management and, 70–72
radiographs of, 75
rotating platform, 316
scoring techniques for, 252–253
surgical principles
extensor mechanism, 282
incisions for, 281–282
knee alignment via ligament balancing, 282–285
unicompartmental knee arthroplasty (UKA), 301–303
Tourniquet use
during knee surgery, 70
vascular complications and, 333
Transforming growth factor-ß (TGF-ß)
bone graft substitution and, 43
osteoinduction and, 46–47
osteoinductive coatings and, 49
Transfusion-related acute lung injury (TRALI), 58
Transfusions. *See also* Allogeneic transfusion alternatives
allogeneic blood
benefits and risks of, 57–59
allogeneic blood and
bacterial contamination of, 58
indications for, 56–57
legal considerations, 63–64
mortality rates and, 61
Transient ischemic attack (TIA), 52
Transplantation
cartilage, 261
chondrocyte, 262–263
Trauma
arthritic knees and, 250
cortical strut grafts (osteonecrotic) and, 132–133
dislocation and, 151
magnetic resonance venography (MRV) and, 80
neuropathy and, 165–166
revision TKA and, 341
supracondylar femoral osteotomy and, 259
thrombogenesis following, 15
wound healing and, 333
Treatments
clinical care pathway, 54–55
deep vein thrombosis (DVT), 290–292
dislocation, 151–152
for infection, 143–147
periprosthetic fracture and, 332–333
Triamcinolone, 255
Triamcinolone acetonide, 255
Tribology. *See* Articulation
Tricalcium phosphate (TCP)
in ceramic osteoconduction, 44–46
as osteoconductive/inductive coating, 48–49
Tricompartmental knee replacement, 314–316
Trochanteric nonunion, 160–162
Trochanteric slide surgical approach, 93
dislocation and, 149, 152
Trochlea, 243–245

U

Ultrahigh molecular weight polyethylene (UHMWPE), 265, 267–270, 272
Ultrasound
assessment using, 78
deep vein thrombosis (DVT) and, 290
deep vein thrombosis (DVT) diagnosis using, 16–17, 79–80
infection and, 141
Uncemented acetabular components. *See also* Uncemented total hip arthroplasty (THA)
hybrid THR and, 210–213
reconstruction and, 231
Uncemented femoral components. *See also* Uncemented total hip arthroplasty (THA); Uncemented total knee arthroplasty (TKA)
extractability/ease of revision, 122
geometry of, 117–119, 123–124

initial stem stability, 117–119, 123
long-term stability, 119–121
modularity and, 118–119
revision THR and, 222, 231–232
Uncemented total hip arthroplasty (THA)
acetabular components
coatings of, 201
fixation, 201
implant material, 199–200
modularity, 201–202
results, 199–200
femoral components
coatings of, 198–199
implant material, 196–197
implant shape, 197–198
modularity, 199
results, 195–196
future trends, 204
select patient subgroups and, 202–203
Uncemented total knee arthroplasty (TKA)
clinical results, 276–277
fixation and, 350–351
long-term TKA results and, 307–308
mobile bearing designs and, 314–316
Unicompartmental knee arthroplasty (UKA), 301–303, 349–350
Urinary tract infections, 155
Uropathy, 53. *See also* Diabetes

V

Vacuum mixing. *See* Porosity reduction
Vancomycin, 144, 325–326
Vancomycin resistant *Enterococcus* (VRE), 137, 139
Vascular system
arthritic knees and, 250
and bone grafts, 35–36
cardiovascular disease, 51–52, 127
complications of, 165–166, 333
revision THR and, 228
Vastus slide surgical approach, 93–94
Vena cava filters, 291–292
Venography, 290. *See* Magnetic resonance venography (MRV)
Venous thromboembolic disease (VTED). *See also* Pulmonary embolism (PE)
description, 13
diagnosis of, 16–17
epidemiology, 13–14
pathogenesis of, 14–16
prophylaxis of, 17–21
treatment of established, 22
Virchow's triad, 14–15
Viscosupplementation therapy, 256

W

Warfarin, 13–14, 17–18, 20, 22, 290–291
Watson-Jones surgical approach, 91
Wear of implant devices. *See* Corrosion/wear of implant devices; Mechanical failure
Western Ontario and McMaster University Osteoarthritis Index (WOMAC), 84–85, 252, 296–297
White blood cell (WBC) scanning, 78, 141, 324
Wolff's Law
bone remodeling and, 9
bone stresses and, 99
Wound healing, 333. *See also* Infection

X

X-ray. *See* Imaging; Radiographs
Xenografts, 35

Y

Yersinia enterocolitica, 58